# CLINICAL MANAGEMENT OF MELANOMA

# DEVELOPMENTS IN ONCOLOGY 5

*Previously published in this series:*

1. F. J. Cleton and J. W. I. M. Simons, eds., Genetic Origins of Tumor Cells
   ISBN 90-247-2272-1
2. J. Aisner and P. Chang, eds., Cancer Treatment Research
   ISBN 90-247-2358-2
3. B. W. Ongerboer de Visser, D. A. Bosch and W. M. H. van Woerkom-Eykenboom,
   eds., Neuro-Oncology: Clinical and Experimental Aspects
   ISBN 90-247-2421-X
4. K. Hellmann, P. Hilgard and S. Eccles, eds., Metastasis: Clinical and Experimental Aspects
   ISBN 90-247-2424-4

*Series ISBN: 90-247-2338-8*

# CLINICAL MANAGEMENT OF MELANOMA

*edited by*

H. F. SEIGLER
*Duke University Medical Center*
*Durham, North Carolina, USA*

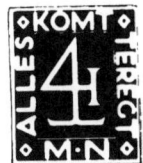

1982

SPRINGER-SCIENCE+BUSINESS MEDIA, B.V.

**Library of Congress Cataloging in Publication Data**   ⊂ℙ

Main entry under title:

Clinical management of melanoma.

   (Developments in oncology ; v. 5)
   Includes bibliographical references and index.
   1. Melanoma--Treatment.  2. Melanoma--Surgery.
I. Seigler, Hilliard F.  II. Series.  [DNLM:
1. Melanoma--Therapy.  W1 DE998N v. 5 / QZ 266
C6417]
RC280.S5C56    616.99'4    81-18987
AACR2

ISBN 978-94-009-7495-1        ISBN 978-94-009-7493-7 (eBook)
DOI 10.1007/978-94-009-7493-7

# Contents

# Preface

Melanoma is a disease entity that has the capability of involving all organ systems of the human body. During the last decade a dramatic increase in the incidence of this disease has been noted. It is surpassed in this dreadful statistic only by carcinoma of the lung. During this time frame, much has been defined and written concerning the histopathology and prognostic factors of this neoplastic disorder. The relative ease of maintaining this malignant cell in tissue culture has permitted the cellular biologist, tumor immunologist, immunochemist and geneticist an ideal in vitro experimental model for advancing our understanding of human malignancy. Histopathologic features, prognostic factors, membrane antigenic expression and host–tumor relationship in this disease have all been extensively studied and it has thus become evident that melanoma can and does serve as a prototype for the study of human malignancies in general. Basic scientists including embryologists, immunologists, virologists, immunochemists, geneticists, biostatisticians and cellular biologists, should find this monograph of interest. Bridging clinical specialists including the pathologist, diagnostic and therapeutic radiologist and epidemiologist will also find areas of interest in these writings. Because of the fact that melanoma can involve all organ systems, clinicians ranging from family practitioners to the subspecialists should become thoroughly familiar with the clinical aspects of this disease, which are fully covered in this book.

Locoregional therapies are discussed in some depth. Chemotherapy, immunotherapy and the hormonal aspects of melanoma are also dealt with in detail. Clinical manifestations as they relate to the head and neck, bone disease, central nervous system, genitourinary, ocular as well as skin are covered by specialists in each of these areas. The prognostic factors and basic biologic behavior of the disease is clearly discussed in such a manner as to permit the responsible physician to be able to outline a reasonable treatment plan for the patient involved with this disease.

# Contributors

BULLARD, Dennis E., M.D., Department of Surgery, Duke Medical Center, Durham, North Carolina

CHANDLER, Arthur C., Jr., M.D., Associate Professor, Department of Ophthalmology; Associate, Department of Anatomy, Duke Medical Center, Durham, North Carolina

CLINE, Wayne A., Jr., M.D., Chief Resident, Division of Urology, Duke Medical Center, Durham, North Carolina

COLE, T. Boyce, M.D., Associate Professor, Division of Otolaryngology, Department of Surgery, Duke Medical Center, Durham, North Carolina

COOK, Wesley A., M.D., Department of Surgery, Duke Medical Center, Durham, North Carolina

COX, Edwin B., M.D., Associate, Hematology and Medical Oncology, Department of Medicine, Duke Medical Center, Durham, North Carolina

GILGOR, Robert S., M.D., Associate Professor, Division of Dermatology, Department of Medicine, Duke Medical Center, Durham, North Carolina

GRAHAM, Sam D., Jr., M.D., American Urological Association Fellow in Oncology, Duke Medical Center, Durham, North Carolina

HARRELSON, John M., M.D., Assistant Professor, Orthopedic Surgery; Assistant Professor, Department of Pathology, Duke Medical Center, Durham, North Carolina

HEASTON, Dennis K., M.D., Assistant Professor, Division of Imaging, Department of Radiology, Duke Medical Center, Durham, North Carolina

HUANG, Andrew T., M.D., Associate Professor, Hematology and Medical Oncology, Department of Medicine, Duke Medical Center, Durham, North Carolina

KLINTWORTH, Gordon K., M.D., Ph.D., Professor, Department of Pathology, Duke Medical Center, Durham, North Carolina

LUCAS, Virgil S., Jr., Clinical Pharmacist, Hematology and Medical Oncology, Department of Medicine, Duke Medical Center, Durham, North Carolina

McCARTY, Kenneth S., Jr., M.D., Ph.D., Assistant Professor, Department of Pathology; Assistant Professor, Department of Medicine, Duke Medical Center, Durham, North Carolina

McCARTY, Kenneth S., Sr., Department of Biochemistry, Duke Medical Center, Durham, North Carolina

PAULL, Douglas E., Department of Pathology, Department of Medicine, Duke Medical Center, Durham, North Carolina

PUTMAN, Charles E., M.D., Professor and Chairman, Department of Radiology, Duke Medical Center, Durham, North Carolina

SCHOLD, S. Clifford, Jr., M.D., Department of Medicine, Duke Medical Center, Durham, North Carolina

SEIGLER, Hilliard F., M.D., Professor, Department of Surgery; Associate Professor, Department of Immunology, Duke Medical Center, Durham, North Carolina

STUHLMILLER, Gary M., Ph.D., Assistant Medical Research Professor, Department of Surgery, Duke Medical Center, Durham, North Carolina

SULLIVAN, Daniel C., M.D., Assistant Professor, Division of Imaging, Department of Radiology, Duke Medical Center, Durham, North Carolina

THOMPSON, William M., M.D., Associate Professor, Division of Imaging, Department of Radiology, Duke Medical Center; Chief of Radiology, Durham V.A. Hospital, Durham, North Carolina

VOLLMER, Robin T., V.A. Medical Center and Department of Pathology, Duke Medical Center, Durham, North Carolina

WEINERTH, John L., M.D., Associate Professor, Division of Urology, Department of Surgery, Duke Medical Center, Durham, North Carolina

# 1. Surgical considerations for cutaneous melanoma

HILLIARD F. SEIGLER

## Introduction

Primary cutaneous melanoma represents the most frequent clinical presentation of this disease entity. Before the surgeon can adequately plan for operative control of the primary, he must be aware of the biologic differences associated with the different histopathological types. Lentigo maligna occurs most commonly in the older age population. This lesion has a tendency to remain for long periods of time in a radial growth phase with little or no tumor invasion and thus metastatic potential. It is usually on the exposed surfaces of the body with the majority being found on the head and neck. This lesion is usually nonpalpable until a vertical growth phase has begun. Superficial spreading melanoma also has an intraepithelial component with early growth being in a radial direction. This portion of the growth phase may reach 2–3 cm in width before the invasive vertical growth begins. If either lentigo maligna or superfical spreading melanoma were to be recognized early during their radial growth phase, essentially all of these lesions could be cured by adequate surgical excision alone. The vertical growth phase reflects invasion and its degree can be clearly correlated with the incidence of metastatic disease and eventual patient survival. The vertical growth phase is usually quite rapid and the lesion may vary in color from pink to brown, to blue, to black. It is during this phase of growth that ulceration usually occurs. Nodular melanomas develop by direct tumor progression and do not clinically present a true radial growth phase. An intraepithelial component is absent. The tumor nodule is easily palpable and is sharply delineated from the normal surrounding tissue. Acral lentiginous melanoma usually occurs on the palmar and plantar surfaces of the body, in the nail beds and on mucous membranes. These lesions seem to behave quite differently and are associated with a high metastatic rate and poor patient survival. Local control using surgical means of the plantar, palmar and mucous membrane locations is difficult to attain.

Both the prognosis and the presence or absence of regional lymph node metastasis can be correlated with the level of invasion of the primary tumor, the location of the primary and tumor thickness [1, 2]. Before the primary surgery can be planned, an accurate diagnosis is paramount. The pathologist

*Seigler, H. F. (ed.), Clinical Management of Melanoma. ISBN 978-94-009-7495-1*
© *1982, Martinus Nijhoff Publishers, The Hague/Boston/London.*

must be provided an optimal surgical specimen on which to measure tumor thickness, determine the level of tumor invasion, determine microscopic satellitosis, gauge host reaction as reflected by the lymphocytic response, as well as comment on the presence or absence of tumor ulceration. Electro-coagulation, curettage and shave biopsies should be discouraged for suspicious cutaneous lesions.

## The biopsy

The entire gross lesion should be excised if the wound can be easily closed in a primary fashion. Presentation of the entire lesion to the pathologist for evaluation permits a more complete study of the histopathologic features. If the lesion is large, or in an anatomical position that would result in a disfiguring procedure, incisional biopsy should be considered. The incisional biopsy should be very carefully selected by the surgeon. The most nodular area, representing the vertical growth potential of the primary, should be selected and the biopsy should include subcutaneous fat so that the greatest accuracy as to the actual depth of penetration can be determined. Once the depth of penetration, tumor thickness and microscopic satellitosis have been accurately documented, the definitive surgical procedure can be more accurately planned.

## Surgical management of the primary lesion

Surgical management of primary cutaneous melanoma has varied from inadequate local excision to removal of large areas of tissue followed by extensive skin grafting procedures. Obviously both of these extremes are based on poor surgical practice and almost always result from a lack of knowledge of the biologic potential and behavior of the particular type of cutaneous melanoma under consideration. As a general guideline, removal of an area twice the size of the primary has been proposed. A knowledge of the type of primary coupled with tumor thickness can, however, provide a more accurate basis for planning surgical margins. A 2 cm margin from the gross lesion for melanomas that are less than 0.76 mm in thickness is adequate. A 3–5 cm margin beyond all clinically visible tumor in those lesions greater than 0.76 mm in thickness is a reasonable guideline. In all cases the subcutaneous fat should be included in the surgical specimen if the proper depth of invasion and adequate surgical margins are to be determined. The surgeon can easily include the deep fascia as an anatomical guideline for depth of removal. The fascia becomes an easily recognized tissue envelope for the area to be removed. Using these predetermined measurements local control of disease can be accomplished in virtually all patients with cutaneous melanoma. Thin lesions can thus be managed, for the most part, by primary wound closure and, depending upon the primary site, many thick lesions can be adequately handled by the same operative technique. The more advanced lesion, and those in special anatomical sites, will usually be best managed by skin graft closure.

### Local recurrent disease

Local recurrent disease is defined as a lesion that recurs within 5 cm of the primary. The lesion should be so defined only if it appears in skin, subcutaneous tissue or soft tissue and is not in a lymph node. Local recurrent disease should be considered for surgical management. In view of the fact that local recurrence is usually associated with microscopic satellitosis or vascular involvement, be it lymphogenous or hematogenous, in the primary, a more aggressive approach should be accomplished by the surgeon. Excision with 5 cm margins and application of the same principles as has been described for management of primary lesions should be entertained. Addition of a regional node dissection with management of the recurrent primary continues to be an arguable point. Most of the published data concerning this topic would favor including a regional node dissection with the procedure.

### Subungal melanoma

Subungal melanomas represent one of the presentations of acral lentiginous melanoma. Any pigmented lesion beneath the nail that cannot be accurately determined to be a hematoma should be diagnosed by adequate biopsy. If melanoma has been the determined diagnosis, management should be accomplished by amputation with no attempt at local excision or coverage. Subungal melanomas of the toes should be managed by amputation at the metatarsal joint. For finger or thumb lesions, unless they are quite extensive proximally, the amputation should be carried out at the level of the distal interphalangeal joint. This procedure provides adequate local control and permits very reasonable functional results.

### Plantar or palmar melanoma

Melanomas that occur on the plantar or palmar surfaces most commonly are of the acral lentiginous type. In view of the broad radial potential of this type of primary, local control may be difficult to attain. Because of the site of the primary, the type of tissue coverage is very important. Stress associated with or weight bearing and other similar challenges dictate either thick split-thickness or full-thickness skin grafting. Very wide local excision without exposure of tendon in the base of the wound must be accomplished. Full-thickness skin coverage can be provided with very reasonable functional results for the patient that uses reasonable care.

## Regional lymph node dissection

Most large clinical series provide data indicating that approximately 40% of patients with melanoma involving a single regional lymph node have an approximate one out of three chance of surviving their disease, whereas those patients with more extensive nodal involvement have a progressively poorer prognosis depending upon the number as well as the extent of disease in the lymph nodes involved with a tumor. It seems reasonable to assume that some patients, who are carefully selected for elective regional lymph node dissection, may indeed derive therapeutic benefit. Das Gupta [3] has reported that approximately one half of 88 patients with lower extremity disease had nodal metastasis. Therapeutic benefit, with both three- and five-year survival of patients with metastatic disease, was realized by this author. The World Health Organization's clinical trial [4] in patients with Stage I melanoma of the extremities involved wide excision of the primary lesion and immediate lymph node dissection compared with wide excision alone. Delayed node dissections were performed when clinically evident regional lymph node metastasis occurred. The survival curves for the two groups at five years were superimposable. The Mayo clinic group [5] data supported this study in that they also realized no difference in the survival of patients with Stage I melanomas whether immediate or delayed node dissection was performed. These data are not completely supported by other series in which survival correlates directly with the extent of nodal disease and in which patients with gross nodal metastasis had severely impaired survival compared to those with microscopic metastasis [3]. Fortner et al. [6] report a five-year cure rate of 60% in patients with a single microscopic focus, 50% with one lymph node involved and 15% with multiple nodes involved. The five-year cure rate in patients treated by wide excision alone and who subsequently developed nodal metastasis was only 12%. Balch et al. [7] have analyzed their data on the basis of tumor thickness. Patients with primary lesions of 0.76–3.99 mm had a significantly better five- and eight-year survival, 86% and 82% respectively, than those who had excision only, 58% and 25% respectively. Their investigations have also suggested that lesions that exceed 4.0 mm in thickness reflect patients with a high risk of distant metastasis at the time of initial diagnosis and that the benefit of prophylactic node dissection in this group will be less apparent. Balch's studies likewise indicate that patients with primary lesions of 0.76 mm in thickness or less experience a very low risk of nodal metastasis and therefore elective node dissection in this group should be discouraged. Data accumulated from the Melanoma Clinical Cooperative Group have been extensively analyzed and reported by Day et al. [8–10]. They have elected to separate their groups into three subdivisions divided according to the breakpoints calculated from the natural history of the disease. Those patients with thin lesions include tumor thickness from 0.76 mm to 1.65 mm; intermediate patients with tumor thickness from 1.51 mm to 3.99 mm; and patients with thick lesions greater than 3.6 mm. Analysis of this very large cooperative patient population has shown that individuals with clinical Stage I disease with tumor thickness from 0.76 to 1.5 mm have a 90% chance of cure by wide local excision of the primary tumor alone. The high risk group for this subsegment of patients include those with upper back, posterior arm, posterior neck and posterior scalp primary locations. These authors suggest a randomized study concerning elective node dissection in patients with these locations as a means of assessing elective versus delayed lymph node dissection. Patients with intermediate tumor thickness also could be divided into high and low risk groups for developing lymph node metastasis. Criteria for the high risk group were reported as those patients having greater than 6 mitoses/mm$^2$, primary tumor sites other than the forearm or leg and histologic evidence in the primary tumor of either ulceration greater than 3 mm wide or microscopic satellites. The low risk group was identified as those patients having fewer than 6 mitoses/mm$^2$ and a location on the leg or forearm with absence of both microscopic satellites and ulceration greater than 3 mm wide of the tumor. Patients with thick primaries were all at significant risk for developing systemic disease. All patients with a primary of the hands or feet died secondary to their melanoma. Other variables that would best predict eventual bony or visceral metastasis included an absent or minimal lymphocyte response at the base of the tumor, histologic type other than superficial spreading melanoma, primary tumor location on the trunk and clinically positive nodes or no initial elective node dissection.

In our own very large clinical series, it is evident from a multivariate analysis that the prognosis in this patient population is highly variable but that much of this variation can be explained by differences in primary site, thickness of the primary lesion and presence or absence of microscopic ulceration. Maldistribution of prognostic factors between treatment groups may indeed obscure treatment effects. For example, if elective lymph node dissection is completed on patients with a high risk for more advanced disease, a benefit due to the treatment may be counterbalanced by the underlying worse prognosis of the patients, so that no difference overall may be seen between such treatment groups. It is our belief that the most sensitive evaluation of the effect of elective node dissection can be done only with multiple regression techniques. Survival regression analysis allows adjustment for the effects of important prognostic factors in the comparison of treatment groups. Tumor thickness and ulceration greater than 3 mm are the dominant factors until time of recurrence in our patient population. Only patients with clinical Stage I disease of the trunk or extremity with tumor thickness between 0.77 and 3.9 mm are considered for elective node dissection. This last restriction is based upon the near uniform good outcome in patients with thin lesions and the very high likelihood of occurrence of distant metastasis in patients with lesions 4 mm in thickness or greater. Only 11 % of the patients who underwent elective lymph node dissection have had metastatic disease, all identified as such by the finding of positive nodes in the surgical specimen. No recurrence has been observed in pathologically confirmed Stage I patients. Only a single patient in the elective lymph node group has subsequently experienced systemic recurrence and died secondary to melanoma. Twenty-three percent (23%) of the patients who did not undergo elective lymph node dissection have had tumor recurrences and just over $\frac{1}{3}$ of these patients have died secondary to their disease. The trend towards better disease-free interval among elective lymph node dissection patients is thus suggested in our patient population. The mean tumor thickness of the elective lymph node dissection group was 1.93 mm while that of the no elective lymph node dissection group was 1.67 mm. Once thickness and ulceration had been accounted for, patients with elective lymph node dissection faired significantly better than patients who had only local excision. This result deserves continued close attention using the guidelines as described.

Cutaneous melanoma that invades the lymphatic system courses to regional lymph nodes in the preponderance of cases. The three main lymph node chains involved include cervical, axillary and ileoinguinal. Antecubital, popliteal, other superficial and deep lymph node groups are affected very rarely. When the surgeon is faced with ambiguous lymph node drainage as certain cutaneous melanomas of the trunk pose, technetium-labeled antimony trisulfide injected around the primary lesion is a predictive and feasible diagnostic tool for documenting lymphatic drainage patterns [11]. This particular technique of lymphoscintography is a valuable adjunct to the physician. If an axillary dissection is to be considered then this lymph node group with or without en bloc removal of the pectoralis minor muscle should be entertained. The incision should follow the skin lines and thus a linear scar with the resultant loss of range of motion in the upper extremity can be avoided. There is continued question concerning the therapeutic benefit of deep pelvic node dissection. There is little question that if pelvic lymph nodes are involved then the prognosis is quite poor. Very few patients with positive iliac nodes will survive greater than three years. It has been our posture to consider the overall benefit–risk ratio to patients being considered for only superficial groin dissection. There is limited wound morbidity with this procedure and very little in the way of lymphadema is resultant from the dissection. Patients with cutaneous melanoma involving the head and neck are considered in Chapter 9 and thus will not be discussed in this review.

**Surgery for distant metastatic disease**

Surgical management of distant lesions may be indicated in selected patients with symptomatic distant disease. Resectable bowel lesions that are associated with performation, obstruction or bleeding should be considered surgical candidates. Not only are the visceral complaints relieved but, if followed by aggressive adjuvant therapy, significant palliation may indeed be realized. Patients, who by CT scan have demonstrable solitary brain lesions that are surgically resectable, should also be considered for operation. This subject is dealt with in some detail in Chapter 7. Many such patients will experience a prolonged disease-free interval if lesions are surgically removed and if this procedure is followed by postoperative whole head irradiation and prolonged chemotherapy and/or immunotherapy are administered. Morton et al. [12] have reported the results of surgical treatment in 60 patients with multiple pulmonary metastases. Their series reveals an approximate 60% patient survival at five years after operation if aggressive surgical resection is completed in those patients who demonstrate a tumor doubling time greater than 40 days for a metastatic lesion. These data were applicable even in patients requiring bilateral thoracotomy. Our own experience would support their approach for patients with a solitary primary lesion in the lung. Our posture has been to observe the tumor doubling time for one month, then to place patients with a tumor doubling time of greater than 30 days on a four drug combination chemotherapy regimen and if additional lesions do not develop during the next sixty days, to follow this by resection of the solitary metastatic pulmonary lesion. The chemotherapeutic regimen is then empirically continued for 24 months. Cytoreductive procedures may be indicated in patients with peripheral disease prior to instituting chemotherapeutic or immunotherapeutic regimens, even though the surgeon must be aware that this will not be a curative operation. Hemipelvectomy and forequarter amputation for melanoma should be discouraged. Experience has shown that most of these patients will have early systemic recurrences thus not justifiying this magnitude of mutilating surgery attendant with a very poor benefit–risk ratio. Extremity amputation for bulky or diffuse local recurrent disease has been associated with a 20% five-year survival rate and this may provide an additional option for the surgeon managing this complicated problem [13].

## References

1. Clark WH, Jr, From L, Bernardino EA et al: The histogenesis and biologic behavior of primary human malignant melanomas of the skin. Cancer Res 29:705, 1969.
2. Breslow A: Thickness, cross-sectional areas and depth of invasion in the prognosis of cutaneous melanoma. Ann Surg 172:902, 1970.
3. Das Gupta TK: Results of treatment of 269 patients with primary cutaneous melanoma: a five year prospective study. Ann Surg 186:201, 1977.
4. Breslow A, Cascinelli N, Van der Esch EP and Morabito A: WHO collaborating centers for evaluation of methods of diagnosis and treatment of melanoma: Stage I melanoma of the limbs: assessment of prognosis by levels of invasion and maximum thickness. Tumori 64:273, 1978.
5. Sim FH, Taylor WF, Ivins JC, Pritchard DJ and Soule EH: A prospective, randomized study of the efficacy of routine elective lymphadenectomy in management of malignant melanoma: preliminary results. Cancer 41:948, 1978.
6. Forther JG, Booher RJ and Pack FT: Results of groin dissections for malignant melanoma in 220 patients. Surgery 55:485, 1964.
7. Balch CM, Soong S, Murad TM and Ingalls AL: A multifactorial analysis of melanoma. III: prognostic factors in melanoma patients with lymph node metastases (Stage II). Ann Surg 193:377, 1981.
8. Day CL, Jr, Mihm MC, Sober AJ et al: Prognostic factors for melanoma patients with lesions 0.76 to 1.65 mm in thickness: an appraisal of "thin" Level IV lesions. Ann Surg (submitted).
9. Day CL, Jr, Mihm MC, Lew RA et al: Prognostic factors for patients with clinical Stage I melanoma of intermediate thickness (1.51–3.99 mm): a conceptual model for tumor growth and metastasis. Ann Surg (submitted).
10. Day CL, Jr, Lew RA, Mihm MC et al: A multivariate analysis of prognostic factors for melanoma paients with lesions greater than 3.6 mm in thickness: the importance of revealing alternative Cox models. Ann Surg (submitted).
11. Sullivan DC, Croker BP, Jr, Harris CC, Deery P and Seigler HF: Lymphoscintography with $^{99m}$Tc antimony sulfur colloid in malignant melanoma. Am J Roentgenol (in press).
12. Morton DL, Joseph WL, Ketcham AS et al: Surgical resection and adjuvanctive immunotherapy for selected patients with pulmonary metastases. Ann Surg 178:360, 1973.
13. Fortner JG, MacLean B and Mulcare RJ: Treatment of recurrent malignant melanoma. In: McCarthy WH (ed) Melanoma and Skin Cancer, p 453. 1972.

# 2. Pathology of melanoma

ROBIN T. VOLLMER

## Introduction to histologic diagnosis of malignant melanoma

In most cases the diagnosis of malignant melanoma rests upon histology, and in most cases the histologic definition of melanoma is adequate enough for an easy diagnosis. Nevertheless, there remain patients with pigmented lesions that defy both expert pathologists and defy our general definition of melanoma. For these the diagnosis depends upon both clinical and histological information, and it probably incorporates some degree of uncertainty, but fortunately lesions of this type are uncommon in the skin and they have the best prognosis even when considered malignant.

Difficulties in histologic diagnosis of cutaneous melanoma come from two sources. First, the pathologist sees only a few vertical planes through a lesion, which otherwise has a complex three-dimensional anatomy—its surface geography in itself goes a long way toward making the diagnosis. Second, and probably more important, is the fact that the biopsy is only a snapshot of a kinetic process. At the time of biopsy many of these lesions are in an unbalanced state between tumor growth and tumor regression, and since both the diagnosis and the prognosis rest upon the determination of the bulk of the tumor mass, partial tumor regression or early growth can render the pathologist impotent for deciding either.

For example, dynamic and geographic factors can combine to produce a section plane that includes only a regression focus. Dynamic and geographic factors can combine to cause a special problem with the definition of early melanoma. In its early stages or at its perimeter, melanoma can mimic the morphology of a benign nevus so closely that, in my opinion, there is a morphological continuum from benign junctional nevus to borderline melanoma and to malignant melanoma. I believe that those who expect sharp morphological discrimants will be frustrated by this tumor and that patients with such gray zone lesions will require evaluation from several viewpoints before choice of therapy and follow-up regimen can be made.

*Seigler, H. F. (ed.), Clinical Management of Melanoma. ISBN 978-94-009-7495-1*
© *1982, Martinus Nijhoff Publishers, The Hague/Boston/London.*

## Classification of melanoma

Melanoma can be classed first as muco-cutaneous and extra-muco-cutaneous. Muco-cutaneous melanoma can then be subclassed as those with a junctional component (including intraepithelial) or those that are entirely subjunctional (nodular), and junctional melanomas can be further classed as in situ and invasive. It is now generally accepted that most cutaneous melanomas first appear as junctional melanomas [1–7]. They spread along the junction and within the epidermis to produce a clinically flat zone of pigmentation. This phase is called radial or horizontal growth phase. Melanomas can remain in this stage for an indefinite period and, as long as they do, they can be cured by simple excision. Some, however, after variable delay invade into the dermis and thus enter a vertical growth phase. The deeper they go the worse the patient's prognosis. Because horizontal growth continues in an invasive junctional melanoma the invasive portion may represent only a portion of the entire pigmented lesion, and a biopsy, or the section plane, may miss the invasive part (Figure 1).

## Melanomas with a junctional component

In this category I group superficial spreading melanoma (SSM), lentigo maligna melanoma (LMM), acral lentiginous melanoma (ALM) and their invasive

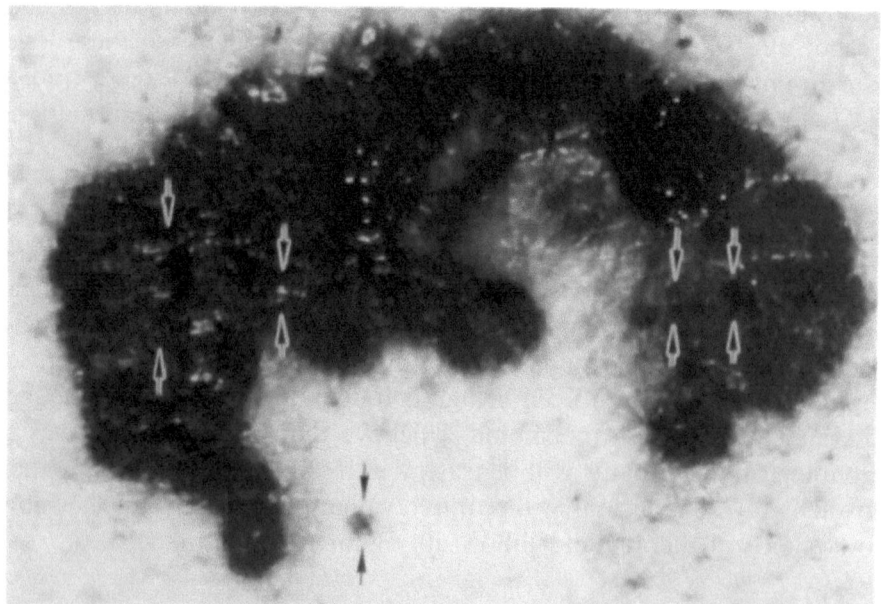

*Figure 1.* Melanoma studied with serial blocking. Zones between arrows indicate invasion. The remaining areas showed in situ melanoma or regression.

counterparts for three reasons. Morphologically, they appear quite similar. For me one of the most difficult discriminations in melanoma is to decide from the biopsy whether a tumor is a LMM, a SSM or a ALM, and many seem to share features of several of the classic morphological prototypes. Second, the rules for discriminating between these tumors and benign nevi are the same. Third, histological prognosis is determined in the same way for each, and in fact tumor thickness, presence of ulceration, lymphocytic infiltrate and status of margins are probably more important to prognosis than the determination of subtype.

Let us define junctional melanoma by comparing it to the benign nevus with a junctional component and to "borderline" melanoma. The three differ primarily by their locations along four morphological scales. These four are: mass of junctional melanocytes, departure of junctional morphology from convex spherical and separate groups, cytological atypia, and loss of maturation of any dermal component present (Table 1).

Junctional melanoma differs from the benign nevus first because it has a significantly greater mass of junctional melanocytes. In fact this feature reflects the rapid growth rate of the tumor. The greater mass is due both to a greater breadth (Figure 2) of junctional involvement and to an increased thickness of melanocytes at any point (Figure 3). Junctional melanocytes appear either singly or as groups beyond the edges of the 4 mm punch biopsy, and the density of melanocytes per unit length of the junction is high. There is a tendency toward continuity of melanocytes along the entire junction (Figure 4) with involvement of both rete ridge tips and the suprapapillary junction, and the junctional groups contain several cell layers of melanocytes. Finally, the mass is greater because melanocytes appear at all levels of the epidermis including the keratin layer.

Junctional melanoma differs from the benign nevus because its junctional groups no longer tend to be separate, convex spheres located only at the rete tips. Instead they form plaques that span several rete processes (Figure 5) and the groups are less uniform in size and shape.

*Table 1.* Light microscopic features of melanomas with junctional component

1. Increased mass of junctional/epidermal melanocytes
       increased breadth
       increased continuity (confluence of groups)
       increased cell layers
       increased intraepidermal cells

2. Departure from convex and separate junction
       morphology

3. Cytologic atypia

4. Loss of dermal melanocyte maturation

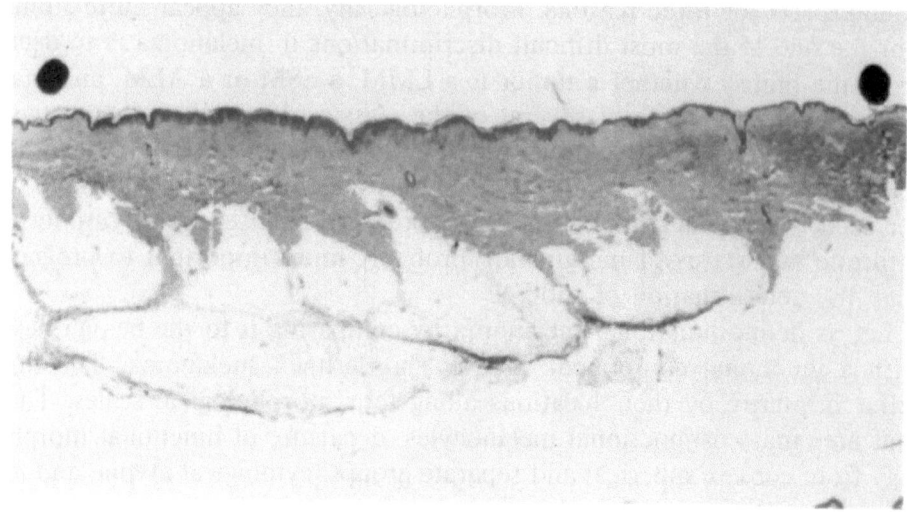

*Figure 2.* Invasive melanoma with a breadth of melanocytic atypia measuring 1.8 cm between dots.

Some junctional melanomas show striking cytological atypia (Figure 6), which I define here as: nuclear and cell enlargement, nuclear and cell pleomorphism, nuclear hyperchromasia and/or pallor, more prominent nucleoli and increased mitotic figures, but unfortunately many junctional melanomas also exhibit little more cytological atypia than occurs in benign junctional nevi.

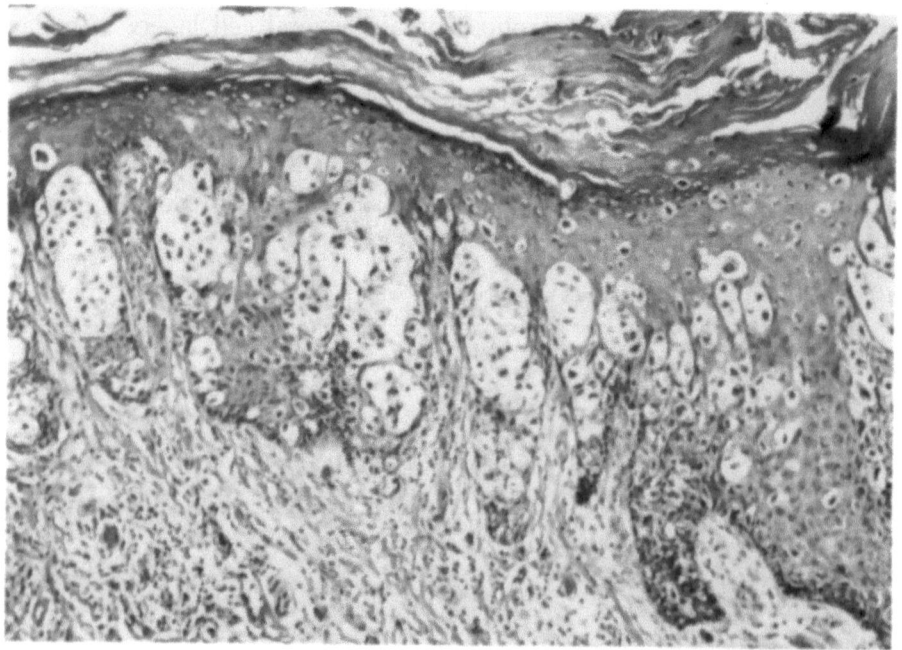

*Figure 3.* Melanoma of toe, SSM pattern.

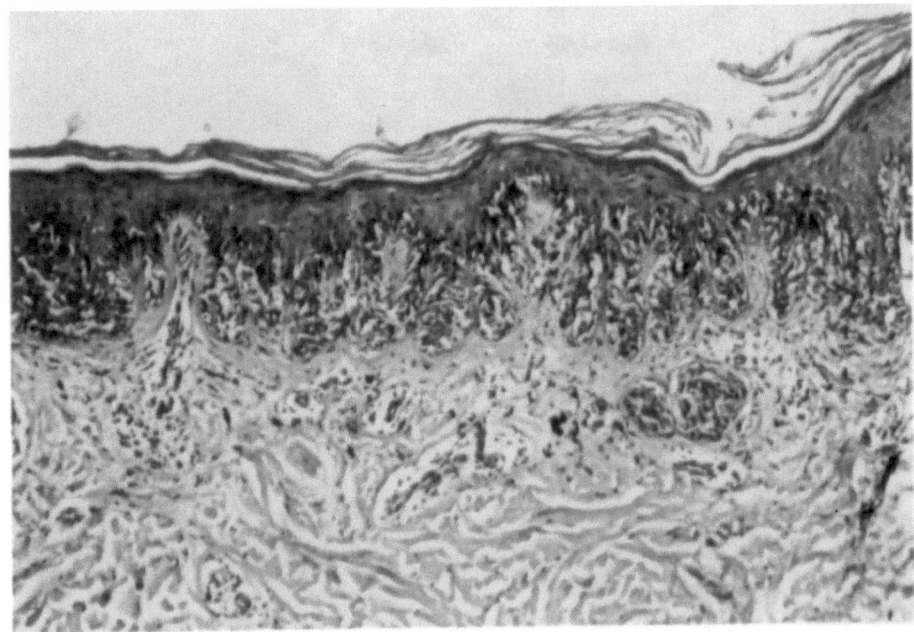

*Figure 4*. Melanoma of thigh, LMM pattern.

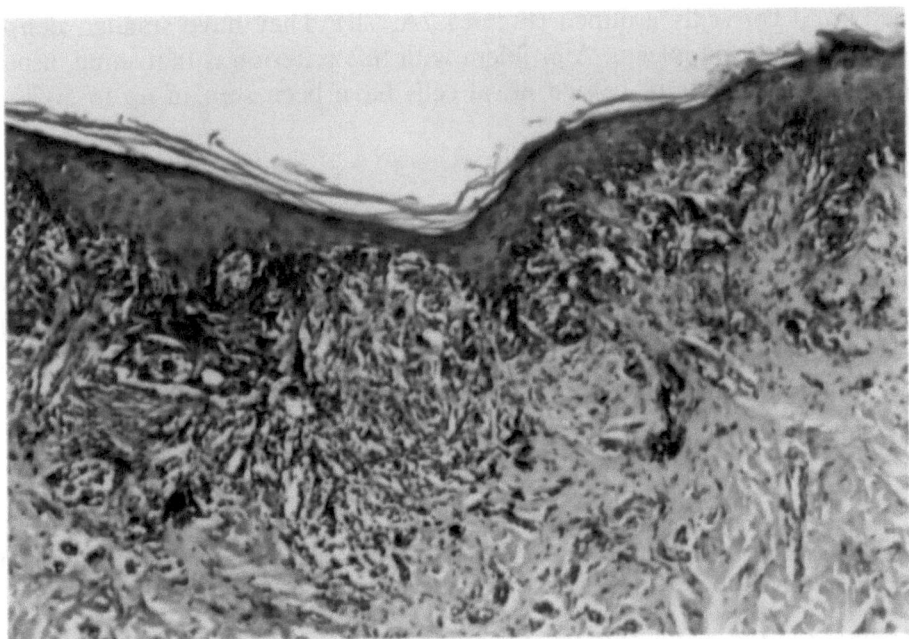

*Figure 5*. Pleomorphic junctional groups in melanoma.

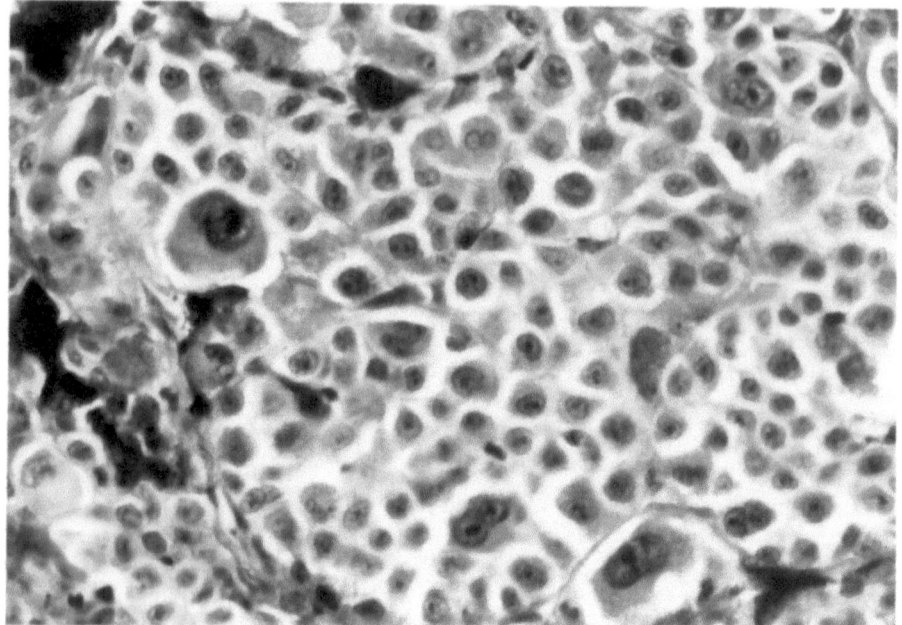

*Figure 6.* Cytologic atypia in melanoma.

Invasive junctional melanomas continue to exhibit cytological atypia to the depth of the tumor; whereas compound nevi show lessening atypia at increasing depths of the dermis, and the benign neval cells become more compactly and convexly grouped (Figures 7A, 7B). They have smaller, denser nuclei and less cytoplasm. A problem with this criterion is that some, usually small, collections of benign neval cells have been seen in up to 50% of malignant melanomas [3].

## Borderline melanoma

The most persuasive argument for morphologic continuity between junctional melanoma and the benign junctional nevus comes from the well established, but poorly defined, and controversial concept of borderline melanoma. Reed et al. [8, 9] coined this entity "minimal deviation melanoma" and define it as:

1) uniform minimal deviation melanoma (uniform population of cells whose cytologic features deviate minimally from nevus cells); and
2) polymorphic melanoma with focal minimal deviation patterns (focal, minimally deviant population of cells whose cytologic features deviate minimally from nervus cells) [8].

He also divides minimal deviation melanoma into epithelioid and spindle cell variants.

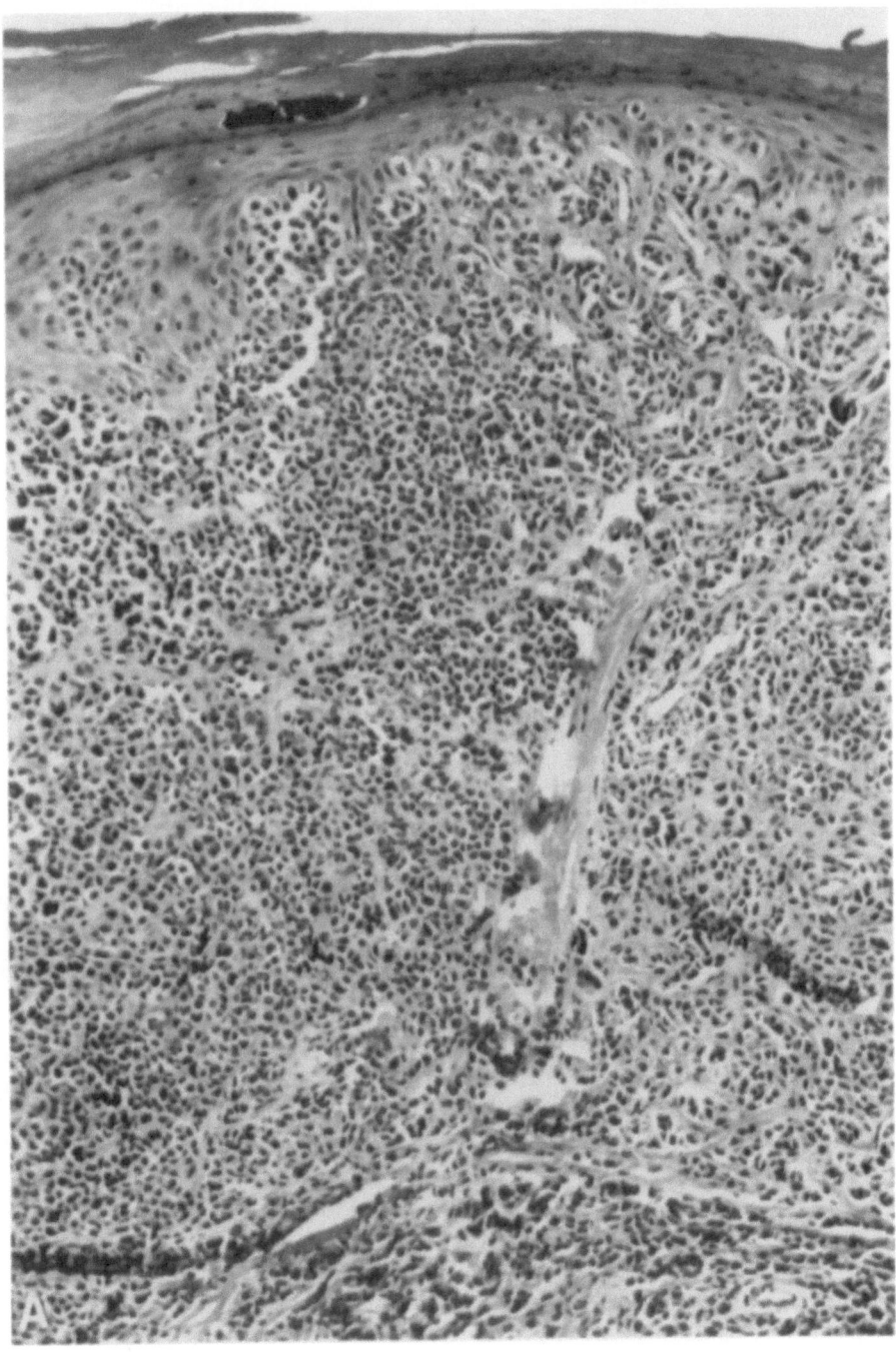

*Figure 7A.* Invasive melanoma.

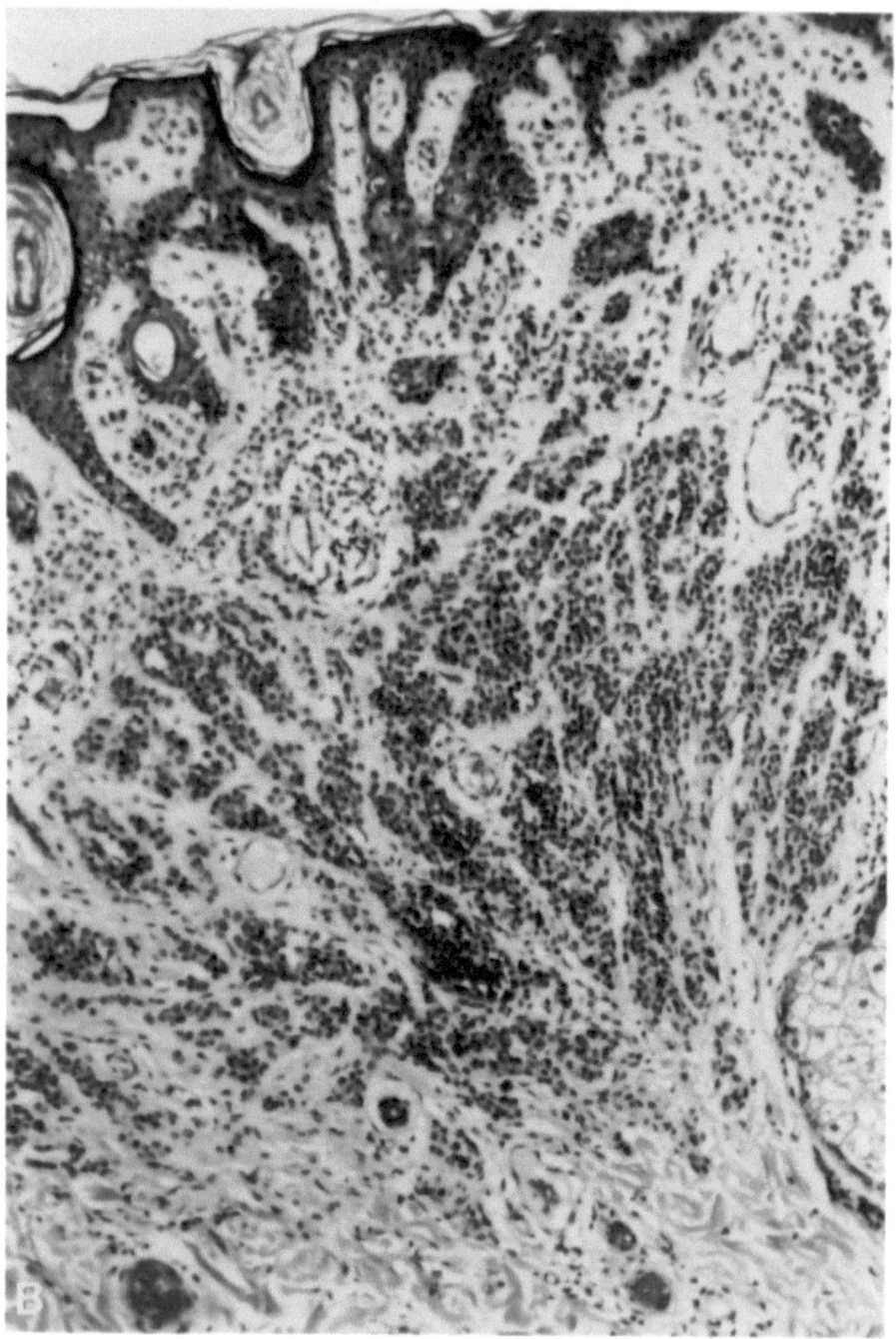

*Figure 7B.* Compound nevus.

Clark uses the term dysplastic nevus and describes it as:

The cytologic appearances that were common to all dysplastic nevi were nuclear pleomorphism and hyperchromatism, seen in a few or many cells of each lesion. Mitotic figures were not frequent. These dysplastic nevi also demonstrated a growth disorder of intraepidermal melanocytes that presented two variants. The most common sub-type, lentiginous melanocytic dysplasia, was seen in all the dysplastic lesions. There was hyperplasia of irregularly-oriented, basally-situated intraepidermal melanocytes. Though some cells were aggregated into small nests, the classical discrete theques of the "junctional nevus" were not present. As a rule, the dysplastic melanocytes were disposed at the periphery of elongated rete ridges. Such elongation of rete with basal melanocytic hyperplasia is similar to that seen in lentigo simplex, and it is for this reason that the histologic appearance is termed lentiginous.

The second pattern of disordered growth, epithelioid-cell melanocytic dysplasia, was present in two of the lesions, in addition to lentiginous dysplasia. Epithelioid-cell dysplasia was characterized by rather well-defined nests of large cells with abundant pale cytoplasm that contained finely-divided "dusty" melanin pigment. The nests tended to confluence and to lateral extension with horizontal orientation across adjacent rete ridges. Although the cytology of this pattern of dysplasia resembles that of classical SSM, pagetoid intraepidermal spread of cells was absent, and mitoses were infrequent [10].

Thus Clark draws the line between dysplastic nevus and melanoma at mitotic figures and intraepidermal melanocytic invasion. He also indicates that these dysplastic changes are found in the benign nevi occurring in patients with familial melanoma (B-K moles) and in patients with melanoma without a familial history.

Sagebiel prefers the term atypical melanocytic hyperplasia (AMH) which he describes as:

Initially, the cells exhibit irregularity, both in manner of spreading and cytological appearance. At low magnification, the process is not sharply circumscribed laterally within the epidermis, nor do the cells reveal the uniform increase in the ridge pattern observed in benign lentigo. The hyperplasia may consist of individual cells or junctional nests; usually, there is a disordered combination of both nests and single cells. At first, the lesion is primarily located in the lower epidermis near the dermal-epidermal junction, with only occasional cells migrating upward. A spectrum of increased numbers of atypical single cells and junctional nests is seen. These nests show greater variation in size and less cohesion than do those of the usual junctional nevus. Nuclear outlines may be pleomorphic, and generally the nucleoli are prominent. Retraction of the cytoplasm separates junctional nests as well as individual melanocytes from adjacent epidermal cells. Pigmentation is commonly irregular, and there is a loss of pigment into the underlying papillary dermis [12].

He found a 16% association between atypical melanocytic hyperplasia and melanoma in the same patients. He allows some intraepidermal invasion within his category of atypical melanocytic hyperplasia, but he also says that the more severe forms of AMH are equivalent to in situ melanomas.

Ackerman says that there is no such lesion truly intermediate between a melanocytic nevus and melanoma and that for some the intermediate desig-

nations are only euphemisms for melanoma in situ [3]. Lesions in the morphological gray zone (for others) he would call benign if they did not fulfill
his criteria for melanoma, malignant if they did, or otherwise he would
simply admit that he did not know:

To us, "borderline" implies that the lesion lies somewhere in between a melanocytic nevus and
a malignant melanoma rather than being one or the other, as it actually is. For that reason we
advocate acknowledging uncertainty directly, without diagnoses such as "borderline melanoma," "minimal deviation melanoma," and "melanocytic dysplasia."

and

Therefore, if the descriptive diagnosis of "atypical melanocytic hyperplasia" is made, it should
be followed in every instance by an explanatory note in which the pathologist conveys that the
lesion is probably benign or potentially malignant, or that he simply does not know for sure.

Finally,

In rare instances, it may be impossible to certify that a particular melanocytic lesion is a junction
nevus or a malignant melanoma in situ. In such cases, a morphologic descriptive diagnosis may
be made with an appended note to explain the difficulties in interpretation to the clinician and
to advise that the lesion should be excised completely rather than "be watched." [3]

Tucker and his colleagues use the older term "activation" of nevi [13].
The histologic features they used were:
1. Noncohesive nests of melanocytes at the dermo–epidermal junction with
fine pigment dispersion
2. Lack of sharp margination of melanocytic activity at lateral margins (>2
rete ridges lateral to dermal nevic component and/or main junctional
activity)
3. Intraepidermal migration of melanocytes
4. Mitotic activity
5. Lack of maturation of melanocytes in lower dermis
6. Atypical cytologic changes of melanocytes
7. Marked pigment production
8. Marked inflammatory infiltrate
Their study went further toward emphasizing the continuity between benign
and malignant morphologies, because they introduced a scoring system for
degree of atypia and applied a probabilistic approach for the presence or
absence of these features in the collection of nevi studied. They found a
spectrum both in activation scores and in frequencies of phenomena across
the nevi and found more atypia in nevi selected clinically, as suspicious,
clinically, or removed from patients with melanoma at other sites.
In summary, there are melanocytic lesions that defy the morphologic definitions of melanoma. Fortunately, they are junctional, superficial and cur-

able by simple excision. That such lesions exist is best demonstrated by the foregoing and other treatments of borderline melanomas, but the frequency of these lesions may vary from time to time, from center to center and from pathologist to pathologist, because, although there is general agreement about which morphologic phenomena are important for the recognition of melanoma, there is no agreement on the exact dividing point between benign and malignant. Most agree that the mass and pattern of junctional and intraepidermal melanocytes are more important than cytologic atypia, but when it is present severe cytologic atypia can make a malignant diagnosis easy to reach. In my opinion these morphological, if not biological, phenomena are continuous so that any dividing points we impose will be artificial. Like severe dysplasias and carcinomas of the cervix some of these atypical lesions will disappear naturally. Others if left alone will become invasive melanoma. In particular cases the best diagnosis and treatment will incorporate the opinions of both clinicians and pathologist.

Several have now established that these atypical and borderline nevi occur more frequently in patients already diagnosed with melanoma [10–13]. This fact raises the possibility of a systemic melanocytic disease in some melanoma patients and suggests a careful search for melanoma in the undiagnosed patient who presents with atypical, especially multiple atypical, nevi. The situation may be similar to adenocarcinoma in situ in a colon polyp. Here also simple excision is curative, but the patient has a greater than usual chance for invasive adenocarcinoma elsewhere in the colon.

## Lentigo maligna vs superficial spreading pattern of junctional melanoma

The discrimination between SSM and LMM types of junctional patterns can be difficult, and Ackerman has said: "Without knowing the anatomic site of a lesion, there are no repetively seen histologic criteria for classifying a malignant melanoma as superficial spreading, lentigo maligna, or acral lentiginous." [4] Clark adds:

Difficulty may be encountered from time to time in histologic distinction among the various forms of melanoma categorized above, but if clinical as well as histologic parameters are assessed, differentiation is not usually a problem. [2]

Nevertheless, few can deny that some melanomas mimic Paget's disease closely; others do not at all; and still others (most?) have intermediate morphologies. I suspect that melanomas comprise a continuum of similarity to Paget's disease morphology.

The histologic discrimination between these two types of junctional and epidermal patterns is best conceptualized as pagetoid (SSM) and nonpagetoid (LMM), and the pagetoid, or epitheloid, melanoma cell is the key feature (Table 2). This cell appears round in section with abundant pale or light and dusty cytoplasm and with a central relatively convex, lightly stained nucleus with moderately prominent nucleolus. These cells are prototypic of SSM but are uncommon in LMM. The best examples of SSM are composed almost entirely of pagetoid melanocytes, and they appear singly or in convex groups throughout the epidermis to mimic Paget's disease completely at scanning magnification (Figure 3).

*Table 2.* Histologic discrimination between SSM and LMM

| Feature | SSM | LMM |
|---|---|---|
| pagetoid cell | prototypic | uncommon |
| pleomorphic spindle cell horizontally arranged | present | present |
| location | junctional and higher | mostly junctional |
| tissue/cell pleomorphism | uniformly atypical | nonuniformly atypical |
| solar elastosis | variable | prominent |
| epidermis | variable or hyperplastic | atrophic |

On the other hand, the best examples of LMM have no pagetoid mela-nocytes (Figure 4) but instead are composed of much more pleomorphic, frequently fusiform melanoma cells with retracted cytoplasmic edges that make the perinuclear zones appear lightly pigmented, clear or webb like with plasma membrane material. There is little or no epidermal invasion above the junction, and the tumor produces plaque like junctional growths rather than convex, more separate groupings. Finally, Clark says that LMM typically shows epidermal atrophy, whereas SSM shows epidermal hyper-plasia and that LMM has more solar elastosis.

This distinction between LMM and SSM may not be entirely academic, since recently McGovern and his colleagues [14] found that those with LMM of the face and neck had a greater five-year survival rate than did those with other types of melanoma, and the two groups had the same overall degree of tumor thickness. In my opinion this is only a preliminary result because there was too little data for a more complete analysis that would have accounted for other prognostic factors such as ulceration and possibly sex. Using a more appropriate multivariate statistical survival model, Balch et al. were unable to show that tumor type was important to prognosis [15].

## Acral lentiginous melanoma

The histologic distinction of melanomas of the palm, sole and nailbed is also a controversial subject. Although there is general agreement that these melanomas are distinctive because of their site and more advanced stage with poorer prognosis, there is disagreement about whether the histologic features of these junctional melanomas are distinctive. Both Arrington et al. [16] and Clark et al. [17] say that these melanomas are all or mostly lentiginous in that they are nonpagetoid with a predominance of junctional proliferation of atypical melanocytes, that these atypical melanocytes have unusually long and prominent dendritic processes, that the epidermis is often hyperplastic and that there is no solar elastosis. But Arrington more than Clark emphasizes epidermal invasion as distinctive from LMM and Clark emphasizes more the bulging junctional nests as distinctive from LMM. Feibleman and his colleagues [18] suggest the following criteria: "atypical spindle-shaped melanocytes with prominent dendrites extending diffusely along the dermal–epidermal junction, epidermal hyperplasia, occasional junctional nesting, little infiltration into the granular layer and stratum corneum, and dermal invasion by fascicles, which often produce a desmoplastic reaction," but they also found that 26% and 3% of melanomas at these sites were respectively SSM (Figure 3) and nodular melanoma (NM) types, and Patterson and Helwig [19] found that 38% of nailbed melanomas were nodular. Clark had indicated that SSM and NM were rare on the palms, soles or nailbeds.

## Melanoma of mucous membranes

Probably less than 5% of melanomas begin in mucosal sites, but those that do devastate the patient. The most common site is the vulva, but other sites include the vagina, anus, penis, oral cavity, nose, sinuses, esophagus and conjunctiva [20]. Clark indicates that their histology is similar to that of ALM, but NM and SSM forms have also been reported. Some have a junctional component; others do not, but submucosal invasion is almost always present (Figures 8, 11). Aside from their occurrence in a mucosa and their more advanced growth, these melanomas differ little with respect to pathology than those from other sites.

## Nodular melanoma

Nodular melanoma is defined as melanoma without a junctional component, but there is debate about whether this always results simply from a junctional melanoma with a predominating and fast vertical growth or

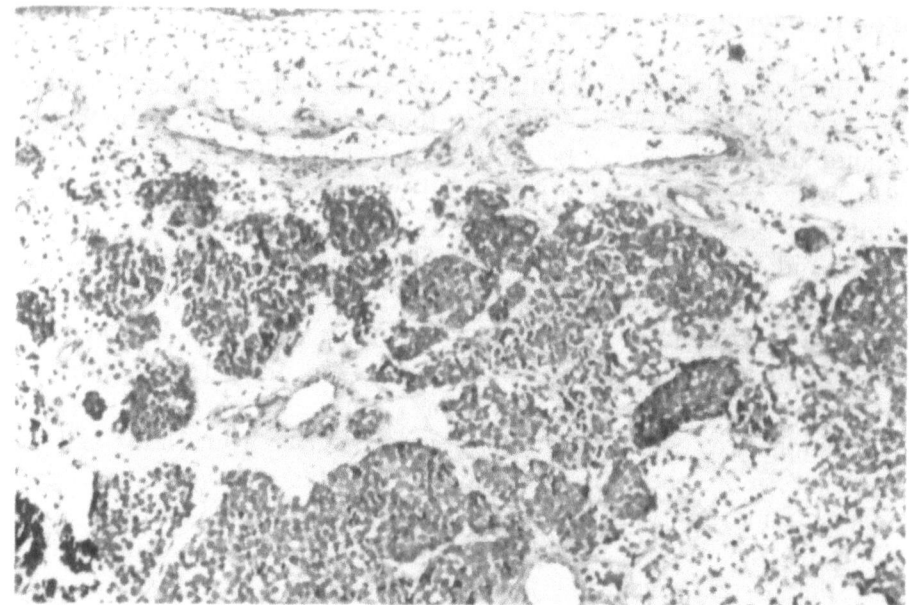

*Figure 8.* Melanoma of nasal mucosa.

whether melanoma can indeed arise de novo in the dermis. The definitions that have allowed up to three adjacent rete ridges of junctional involvement in NM have only weakened the concept [2], but the snapshot biopsy information available tells too little about the evolution of melanoma to decide the issue. My experience has included at least one melanoma without a junctional component even in the overlying intact epidermis (Figure 9), and

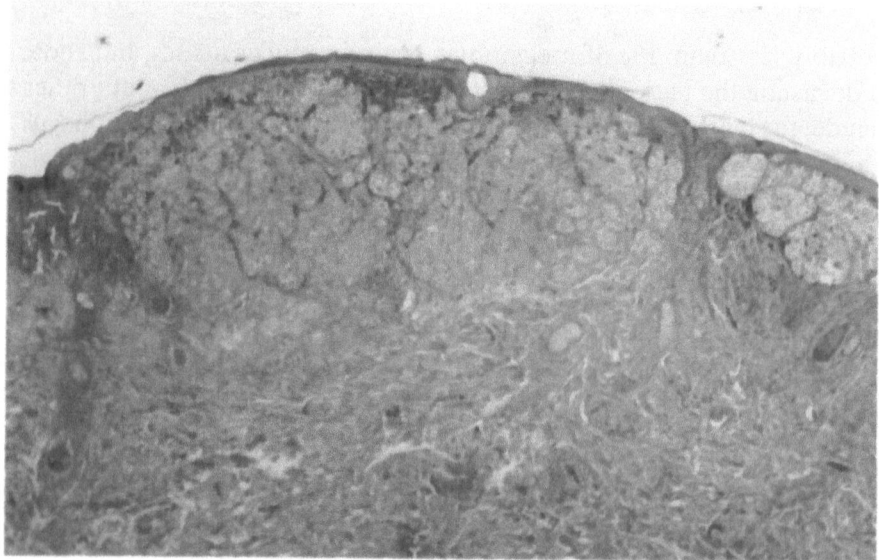

*Figure 9.* Nodular melanoma. The patient had this single cutaneous lesion for several years.

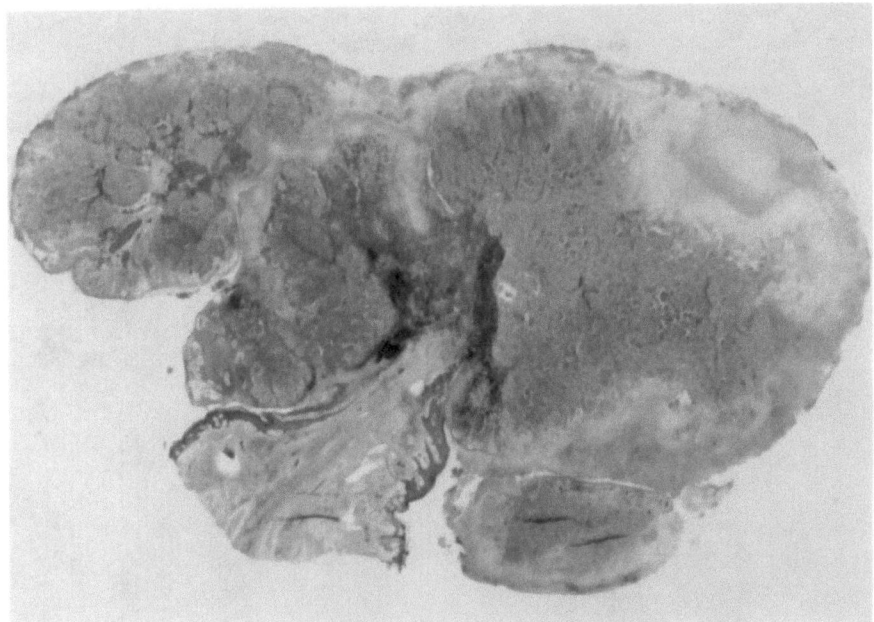

*Figure 10.* Polypoid melanoma.

I am sure this is not an uncommon phenomenon. Who feels they know enough of the biology of melanoma to restrict it to arising at the junction? I certainly do not. Fortunately, the issue is not of prognostic importance, since NM has the prognosis of a SSM of the same tumor thickness [21].

Polypoid melanomas have a distinctive appearance (Figure 10), because they are exophytic growths attached to the skin by relatively thin stalks of dermis. Many can be classed as NM, since they are always thick tumors and since they often have little junctional component. Others show significant adjacent junctional melanoma. They have a prognosis straitforwardly explained by their thickness and thus are not distinctive enough to be placed in a separate class.

## Histochemistry of melanin

In H & E stained sections melanin appears as brown granules of low refractivity, which fail to stain blue with the Prussian blue stain for iron. Although many melanomas can be safely diagnosed without a stain for melanin, there remain "amelanotic" melanomas whose nature is less clear with just the H & E stain and there are soft tissue or neural tumors, whose pigment in H & E sections is not sufficiently specific for the unusual diagnosis of soft tissue melanoma. Thus, it becomes important to have special techniques to stain melanin.

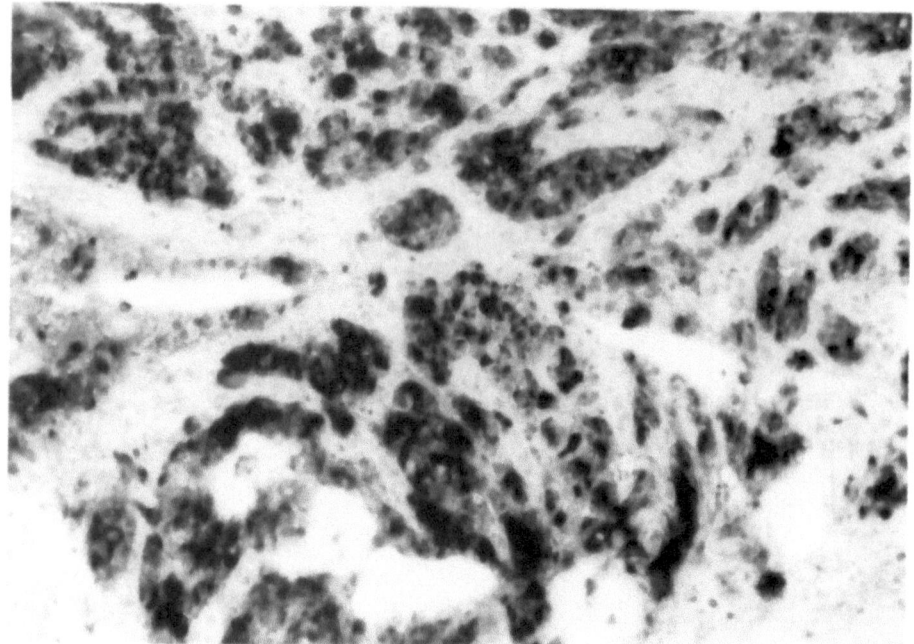

*Figure 11.* Dopa-oxidase stain on nasal melanoma (same case as Figure 8).

Melanin is a partly understood complex of protein and polymerized 5,6-indolequinone, which in turn is synthesized from tyrosine by the enzyme tyrosinase (DOPA oxidase). Melanin is poorly soluble and has the ability to reduce silver nitrate to silver, and this is the basis for the two most important stains: the Fontana-Masson and the modified Warthin-Starry [22, 23]. Both methods result in black silver deposits at melanin sites, but Warkel and his colleagues [23] at the AFIP have demonstrated that the Warthin-Starry stain at pH 3.2 is both more sensitive and more specific for melanin than is the Fontana-Masson stain, which is notorious for staining argentaffin, chromaffin and some lipofuscin pigments.

The presence of D tyrosinase and melanin production capability can also be demonstrated histochemically by incubating unfixed cryostat cut sections of tissue in a medium containing 3,4-dihydroxyphenylalanine (DOPA). After several hours the produced melanin will appear as brown to black granules (Figure 11) [22].

Neuromelanin is also a brown pigment that is present in both the peripheral and central nervous system tissues as well as in rare pigmented central nervous system tumors. With the H & E stain alone it is identical to melanin, but unlike melanin it does not stain with the Warthin-Starry stain, and it does stain with acid fast and oil red O stains.

## Ultrastructure of melanoma

The specific ultrastructural feature for melanoma is the premelanosome—a round to oval body with internal filaments that possess electron dense periodicity (Figure 12) [24, 25]. Their minor diameters range from 0.1 to 0.5 µm, and their major diameters range from 0.4 to 1.0 µm. They have a relatively simple external membrane, but their internal filaments are arranged in a lattice with a planar pattern similar to Venetian blinds and with a 90 A period or as lamellae. The greatest problem with the ultrastructural diagnosis of melanoma is that these classical premelanosomes are often infrequent, and thus may require exhaustive search. In addition to this sampling problem, dense deposits of melanin obscure the lattice in more "mature" melanosomes (Figures 12, 13), so that the organelle cannot be reliably discriminated from a lysosome.

Variant forms of premelanosomes may be more numerous in melanoma, and, taken together with other less specific features, can allow a diagnosis of melanoma [26]. These include particles with less well-ordered lamellar fila-

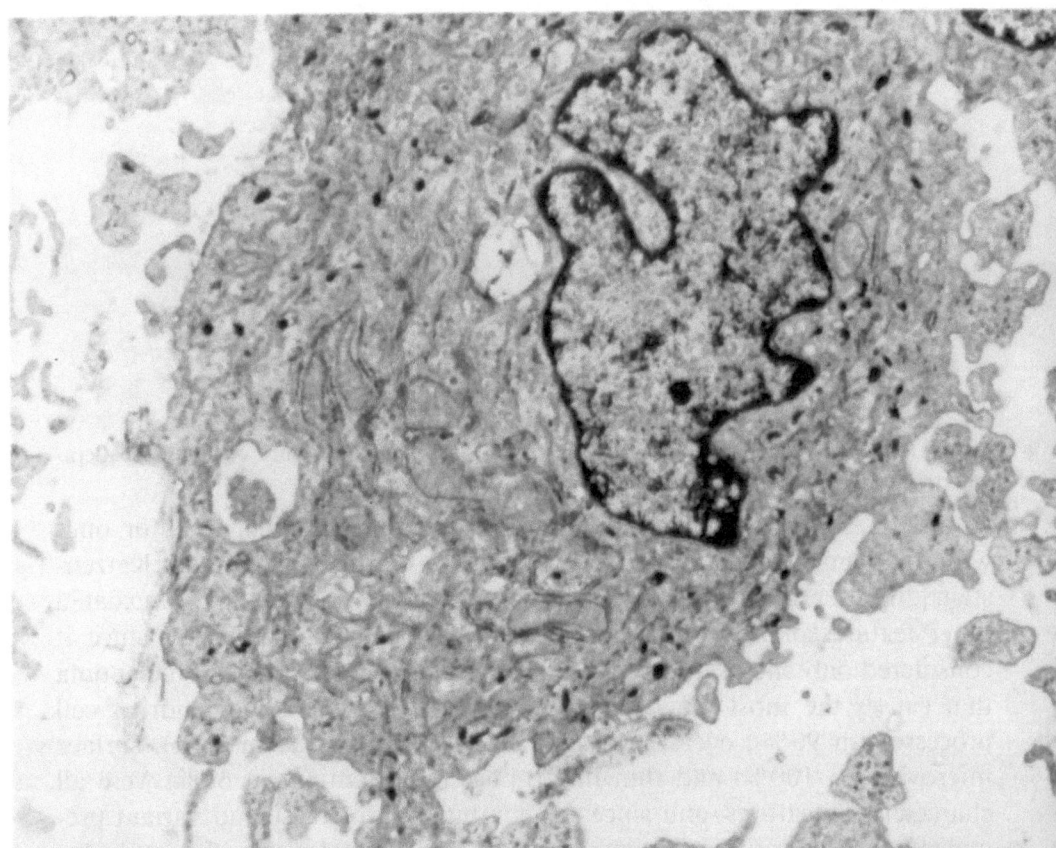

*Figure 12.* Melanoma cell with numerous mature melanosomes (courtesy of Dr. John D. Shelburne)

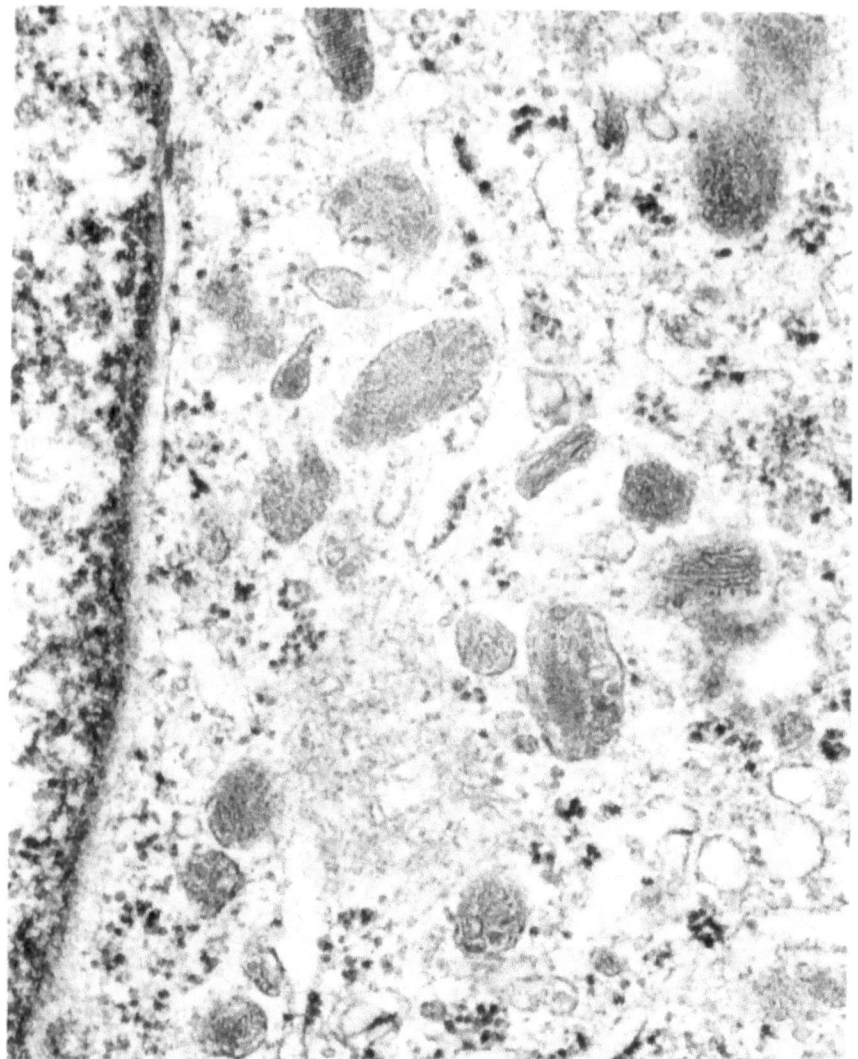

*Figure 13.* Cytoplasm of melanoma cell showing several premelanosomes with lattice pattern (courtesy of Dr. John D. Shelburne).

ments, ones with a single or several peripheral ringed filaments, or ones with filaments partly obscured by granular matrix. Mazur and Katzenstein [26] recently have emphasized these variant forms and have elucidated other features of melanoma. Their study is particularly relevant, since it considered only metastatic melanoma, and it is the metastasis of melanoma that causes the most diagnostic difficulty. They found that dendritic cell processes (in 96%), occasional tight 3–6 cell groupings (in 69%), surface microvilli (in 100%) and thin interrupted basal lamina (in 62%) were all characteristic features, and since the combination of these and variant premelanosomes is probably never seen outside of melanoma they may together provide a diagnosis.

## Histologic prognosis of cutaneous melanoma

Histologic analysis is necessary not only for the diagnosis of melanoma, but also for at least four important determinants of prognosis: tumor thickness, tumor ulceration of surface epidermis, degree of lymphocytic infiltrate and percent of regional lymph nodes involved by tumor.

The initially popular Clark method of determining tumor level of invasion has now been shown to be a weaker prognosticator than tumor thickness [15], and it is a more difficult and inconsistent measure than the Breslow thickness, since it requires two subjective evaluations: one for the point of greatest tumor depth and one for the tissue milieu of that point [27–29]. The Breslow method utilizes only the point of maximum tumor thickness (usually also the maximum tumor depth). This measure is made with a calibrated eyepiece micrometer from the granular cell layer to the deepest tumor point, but care should be taken to block the entire excised lesion so that the thickest point may be seen. Tumor collections that appear to follow adnexal structures into the deeper layers are not used, and all measurements are made from the surface. If the epidermis is ulcerated, then the surface of the ulcer bed is used instead of the granular cell layer. The presence of tumor regression invalidates any conclusions of the measurement, but regression itself is not an important prognostication [30].

Tumor thickness reflects factors other than just tumor bulk. It can be artifactually *increased* by "suboptimal (tissue) processing, slightly higher temperatures in (the histotechnician's) floatation bath, and the use of more concentrated alcohol solutions during the 'floating out' stage" [31], by thinner than usual sections, and by departure from a vertical tissue section plane. It can be artifactually *decreased* by altering the facet "by tilting the angle of the microtome knife or altering the facet at the time of sharpening" [32]. These artifacts have been worked to produce measurement errors ranging from 20% to 40% [31, 32], but Breslow effectively silenced critics by simply pointing out that the method works, and it works well, in spite of whatever variations there might be [33]. I presume that the explanation is that histologic laboratory techniques are sufficiently uniform from day to day, from technician to technician, and from lab to lab to allow comparable results.

Because the Breslow thickness is a linear measurement, it emphasizes the continuous nature of melanoma and because melanoma is a continuous process, I believe any discrete dividing points in the thickness such as 0.76 mm or 1.5 mm may be too arbitrary. Particular patients may not follow such divisions, but certainly as their tumor thickness increases continuously one should expect their survival probability to decrease continuously. Only in the average will their survival follow the published formulas for specific tumor thicknesses.

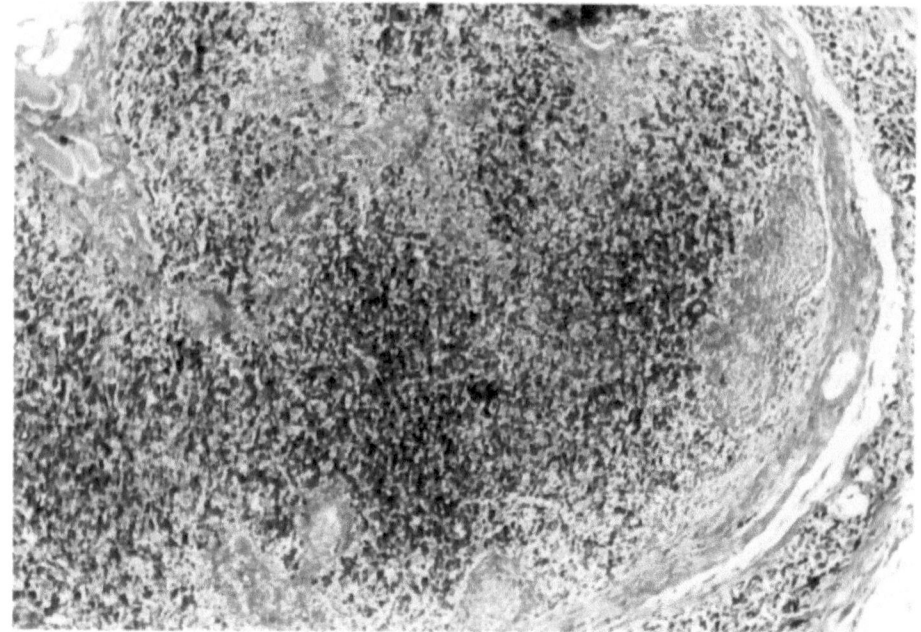

*Figure 14.* Melanosis of lymph node.

The second histologic prognostic feature, ulceration, is defined as necrosis of the surface epidermis overlying the melanoma exclusive of simple tumor invasion of the epidermis. Balch found that the width, but not the depth, of the ulcer was a correlate to survival, and found that those with ulcer widths from 0.25 to 6.0 mm had a 44% five-year survival, whereas those with widths from 6.2 to 28.0 mm had a 5% survival [34].

Lymphatic infiltrate is determined only at the base of the tumor and is divided into two categories: *low,* i.e., "absent to minimal" infiltrate and *high,* i.e., "moderate to marked" infiltrate. In a recent report [35] Day et al. proved that this parameter was an important prognosticator. They found that patients with thick melanomas (>3.5 mm) and with less than 20% of nodes involved by tumor, had a poorer survival if there was a low level of lymphocytic infiltrate at the base of their tumors.

Percentage of lymph nodes involved by a tumor is defined simply as the number of histologically positive nodes divided by the total number of dissected nodes multiplied by 100, and in the same study Day et al. found that this prognosticator outweighed the others, because patients with greater than 20% of their lymph nodes involved had a poor survival rate regardless of tumor thickness or lymphocytic infiltrate.

Determination of the percentage of positive lymph nodes is not entirely straightforward because of two potential problems. First, the regional lymph

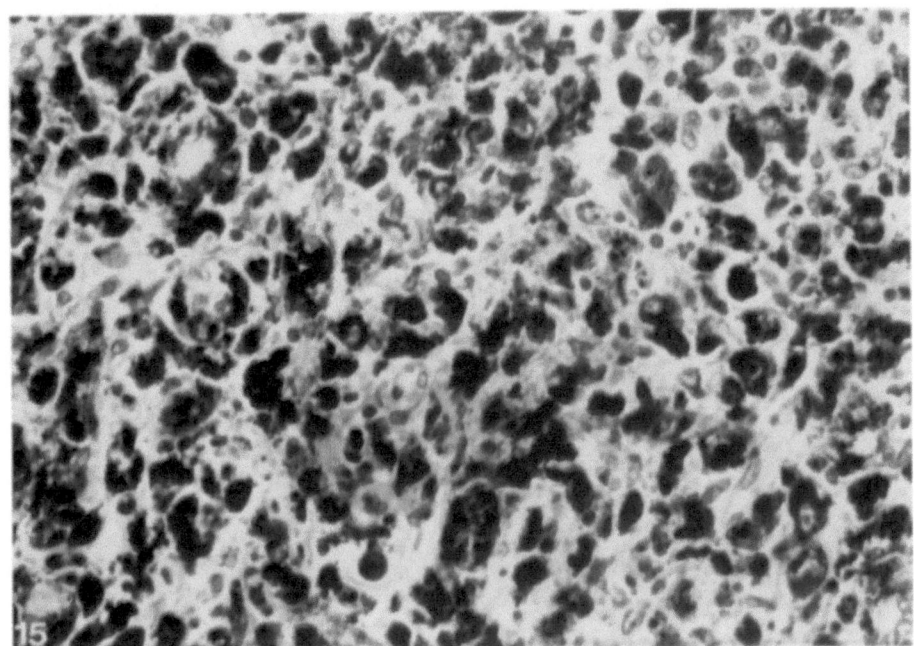

*Figure 15.* Melanosis of lymph node.

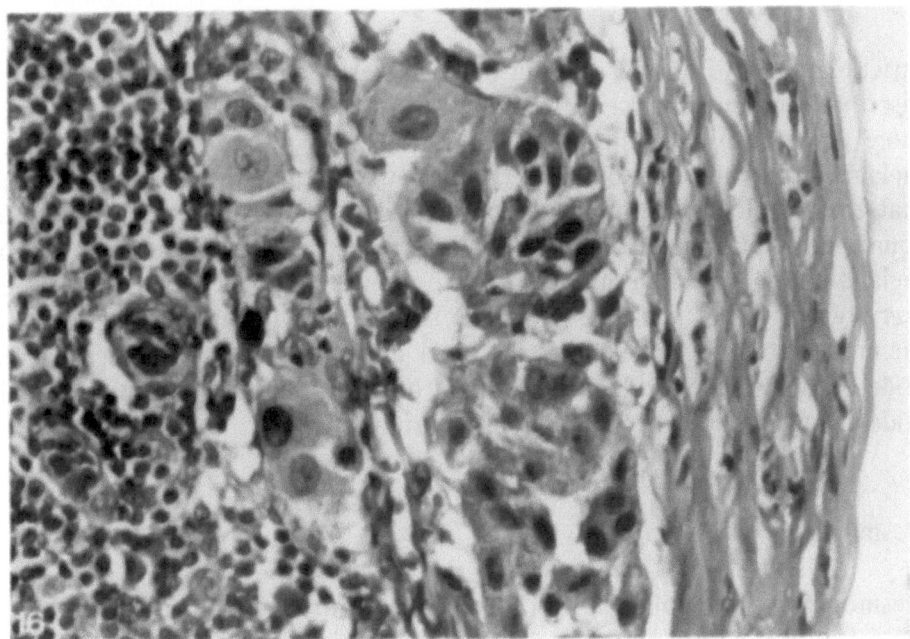

*Figure 16.* Melanoma in lymph node.

nodes draining melanoma can develop an intense melanosis—filling of the nodes with benign melanophages (Figures 14, 15)—that results in many black nodules and makes difficult any gross or microscopic conclusions.

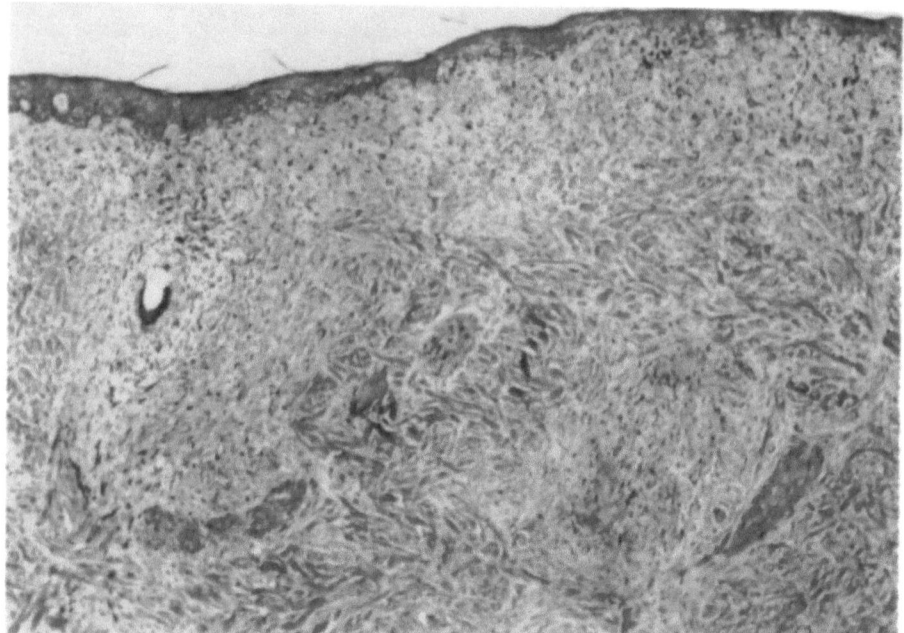

*Figure 17.* Desmoplastic melanoma.

Strict attention to nuclear criteria for malignancy should be most helpful in discriminating melanoma from melanosis. Melanoma cells will have larger more pleomorphic and more visible nuclei and will contain less and finer melanin than the melanophages (Figure 16). Second, the method requires that the histologic sampling of lymph nodes be accurate with respect to counting lymph nodes and sensitive with respect to detecting small foci of melanoma. In my opinion it is best to submit for histologic exam *all* of *every* lymph node. The prosector then should keep careful gross records of the number of nodes placed in each block and of the occasions when a large node occupies several blocks. The final histologic count of positive lymph nodes should then reflect this gross information.

## Desmoplastic melanoma

Desmoplastic melanoma (DM) [36–41] is a dermal and subcutaneous spindle cell tumor whose name, melanoma, comes largely from a chronological association with a junctional melanoma at the same site. Months to years after removal of a junctional melanoma, a nodule occurs at the same site. The biopsy typically shows a deep pleomorphic spindle cell tumor that is both amelanotic and contains many cells with enlarged hyperchromatic nuclei (Figures 17, 18). The tumor fills the dermis, but attachment to the

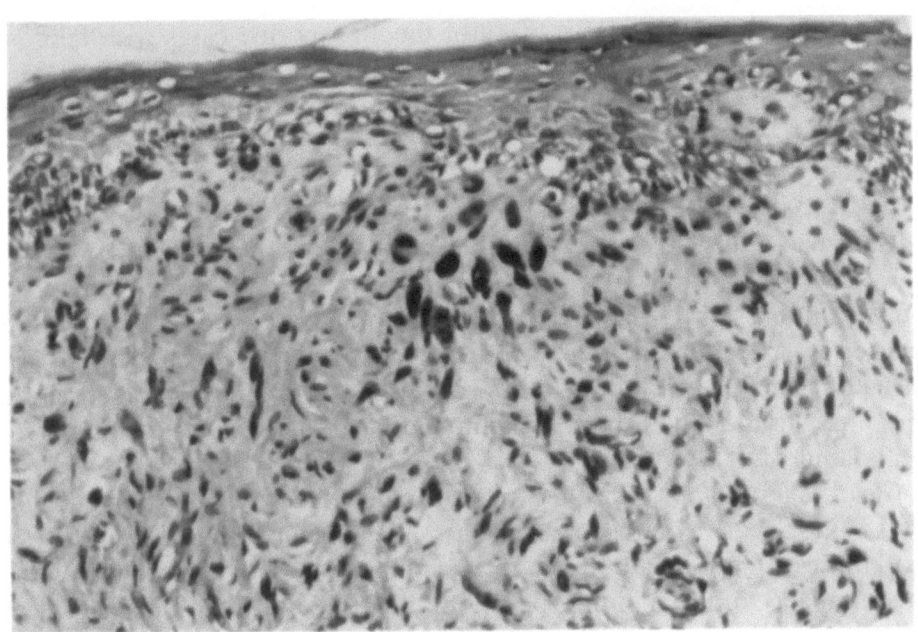

*Figure 18.* Desmoplastic melanoma.

epidermis is either absent or subtle, and a junctional component is usually missing. Special stains for melanin or dopa-oxidase are usually negative, and electron microscopy usually shows no melanosomes. Consequently, unless they are aware of the prior pigmented lesion, pathologists are likely to mistake the lesion for an atypical fibroxanthoma on the one hand or a spindle squamous cell carcinoma or soft tissue sarcoma on the other. Thus the key to both the definition and recognition of DM is the prior or concurrent pigmented lesion. To establish the diagnosis one must confirm that a junctional melanoma either precedes or coexists with the lesion or demonstrate melanin production by the tumor cells with special stains or electron microscopy. Less distinctive features include more tissue and cellular pleomorphism with more collagen than is typical for either dermatofibrosarcoma protuberans or fibrosarcoma, occasional grouping of tumor cells into cohesive epithelial units without interspersed reticulum, a tendency for tumor cells to either involve or mimic nerves, and by electron microscopy tumor cells with primitive intercellular junctions, lack of tonofilaments and with dilated endoplasmic reticulum and extracellular collagen.

Desmoplastic melanoma rarely occurs de novo, but more commonly is a recurrence at the site of a lentigo maligna, a borderline melanoma, an unspecified melanoma or unspecified pigmented lesion. It occurs after a time lapse of from several to many months (minimum 3 months, maximum 20 years, average approximately 50 months). DM is an aggressive tumor. It recurs in greater than 50% of patients and metastasizes in a little less than

50%. It has caused the death of 19 of the 48 reported cases with approximately a 30% five-year survival from the time of the initial lesion. Thus wide excision and regional lymph node dissection have been recommended as routine treatment.

## Melanoma of soft tissue and neural origins

For this discussion I group the melanomas of extraordinary sites into three categories: melanin producing clear cell sarcoma arising in soft tissues, melanotic spindle cell tumors that occur within or around neural structures and finally tumors with both melanin and small dense core "neurosecretory" granules.

Clear cell sarcoma [42–49] is a term coined in 1965 by Enzinger [42]. This tumor nearly always arises in the subcutaneous tissue and mostly on extremities. Histologically it is a mix of spindle and epithelioid cells with a predominance of the spindle type, and it is distinguished by unusually clear-staining cytoplasm due to abundant glycogen and by the presence of brown pigment that in some cases stains for iron and in some cases stains for melanin with the Fontana-Masson stain [47]. Furthermore, a number of investigators have found it to contain melanosomes [43–45, 47, 48]. It is usually only locally aggressive—sometimes with a long history of local growth—and it can be cured by local wide excision or amputation, but some patients have died of recurrent and metastatic growths. Several authors emphasize that clear cytoplasm is not a specific tumor feature, since it also occurs in renal cell carcinomas, synovial sarcomas, leiomyosarcomas and giant cell tumors [45]. Furthermore, some of these clear cell sarcomas have electron microscopic features of schwannomas: interdigitating cytoplasmic processes, basement membranes and rudimentary cell junctions [48]. Thus, although clear cell sarcoma may not be a single homogeneous entity, it includes a malignant melanin-producing tumor of soft tissue origin.

The next group of melanotic tumors may be related to the clear cell sarcomas, because they have also shown Schwann cell differentiation, but they are distinguished because of their obvious association with either nerves or ganglia [50–58]. These are the melanotic nerve sheath tumors or melanotic schwannomas. Their locations have included the spinal nerve roots—both intradural and extradural, paravertebral sympathetic ganglia, the acoustic nerve, the adrenal gland, the mandible—and such nonspecific sites as subcutaneous and peritoneal tissues. Histologically, they have been comprised of spindle stromal type cells with melanin pigment, premelanosomes and mature melanosomes (by EM) and with variable degrees of cellularity, mitotic figures, and atypia. Most of the reported tumors have had a nonspecific interlacing fasicular pattern of spindle cells, but a case that we saw

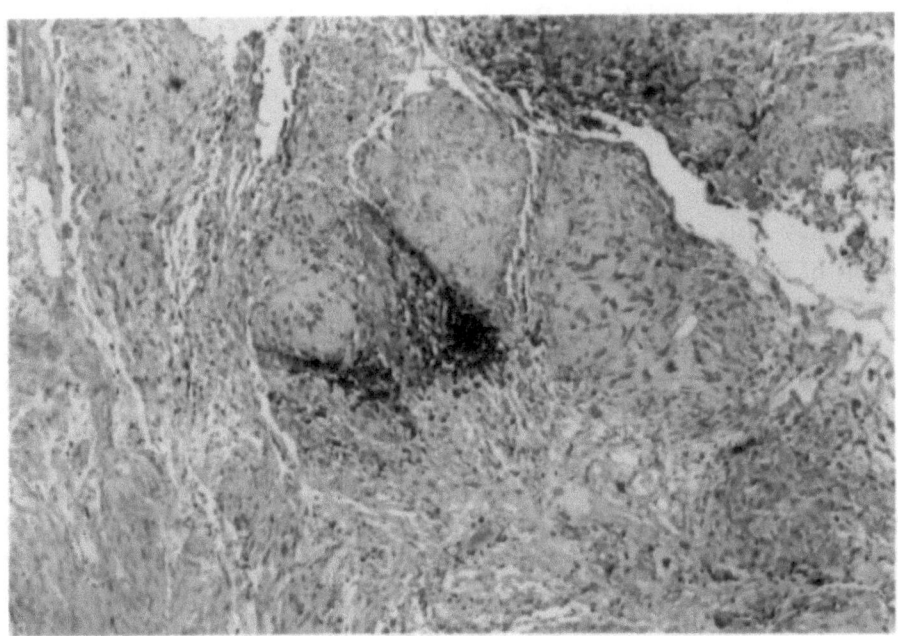

*Figure 19.* Melanotic schwannoma. The tumor was a circumscribed nodule in the paravertebral location of the thorax. Abundant melanin was present.

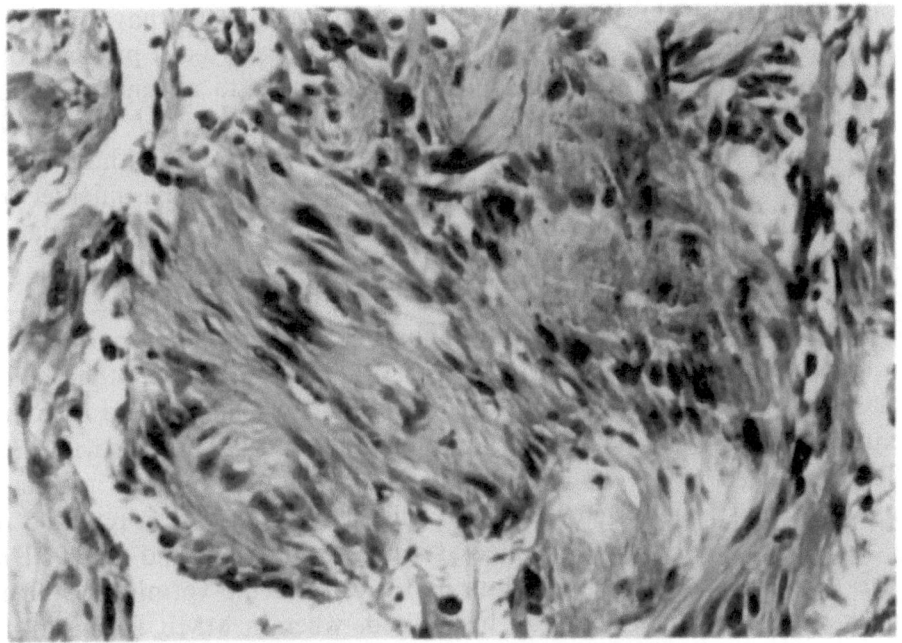

*Figure 20.* Melanotic schwannoma. Melanin pigment in tumor cells (Verocay formation).

showed typical antoni A and B stromal patterns with verocay bodies as well as melanin (Figures 19, 20). They present as relatively circumscribed growths so that surgical excision has been curative for some of these patients, but the prognosis has been variable with some patients dying of disseminated tumor quickly or after 8 years and with some patients surviving over 17 years without recurrence. This variability suggests that this group may also be heterogeneous and be composed of a spectrum from benign to malignant.

The most widely reported central nervous system melanoma is that arising in the soft tissue coverings of the brain and spinal cord: the meningeal melanoma [59-61]. This tumor characteristically occurs in younger patients than does cutaneous melanoma. Its peak incidence spans the years from 20 to 50, and 45% of the reported cases have been in their first three decades. It usually produces a diffuse indurated growth in the meninges, although some localized tumors have been reported, and it usually cannot be resected, so that it is nearly always fatal and in a time period characteristically less than a year. It can involve the coverings of any part of the brain or spinal cord. Histologically, meningeal melanoma shares features with cutaneous melanoma, but spindle cell morphology is probably more common. Electron microscopy has shown both premelanosomes and melanosomes. The greatest controversy about meningeal melanoma centers about the concurrence of pigmented lesions in the skin or other organs. Some patients have had concurrent giant pigmented nevi or multiple cutaneous nevi— perhaps in a manner similar to the dysplastic nevus or activated mole syndromes—and there are reports of meningeal melanomas that have metastasized outside the CNS. Generally, when melanoma has been present both inside and outside the CNS, the prejudice has been to assign the tumor origin to the extraneural sites, and one author has suggested that the criteria for meningeal melanoma require diffuse meningeal melanosis without a history of extraneural pigmented lesions [61]. Nevertheless, Pasquier et al. reported one case and found 13 other acceptable examples of CNS melanoma with metastases to other organs—most commonly the liver [62].

There have been two tumor types in which both neural differentiation and melanin production have been established. They are the melanotic neuroectodermal tumor of infancy (MNTI) [63-67] and the melanotic medulloblastoma (MMB) [68-73]. Both occur in infants or children and both are comprised in part by small central undifferentiated cells together with peripherally located larger cuboidal to columnar cells with melanin pigment. The MNTI most often occurs in the maxilla, but has also been reported in the mandible, skull, shoulder, mediastinum, epididymis and thigh. The MMB occurs only in the cerebellum and mostly in the vermis. MMTI is usually a benign tumor that can be excised, whereas MMB is uniformly lethal due to early and widespread dissemination through the CSF. Electron microscopy of at least one case has demonstrated dense core granules in the central cells and premelanosomes and melanosomes in the peripheral cells [66].

## Melanoma of unknown primary site

In clinical practice and in reported series of melanoma patients, there are some who have metastatic melanoma without an obvious primary site [74–78]. The prevalence of these is 4% among all melanoma patients, and they fall into two roughly equally numbered categories: those with tumors in a single regional lymph node group, and those who have either regional lymph nodes and regional cutaneous and subcutaneous tumor nodules or who have distant or disseminated tumor. The latter group has uniformly poor prognoses, and most die within a year, but the first group are special, because between 25% and 50% of them will survive ten years after node dissection and because they spark a controversy about whether melanoma arises in lymph nodes.

In this regional lymph node group the axilla is the most common site (50%), and the neck and groin have a lower prevalence (approximately 25% each), although Baab and his colleagues have also found that for women the groin may be the most common site (58%) [78].

Two hypotheses have been offered to explain melanomas presenting in lymph nodes without cutaneous or visceral primary sites [75]. The favored one is that most of these tumors are metastases from regressed cutaneous primaries. The unfavored one is that melanoma can arise in lymph nodes.

Certainly regression of both moles and melanoma is an established phenomenon. Some have found that the presence of regression in a thin melanoma indicates a greater chance for regional metastasis [79]. Others have found that regression is not a prognostic factor [30], but I believe everyone's experience would verify that at least partial regression of cutaneous melanomas is a common finding so that it seems reasonable that some melanomas could first metastasize and then regress. The most compelling argument for this mechanism is Smith and Stehlin's observation of eight patients with metastatic melanoma and no obvious primary site [77]. Careful questioning and examination of these eight revealed that all had had an atypical pigmented skin lesion in the area drained by their respective involved lymph nodes, and that all had retained clinical and histologic evidence of a regressed pigmented lesion at the site.

The arguments that favor melanoma arising in lymph nodes are three: benign pigmented neval cells occur in lymph nodes [80–82]; there remain patients who have tumors in lymph nodes, who have not had current or previous atypical pigmented lesions, even after careful scrutiny [77] and who achieve long survival after excision of just the lymph nodes; and finally nothing in the arguments that favor the regression hypothesis excludes the possibility that *both* mechanisms can work in different patients to produce a lesion with "unknown primary."

Das Gupta and his colleagues [75] prefer to consider the neval cells in lymph nodes as embolic, but this is an opinion—no one really knows. They also state that these neval collections are only rarely found, but who can say that they are too rare to account for another rare event, occult melanoma [82]? Just as Smith and Stehlin's eight patients provided support for the regression hypothesis, the 31, for whom their scrutiny failed to uncover pigmented skin lesions, leave open the issue of tumor origin. Finally, the most general starting assumption is that both mechanisms may work, and until there exists evidence that one is unlikely the safest assumption is the most general.

All these arguments are of lesser importance, since they affect only how we conceptualize melanoma. The important and established fact about occult melanoma is that some of these patients who have melanoma in regional lymph nodes will achieve a long survival after lymph node resection.

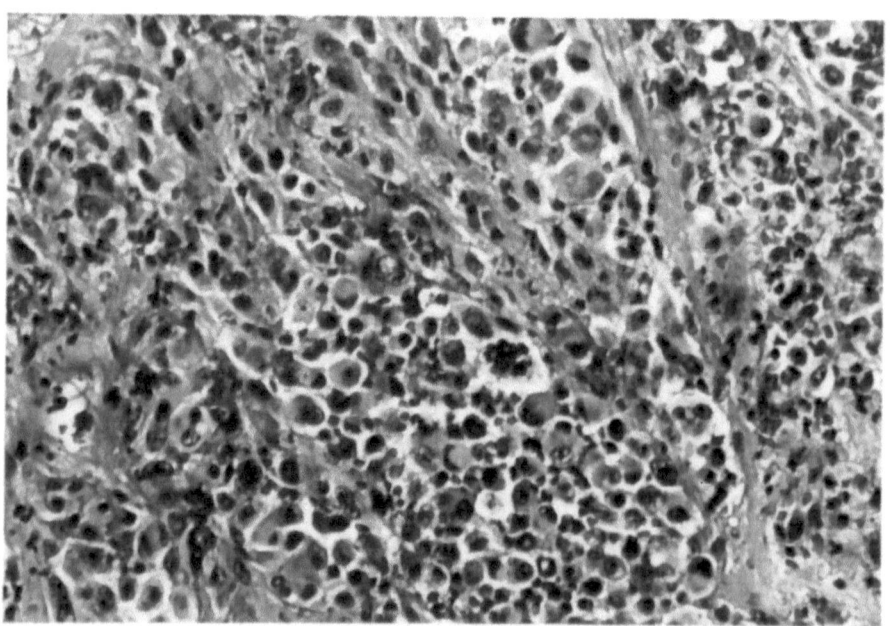

*Figure 21.* Amelanotic melanoma.

## Amelanotic melanoma

In the total collection of human tumors there are some that histologically resemble melanoma but do not contain sufficient melanin to be recognized even with special stains. Since electron microscopy and dopa-oxidase techniques are not routinely used for undifferentiated tumors, the diagnosis of amelanotic melanoma is probably made in a non-uniform and rough way by most pathologists. The histologic setting is that of a large cell undifferentiated carcinoma with abundant either densely eosinophilic or lightly granular cytoplasm, atypical nuclei with prominent nucleoli, and a loose cohesiveness to the cells (Figure 21). The arrangement of the tumor cells at the junction and in the dermis will suggest melanoma, but some pathologists can recognize amelanotic melanoma in lymph nodes and in cytologic preparations. Nevertheless, the diagnosis is never certain without electron microscopic demonstration of melanosomes.

Huvos, Shah and Goldsmith [83] have estimated amelanotic melanoma to comprise approximately 2% of all melanomas, and their study indicates that this tumor is distinctive in several ways. First, it appears more often in females than males. Second, it more often presents in a later stage of disease than does pigmented melanoma. Third, for any stage of disease it has a worse prognosis than does pigmented melanoma, and finally it presents as tumor with an occult primary more often than does pigmented melanoma (approximately 29% of cases).

## References

1. Clark WH, Jr, Folberg R and Ainsworth AM: Tumor progression in primary human cutaneous malignant melanomas. In: Clark WH, Jr, Goldman LI and Mastrangelo NJ (eds) Human Malignant Melanoma, pp 15–32. Grune & Stratton, New York, 1979.
2. Elder DE, Ainsworth AM and Clark WH, Jr: The surgical pathology of cutaneous malignant melanoma. In: Clark WH, Jr, Goldman LI and Mastrangelo NJ (eds) Human Malignant Melanoma, pp 55–108. Grune & Stratton, New York, 1979.
3. Ackerman AB and Su WPD: The histology of cutaneous malignant melanoma. In: Kopf AW, Bart RS, Rodriquez-Sanas RS and Ackerman AB (eds) Malignant Melanoma, pp 25–147. Masson, 1979.
4. Ackerman AB: Malignant melanoma: a unifying concept. Am J Dermatopathol 2:309–313, 1980.
5. Elder DE, Jucovy PM, Tuthill RJ and Clark WH, Jr: The classification of malignant melanoma. Am J Dermatopathol 2:315–320, 1980.
6. McGovern VJ et al: The classification of malignant melanoma and its histological reporting. Cancer 32:1446–1457, 1973.
7. Kopf AW, Bart RF, Rodriquez-Sanas RS and Ackerman AB: Malignant Melanoma, pp 7–24. Masson, 1979.
8. Reed RJ, Ichinose H, Clark WH, Jr and Mihm MC, Jr: Common and uncommon melanocytic nevi and borderline melanomas. Sen Oncol 2:119–147, 1975.
9. Reed RJ: Consultation case. Am J Surg Path 2:215–220, 1978.

10. Elder DE, Goldman LI, Goldman SC, Greene MH and Clark WH, Jr: Dysplastic nevus syndrome: a phenotypic association of sporadic cutaneous melanoma. Cancer 46:1787–1794, 1980.

11. Clark WH, Jr, Reimer RR, Greene MH, Ainsworth AM and Mastrangelo MJ: Origin of familial malignant melanomas from heritable melanocytic lesions. Arch Dermatol 114:732–738, 1978.

12. Sagebiel RW: Histopathology of borderline and early malignant melanomas. Am J Surg Pathol 3:543–552, 1979.

13. Tucker SB, Horstmann JP, Hertel B, Aranha F and Rosai J: Activation of nevi in patients with malignant melanoma. Cancer 46:822–827, 1980.

14. McGovern BJ, Saw HM, Milton GW and Farago GA: Is malignant melanoma arising in a Hutchinson's melanotic freckle a separate disease entity? Histopathology 4:235–242, 1980.

15. Balch CM, Murad TM, Soong S, Ingalls AL, Halpern NB and Maddox WA: A multifactorial analysis of melanoma. Ann Surg 188:732–742, 1978.

16. Arrington JH, Ill, Reed RJ, Ichinose H and Krementz ET: Planter lentiginous melanoma: a distinctive variant of human cutaneous malignant melanoma. Am J Surg Pathol 1:131–143, 1977.

17. Clark WH, Jr, Bernardino EA, Reed RJ and Kopf AW: Acral lentiginous melanomas. In: Clark WH, Jr, Goldman LI and Mastrangelo MJ (eds) Human Malignant Melanoma, pp 109–124. Grune & Stratton, 1979, New York.

18. Feibleman CE, Stoll H and Maize JC: Melanomas of palm, sole and nailbed. Cancer 46:2492–2504, 1980.

19. Patterson RH and Helwig EB: Subungual malignant melanoma: a clinical-pathologic study. Cancer 46:2074–2087, 1980.

20. Das Gupta TK, Brasfield RD and Paglia MA: Primary melanomas in unusual sites. Surg Gynecol Obstet 12B:841–848, 1969.

21. McGovern BJ, Shaw HM, Milton GW, Farago GA: Prognostic significance of histological features of malignant melanoma. Histopathology 3:385–393, 1979.

22. Stevens A: Pigmants and minerals. In: Bancroft JD and Stevens A. Theory and Practice of Histological Techniques, pp 194–197. Churchill-Livingstone, 1977.

23. Warkel RL, Luna LG and Helwig EB: A modified Warthin-Starry procedure at low pH or melanin. Am J Clin Pathol 73:812–815, 1980.

24. Zelickson AS: Melanocyte, melanin granule and Langerhans cell. In: Zelickson AS. Ultrastructure of Normal and Abnormal Skin, Ch 8. Lea & Febiger, Philadelphia, 1967.

25. Wellings SR and Siegel BV: Electron microscopy of human malignant melanoma. J Nat Cancer Inst 24:437–461, 1960.

26. Mazur MT and Katzenstein AA: Metastatic melanoma: the spectrum of ultrastructural morphology. Ultra Pathol 1:337–356, 1980.

27. Suffin SC, Waisman J, Clark WH, Jr and Morton DL: Comparison of the classification by microscopic level (stage) of malignant melanoma by three independent groups of pathologists. Cancer 40:3112–3114, 1977.

28. Breslow A: Thickness, cross-sectional areas and depth of invasion in the prognosis of cutaneous melanoma. Ann Surg 172:902–908, 1970.

29. Breslow A: Problems in the measurement of tumor thickness and level of invasion and cutaneous melanoma. Hum Pathol 8:1–2, 1977.

30. McLean DI, Lew RA, Sober AJ, Mihm MC and Fitzpatrick TB: The prognostic importance of white depressed areas and the primary lesion of superficial spreading melanoma. Cancer 43:157–161, 1979.

31. Weedon D: Measurements of tumor thickness. Hum Pathol 9:124, 1978.

32. Bhagavan BS: Measurements of tumor thickness. Hum Pathol 8:711–712, 1977.

33. Breslow A: Measurements of tumor thickness. Hum Pathol 9:238–239, 1978.

34. Balch CM, Wilkerson JA, Murad TM, Soong S, Ingells AL and Maddox WA: The prognostic significance of ulceration of cutaneous melanoma. Cancer 45:3012–3017, 1980.
35. Day CC et al: Malignant melanoma with positive nodes and relatively good prognoses: micro staging retains prognostic significance in clinical Stage I melanoma patients with metastases to regional nodes. Cancer 47:955–962, 1981.
36. Conley J, Lattes R, Orr W: Desmoplastic and malignant melanoma ( rare variant of spindle cell melanoma). Cancer 28:914–936, 1971.
37. Labrecque PG, Hu C and Winkelmann RK: The nature of desmoplastic melanoma. Cancer 38:1205–1213, 1976.
38. Valensi QJ: Desmoplastic and malignant melanoma: a report on two additional cases. Cancer 39:286–292, 1977.
39. Valensi QJ: Desmoplastic and malignant melanoma: a light and electron microscopic study of two cases. Cancer 43:1148–1155, 1979.
40. Reed RJ, Leonard DD: Neurotropic melanoma: a variant of desmoplastic melanoma. Am J Surg Pathol 3:301–311, 1979.
41. Yannopoulos K: Desmoplastic malignant melanoma. In: Fenoglio CM and Wolff M (eds) Progress in Surgical Pathology, Vol 2, pp 269–289. Masson, 1980.
42. Enzinger FM: Clear cell sarcoma of tendons and aponeuroses and analysis of 21 cases. Cancer 18:1163–1174, 1965.
43. Hoffman GJ and Carter D: Clear cell sarcoma of tendons and aponeuroses with melanin. Arch Pathol 95:22–25, 1973.
44. Mackenzie DH: Clear cell sarcoma of tendon and aponeuroses with melanin production. J Pathol 114:231–234, 1974.
45. Bearman RM, Noe J and Kempson RL: Clear cell sarcoma with melanin pigment. Cancer 36:977–984, 1975.
46. Toe TK and Saw D: Clear cell sarcoma with melanin: a report of two cases. Cancer 41:235–238, 1978.
47. Boudreaux D and Waisman J: Clear cell sarcoma with melanogenesis. Cancer 41:1387–1394, 1978.
48. Tsuneyoshi M, Enjoji M and Kubo T: Clear cell sarcoma of tendons and aponeuroses: a comparative study of 13 cases with a provisional subgrouping into the melanotic and synovial types. Cancer 42:243–252, 1978.
49. Raynor AC, Vargas-Cortes F, Alexander RW and Bingham HG: Clear cell sarcoma with melanin pigment: a possible soft-tissue during a malignant melanoma. J Bone Joint Surg 61A:276–280, 1979.
50. Mallar WG: A malignant melanotic tumor of ganglion cells arising from a thoracic sympathetic ganglion. J Pathol Bacteriol 35:351–357, 1932.
51. Kniseley RM and Baggenstoss AH: Primary melanoma of the adrenal glands. Arch Pathol 42:345–349, 1946.
52. Dick JC, Titchie GM and Thompson H: Histological differentiation between pheochromocytoma and melanoma of the suprarenal gland. J Clin Pathol 8:89–98, 1955.
53. Mandybur TI: Melanotic nerve sheath tumors. J Neurosurg 41:187–192, 1974.
54. Fu Y, Kaye GI and Lattes R: Primary malignant melanotic tumors of the sympathetic ganglia, with an ultrastructural study of one. Cancer 36:2029–2041, 1975.
55. Graham DI, Paterson A, McQueen A, milne JA and Urich H: Melanotic tumours (blue naevi) of spinal nerve roots. J Pathol 118:83–89, 1976.
56. Mennemeyer RP, Hammar SP, Tytus JS, Hallman KO, Raisis JE and Bockus D: Melanotic schwannoma. Am J Surg Pathol 3:3–10, 1979.
57. Lowman RM and Livolsi VA: Pigmented (melanotic) schwannomas of the spinal canal. Cancer 46:391–397, 1980.
58. Parker JB, Marcus PB and Martin JH: Spinal melanotic clear-cell sarcoma: a light and electron microscopic study. Cancer 46:718–724, 1980.

59. Gibson JB, Burrows D and Weir WP: Primary melanoma of the meninges. J Pathol Bacteriol 74:419–438, 1957.

60. Limas C and Tio FO: Meningeal melanocytoma ("melanotic meningioma"): its melanocytic origin as revealed by electron microscopy. Cancer 30:1286–1294, 1972.

61. Savitz MH and Anderson PJ: Primary melanoma of the leptomeninges: a review. Mt Sinai J Med N Y 41:774–791, 1974.

62. Pasquier B, Coudere P, Pasquier D, Panh MH and Arnold JP: Primary malignant melanoma of the cerebellum: a case with metastases outside the nervous system. Cancer 41:344–351, 1978.

63. Stowens D: A pigmented tumour of infancy: the melanotic progonoma. J Pathol Bacteriol 73:43–51, 1957.

64. Misugi K, Okajima H, Newton WA, Kmatz DR and DeLorimier AA: Mediastinal origin of a melanotic progonoma or retinal anlage tumor: ultrastructural evidence for neural crest origin. Cancer 18:477–484, 1965.

65. Hayward AF, Fickling BW and Lucas RB: An electron microscope study of a pigmented tumour of the jaw of infants. Br J Cancer 23:702–708, 1969.

66. Palacios JJN: Malignant melanotic neuroectodermal tumor: light and electron microscopic study. Cancer 46:529–536, 1980.

67. Mullins JD: A pigmented differentiating neuroblastoma: a light and ultrastructural study. Cancer 46:522–528, 1980.

68. Fowler M and Simpson DA: A malignant melanin-forming tumour of the cerebellum. J Pathol Bacteriol 84:307–311, 1962.

69. Best PV: A medulloblastoma-like tumour with melanin formation. J Pathol 110:109–111, 1973.

70. Sung JH, Mastri AR and Segal EL: Melanotic medulloblastoma of the cerebellum. J Neuropathol Exp Neurol 32:437–445, 1973.

71. McCloskey JJ, Parker JC, Brooks WH and Blacker HM: Melanin as a component of cerebral gliomas: the melanotic cerebral ependymoma. Cancer 37:2373–2379, 1976.

72. Hahn JF, Sperber EE, Netsky MG: Melanotic neuroectodermal tumours of brain and skull. J Neuropathol Exp Neurol 35:508–519, 1976.

73. Boesel CP, Suhan JP and Sayers MP: Melanotic medulloblastoma: a report of a case with ultrastructural findings. J Neuropathol Exp Neurol 37:531–543, 1978.

74. Pack GT and Miller JR: Metastatic melanoma with inderterminate primary site. J Am Med Assoc 176:55–56, 1961.

75. Das Gupta T, Bowden L and Berg JW: Malignant melanoma of unknown primary origin. Surg Gynecol Obstet 117:341–345, 1963.

76. Mundth ED, Guralnick EA and Raker JW: Malignant melanoma: a study of 427 cases. Ann Surg 162:15–28, 1965.

77. Smith JL and Stehlin JS: Spontaneous regression of primary malignant melanomas with regional metastases. Cancer 18:1399–1415, 1965.

78. Baab GH and McBride CM: Malignant melanoma: in patient with an unknown site of primary origin. Arch Surg 110:896–900, 1975.

79. Gromet MA, Epstein WL and Blois MS: The regressing thin melanoma: a distinctive lesion with metastatic potential. Cancer 42:2282–2292, 1978.

80. Johnson WT and Helwig EB: Benign nevus cells in the capsule of lymph nodes. Cancer 23:747–753, 1969.

81. Hart WR: Primary nevus of a Lymph node. Am J Clin Pu 551:88–92, 1971.

82. Ridolfi RL, Rosen PP and Thaler H: Nevus cell aggregates associated with lymph nodes: estimated frequency and clinical significance. Cancer 39:164–171, 1977.

83. Huvos AG, Shah JP and Goldsmith HS: A clincopathologic study of amelanotic melanoma. Surg Gynecol Obstet 135:917–920, 1972.

# 3. Melanoma of the genitourinary tract

SAM D. GRAHAM, Jr., WAYNE A. CLINE, Jr. and
JOHN L. WEINERTH

## Introduction

Malignant melanoma of the genitourinary tract is a very uncommon disease. Less than 200 primary melanomas of the genitourinary tract have been
described in the world literature. Even fewer secondary melanomas of this
system have been discovered prior to autopsy. The presenting symptoms of
genitourinary melanoma are similar to symptoms of all other genitourinary
neoplasms, and, as in other urologic neoplasms, these are usually tumors of
the aged. Due to the small number of cases, there is no single large series of
patients, and thus no controlled clinical studies of therapeutic modalities
versus stage of disease. Despite the lack of such series, the results of most
treatments have resulted in uniform failures, and the discovery of this disease usually carries a grim prognosis. This chapter will examine the world's
literature regarding this disease and summarize the collective experiences of
all authors in regards to treatment and prognosis.

## Primary melanoma

Primary malignant melanoma is described in the urologic literature in various synonymous terms including melanocarcinoma, melanosarcoma, melanoepithelioma or melanoblastoma. The first reported cases of genitourinary
melanoma were all in the latter half of the 19th century. Since then, there
have been scattered case reports and small series in the literature. Unfortunately, the treatment and prognosis for genitourinary melanoma has not
appreciably changed in the last 100 years. It is hoped that recent therapeutic
advances such as immunotherapy will make a difference in the prognosis of
this disease. Primary melanoma has been reported in the penis, urethra,
scrotum, vulva, adrenal and possibly the prostate. The remaining organs of the
genitourinary tract are almost always the sites of secondary, metastatic,
melanoma.

The incidence of malignant melanoma is rare in the genitourinary organs.
Long et al. [1] examined 700 000 women at the Mayo Clinic and found only
three melanomas of the genitourinary tract. Allen and Spitz [2], in their

*Seigler, H. F. (ed.), Clinical Management of Melanoma. ISBN 978-94-009-7495-1*
© *1982, Martinus Nijhoff Publishers, The Hague/Boston/London.*

series of 934 melanomas, found only four (0.4%) involved the male and 34 (3.7%) involved the female genitalia, with respective survivals of 25% and 20%. Pack et al. [3] examined and recorded the incidence of distribution of moles in 1000 otherwise healthy patients. Of 14 609 benign nevi found, only 14 (0.1%) were found on the male or female genitalia, versus 35 of the 1225 melanomas seen at their institution. Their conclusion was that any pigmented genital lesion of the genitalia should be closely followed.

Diagnosis of melanoma is by excisional biopsy. Most lesions are blue or blue-black in color, but, especially in the female urethra, may be red, polypoid and friable. The presenting symptoms vary according to the site affected, but are usually dramatic only in the rapidity of progression. A high index of suspicion should be held for any rapidly changing lesion and the clinician should be ready to proceed quickly once the diagnosis has been established. Treatment of primary genitourinary melanoma is surgical, with the longer survivals usually following radical excision.

## Penis

The penis is the most frequent site of primary malignant melanoma of the male genitalia. As opposed to other types of penile malignancies, melanoma of the penis is almost exclusively limited to whites [4]. The age range for reported cases is 23 to 77 years with the most occurring in the 6th and 7th decades (Table 1). The first case reported was by Murchison in 1851 [5].

The incidence of penile melanoma is quite rare with only 53 reported cases in the world literature. The true incidence, however, may be somewhat higher. In Wheelock and Clark's series of 59 793 surgical and 2822 autopsy specimens, there were 31 squamous cell carcinomas and two melanomas of the penis [6]. While uncommon in humans, penile melanoma is relatively common in horses, again being limited primarily to white and gray horses [4].

The usual presenting symptom of penile melanoma is a nodule or a lesion which has undergone recent change. Most lesions described are blue or blue-black and nontender. The usual duration of symptoms is three or four months with a range of two weeks to eight years (Table 1). The most common site of occurrence is the glans penis (88%). Of all patients presenting with penile melanoma, 57.5% have palpable inguinal adenopathy at the time of presentation.

The usual clinical course of a patient with penile melanoma is a rapid demise due to widespread disease. Of the patients with reported follow-ups, only two of 33 are alive and well with no evidence of disease over five years from presentation [6, 7]. A third patient died at 12 years of disseminated

*Table 1.* Penile melanoma

| Author | Reference | Patient age | Presenting symptoms | Site | Nodes |
|---|---|---|---|---|---|
| Murchison | 5 | 54 | ? | glans | + |
| Holmes | 38 | 52 | ? | glans | ? |
| Gould | 39 | 75 | dysuria | glans | − |
| Bird | 40 | ? | ? | ? | ? |
| Battle | 25 | 60 | penile enlargement | glans | − |
| Fischer | 36 | 53 | ? | glans & shaft | + |
| Miner | 26 | 55 | ? | glans | + |
| Payra | 30 | 63 | ? | glans | + |
| Frick | 21 | 33 | ? chancre | glans | + |
| Peters | 31 | 72 | ? | glans | + |
| Isnardi | 32 | 56 | ulcer & enlargement | glans | + |
| Coley | 41 | 48 | ? | glans | − |
| Noordenbos | 33 | 79 | ? | glans | − |
| Wheelock | 6 | 49 | | glans | + |
| | | 78 | | glans | + |
| Harrison | 34 | 59 | | glans | + |
| Roberts | 27 | 62 | | glans | − |
| Abrams | 42 | 60 | | ? | ? |
| MacDermott | | 33 | | glans | + |
| Stefan | 35 | 65 | | glans & meatus | + |
| Reid | 8 | 65 | | meatus | ? |
| Batolo | 43 | 50 | ? | meatus | ? |
| Shanin | 10 | ? | ? | ? | ? |
| Svendezov | 28 | 52 | increase size of lesion | prepuce | + |
| Buddington | 22 | 67 | lesion of coronal sulcus | glans | ? |
| Cerimele | 23 | 66 | ? | glans | − |
| Das Gupta | 29 | 53 | none | prepuce | − |
| | | 77 | ulcer | glans & shaft | ? |
| Schneiderman | 11 | 50 | lesion | glans | ? |
| Sirsat | 19 | 65 | lesion | glans | ? |
| | | 55 | lesion | glans | − |
| Patoria | 20 | 35 | lesion | glans | − |
| Thomas | 24 | 36 | | glans | + |
| Ellis | 16 | 44 | | glans | − |
| Cascinelli | 45 | 43 | ? | ? | ? |
| Cochran | 46 | 37 | ? | ? | ? |
| Frontsin | 12 | 70 | | glans | − |
| | | 66 | | glans | − |
| Trotskii | 47 | ? | ? | ? | ? |
| Banchein | 48 | ? | ? | ? | ? |
| Gojasejni | 13 | 54 | black lesion, ulcer | glans | + |
| Girgis | 14 | 51 | blood-stained shorts | glans, meatus | − |
| Johnson | | 23 | mole | prepuce | − |
| | | 67 | lesion | glans | + * |
| | | 66 | balanitis | glans | − |
| Bracken | 15 | 45 | lesion | glans | − |

*Table 1 continued.*

| Author | Reference | Patient age | Presenting symptoms | Site | Nodes |
|--------|-----------|-------------|---------------------|------|-------|
| Baruah | 49 | 70 | ulcer | glans | + |
| Shanik | 50 | 51 | swollen, tender penis | glans, prepuce | + |
| Tallerman | 37 | 63 | pain, swelling | glans & corpora | + |
| | | 56 | phimosis, difficulty voiding | prepuce | ? |
| Kherzi | 17 | 72 | swelling, change in color | glans | + |
| | | 42 | lesion | prepuce | + |

* History previous melanoma of knee—probably secondary penile melanoma.

disease [8]. Eight other patients are reported alive at two years [5, 9–15], of whom five eventually succumbed to their disease [5, 9, 10, 12, 14].

There are very few effective treatment modalities for melanoma of the penis. Radiation therapy, both local and external beam, has been unsuccessful, resulting in uniform treatment failure and further attempts at salvage therapy [9]. Preoperative radiation was tried by MacDermott and Kennedy [9] with the patient dying at 28 months post-treatment. A few isolated reports of chemotherapy with or without combined surgery has had some success. Ellis and White [16] used endolymphatic $^{131}$I lipiodol combined with partial penectomy on one patient and reported the patient alive at 21 months post-treatment. Johnson and Ayala [7] used local excision of a melanoma of the prepuce combined with pelvic infusion of phenylalanine mustard and nitrogen mustard for a survival of $12\frac{1}{2}$ years. A second patient of Johnson's received BCG, DTC, cytoxan and methyl-CCNU, but exhibited progression of his disease. Attempts at salvage with total penectomy and lymphadenectomy were unsuccessful in halting the progression. Alkeran was used by Gojasejni and Nitigant [13] in addition to total penectomy and bilateral lymphadenectomy with a reported two-year survival. Khezri [17] used BCG in addition to partial penectomy in a patient with clinically positive nodes and achieved a four-month survival.

The most successful form of therapy has been surgical excision of the lesions (Table 2). Partial penectomy has been performed in seven patients [6, 7, 14, 17, 18, 19, 20]. Five of these died from disease, one survived for over ten years with no evidence of disease, despite palpable nodes prior to surgery [6]. The second survivor is MacDermott's patient who also received $^{131}$I lipiodol [9]. The average survival period was 27 months.

Partial penectomy and inguinal lymphadenectomy were performed in five patients [11, 21–24] with adequate follow-up. The addition of lymphadenectomy to partial penectomy resulted in a slightly improved mortality rate (60% vs. 71%), but follow-up on these patients was not as long. The average survival

*Table 2.* Treatment of penile melanoma

| Treatment | Number patients | Mortality rate | Avg. survival (mo.) | NED * |
|---|---|---|---|---|
| None | 2 | 2 (100%) | 22 | 0 |
| Partial penectomy | 7 | 5 (71%) | 27 | 1 |
| Partial penectomy + nodes | 5 | 3 (60%) | 19 † | 0 |
| Total penectomy | 5 | 4 (80%) | 7.35 †† | |
| Total penectomy + nodes | 11 | 6 (54%) | 11.5 | 2 |
| Chemotherapy alone | 1 | – | 150 | 1 |

† Includes 1 perioperative death.
†† Includes 2 perioperative deaths.
* Over 2 years.

of patients undergoing partial penectomy and inguinal lymphadenectomy was 19 months, including one patient dying on the second postoperative day [24].

Total penectomy was the most commonly used surgical procedure, with or without concomitant lymphadenectomy. Follow-up is available in five patients who underwent total penectomy alone [25–29] with only one surviving with no evidence of disease [27]. There were two peri-operative deaths [25, 26] and two patients later died of disease [28, 29] for an 80% mortality rate. Lymphadenectomy was performed in addition to total penectomy in 11 patients with follow-up [6, 13, 15, 30–37]. Of these, five patients were still alive and two patients were survivors for periods exceeding two years from surgery. The overall mortality rate following this procedure is 54%.

Prognosis of penile melanoma, as in most genitourinary melanomas, is poor. Of 34 patients with any follow-up reported, 20 were dead at the time of the reports. Only three lived over ten years, one of whom died of disease at $12\frac{1}{2}$ years. Ten lived at least two years, half of whom later succumbed. As expected, the extent of the patient's disease at presentation had a direct bearing on patient survival. No patient presenting with visceral or corporal involvement survived more than two years, regardless of treatment modality. Patients with glandular involvement alone experienced slightly improved gross survival (54%) than those with clinically apparent nodal disease (41%). Patients with isolated prepuce lesions did the best with 66% surviving (Table 3).

Treatment variations had effect only in those patients with nodal disease. No patient with clinically positive disease survived if treated by penectomy alone, whereas three (43%) of the patients with solitary glandular disease who had penectomy alone survived. Addition of lymphadenectomy to either total or partial penectomy produced four survivors (Table 4).

*Table 3.* (penile melanoma) Stage of disease vs. gross survival rate

| Site | Number patients | Number survivors | Avg. survival (mo.) |
|------|-----------------|------------------|---------------------|
| Prepuce | 3 | 2 | 61 |
| Glans | 13 | 7 | 25.5 |
| Glans+corpora | 1 | – | 14 |
| Nodes * | 12 | 5 | 19.5 |
| Distant mets | 5 | – | 7 |

* Clinically evident.

Prognosis, regardless of stage of the disease or therapy is guarded, however. Buddington [22], for example, performed a partial penectomy and bilateral lymphadenectomy with all nodes negative, yet the patient developed metastatic disease and died two years postoperatively. No patient can be considered cured despite lack of clinically or pathologically evident disease. Recurrences have been reported after five to ten year disease-free intervals, making follow-up of these patients a lifetime affair.

## Urethra

Primary melanoma of the urethra is more common in females than males. Abeshouse [51] found 24 primary urethral melanomas, with a male to female ratio of 1:4. The racial incidence, as in most melanomas, shows a 3–4:1 white to black incidence. This form of melanoma in both males and

*Table 4.* (penile melanoma) Stage of disease vs. treatment vs. gross survival rate

| Site | Number | None | local excision | Partial penectomy | Partial penectomy +nodes | Total penectomy | Total penectomy+ nodes |
|------|--------|------|----------------|-------------------|--------------------------|-----------------|------------------------|
| | | Treatment–survivors/total no. patients | | | | | |
| Prepuce | 3 | 0/1 | 1/1 | — | — | — | 1/1 |
| Glans | 13 | — | 0/1 | 2/2 (67%) | 2/4 (50%) | 1/3 (33%) | 2/2 (100%) |
| Glans+corpora | 1 | — | — | 0/1 (0%) | — | — | — |
| Nodes | 12 | — | — | 0/1 (0%) | 1/3 (33%) | — | 3/8 (37.5%) |
| Distant mets | 5 | 0/1 | 0/1 | — | 0/1 | — | 0/2 |

* Clinically evident.

females is more common in the distal portion of the urethra. The disease is usually progressive and fatal.

In the male, the urethra is the second most common site of occurrence of primary melanoma. In Abeshouse's review [51], he found only five genuine cases [21, 52–55] as opposed to 17 penile melanomas. Since Abeshouse, there have been seven additional cases reported [9, 15, 56–60], bringing the total reported cases in the world literature to 12. The first reported case was in 1906 by Albrecht [52]. All cases have been anecdotal with age range, treatment and prognosis basically the same as in penile melanomas.

As opposed to penile melanoma, however, urethral melanomas are more likely to be symptomatic. Symptoms include hematuria, both spontaneous and following intercourse, urethral discharge, dysuria, meatal mass, and various obstructive symptoms (Table 5). Most melanomas occur in the distal urethra (seven cases), followed by the bulbar urethra, penoscrotal junction, and one case [52] in the prostatic urethra. Also, as opposed to penile melanoma, nodal involvement is not clinically apparent on presentation, with only two of eight patients having positive nodal disease. One of the remaining six, however, was later found to have pathologically positive nodes.

Of the nine patients with follow-ups reported, six underwent subsequent partial or total penectomy, only one survived two years with no evident disease (partial penectomy with postoperative radiation). A second patient of Guinn et al. [59] survived for 28 months following radical surgery, and

Table 5. Melanoma of the male urethra

| Author | Reference | Patient age | Presenting symptoms | Site | Nodes |
|---|---|---|---|---|---|
| Albrecht | 52 | ? | ? | prostatic | ? |
| Frick | 21 | 33 | ulcer | distal | ? |
| Campbell | 53 | 76 | dysuria | penoscrotal | + |
| McKenna | 54 | 65 | erosion glands | distal | + |
| Shih | 55 | 70 | deviation stream | distal | + |
| MacDermott | 9 | 33 | hematuria post-intercourse | meatus | – * |
| Signorelli | 56 | ? | ? | ? | ? |
| Chiappino | 57 | ? | ? | ? | ? |
| Salm | 58 | 53 | meatal mass | distal | – |
| Guinn | 59 | 43 | hemturia | penoscrotal junction | – |
| Geelhoed | 60 | 58 | spraying | distal | – |
| Bracken | 15 | 71 | outlet obstruction | distal & peno- scrotal junction | – |

* Previous penoscrotal junction urethral melanoma treated with radiation – tumor disappeared. Nodes negative clinically, positive pathologically.

*Table 6.* Melanoma of the female urethra

| Author | Reference | Patient age | Presenting symptoms | Site | Nodes |
|--------|-----------|-------------|---------------------|------|-------|
| Reed | 62 | 64 | hematuria, discharge | distal | |
| Mundell | 63 | 46 | ? | ? | |
| Kustner | 64 | – | discharge, dysuria | ? | |
| Hermann | 65 | 58 | urethral mass | distal | |
| Kauffman | 66 | 55 | | | |
| Basler | 67 | 55 | | | |
| Saenger | 68 | 72 | discharge, dysuria, mass | orifice | |
| Koerner | 69 | 75 | discharge, mass | orifice | |
| Fornero | 70 | 75 | discharge, mass | meatal | |
| Shaw | 72 | 63 | irritation | orifice | |
| Rosenthal | 73 | 75 | discharge, mass | orifice | |
| Newell | 74 | 64 | mass | orifice | |
| Kyrle | 75 | 52 | | | |
| Long | 1 | 70 | discharge, mass | meatus | |
| | | 78 | discharge, perineal drop | orifice | |
| | | 72 | | meatal & vaginal | + |
| Savran | 76 | 70 | discharge | meatus | |
| Glenn | 77 | 45 | dysuria | orifice | |
| McBurney | 78 | 77 | hematuria, discharge | orifice | |
| Abrams | 42 | 60 | mass | meatal | |
| Limburg | 79 | 68 | ? | ? | ? |
| Abeshouse | 51 | 60 | hematuria, irritability | meatal | |
| Woodruff | 80 | 60 | hematuria, incontinence | orifice | + |
| | | 68 | dysuria | orifice | – |
| Letzerukov | 81 | 80 | ? | ? | |
| Sokal | 82 | 80 | hematuria | ? | |
| Rabon | 83 | 63 | dysuria, frequency caruncle | orifice, clitoris, labia | |
| Grabstald | 85 | 65 | terminal hematuria, dysuria, mass | entire | + |
| | | 68 | terminal hematuria, mass | distal | |
| | | 73 | terminal hematuria, mass | meatal | |
| | | 75 | terminal hematuria, mass | meatal | |
| Gillenwater | 84 | 56 | discharge, irritability | distal | |
| Block | 61 | 54 | mass | distal | |
| Cochran | 46 | 5 * | | | |

* Five cases all over 50 years of age, details not stated.

interestingly had had a previous bulbar urethral melanoma irradiated with disappearance for ten years. One patient underwent radical perineal prostatectomy and bilateral node dissection [9] and died of his disease at two years. The final patient underwent radical cystoprostectomy and urethrectomy for a local recurrence 16 months following an excisional biopsy. Following the salvage procedure, he was noted to have a 22 month disease-free interval [60].

Melanoma of the female urethra is more common than its male counterpart. In the series reported by Pack et al. [3], female genital melanomas were found to be nine times more common than male. Abeshouse [51], in his review, found the ratio to be 4:1. To date, there have been 38 reported cases in the world literature, beginning with Reed's case in 1896 [62] (Table 6). The majority of cases (25/28) in which the site of the melanoma was stated occurred in the distal urethra. Presenting symptoms included discovery of a mass, vaginal discharge, which was usually bloody and occasionally foul smelling, various irritative symptoms, especially dysuria, and hematuria. One patient complained of incontinence and one of perineal discomfort. No patient complained of obstructive symptoms. Often a patient's melanoma was discovered during the course of treatment for a urethral caruncle. The mistaken diagnosis of caruncle frequently caused delay in treatment and advance of the disease with concomitant poor survival.

As in its male counterpart, melanoma of the female urethra is best treated by radical surgery [61]. Of eight patients who underwent local or "wide" excision of urethral melanoma [42, 62, 75, 76, 78, 80, 84], seven had recurrences and only two of these lived more than 24 months from first diagnosis [42, 80]. The one patient without a recurrence only had a seven-month follow-up [75]. Radiation therapy was used alone or in combination with surgery in seven patients and all experienced recurrences [51, 68–73]. Urethrectomy or cystectomy combined with node dissection was performed in six patients [77, 86, 61, 83, 85] with less recurrence (3/6, 50%), and longer survival (three over five years). Another patient had a myocardial infarction and died at one year with no evident disease [85]. A seventh patient [79] had no details of recurrence or follow-up. The node dissection in these patients should be primarily the superficial inguinal nodes. If the primary tumor is deeply invasive, the clinician should suspect deep inguinal secondary deposits and subsequent hematogenous spread. Most recurrences initially were either local or nodal, but distant subcutaneous and visceral recurrences usually preceded the terminal event. Interestingly, one of Grabstald's patients had clinically evident spread of her disease found at laparotomy and was managed only with suprapubic cystostomy [85]. She survived $5\frac{1}{2}$ years before succumbing to widespread disease.

The ultimate survival is, however, correlated to the spread of disease on presentation. Early misdiagnosis of caruncle, prolapsed mucosa, fibroma, carcinoma, sarcoma or chancre only leads to delay in therapy [1]. Therefore, any lesion of the female urethra which is in any way suspicious should be biopsied.

## Scrotum and vulva

Though these areas of the genitalia have a common embryological origin, the comparative incidence of melanoma is vastly different. Melanoma of the scrotum is very rare [51, 90, 91], whereas melanoma of the vulva is the most commonly reported site in the female genitourinary tract [80, 86–89]. The occurrence of primary melanomas in these areas follows the same pattern as any other genitourinary melanoma, being predominantly in white and aged patients. Prognosis is again poor and radical surgery combined with node dissection is the treatment of choice [80]. Symptoms of lesions in these areas are primarily discoloration, mass or change in a preexisting lesion.

## Miscellaneous

Other genitourinary organs involved with primary melanoma include the one case of melanoma of the prostate [92], one in the testes [41], one in the bladder [93] and the adrenal glands [94]. The case of Berry et al. [92] has been challenged by other authors [51] as having originally been of the prostatic urethra and not of the prostate itself. Though blue nevi of the prostate have been reported and the prostate is a known site of melanin production [95, 96], no unequivocal primary melanoma has been reported. Melanoma of the testicle is also very rare. One case of true primary melanoma has been reported by Coley and Hoguet [41]. The one case of primary bladder melanoma presented with gross painless hematuria and complete examination revealed a melanoma of the bladder with no primary lesion [93]. Another case by Su and Prince [97] of bladder melanoma has been reported, but an examination for a possible cutaneous primary was not thorough and scalp lesions "developed" three weeks later.

Primary adrenal melanomas differ from most other primary genitourinary melanomas. Most appeared in the early 20th century literature and were "unassociated" with any primary tumor [98–101]. No patient, however, was examined with Wood's light, etc. for a primary melanoma which had regressed, and over half of the reported cases were bilateral and symmetrical. The adrenal glands usually retained a "normal configuration," but were black and several times normal size. All patients rapidly succumbed to widespread disease. One case of a pigmented adenoma has been described by Baker [103] in which the histologic morphology differed from that of a melanoma. If one accepts the mesoblastic chromatophore theory [1] of the origin of melanoma, then the predicted incidence of adrenal melanomas should be much higher.

## Secondary melanomas

Secondary melanomas comprise over half of all genitourinary melanomas, yet most are discovered at autopsy. If symptoms occur, they are usually of shorter duration, but may not appear until ten or more years following removal of a melanoma from an area remote to the genitourinary tract. The genitourinary organs usually involved are aso completely different from those involved with primary melanoma. Most secondary melanomas occur primarily in the adrenals, bladder, kidneys and ureters. Also, in contrast to primary melanoma, treatment of these lesions is usually palliative rather than radical surgery. The prognosis for patients with secondary genitourinary melanoma is even worse than in those patients with primary melanoma. This is related to the fact that rarely, if ever, is the genitourinary tract solely involved. In almost all cases, there is widespread disease.

The more recent literature recommends that patients with melanoma should undergo excretory urography and cytoscopy to establish the diagnosis of metastasis and prevent exploration [104, 105]. Goldstein, for example, found 14/20 patients with metastatic melanoma to have urographic evidence of involvement.

Another method of diagnosis showing some promise is urinary cytology, which shows a characteristic pattern [106–108]. The most important findings are intranucleolar vacuolation and, occasionally, an intranuclear eosinophilic mass (Kernsecretion). Cytologic diagnosis also depends on finding cells with fine-scattered chromatin, unusual nucleolar enlargement, faint nucleolar membranes, cohesive epitheliod clumps and fine melanin granules in the cytoplasm. Using this technique, Hajdu and Savino found 5% of 239 patients with melanomas to have positive urinary cytology [108]. Detection of melanin or promelanin in the urine has not been especially helpful.

## Bladder

Though primary melanoma of the bladder is very uncommon [109, 110], the bladder is one of the most common sites of secondary genitourinary melanoma. Abeshouse's review of the literature found the bladder to be the most common site of secondary melanoma [51]. Later large autopsy series, such as that of Das Gupta and Grabstald, found bladder metastasis to be the third most common site, occurring in 18% of all patients with metastatic melanoma [111]. Melanoma is also the second most common type of all secondary bladder tumors, with gastric tumors being slightly more common [112, 113]. Some authors, however, found no melanomas occurring as secondary bladder tumors [114]. In Sheehan's series of 5 200 autopsies, eight of 37 patients with primary cutaneous melanoma had bladder metastasis [113]. Interestingly, as opposed to primary melanoma of the genitourinary tract, these lesions occurred in patients much younger, ranging from 22 to 60 years (average 40).

Metastatic melanomas of the bladder are more commonly discovered ante mortem than any other genitourinary site. This is due to the continuous expansion and contraction of the bladder, and the friability of bladder lesions, resulting in the relatively early symptoms of hematuria and irritability [99, 115–117, 119, 120]. Some authors [114, 121] challenge this, stating that secondary metastasis are submucosal, and thus bleed infrequently. Ganem and Batal [112] state that the appearance of symptoms is related to the rapidity with which the tumor grows. Other reported symptoms include bladder outlet obstruction with urinary retention [122]. The diagnosis of secondary bladder melanoma is made cytoscopically and usually presents as blue-black patches or nodules found in any portion of the bladder. The lesions may be single or multiple. No case of secondary bladder melanoma has been a single isolated lesion, but rather is only a sign of widespread disease. Attempts at curative surgery have uniformly resulted in failure [118]. Most authors recommend transurethral resection for diagnosis and localized therapy [51, 53, 111, 119, 123, 124]. Recent reports of intralesional BCG injection have shown some early success [125, 126].

The overall age of patients with bladder melanoma was 22 to 71 [107]. The duration of the disease-free interval from time of removal of the primary melanoma—usually cutaneous—to the appearance of secondary metastasis was up to 12 years [122]. The case reported by Amar [120] illustrates the usual pattern of disease with symptomatic metastatic bladder melanoma. A 33-year-old patient had a melanoma of the neck removed seven years previously and presented with gross hematuria. Cytoscopy revealed a lesion in the dome of the bladder. Subsequent exploratory laparotomy revealed multiple metastasis. The patient underwent a partial cystectomy, but four weeks later developed even more widespread disease, with a large submandibular mass and soon expired.

## Adrenals

Metastatic melanoma to the adrenal is far more common than originally thought. Abeshouse [51] found only 12 cases in the literature, but subsequent large autopsy series have shown the incidence of adrenal metastases to be quite high. Das Gupta and Brasfield found 63 of 125 autopsy cases to have adrenal metastasis [111] and, of the 49 melanoma patients with thyroid metastasis, 42 had adrenal metastasis. Willis [127] in his series of 323 patients dying of malignancy found 27 (8.3%) had adrenal metastasis, with lung carcinoma and melanoma being the most common. Clark and Rowntree [128] in 25 000 autopsies found 202 adrenal tumors, 42 of which were metastatic and 10% of these were melanomas. Glomset [129] in 4000 autopsies, which included 821 patients dying of malignancy, found 110 adrenal metastases. Sixty percent of these were due to melanoma, and were usually bilateral, very few metastatic adrenal melanomas are discovered ante mortem, and if found, all usually seen on routine pyelography. The treatment, as in all other metastatic melanomas, is palliative.

## Kidney

The kidney is the third major genitourinary site of metastatic melanoma, being only second in frequency behind the adrenal in Das Gupta and Bresfield's series [111]. As in other metastatic melanomas, it is more frequently found to be involved at autopsy than clinically [130]. Due to its continuity with the urinary tract, however, patients more often may exhibit symptoms, such as melanuria and hematuria, or have positive urinary cylology. The kidney differs from most organs involved in metastatic disease in that its involvement can occur in two forms. Some kidneys will exhibit mass lesions within the parenchyma, probably secondary to hematogenous spread. Others will become diffusely involved with the entire parenchyma being black, with or without renal enlargement [131]. Furthermore, a syndrome of melanuric nephrosis has been described [132], leading to acute and chronic renal insufficiency, but no actual invasion of the kidney.

The diagnosis of renal melanoma is rarely made prior to the patient's demise. With the increased emphasis on aggressive follow-up, including routine urography [104, 105], gallium-67 citrate localization [133], or computerized axial tomography [134], the ante mortem diagnosis of renal melanoma should become more common. The treatment, however, at this time is still conservative, unless life-threatening complications should occur [135].

## Ureter and renal pelvis

Metastatic melanoma to the upper-collecting system is far less common than involvement of the adrenals, kidneys or bladder. Lesions of the ureter are, however, more common than other genitourinary sites, and have a higher potential for lethality, usually due to complications. The ureteral melanoma is occasionally discovered by the presence of hematuria, hypertension or flank pain [136–138, 140], but most commonly is found on routine urography. The lesion is usually either polypoid or obstructing. It is the tendency for ureteral melanoma to cause obstruction that has led to renal failure sepsis and death [72]. Urographic findings may show complete obstruction and nonfunction, or partial obstruction and hydronephrosis. If the patient has a polypoid lesion of the ureter, there may be a goblet sign [141] with dilation of the ureter distal to the obstruction. This is thought to be pathognomonic for malignancy. The treatment of ureteral melanoma as in all metastatic melanomas is conservative. McKenzie and Bell [140] report a "solitary" metastasis to the ureter ten years following removal of a scapular melanoma. Within four months following a nephroureterectomy, the patient developed a prostatic urethral recurrence and progressive disease.

## Other

Other genitourinary sites of metastatic melanoma which have been reported are the ovary [111], Fallopian tubes [111], uterus [111], labia [111], broad ligament [111], epididymis [29, 132, 143], testicle [29, 111, 142, 144, 147], seminal vesicle [29, 92, 143], prostate [6, 24, 41, 94, 143, 144], penis [146], urethra [29] and scrotum [29]. All patients exhibited widespread metastatic disease, and nearly all were discovered at autopsy.

## Transplantation

With the rising interest in renal transplantation, there has been a similar rise in reports of tumors transplanted with the renal graft. This problem is particularly noteworthy due to the large doses of immunosuppressives used routinely in these patients. Also there have been reports of these patients exhibiting a higher incidence of de novo tumors, again thought to be linked to their immunosuppressive therapy. With melanoma, this becomes especially crucial as this tumor is relatively highly immunogenic and the only nonsurgical therapy available is passive immunotherapy.

The incidence of de novo melanomas is low in renal transplant patients, but higher than in the general population. Three large transplant series have been reported to date. Of 1884 patients receiving renal transplants in Australia and New Zealand, three developed malignant melanoma and only one survived [148]. 12 of 1589 patients in Denmark undergoing renal transplation developed de novo tumors, one of which was a malignant melanoma. This patient was still alive at the time of the report [149]. Penn, in reviewing 5000 renal transplant patients, found nine de novo melanomas, four of whom died of metastasis [150].

There is little the transplant surgeon can do about preventing the occurrence of de novo melanomas. However, the transplantation of melanoma along with the allograft is a particularly preventable and potentially disastrous complication. Two malignant melanomas have been reported as having been transplanted with the renal allograft. Jeremy et al. [151] transplanted two kidneys from a cadaver donor with oligodendroglioma. At necropsy, the donor was found to have unsuspected metastatic melanoma. One recipient died 13 months later with melanoma, but the second recipient had no evidence disease at three years. Another case was reported by Peters and Stuard [152]. This patient received a cadaver allograft from a donor who was found to have an occult spindle cell carcinoma of the spleen. 19 months later, the patient developed widely metastatic melanoma and died. The conclusion of these authors is that consideration in these cases should be given to removing the graft, and stopping all immunosuppressives. Apparent success with this technique has been reported, resulting in rejection of the foreign tumor.

Finally, in regard to transplantation, consideration must be given to the possibility of the immunosuppressive therapy altering the body's defense against previously dormant tumors. Evans and Calne report a case of a 56-year-old woman who received a renal allograft for renal failure due to polycystic kidney and liver disease. Subsequently she developed metastatic melanoma and died. The review of her chart revealed that a previous mole on her thigh had been removed and was "benign."

**Summary**

Malignant melanoma is a very uncommon malignancy in the genitourinary tract. Primary melanomas are most common in the urethra, penis and vulva. The treatment is primarily surgical, with radical excision being preferred. Newer forms of therapy such as immunotherapy may be important in the future.

Secondary genitourinary melanoma is more common than is thought. More careful follow-ups will undoubtedly increase the reported incidence. These usually occur in the bladder, kidney or adrenal. The only therapy currently available is palliative, and the finding of metastatic urologic disease is only a sign of widespread systemic disease and short survival periods.

Melanoma among transplant patients can occur by three methods, all related to the use of immunosuppressive theapy. The first is de novo tumor formation. There is a reported higher incidence of melanomas among transplanted patients than the general population, and thus increased surveillance among transplant recipients should be carried out. Transplantation of melanoma with the renal allograft has occurred in two cases. Possible therapy for this unfortunate event should include consideration of allograft removal.

The final way that melanomas can occur in transplant patients is by activation of a previously dormant tumor, as reported in one case to date.

Hopefully new and efficacious therapy for all melanomas of the genitourinary tract will soon appear. Not enough attention has been paid to immunotherapy and some success has been achieved with chemotherapy. The disease is so uncommon, however, that therapeutic successes are at best anecdotal, and conclusions on the most appropriate therapy cannot be clearly drawn. Until the advent of a second phase of urologic melanoma therapy, radical surgical therapy offers the best hope.

## References

1. Long GC, Counsellor VS and Dockerty MB: Primary melano-epithelioma of the female urethra: review of the literature: report of 3 cases. J Urol 55:520-529, 1946.
2. Allen AC and Spitz S: Melanoma: diagnosis and prognosis. Cancer 6:1-45, 1953.
3. Pack GT, Lenson N and Gerber DN: Regional distribution of moles and melanomas. Arch Surg 65:862-870, 1952.
4. Dean AL: Tumors of penis, urethra, scrotum and testes. In: Campbell MF (ed) Urology, Vol 3, p 177. WB Saunders, Philadelphia, 1952.
5. Murchison as cited in: Gross SD A System of Surgery, 6th ed, Vol 2, p 834. HC Lea's, Philadelphia, 1889.
6. Wheelock MC and Clark PJ: Sarcoma of the penis. J Urol 49:478-481, 1943.
7. Johnson DE and Ayala AG: Primary melanoma of penis. Urology 2: 174-177, 1973.
8. Reid JD: Melanosarcoma of the penis. Cancer 10:359-362, 1957.
9. MacDermott EN and Kennedy JD: A case of melanoblastoma of the penis. Br J Surg 43:213-214, 1955.
10. Shanin AP: Pigmented Tumors, p 229. Medgiz, Leningrad, 1959.
11. Schneiderman C, Semon MA and Levine RM: Malignant melanoma of the penis. J Urol 93:615-619, 1965.
12. Frontsin MH and Hutcheson JB: Malignant melanoma of the penis: a report of two cases. Br J Urol 41:324-326, 1969.
13. Gojasejni P and Nitigant P: Malignant melanoma of the penis. Br J Urol 44:143-146, 1972.
14. Girgis AS, Bergman H, Rosenthal H and Solomon L: Unusual penile malignancies in circumcised Jewish men. J Urol 110:696-702, 1973.
15. Bracken RB and Diokno AC: Melanoma of the penis and the urethra: 2 case reports and review of the literature. J Urol 111:198-200, 1924.
16. Ellis H and White WF: Malignant melanoma of the penis: endolymphatic therapy with 131-I lilipiodol. Br J Surg 55:238-241, 1969.
17. Khezri AA, Dounis A and Roberts JBM: Primary malignant melanoma of the penis. Two cases and a review of the literature. Br J Urol 51:147-150, 1979.
18. Colby FH: Melanotic sarcoma of the penis: report of a case. N Engl J Med 201:924, 1929.
19. Sirsat MV and Shrikande SS: Malignant melanoma of the penis in Indians (a report of two cases). Indian J Pathol Bacteriol 8:237, 1965.
20. Patoria NK and Junnarker RV: Malignant melanoma of the penis: report of a case. Indian J Cancer 3:37-38, 1966.
21. Frick W and Hall FJ: Generalized multiple pigmented sarcoma originating in the skin. J Am Med Assoc 46:1911-1915, 1906.

22. Buddington WT, Kickham CJE and Smith WE: An assessment of malignant disease of the penis. J Urol 89:442–449, 1963.
23. Cerimele D: Melanosi precancerosa circoscitta e melanoma maligno: a proposito di un caso localizzato al pene. G Ital Dermatol Sifalol 105:669–678 (as quoted in [37]).
24. Thomas JA and Fenn AS: Malignant melanoma of the penis: a report of a case and a review of the literature. Indian J Pathol Bacteriol 10:372–378, 1967.
25. Battle WH: Report on primary sarcoma of the penis to the Pathology Society of London. Lancet 1:520, 1885.
26. Miner CH: Primary sarcoma of the penis. Univ Med Mag Pa 9:824–834, 1896 (as quoted in [37]).
27. Roberts DI: Massive malignant melanoma of the penis occurring in a Malayan. Br J Surg 39:561–568, 1952.
28. Svedenzov EP: Melanoma of the penis. Vopr Onkol 7:88–89, 1961 (as quoted in [37]).
29. Das Gupta T and Grabstald H: Melanoma of the genitourinary tract. J Urol 93:607, 1965.
30. Payra E: Melanom des penis. Dtsch Z Chir 33:221–235, 1899 (as quoted in [37]).
31. Peters W: Melanosarcoma of the penis in a man of 72. J Urol 16:1–3, 1922.
32. Isnardi: Epithelioma mélanique de la verge. Loire Med 48:218–222, 1928 (as quoted in [37]).
33. Noordenbos W: Melanoma of the penis. Ned Tijdschr Geneeskd 77:1879–1855, 1933 (as quated in [37]).
34. Harrison FG: Malignancy of the penis and urethra. Clinics 3:20–32, 1944.
35. Stefan H: Melanoblastoma of the penis. Rozhl Chir 34:103–109, 1955 (as quoted in [37]).
36. Fischer G: Melanosarkom des penis. Dtsch Z Clin 25:313–322, 1887 (as quoted in [37]).
37. Tallerman A: Malignant melanoma of the penis. Urol Int 27:66–80, 1972.
38. Holmes T: Melanosis of the penis. Trans Pathol Soc London 23:175–177, 1871.
39. Gould AP: A case of melanotic epithelioma of the penis. Lancet 1:438–439, 1880.
40. Bird G: Primary sarcoma of the penis. Lancet 1:520, 1885.
41. Coley WB and Hoguet JP: Melanotic cancer: a report of 91 cases. Ann Surg 64:206–241, 1916.
42. Abrams M: Primary melanoma of the female urethra. J Urol 74:371–374, 1955.
43. Batolo D and D'Aquino S: Melanoma del glande: sera documentabile origine da elementi della guaina nervosa. Arch Ital Pathol Clin Tumori 2:285–302, 1958 (as quoted in [37]).
44. Gentil F, Lima EW and Abrao A: Melanoma de penis: relato de 2 casos. Rev Bras Cir 50:183, 1965 (as quoted in [15]).
45. Cascinelli N: Melanoma maligno del pene. Tumori 55:313, 1969 (as quoted in [15]).
46. Cochran AJ: Malignant melanoma: a review of 10 years experience in Glasgow, Scotland. Cancer 23:1190–1199, 1969.
47. Trotskii OA: Melanoma polovogo chlena. Urol Nefrol 36:61, 1971 (as quoted in [15]).
48. Bancheri FR, Gallizia G and Grandinetti C: Un cas de mélanom primitif du pénis. J Urol Nephrol 77:138, 1971 (as quoted in [15]).
49. Baruah BD and Dutta A: Malignant melanoma of the penis. J Indian Med Assoc 62:354–356, 1974.
50. Shanik GD and Tagoe SW: Case report: malignant melanoma of the penis. Ir J Med Sci 145:207–208, 1976.
51. Abeshouse BS: Primary and secondary melanoma of the genitourinary tract. South Med J 51:994–1006, 1958.
52. Albrecht H: Verh Deutsch Ges Pathol 14:253, 1910 (as quoted in [60]).
53. Campbell MF and Fein MJ: Malignant melanoma of the penile urethra: with a brief review of urethral sarcoma in the male. J Urol 35:573–582, 1936.

54. McKenna CM: Melanoblastoma of the penile urethra. Trans Am Assoc Genitourin Surg 30:401–404, 1937.
55. Shih HE: Melanoma of the urethra. Am J Cancer 36:243–246, 1939.
56. Signorelli E: Tumori primitivi dell'uretra Maschile. Urologia 29:530, 1962 (as quoted in [15]).
57. Chiappino G, Strada R: Malignant melanoma of the male urethra. Cancer 15:121, 1962 (as quoted in [15]).
58. Salm R and Rutter TE: A double primary malignant melanoma of the fossa navicularis. Br J Urol 36:91–96, 1964.
59. Guinn GA and Ayala AG: Male urethral cancer: report of 15 cases including a primary melanoma. J Urol 103:176–179, 1970.
60. Geelhoed GW and Meyers GH: Primary melanoma of the urethra. J Urol 109:634–637, 1973.
61. Block NL and Hotchkiss RS: Malignant melanoma of the female urethra: report of a case with five-year survival and review of the literature. J Urol 105:251–255, 1971.
62. Reed CAL: Melanosarcoma of the female urethra; urethrotomy; recovery. Am J Obstet Dis Women Child 34:864–867, 1986.
63. Mundell DE: Melanosarcoma of the female urethra. Kingston Med Q 5:75, 1901.
64. Kustner: In: Kurzes Lehrbuch der Gynäkologie 412, 1917 (as quoted in [71]).
65. Hermann: Melanosarcoma of urethra. Wein Med Wochenschr 1:706, 1917 (as quoted in [71]).
66. Kauffman E: Lehrbuch der Speziellen pathologischen Anatomie für Studierende und Arzte, Band 2, S1139. de Gruyter, Berlin, 1922.
67. Basler: (as quoted in [66]). Original translation was of a woman in Basel, but recent reviews of the subject refer to this person as a patient of Basler.
68. Saenger: Melanosarkom. Monatsschr Geburtshilfe Gynaekol 66:177, 1924 (as quoted in [71]).
69. Koerner J: Eineige Geschwürstprobleme an Hand setener (Melanoma urethrae, struma ovarie carcinomatosa, Pseudomyoma peritonei). Centralbl Gynaekol 51:834, 1927 (as quoted in [71]).
70. Fornero: Monit Ostet Ginecol 3:114, 1931 (as quoted in [79]).
71. McCrea LE: Malignancy of the female urethra. Urol Surv 2:85, 1952.
72. Shaw EC: Primary tumor of the female urethra with metastasis to each ureter. J Urol 34:244–253, 1935.
73. Rosenthal AH: Melanoma of the urethra. Am J Obstet Gynecol 30:115–118, 1935.
74. Newell OU and Serivner WC: Melanoma of the female urethra. Am J Obstet Gynecol 35:328–330, 1938.
75. Kyrle P: Zur Kennt der Malignoma Melanoblastoma der Harnröhre. Z Urol Chir Gynaekol 45:287, 1940 (as quoted in [79]).
76. Savran J, Sayer EA and Schradiack CE: Primary malignant melanoma of the female urethra. Am J Surg 75:743–745, 1948.
77. Glenn JF: Malignancy of the female urethra: a report of eight cases. N C Med J 14:201–204, 1953.
78. McBurney RP and Bale GF: Primary malignant melanoma of the female urethra. Surgery 37:973–978, 1935.
79. Limburg VH: Geburtshilfe Frauenheikd 16:75, 1956 (as quoted in [61]).
80. Woodruff JD and Brack CB: Unusual malignancies of the vulvo-urethral region: report of 12 cases. Obstet Gynecol 12:677–686, 1958.
81. Letzerukov MA: Urologiya 27:62, 1962 (as quoted in [61]).
82. Sokal Z: Pol Przegl Chir 34:587, 1962 (as quoted in [61]).
83. Rabon NA: Malignant melanoma developing in a urethral caruncle. J Am Med Women Assoc 19:855–856, 1964.

84. Gillenwater JY and Burros HM: Unusual tumors of the female urethra. Obstet Gynecol 31:617–620, 1968.
85. Grabstald H, Hilaris B, Henschke U and Whitmore WF: Cancer of the female urethra. J Am Med Assoc 197:835–842, 1966.
86. Rutledge FN: Clinical conference on malignant melanoma. Med Times (66):1d–15d, 1977.
87. Kehrer: (as quoted in [80]). Also, see Obstet Gynecol 12:677–686, 1958.
88. Pack GT: The pigmented mole and malignant melanoma. Cancer J Clin 12:11–26, 1962.
89. Taussig FJ: Cancer of the vulva an analysis of 155 cases. Trans Am Gynecol Soc 65:173–188, 1940.
90. Higgins CC and Worden JG: Cancer of the scrotum. J Urol 62:250–256, 1949.
91. Ray B, Huvos AG, Whitmore WF: Unusual malignant tumors of the scrotum: review of 5 cases. J Urol 108:760–766, 1972.
92. Berry NE and Reese L: Malignant melanoma which had its first clinical manifestations in the prostate gland. J Urol 69:286–290, 1953.
93. Ainsworth AM, Clark WH, Mastrangelo M and Conger KB: Primary malignant melanoma of the urinary bladder. Cancer 37:1928–1936, 1976.
94. Knisely RM and Baggentoss AH: Primary melanoma of the adrenal gland. Arch Pathol 42:345–349, 1946.
95. Tannenbaum M: Differential diagnosis in immunopathy III: melanotic lesions of the prostate: blue nevus and prostatic epithelial melanosis. Urology 4:617–621, 1974.
96. Nigogosyan G, de la Pava S, Pickren JW and Woodruff MW: Blue nevus of the prostate gland. Cancer 16:1097–1099, 1963.
97. Su CT and Prince CL: Melanoma of the bladder. J Urol 87:365–367, 1962.
98. Maclachan WWG: Primary melanosarcoma of the adrenal. J Med Res 33:93–106, 1915.
99. McComb RA and Smith DB: A case of melanotic sarcoma of the adrenal glands with secondary tumor in the bladder. J Urol 30:49–59, 1933.
100. Pappenheimer AM: Malignant melanotic tumor, primary in the adrenals. Proc N Y Pathol Soc 14:173–185, 1914.
101. Smith RM: Bilateral melanotic growth of suprarenal gland. Med J Aust 1:683–684, 1927.
102. Shnyronkova OV: Adrenal melanoblastoma with metastases. Arkh Patol 18:111, 1956 (as quoted in [51]).
103. Baker MR: A pigmental melanoma of the adrenal. Arch Pathol 26:845–852, 1938.
104. Weinstock NI, Willscher MK and Novicki DE: Importance of urinary tract investigation in metastatic malignant melanoma. Urology 10:547–549, 1977.
105. Goldstein HM, Kaminisky S, Wallace S and Johnson DE: Urographic manifestations of metastatic melanoma. Radiology 101:801–805, 1974.
106. Yamada T, Itou U, Watanabe Y, Ohashi S: Cytologic diagnosis of malignant melanoma. Acta Cytol 16:70, 1972.
107. Woodard BH, Heker RE and Johnston WW: Cytologic diagnosis of malignant melanoma in urine: a case report. Acta Cytol 22:350–352, 1978.
108. Hajdu SI and Savino A: Cytologic diagnosis of malignant melanoma. Acta Cytol 17:320–327, 1973.
109. Dan AL and Ash JE: Study of the bladder tumors in the Registry of the AUA. J Urol 63:618–621, 1950.
110. Melicow MM: Tumors of the urinary bladder: a clinicopathological analysis of over 2,500 specimens and biopsies. J Urol 74:498–521, 1955.
111. Das Gupta T and Brasfield R: Metastatic melanoma: a clinicopathological study. Cancer 17:1323–1339, 1964.

112. Ganem EJ and Batal JT: Secondary malignant tumors of the urinary bladder metastatic from primary foci in distant organs. J Urol 75:965–972, 1956.

113. Sheehan E, Greenberg D and Scott R: Metastatic neoplasms of the bladder. J Urol 90:281–284, 1963.

114. Klinger ME: Secondary tumors of the genitourinary tract. J Urol 65:144–153, 1951.

115. Morrow RP, Woolner LB and Emmett JL: Metastatic melanoepithelioma of the urinary bladder: report of a case. J Urol 67:92–94, 1952.

116. Pontes JES and Oldford J: Metastatic breast carcinoma to the urinary bladder. J Urol 104:839–842, 1970.

117. Samellas WM and Marks AR: Metastatic melanoma of the urinary tract. J Urol 85:21–23, 1961.

118. Wheelock MC: Sarcoma of the urinary bladder. J Urol 48:628–634, 1942.

119. Walsh EJ, Ockuly GA, Ockuly EF and Ockuly JJ: Treatment of malignant melanoma of the bladder. J Urol 96:472–478, 1966.

120. Amar AD: Metastatic melanoma of the bladder. J Urol 92:198–200, 1964.

121. Hermann HB: Metastatic tumors of the urinary bladder. J Urol 22:257–273, 1929.

122. Weston PAM: Metastatic melanoma in the bladder and urethra. Br J Surg 51:78–79, 1964.

123. Bartone FF: Metastatic melanoma of the bladder. J Urol 91:151, 1964.

124. Milner WA: Conservative treatment of tumors of the bladder:296 cases. J Int Coll Surg 20:566–572, 1953.

125. Silverstein MJ, DeKernion JB and Morton DL: Regression following intratumor injection of BCG vaccine. J Am Med Assoc 229:688, 1974.

126. DeKernion JB, Golub SH, Gupta RK, Silverstein MJ and Morton DL: Successful intralesional BCG therapy of a bladder melanoma. Cancer 36:1662–1667, 1975.

127. Willis RA: The Spread of Tumors in the Human Body, p 287. CV Mosby, St. Louis, 1952.

128. Clark JH and Rowntree LG: Studies of adrenal glands in health and diease: dieases in the adrenal glands as revealed in 25,000 autopsies. Endocrinology 18:256–273, 1934.

129. Glomset DA: The incidence of metastasis of malignant tumors to the adrenals. Am J Cancer 32:57–61, 1938.

130. Abeshouse BS and Goldstein AE: Metastatic malignant tumors of the kidney: a review of the literature and report of 23 cases. Urol Cutaneous Rev 45:163–186, 1941.

131. Goodall P, Spriggs AI and Wells FR: Malignant melanoma with melanosis and with pigmented monocytes and tumor cells in the blood. Br J Surg 48:549–555, 1960.

132. Rosenberg JC: Melanuric Nephrosis. Arch Pathol 62:399–402, 1956.

133. Frankel RS, Richman SD, Levenson SM and Johnston GS: Renal localization of gallium-67 citrate. Radiology 114:393–397, 1975.

134. Lee M: Malignant melanoma: pattern of metastases. Cancer J Clin 30:137–142, 1980.

135. Turner P: Melanotic sarcoma of the kidney. Proc R Soc Med 14:38–40, 1920.

136. Srivastava VK: Secondary melanoma of the ureter. Br J Urol 45:568, 1973.

137. Cohen WM, Freed SZ and Husson J: Metastatic cancer to the ureter: a review of the literature and case presentations. J Urol 112:188–189, 1974.

138. Edson M and Hutchins KR: Metastatic melanoma of ureter. N Y State J Med 73:459–461, 1975.

139. Nakazono M, Iwata S and Kuribayashi N: Disseminated metastatic ureteral melanoma: a case report. J Urol 114:624–625, 1975.

140. McKenzie DJ and Bell R: Melanoma with solitary metastasis to ureter. J Urol 99:399–140, 1968.

141. Bergman H, Friedenberg RM and Sayegh V: New roentgenologic signs of cancer of the ureter. Am J Roentgenol 86:707–717, 1961.

142. Barnes JF and King LS: Malignant melanoma virtually limited to serous surfaces. Ill Med J 96:117, 1949.

143. Lowsley OS: Melanoma of the urinary tract and prostate gland. South Med J 44:487–493, 1951.

144. Johnson DE, Jackson L and Ayala G: Secondary carcinoma of the testis. South Med J 64:1128–1130, 1971.

145. Smith GW, Griffith DP and Pranke DW: Melanospermia: an unusual presentation of malignant melanoma. J Urol 110:314–316, 1973.

146. Pacquin AJ and Roland SI: Secondary carcinoma of the penis: a review of the literature and a report of 9 new cases. Cancer 9:626–632, 1956.

147. Weller CV: Unusual cardiac and cerebral metastasis in melanosarcoma. J Cancer Res 7:313–327, 1922.

148. Sheil AGR: Cancer in renal allograft recipients in Australia and New Zealand. Transplant Proc 9:1133–1136, 1977.

149. Birkeland SA: Malignant tumours following immunosuppression in renal transplantation. Proc Eur Dial Transplant Assoc 10:429–433, 1973.

150. Penn I: Malignancies associated with renal transplantation. J Urol 10 (suppl):57–63, 1977.

151. Jeremy D, Farnsworth RH, Robertson MR, Annetts DL and Murnaghan GF: Transplantation of malignant melanoma with cadaver kidney. Transplantation 13:620–679, 1972.

152. Peters MS and Stuard ID: Metastatic malignant melanoma transplanted via a renal homograft. Cancer 41:2426–2430, 1978.

153. Evans DB and Calne RY: Renal transplantation in patiens with carcinoma. Br Med J 4:134–136, 1974.

# 4. Radiographic manifestations of thoracic malignant melanoma

DENNIS K. HEASTON and CHARLES E. PUTMAN

## Introduction

The importance of the thoracic cavity to the patient with malignant melanoma is rivaled only by that of the integument, since even though most melanomas originate in the skin, such intrathoracic structures as the lungs and heart determine their eventual outcome as they disseminate [85]. The filtering function of the lungs in particular to snare free-floating foci of malignant tissue is well known [31]. Of the 14 100 projected new cases of malignant melanoma to be diagnosed in 1980, approximately 4600, or one person in three, will die of the disease within five years [122]. Half of these people will succumb to cardiorespiratory failure due to replacement of their normal tissue by secondary tumor [100]. Pulmonary infection resulting directly from metastatic disease or its treatment will claim several hundred more individuals. Various autopsy series showing an incidence of cardiac and pulmonary metastases in advanced cases up to 64% and almost 90% respectively suggest an even greater role of the thorax in patient survival [5, 65].

The prognosis of those who develop metastatic malignant melanoma however is not uniformly dismal. Now nearly one patient in five displaying distant disease in the chest may manifest a five-year survival [25, 56]. Survival even up to 42% at five years has been noted when the primary site was unknown [46]. Expectantly, aggressive multidisciplinary approaches to these tumors combining surgical resection, oblative radiation therapy, more effective chemotherapy and specific immunotherapy will increase these gains further.

This makes paramount the importance of accurate diagnosis of thoracic malignant melanomas. Application of newer, more sensitive, diagnostic modalities such as computed tomography to the sites of suspected tumor spread, as well as more optimal utilization of such traditional techniques as plain chest radiography promises to improve existing diagnostic accuracy. Above all for diagnosis of thoracic disease, however, is needed a clear image of the protean presentations and radiographic manifestations of thoracic malignant melanoma.

*Seigler, H. F. (ed.), Clinical Management of Melanoma. ISBN 978-94-009-7495-1*
*© 1982, Martinus Nijhoff Publishers, The Hague/Boston/London.*

## Diagnostic modalities

*Chest plain films*

Due to its uniform availability and low cost, the conventional chest radiograph remains the mainstay of thoracic melanoma diagnosis. Several studies have suggested a high rate of diagnostic accuracy in both symptomatic and asymptomatic individuals being followed for various stages of malignant melanoma [6, 81]. The largest series reviewing routine chest roentgenograms from detection of malignant melanoma comes from Duke University Medical Center where 260 patients of the 1600 treated between 1970 and 1980 were noted to have thoracic metastases [30]. This represents a 16% prevalence of documented thoracic spread for all stages of the disease. Interestingly this prevalence approximately doubled when stereoscopic views, as in the first 600 cases, were replaced by high kilovoltage frontal and lateral views [115].

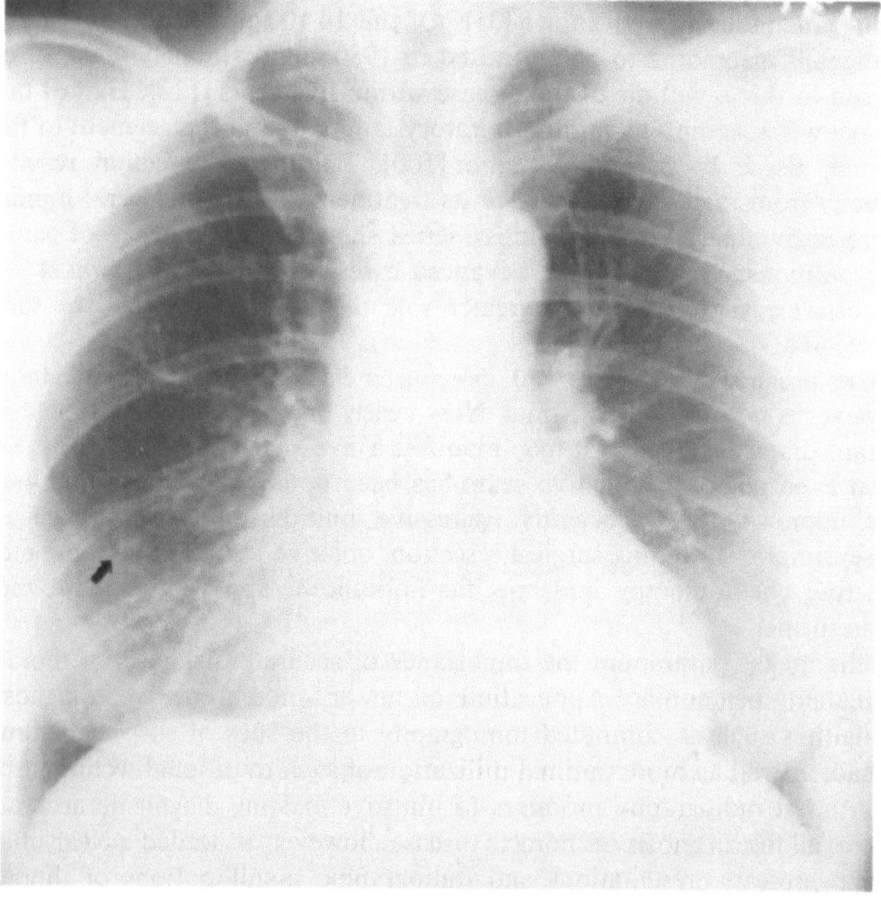

*Figure 1A.* This 56-year-old woman developed a solitary pulmonary nodule (arrow) 3½ years following surgical excision of a lower extremity malignant melanoma.

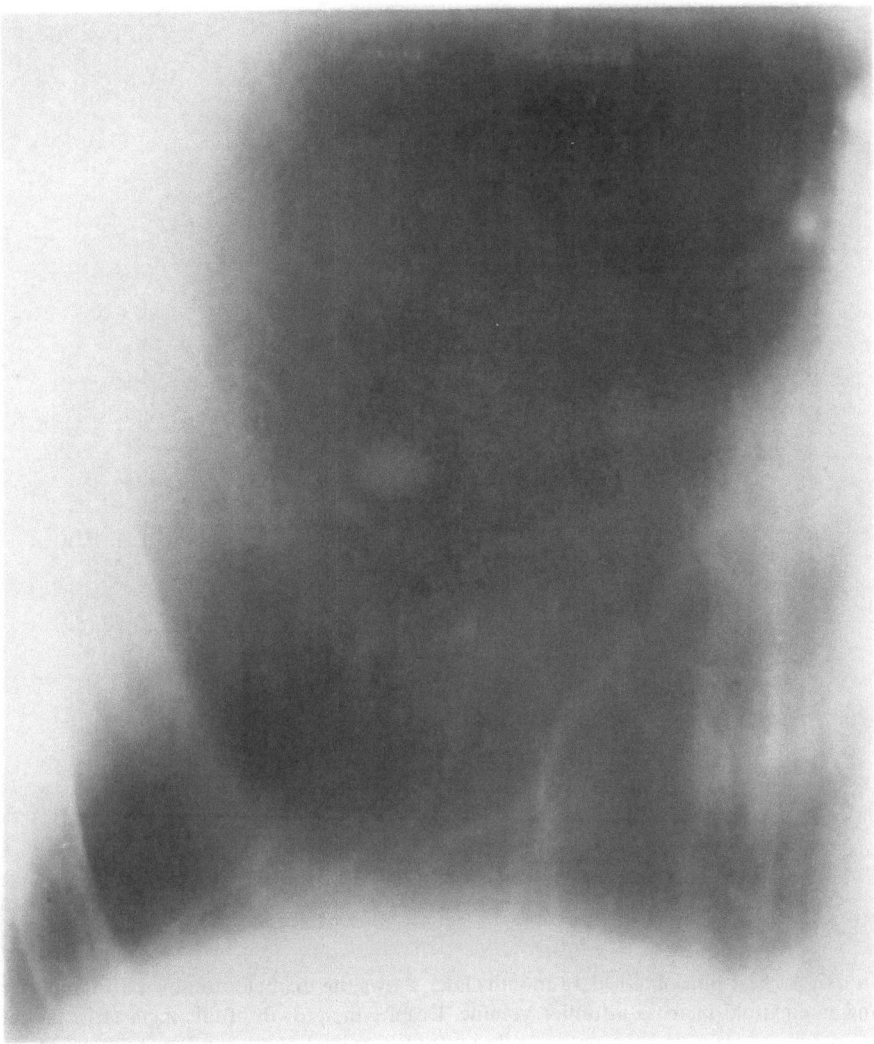

*Figure 1B.* Conventional tomography shows the absence of calcification in the well-demarcated right-middle lobe nodule, which measures 8 mm in diameter.

In the ten-year compilation of the Duke results [30], half of the patients who developed chest disease had evaluable radiographs (130 patients). Eighty-three percent of these displayed evidence of pulmonary metastasis with or without lymphadenopathy or pleural and extrapleural abnormality. The prognostic importance of discovering these metastases was stressed, since overall survival seemed to be related to their specific radiographic presentation and their time of appearance following the original diagnosis. A solitary lung nodule for example was associated with a 51-month average survival (Figure 1), whereas a disseminated miliary pattern yielded only two months of life in two patients (Figure 2). Radiographic evidence of thoracic

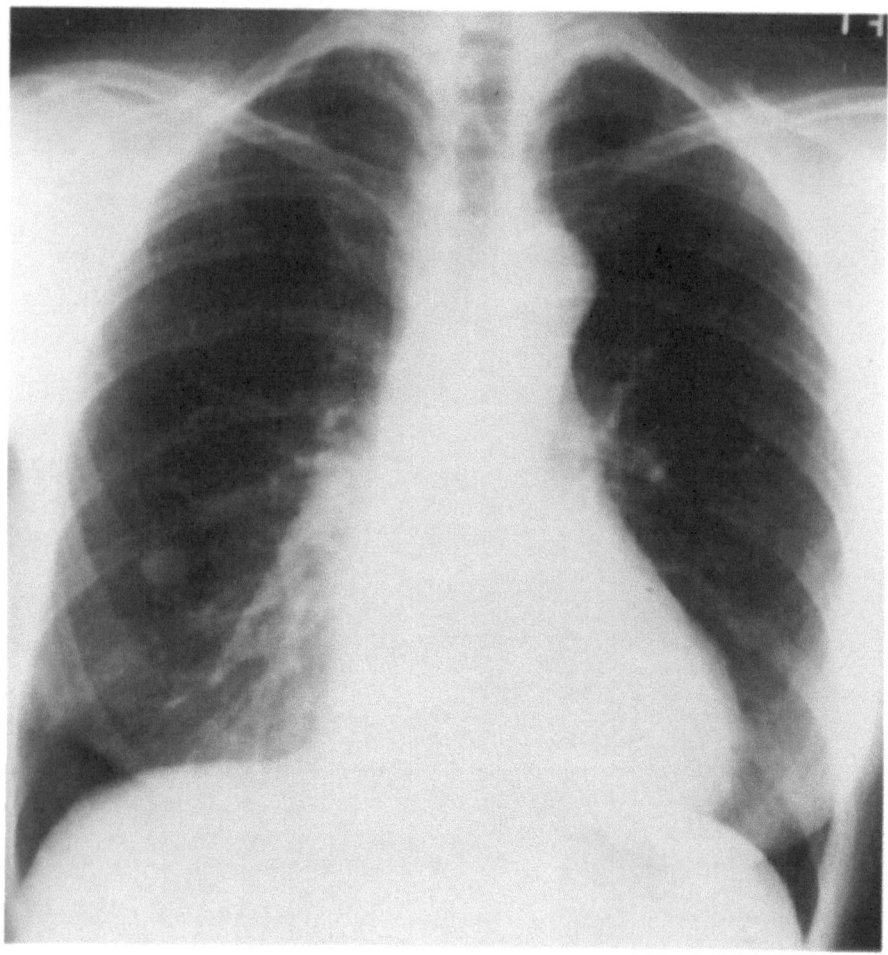

*Figure 1C.* A chest film obtained 18 months later shows the diameter to now be 16 mm, representing an eightfold increase in tumor volume. Despite the growth of this metastasis, the lungs appear otherwise clear and the patient subsequently survived another two years.

metastases was highly dependent upon clinical staging. Of those patients whose tumor caused their demise, the chest x-ray was positive 40% of the time [115].

This same pessimistic prognosis was earlier noted by Webb and Gamsu for eight persons with innumerable miliary (or snowstorm) nodules [145]. In their study 63 of 65 patients purported to have thoracic melanoma displayed chest film abnormalities (pleural or parenchymal nodules or masses, pleural effusion, bronchial obstruction with atelectasis, cardiomegaly). Pulmonary metastases were identified radiographically in nearly 90% of their patients. In 42 of 62 with widespread metastases, the chest x-ray provided the first evidence of dissemination beyond regional lymph nodes. Radiographic identification of pulmonary metastasis was even made in two cases

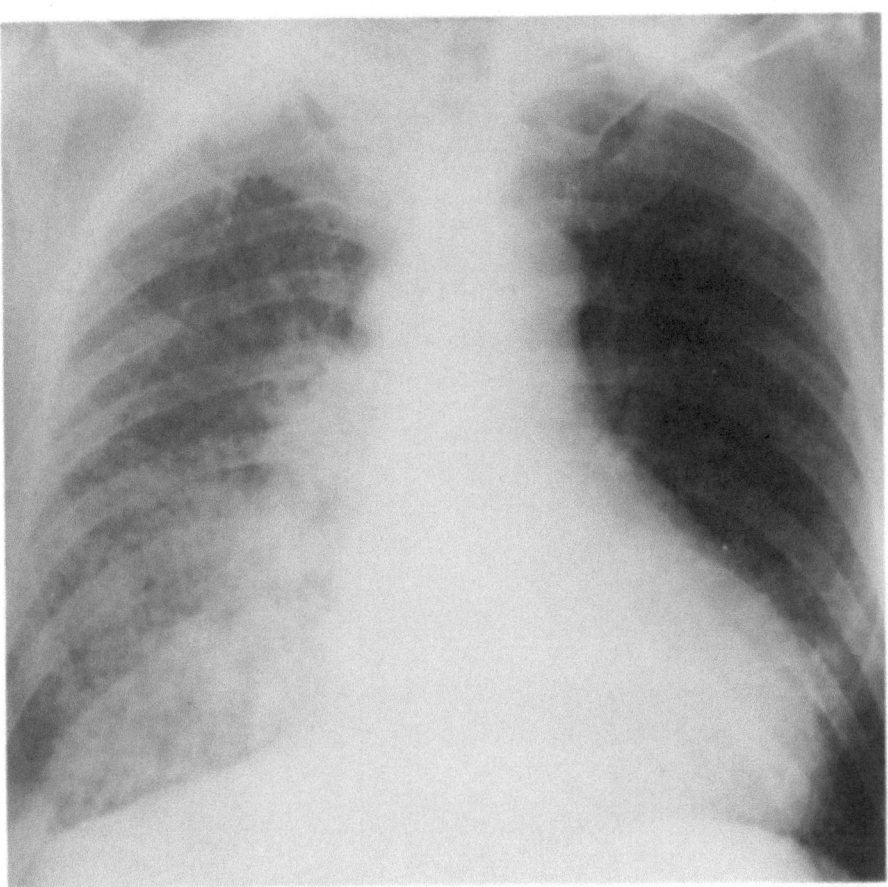

*Figure 2.* This 59-year-old man presented with shortness of breath approximately 3½ years following therapy for his original skin lesion. His chest film shows innumerable tiny nodular densities reminiscent of a snowstorm. Within two months he had expired.

before detection of the primary tumor. Chest films were therefore felt by these authors to be essential in the initial evaluation and follow-up of melanoma patients (Figure 3). Once intrathoracic disease was established however, they felt that radiographic follow-up was of limited usefulness, since the only finding of definite prognostic significance was the snowstorm appearance which proved invariably rapidly fatal [147]. Chest radiographs were stated to also have limited usefulness in detecting nodal melanoma deposits. While almost half of their patients showed lymph node enlargement, more than 50% of those without radiographically enlarged hilar or mediastinal lymph nodes had nodal metastases at autopsy. It is interesting that among the 31 total autopsies reviewed for pathologic correlation in this series were the two patients with negative chest x-rays, both of whom showed small postmortem pulmonary metastases. In all, five patients were

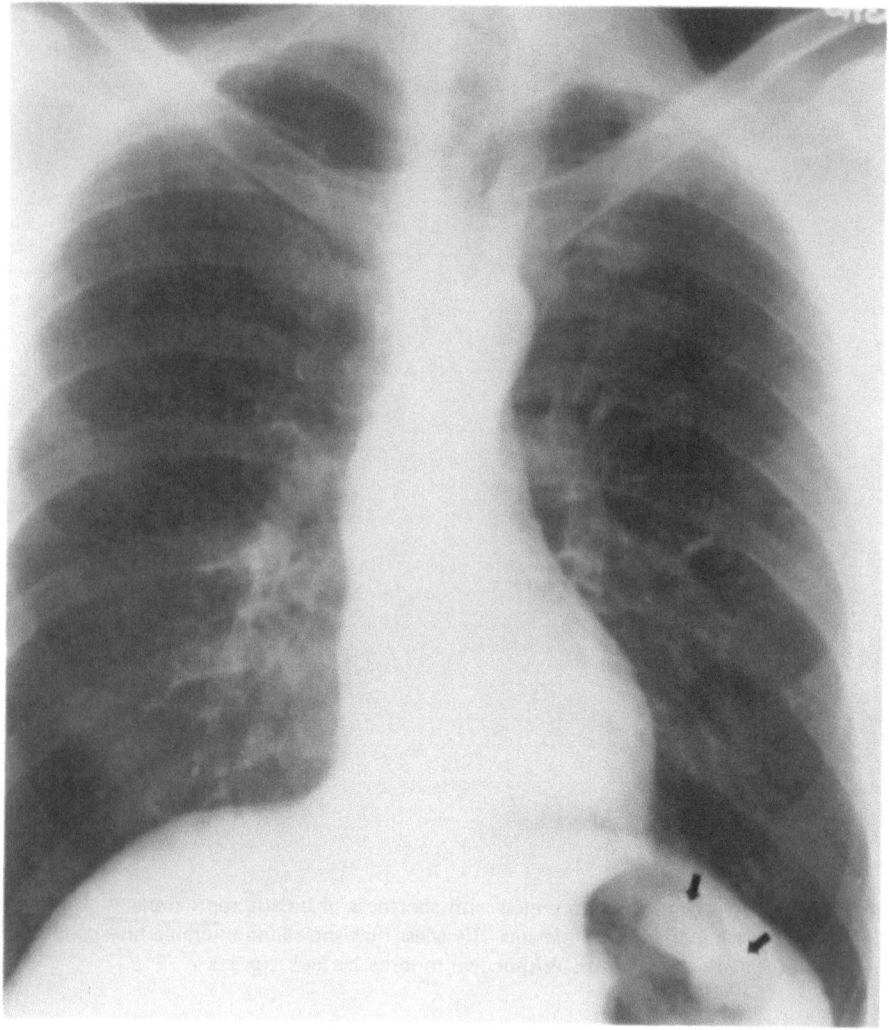

*Figure 3.* Plain chest films are adequate for assessing most metastases to the lungs, the usual site of systemic melanoma spread beyond regional lymph nodes. Even unusual sites of initial relapse may occasionally be uncovered by chest roentgenograms as in this 63-year-old man who had no evidence of melanoma dissemination other than the gastric fundal mass (arrows) first suggested in routine follow-up.

found at autopsy to have multiple nodules without prior radiographic detection.

This discrepancy in roentgenographic and postmortem findings was emphasized by Simeone et al. [123] in reporting on 17 patients with known metastatic malignant melanoma. In nine of the 17, disease not visible on premortem chest films, including nodules, nodes, pleural effusions, heart and bone lesions, was found at autopsy. Likewise Nathanson et al. [94] reported a 30% clinical incidence of pulmonary metastases in 164 patients but an 82% involvement when 32 of these were autopsied. The same was true for diagnosis of heart metastases where autopsy abnormality was eight times higher than that suspected clinically. These statistics correspond to other autopsy data in the literature for lung (70–80%) and heart (40–64%) [5, 65]. They also suggest that means other than the plain chest x-ray are needed to lessen the marked disparity in observed clinical and autopsy metastases.

Meyer and Stolbach [81], on the other hand, followed 53 melanoma patients for a year or more after an extensive pretreatment radiographic examination had been performed. Metastatic disease was said to be proven in 21 of the 53. Asymptomatic metastases visible on chest x-ray without tomography were discovered in nine patients, while symptoms heralded the discovery of metastases in the other 12 patients. In none of these were the radiographic abnormalities retrospectively visible on the original screening studies. These authors concluded that in the asymptomatic patient, a complete history and physical examination, routine laboratory determinations and a chest x-ray were sufficient tools for the initial evaluation of asymptomatic individuals with malignant melanoma.

In contradistinction is the review by Gromet et al. [49] of 13 melanoma patients who experienced systemic relapse during a two-year follow-up of 324 patients. The lung was found to be the initial site of dissemination in ten of the 13 and intrathoracic, extrapulmonary sites were noted in two others. Eight of the 12 had had no prior regional spread of disease. Even though routine chest views first suggested the diagnosis, in each case a retrospective analysis of previous films revealed missed intrathoracic metastates in four (33%). Initial full-lung tomography uncovered more nodules than the plain films in three patients, although it actually altered eventual therapy in only one. Since these five patients who underwent surgical resection of their isolated parenchymal nodules seemed to experience prolongation of survival compared to unoperated patients, the authors concluded that more vigorous radiographic surveillance was necessary to detect systemic relapse while patients were still in an operable stage. The failure of routine chest views to accomplish this suggested that either computed tomography or conventional full-lung tomography be employed in persons at high risk. Included were those with primary tumors thicker than 1.5 mm, noted by Breslow [16] to portend a more ominous prognosis, and those with any microstage who had experienced a local or regional recurrence.

The frequency of optimal radiographic follow-up examinations is directly related to the optimism and aggressiveness with which the patient is treated as well as to calculated tumor doubling times. Based on the six-year, 24% conversion of 638 patient chest radiographic series from negative to positive and a 43-day doubling time for metastatic pulmonary nodules, Seigler has obtained routine chest radiographs at four- to six-month intervals [115].

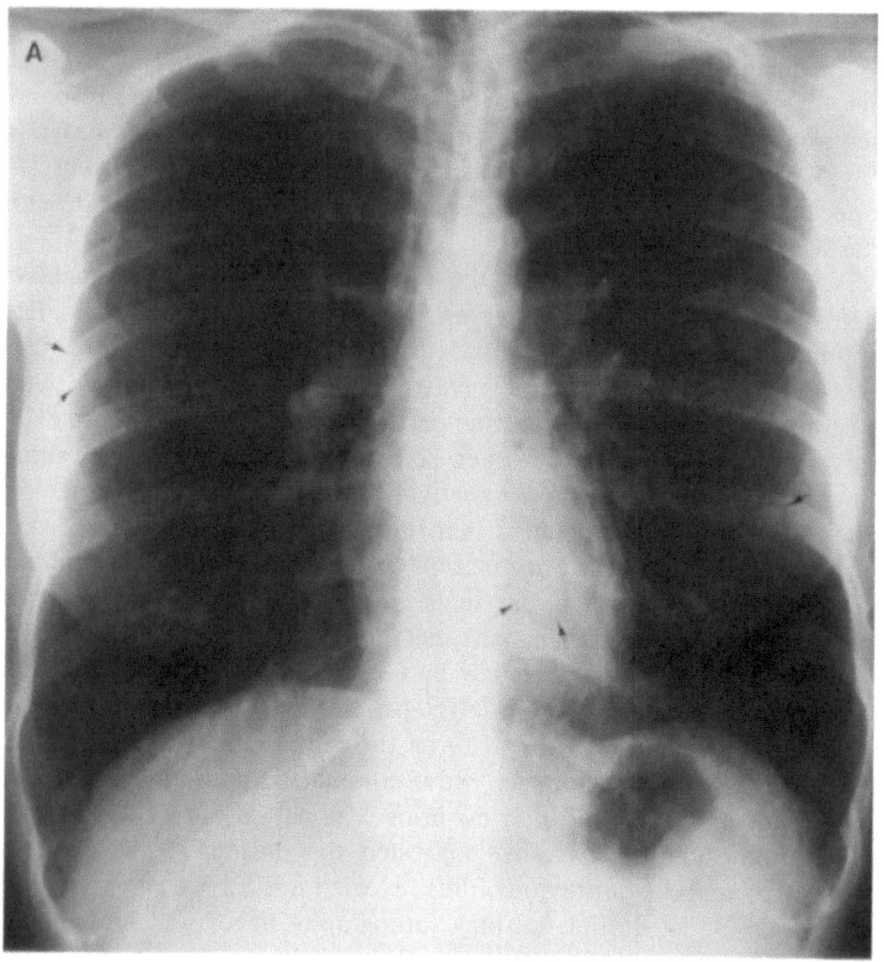

*Figure 4.* Our experience suggests that a pulmonary metastatic response to chemoimmunother-apy or perhaps spontaneous regression [74, 79, 93] is associated with a prolongation of survival. Figure 4A shows the development of bilateral lung metastases (arrows) in this 35-year-old woman 15 months following her original diagnosis of Level four malignant melanoma. Figure 4B, two months later, shows marked resolution following institution of systemic therapy. Plain films and CT scans have failed to disclose any pulmonary nodules during the subsequent 31 months during which time she has remained well.

Others have advocated three-month intervals using data obtained by the in vivo tritiated thymidine technique [119]. Still others recommend short-er [19] or longer intervals [54, 57] or no follow-up [145], once metastases are manifested, feeling that prognosis is not altered by the rate of growth of metastatic lesions nor by the uncommon regression of pulmonary nodules (Figures 4, 5).

Actually the necessary time for doubling the volume of a metastatic mela-noma nodule is variable and appears to be related to its size. Metastases

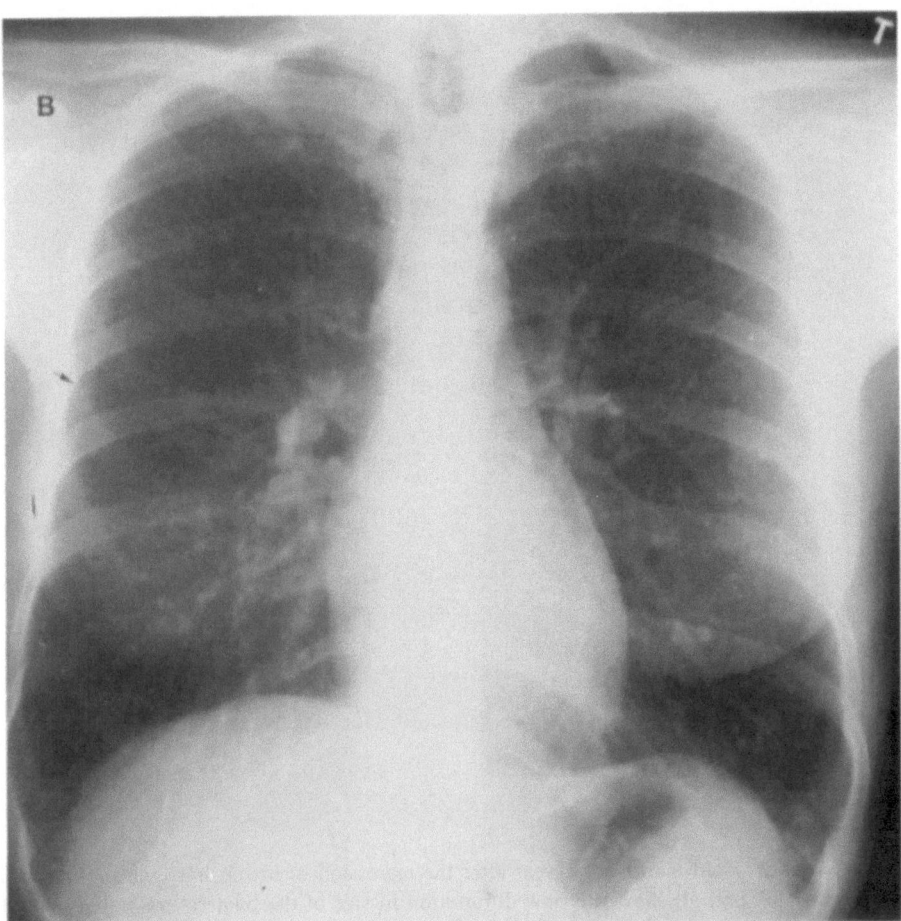

*Figure 4B.*

with diameters less than 15 mm appear to grow roughly twice as fast as those over that dimension. One study reported a subgroup of melanoma metastases, comprising about 10 % of the total, which displayed a doubling time greater than three times that of the mean of 49 days [102]. Others have also placed the mean tumor doubling time at seven weeks while noting that metastatic melanoma growth may vary from one week to five months (Figures 6, 7).

The importance of these biological variations is in their application to patient management. Both Seigler and Fetter [115] and Morton and coworkers [90] have advocated eventual surgical resection of pulmonary nodules which demonstrate tumor doubling times greater than 30 or 40 days respectively. Based on such treatment in 60 patients Morton et al. reported an approximately 60 %, five-year survival. Seigler and Fetter have recommanded a 60-day waiting period prior to thoracotomy during which time additional occult lesions or those possessing significantly different growth patterns may manifest themselves.

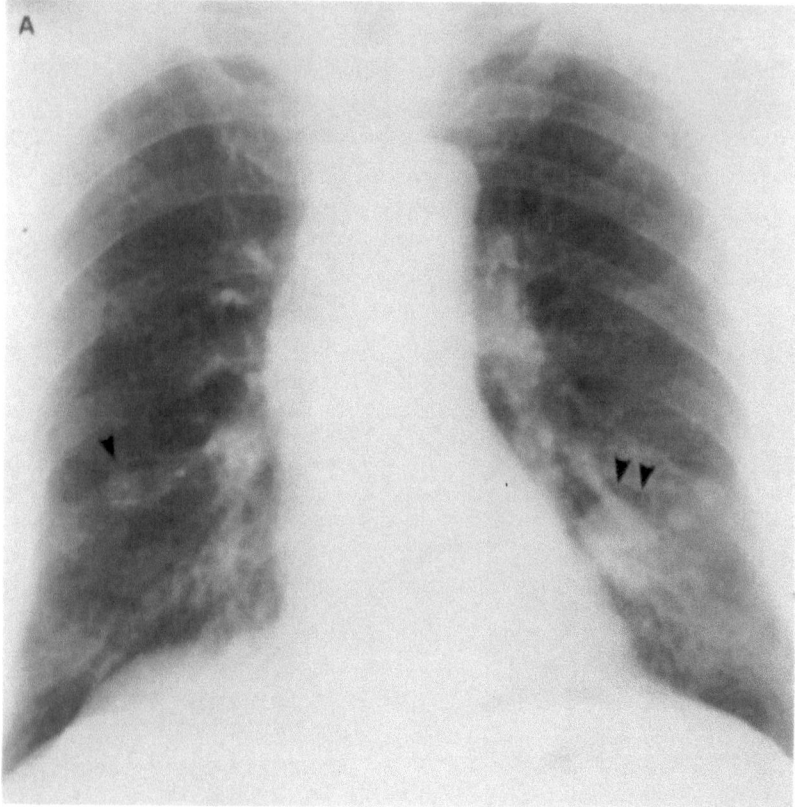

*Figure 5.* This-year-old man lived a year after the regression of his primary melanoma metastases. Figures 5A and 5B show the slow diminution in size of the bilateral pulmonary nodules during an 8-month period.

## Conventional tomography

Sporadic accounts of scanty cases are all that attest to the superiority of conventional tomography over plain chest radiography in the detection of disseminated malignant melanoma. While it is known that tomography can detect abnormalities undetectable on routine chest x-ray [27, 69, 104], a comprehensive series specific for melanoma is unpublished to our knowledge. To this end a three-year project to "determine and compare the utilization of full-chest tomography, stereoscopic radiography and 350 KV radiography in detecting metastatic deposits in the lung not visible by standard chest radiography" was initiated at Yale in 1976. Preliminary results suggested that full-chest tomography was indicated in patients with locally invasive melanoma when chest radiographs were normal. Webb and Gamsu [145] described 12 tomographic examinations in 11 patients of which

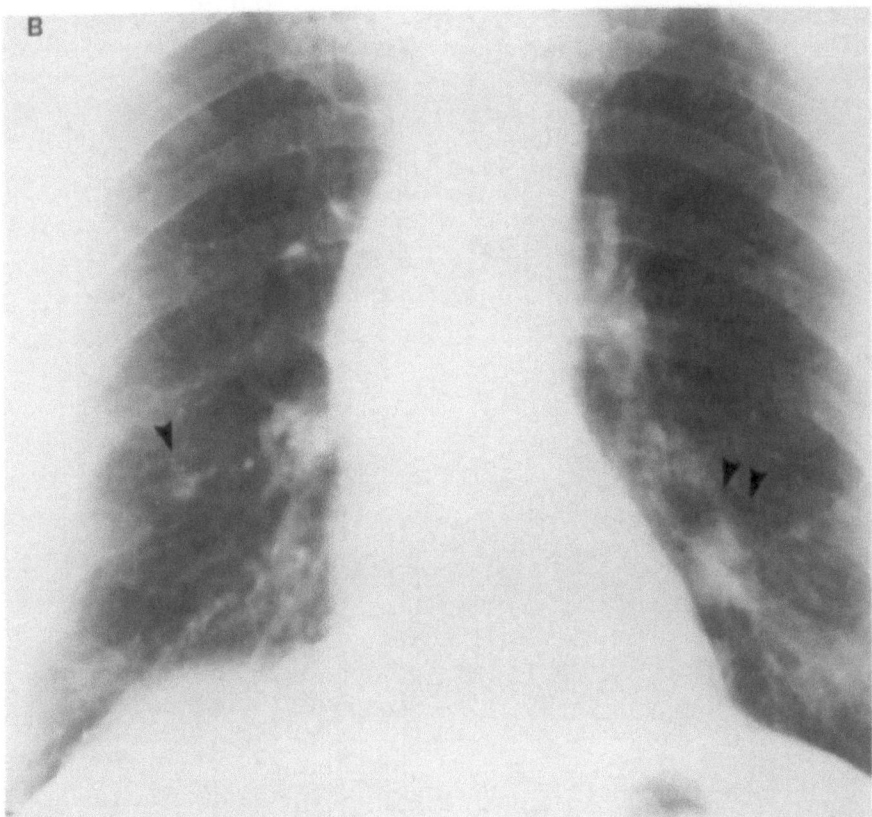

*Figure 5B.*

they felt ten were helpful in determining the extent of thoracic melanoma. Better definition of bronchial narrowing was noted in two studies and clarification of pulmonary nodules occurred in the others. Tomography revealed pulmonary nodules previously unnoticed in seven patients, for the first time in two of these. In the series of Gromet et al. [49] full-lung tomography was used to verify plain chest findings in patients to undergo further radical surgery or whose tumor microstage placed them at high risk. Thus, tomography disclosed isolated nodules in the five patients who underwent subsequent surgical resection and verified inoperability due to widely disseminated disease in their other seven.

Suspected malignant melanoma metastases comprised 22 of the 182 thoracotomies performed at the Surgery Branch of the National Cancer Institute from 1955 to 1975 [95]. Results were compared with conventional preoperative radiographs and full-chest linear tomograms (15 to 18 films) obtained at 1 cm intervals utilizing a grooved filter to allow combined visualization of mediastinum and peripheral lung fields. The addition of coned views of suspicious areas permitted diagnostic spatial resolution of

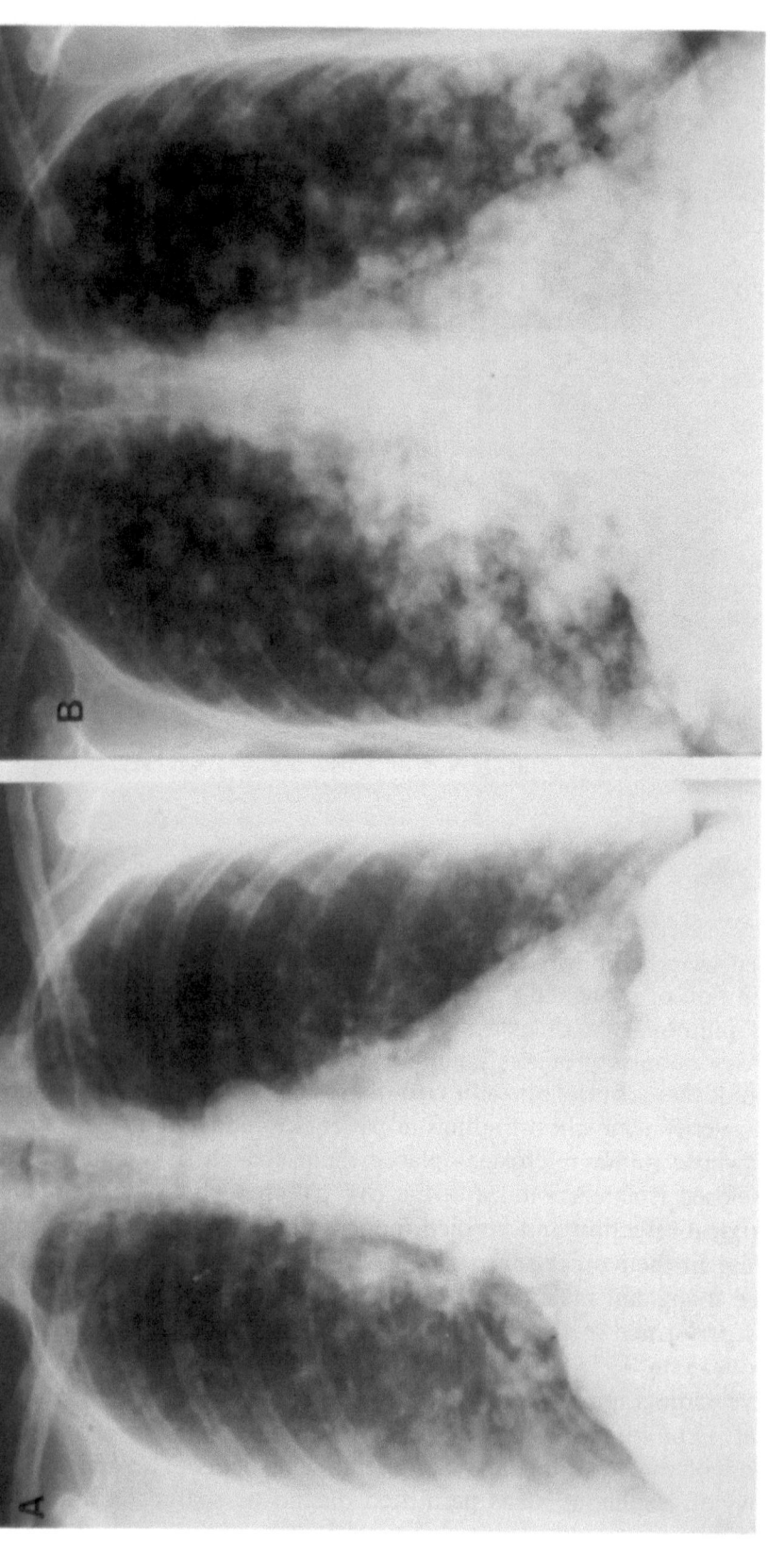

*Figure 6.* The tumor doubling time in malignant melanoma may be highly variable. Pulmonary metastases first appeared in this 54-year-old woman 10 years after her original skin lesion. Figure A shows her lung fields two years later and in Figure B another two-year interval has elapsed.

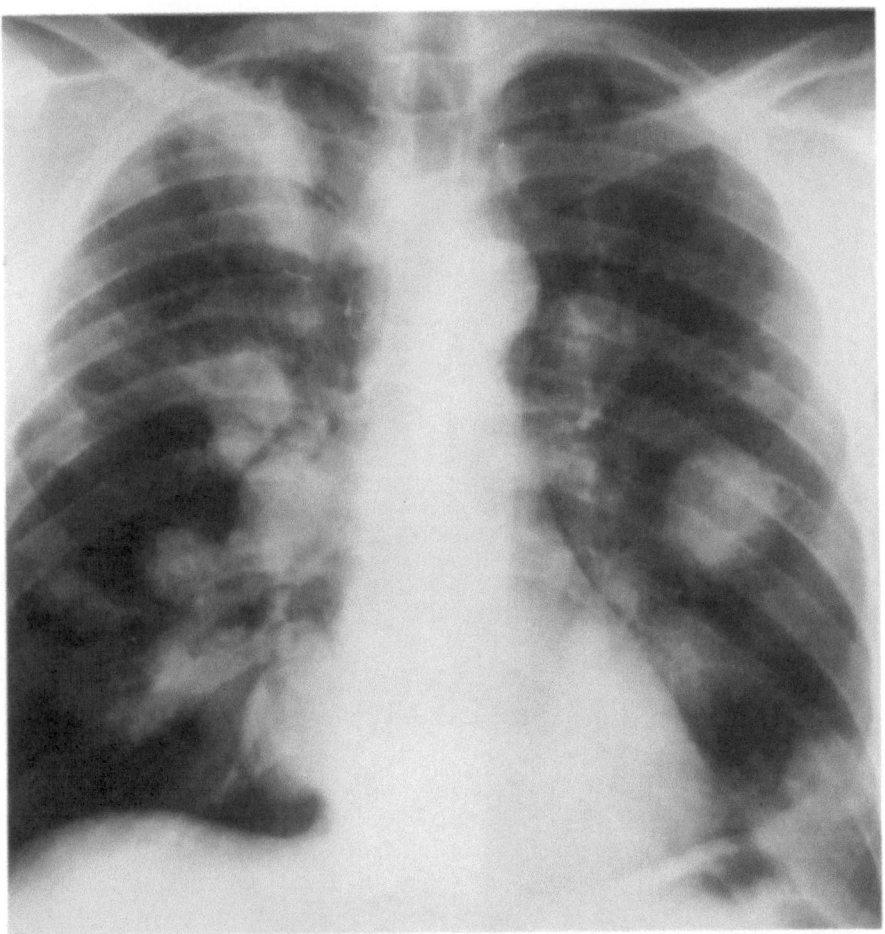

*Figure 7.* A rapid tumor doubling time was evident in this 44-year-old man who developed lung metastases one month following resection of his original malignant melanoma. This PA chest film taken six months later, shortly before his death, demonstrates multiple bilateral well-demarcated melanoma masses.

approximately 3 to 4 mm. Among the 19 patients with melanoma operated on, six proved to have benign disease, seven were unresectable; but none of the six patients undergoing resection of all known tumor had survived longer than 12 months at the time of the study. The value of tomography was shown in that melanoma metastases were seen when the chest x-ray was normal, multiple nodules were seen in a case when only solitary disease was previously noted, and bilateral nodules were found in two cases thought to have only unilateral metastases by routine radiography. Tomography confirmed plain film findings in the other cases; however, thoracotomy disproved both in one of these (Figures 8, 9).

Although this study was performed at 1 cm intervals, as has been shown to be optimal for detecting melanoma nodules by full-lung linear tomogra-

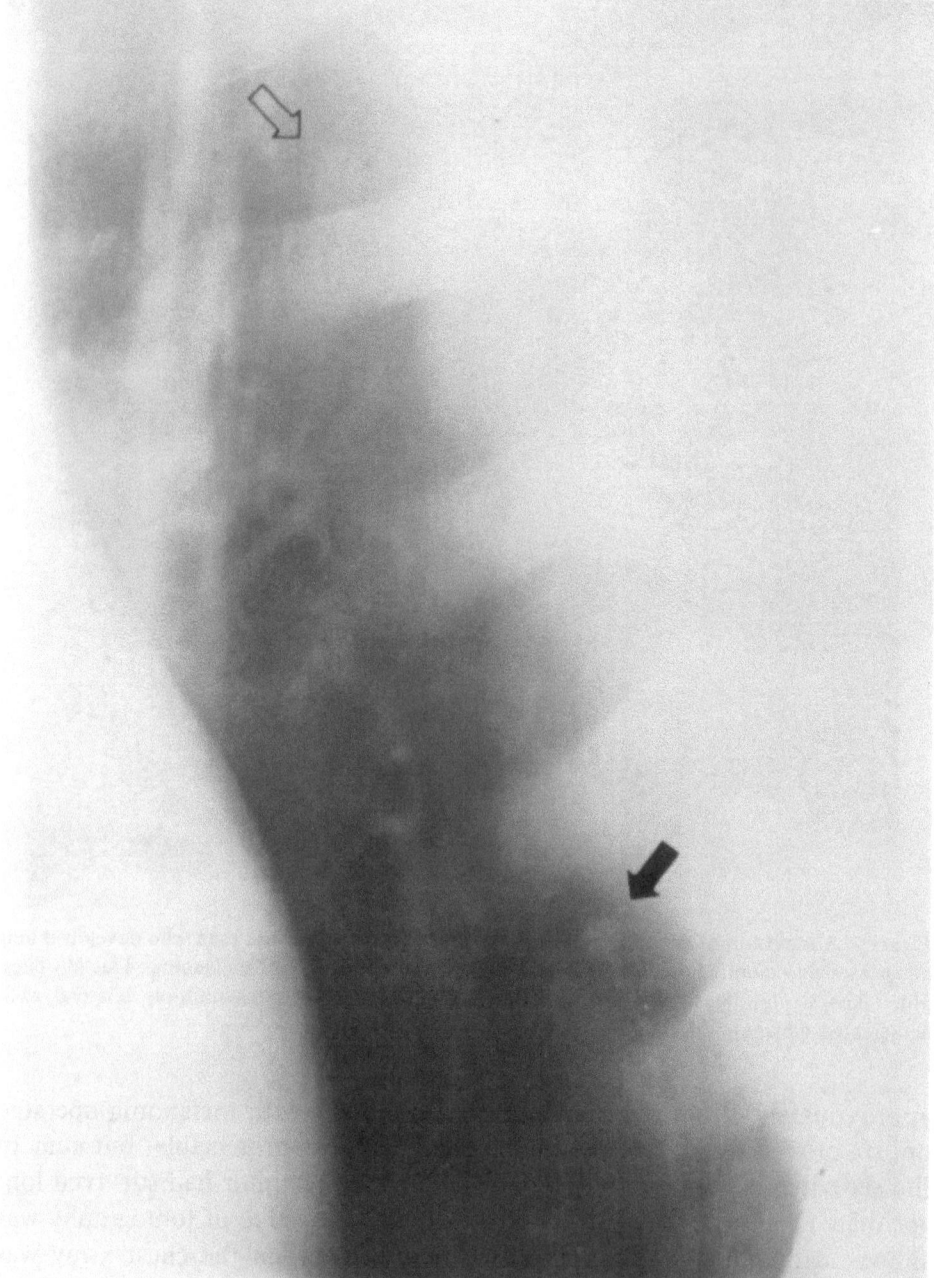

*Figure 8.* Linear tomography in this 21-year-old man disclosed a 5 mm lower lung field metastatic nodule (solid black arrow) not appreciated on chest plain films. The upper lobe nodule (open arrow) which is not in focus on this tomographic section was evident on both studies.

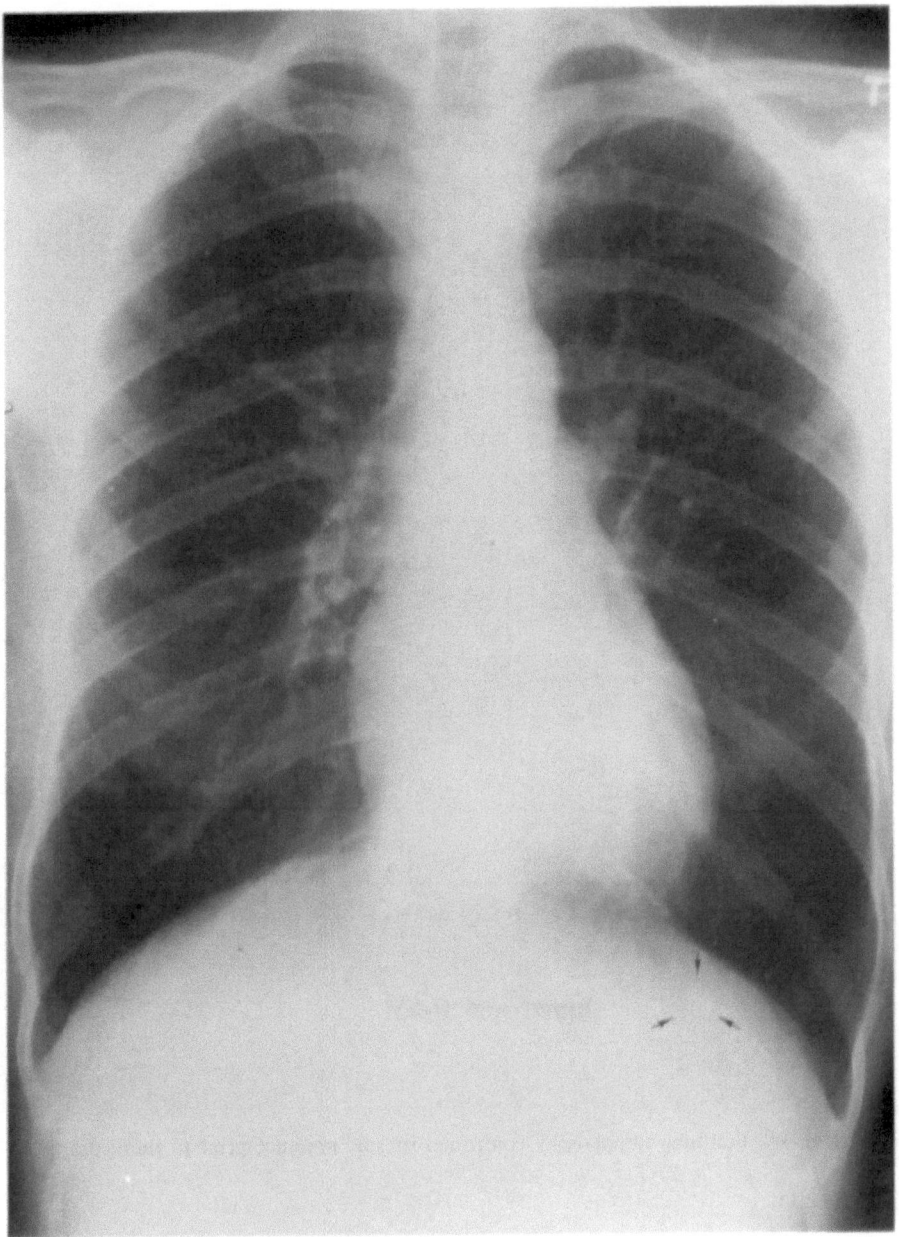

*Figure 9A.* A solitary 1 cm nodule is suggested at the left lung base on the PA chest view of this 38-year-old woman with malignant melanoma.

phy [11, 104], there is evidence that pluridirectional tomography more accurately depicts chest anatomy. Littleton et al. [69] for example feel that a whole-lung series performed with high resolution trispiral motion on a cooperative patient should detect all pulmonary implants larger than 3 mm in

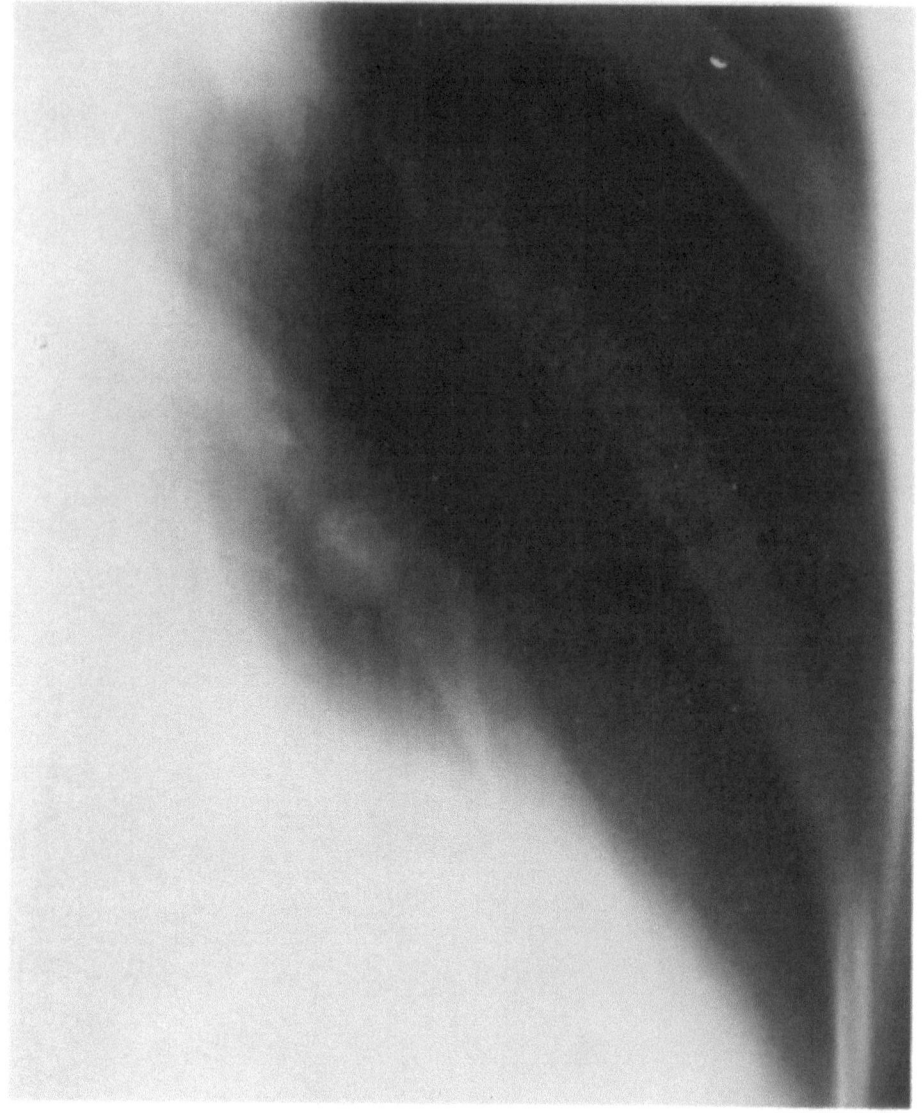

*Figure 9B.* Full-lung tomography confirmed its sole presence prior to thoracotomy.

diameter. Unfortunately large clinical studies comparing full-lung linear and pluridirectional tomography in the detection of pulmonary nodules are not yet available. Information that is extant estimates that whole-lung tomography may detect up to 20% more metastases than will plain chest radiography when secondary tumors in general are considered [120]. When malignant melanoma metastases specifically are in question, that figure may be doubled.

*Computed tomography*

Although indications for thoracic computed tomography (CT) are still evolving, recent reports emphasize its great utility in the diagnosis of malignancy throughtout the thorax [21, 61, 91, 120]. The added sensitivity of this modality can be particularly important for the tumor such as malignant melanoma which so frequently affects the chest.

In the detection of pulmonary nodules computed tomography is to conventional tomography what conventional tomography is to plain chest radiography. Whereas the spatial resolution of plain chest radiography is in the 4–10 mm or greater range, and that of conventional tomography approximates 3–4 mm, CT is thought to be able to resolve 2 mm definition with ease [120]. Differences in density between an individual nodule and its background and an adjustable gray scale allowing optimal display of the nodule combine to give CT inherent advantages. Several studies have shown that up to twice as many nodules can be detected by the computerized versus the standard tomographic study [21]. These tend to be located in the lung apices, in subpleural sites or in the diaphragmatic lung recesses, sites of known diagnostic difficulty for plain tomography (Figure 10). Muhm et al. [91] found more pulmonary nodules by CT than whole-lung tomography or plain chest roentgenography in 44% of the 52 patients in their study. There were three false-positive and four false-negative cases among the 52. In ten of 29 patients (35%) CT detected more nodules than whole-lung tomography. Most of these were 5–10 mm in diameter; a few, however, measured 2–3 mm. The important point of the study was the alteration in therapy for one-fourth of the patients in whom additional pulmonary nodules were demonstrated. Jost et al. [61] likewise reported a significant CT effect on patient management in five patients with lung nodules detected by computed but not by standard tomography.

The applicability of these data to malignant melanoma was shown by Schaner et al. [113] and again by Chang et al. [21]. In their analyses ten of the 25 patients undergoing surgical correlation of the CT and conventional tomographic findings had from one to four melanoma metastases. Overall, CT identified more nodules than plain tomography in nearly half of the cases. These were usually 3–6 mm in diameter and occurred in pleural or subpleural sites (Figure 11). Nodules at the lung apices or along the diaphragm greater than 3 mm in diameter however were not always detected as subsequent surgery disclosed. Nor were malignant metastases in the 3–6 mm range able to be reliably distinguished from granulomas, subpleural lymph nodes or other benign tissue. Only about half of the CT-detected nodules, including the melanoma population, proved to be metastatic, compared to a 66% conventional tomographic specificity. This apparent superiority of plain tomography reflects the fact that it discovered fewer total

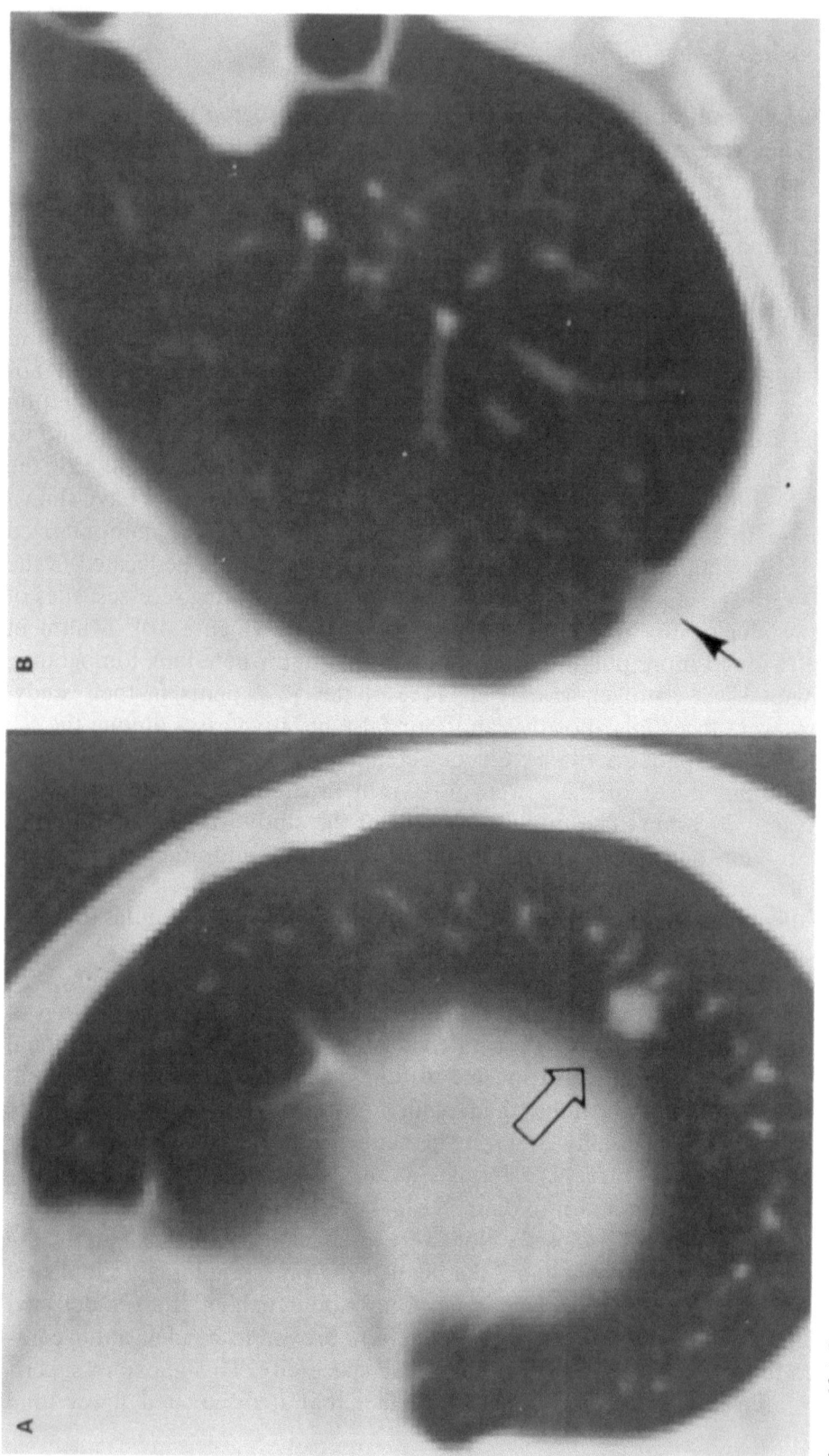

*Figures 10A, B.*

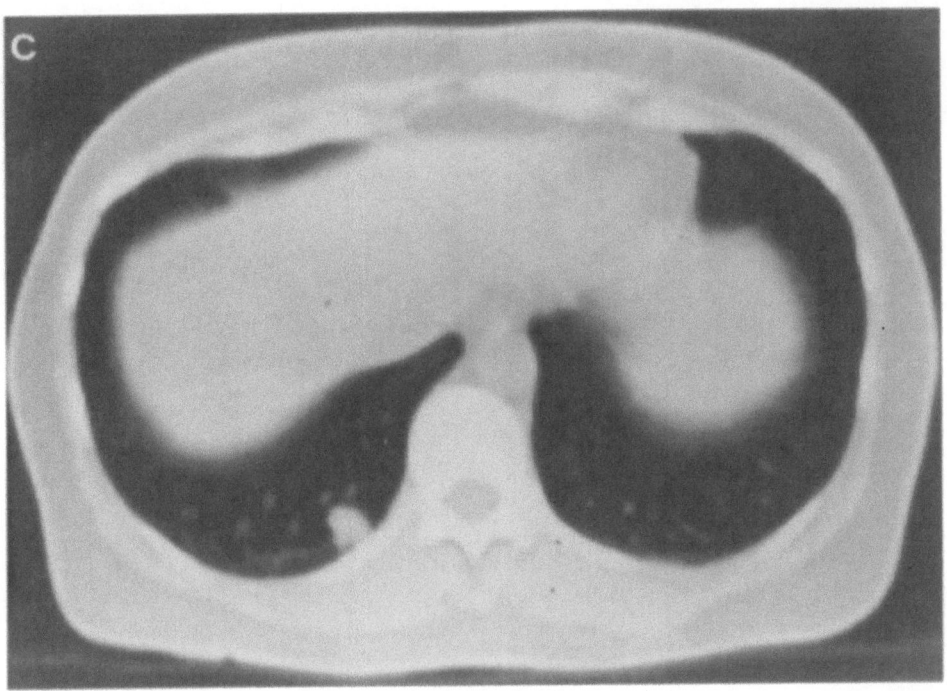

*Figure 10.* CT appearance of typical pulmonary metastases in patients with malignant melanoma. (A, facing page) 1 cm parenchymal nodule in the left diaphragmatic recess (open arrow) in a 32-year-old man. (B, facing page) Pleural based nodule (arrowhead) in same patient as A. (C) 1.5 cm pleuroparenchymal nodule in the right recess of a 52-year-old woman.

nodules. The authors pointed out that even open thoracotomy had its limitations in the accurate assessment of metastatic nodules and hence the true positive rate by which to analyze CT or conventional tomography. Sixteen 3–6 mm nodules identified on CT scans were not found operatively. Six more with diameters greater than 6 mm detected by CT and linear tomography alike could not be palpated at thoracotomy. That these nodules were still present following surgery was verified by CT in three cases. Postoperative anatomic distortion, atelectasis or fibrosis hampered their detection by CT in other attempts.

In view of the increased five-year survival possible when favorable pulmonary melanoma metastases can be resected [49, 75, 78], the importance of their accurate detection is apparent. On the other hand, one strongly hopes to avoid thoracotomy for removal of benign nodules for equally obvious reasons. The earlier resection of tiny nondescript pulmonary lesions therefore seems superfluous if differentiation between benignancy and malignancy cannot be reasonably made a priori. One very promising step in this determination is the association of benign disease with high radiographic density. The presence of calcification within a nodule has been shown in several large series [138] to be a reliable indicator of benignancy. For mela-

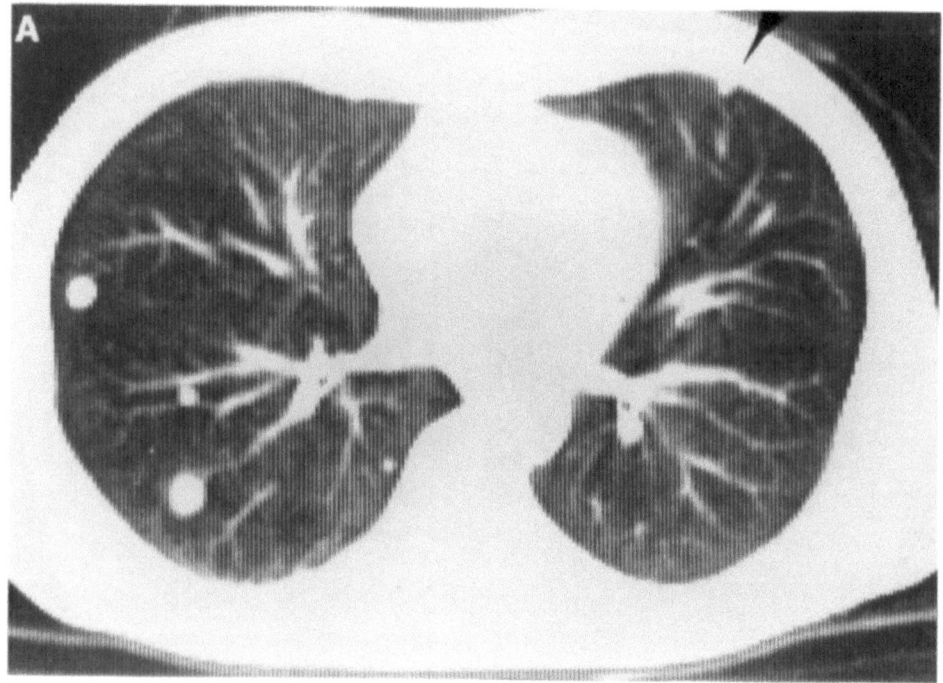

*Figure 11.* Pleural and subpleural melanoma metastases not appreciated on conventional whole-lung tomographic studies (arrows). (A) The four nodules in the right lung were seen tomographically. (B, next page) Lung window settings show a tiny nodule deep at the right lung base. (C, next page) Pulmonary congestion and right pleural effusion accompanying extensive hilar and mediastinal adenopathy is present.

noma in particular the incidence of contained calcification is indeed small. Only two cases have been reported to our knowledge, neither appeared in a pulmonary nodule. One presented on chest x-ray as a calcified dumbbell-shaped mass which eroded ribs and spine at the third thoracic vertebral level [131]. Superior vena caval obstruction and massive pulmonary involvement were apparent at the child's demise. The second melanoma calcification was in an adrenal metastasis [140]. If calcification could therefore be detected within a pulmonary nodule the overwhelming odds would favor that nodule not being a melanoma metastasis. Even though conventional radiography and tomography can detect such calcification, CT, with its capacity for measuring absorption coefficients, is a more precise means of density determination (Figure 12).

Raptopoulos et al. [103] and more recently Siegelman et al. [121] have used CT to collect such data on pulmonary nodules. The first study, using six-minute CT scanning times and 1 cm slice thicknesses, compared imaging modalities in 42 patients with both solitary and multiple nodules [103]. CT predicted the presence of calcification in 24 of these based on a high average attenuation value or CT number. All proved to be benign. This detection

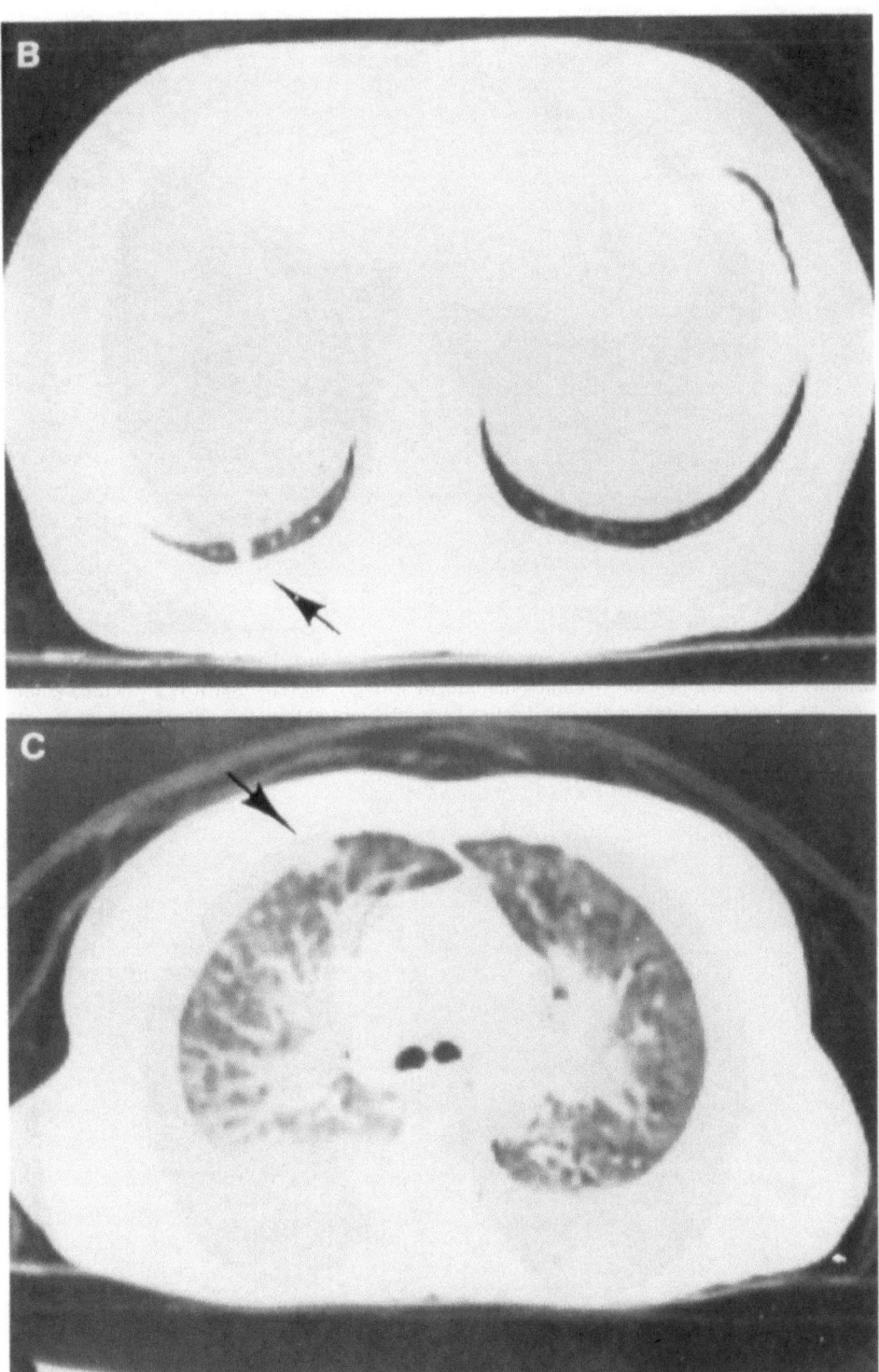

*Figures 11B, C.*

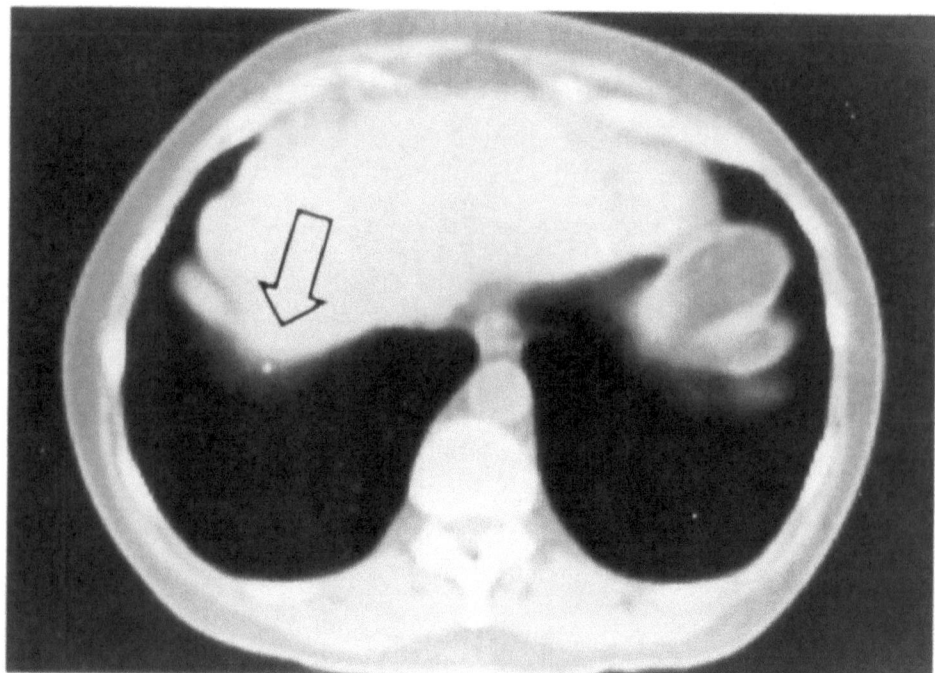

*Figure 12A.* CT defines a tiny 2–3 mm nodule at the right lung base (open arrow). Its ease of visibility against the partially volumed diaphragm strongly suggests that it is a calcified granuloma. Mediastinal lymph node calcification was also present in this 69-year-old man with known metastatic melanoma.

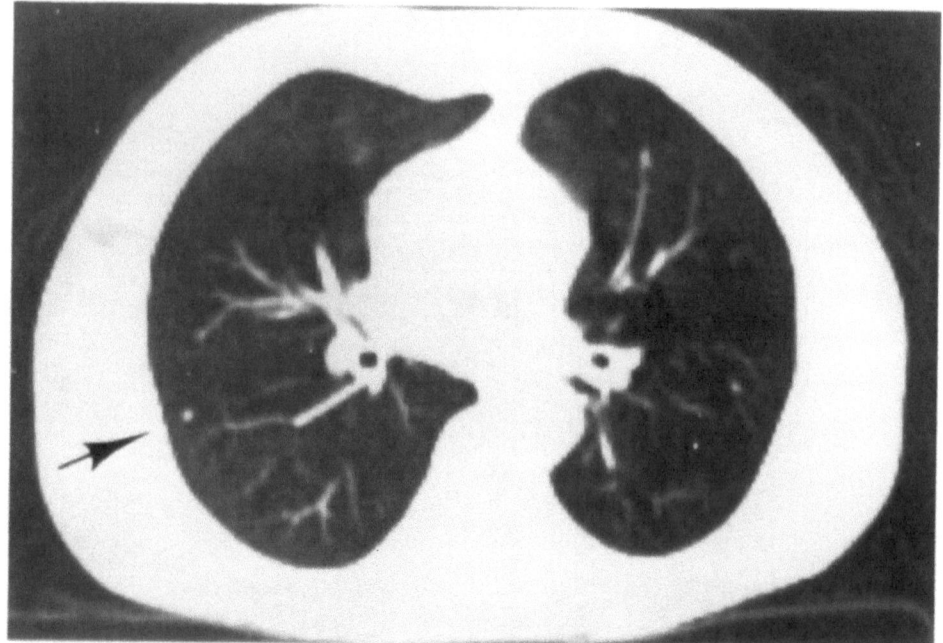

*Figure 12B.* Another scan in the same man shows a similar nodule without recognizable calcification. Further diagnostic follow up was therefore required to exclude malignancy.

rate of calcium by CT was significantly better than that of conventional radiography. The second study utilized ten-second scan times and 2–5 mm slice sections in 91 apparently noncalcified pulmonary nodules [121]. Thirteen of these were known to be metastatic, one from malignant melanoma. The representative CT numbers of this group ranged from 57 to 147 Hounsfield units (H), (mean, 98H). Of the 33 presumed or biopsy proven benign lesions however, 20 had a representative CT number of 164H. This number is the mean representative CT number of their 45 proven lung malignancies (92H) plus four standard deviations, which the authors felt should include all probable malignancies they would encounter. They attributed this higher CT number to the probable diffuse deposition of calcium within the nodule as well as the more tightly organized tissue of granulomas as opposed to malignant neoplasms which would be more likely to have central areas of necrosis with lower attenuation foci. They postulated that benign lesions with lower CT numbers were poorly organized acute inflammatory infiltrates or fat containing lesions. By employing strict attention to technique they suggested that CT number was a reliable indicator of benign or malignant disease for which radiographic follow-up or needle biopsy or thoracotomy could be recommended (Figure 12).

Experience with the radiographic follow-up of malignant melanoma at Duke University Medical Center corroborates the high sensitivity and specificity of CT in the patient with suspected metastases. Thirty-three persons have prospectively received periodic plain chest films, whole-lung linear tomography and computed tomography during the past $1\frac{1}{2}$ years. Examinations have been conducted at four- to six-month intervals as previously reported [115] in keeping with the published doubling time of the average metastasis and the rate of our patient population to convert their chest radiographs from normal to abnormal. CT has been performed with two five-second scanners (Searle and AS & E). Scans are obtained at 1 cm intervals, using standard 1 cm slice widths. An accurate CT number for suspected pulmonary nodules using narrower slice widths has been determined only recently in a limited number of cases. Of the 33 patients evaluable in this ongoing study, seven (21%) have been shown to be normal by all three chest imaging modalities. Another six have shown normal computed and conventional tomography when a metastatic abnormality was suspected on plain chest films. CT has confirmed plain film and tomographic solitary nodules in three cases and verified chest film abnormality in three cases where conventional tomography was nonconfirmatory (Figure 13). In each of the remaining 14 patients CT disclosed more information than was available on review of the other two examinations. This was true not only for the pulmonary parenchyma but also for the mediastinum, pleura and extrapleural chest wall (Figures 14, 15). Others have noted similar CT advantages in evaluating the diaphragm, trachea, heart and pericardium (Figure 16).

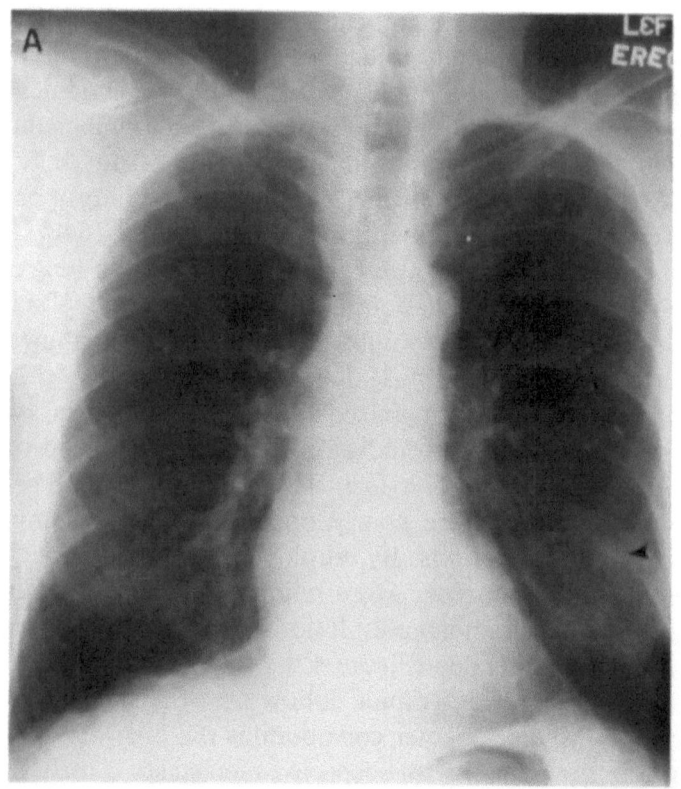

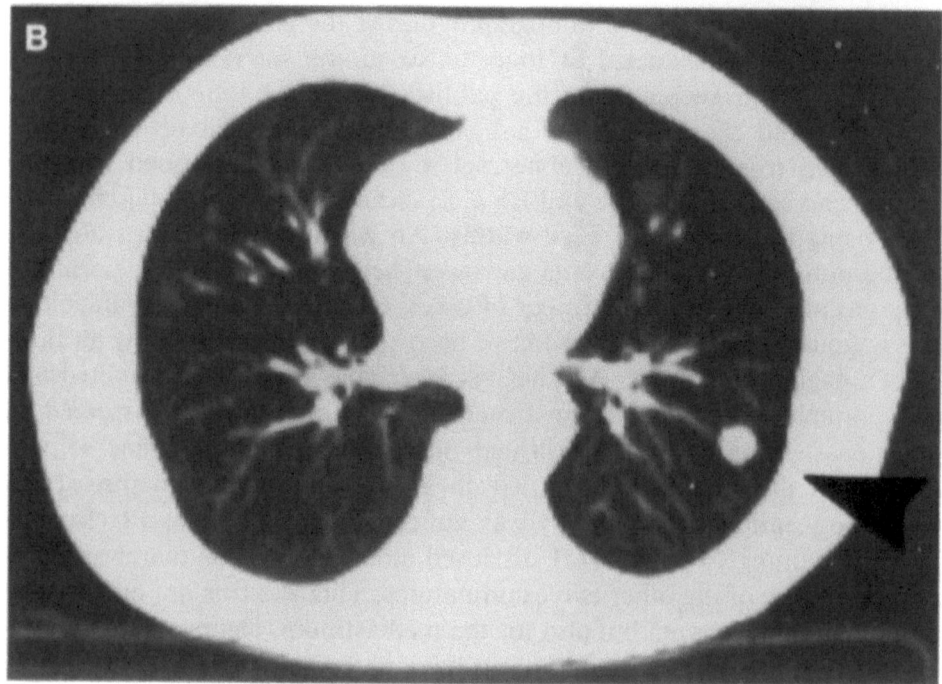

Figures 13A, B.

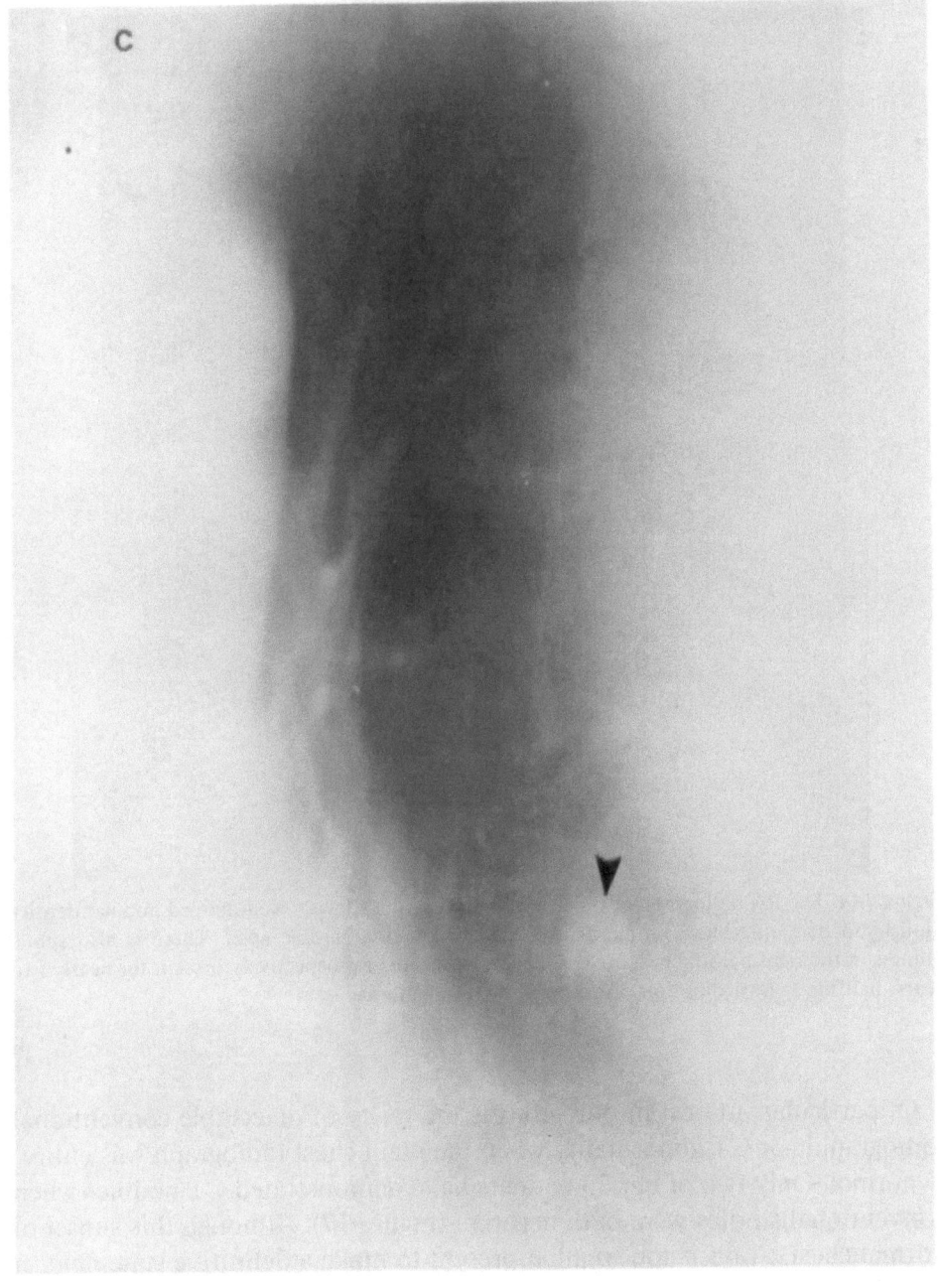

*Figure 13.* Confirmation of a 2 cm solitary pulmonary nodule (arrowhead) in the left lower lobe was made by (A, facing page) PA chest view, (B, facing page) computed tomogram, and (C) linear tomogram.

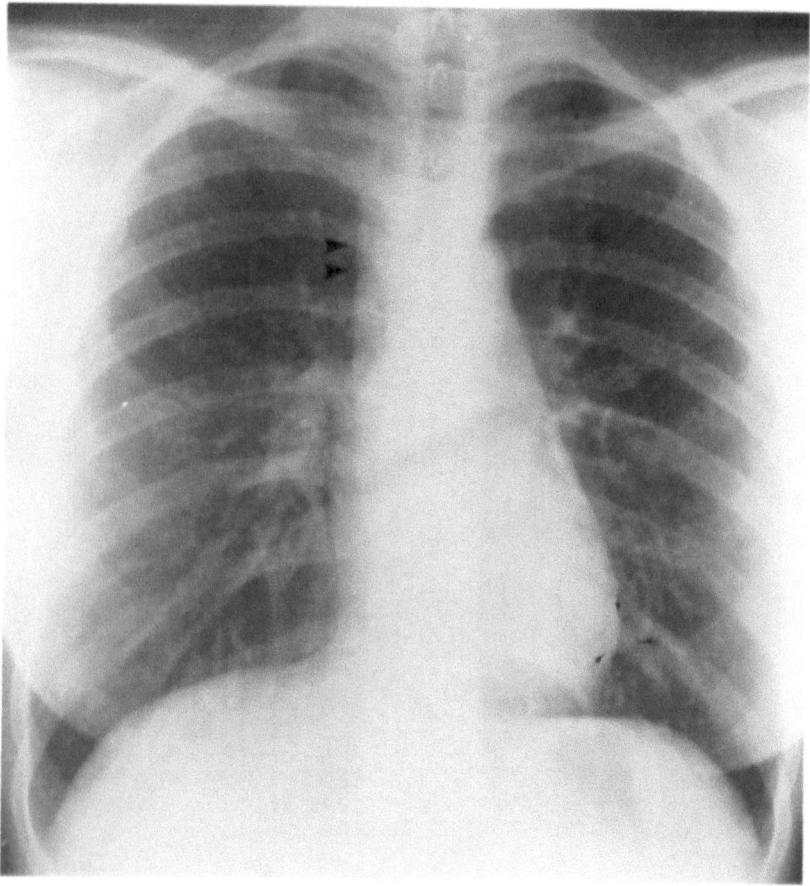

*Figure 14A.* The PA radiograph of this 23-year-old woman shows a well-defined nodular density thought to be a metastasis (triple arrows) adjacent to the cardiac apex. There is also subtle fullness in the right paratracheal area (double arrowheads) retrospectively present for nearly two years, half the known duration of her malignant melanoma.

Of particular interest in our series is the rarity of detectable conventional tomographic or CT abnormality when the plain chest radiograph was entirely normal. Only two of our 33 patients have demonstrated CT nodules when conventional studies were both negative (Figure 17). Although this subset of normal chest x-rays is too small at present to make a definitive statement, it would be highly advantageous to screen melanoma patients with plain chest films rather than considerably more expensive CT scans. In view of the retrospective discovery by Gromet et al. [49], however, of missed intrathoracic metastases in one third of their relapsing patients who were followed by periodic plain chest views, it seems unlikely that this trend will hold. The clinical importance of this problem has already been alluded to in the reports of improved patient survival with early resection of pulmonary

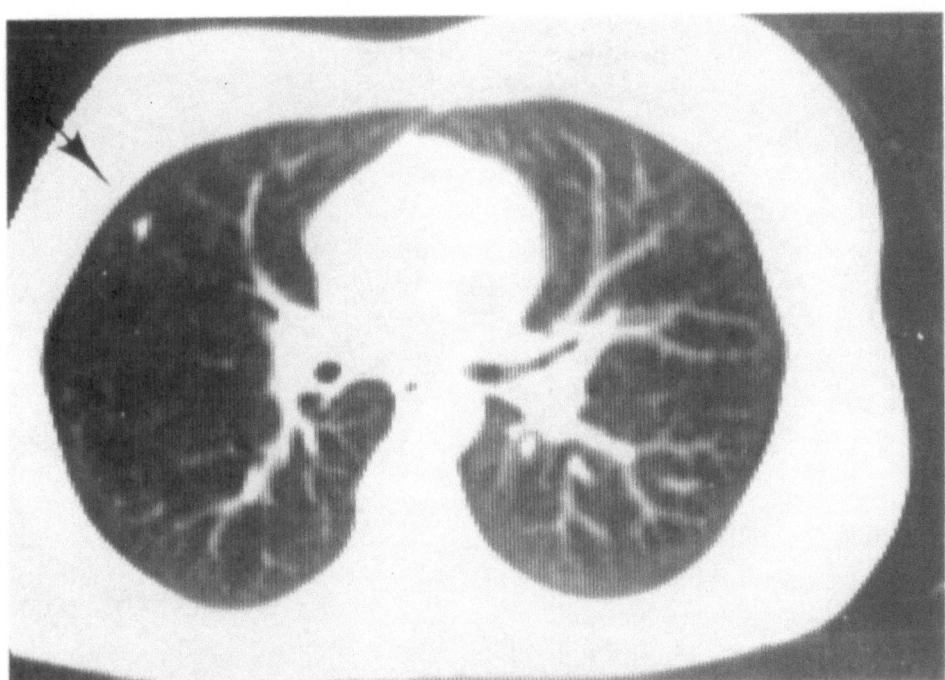

*Figure 14B.* Neither conventional nor computed tomography could confirm the left lung nodule which likewise was no longer present on a subsequent PA chest film. CT however did disclose a probable metastasis in the right lung (arrow) not visualized by conventional radiography.

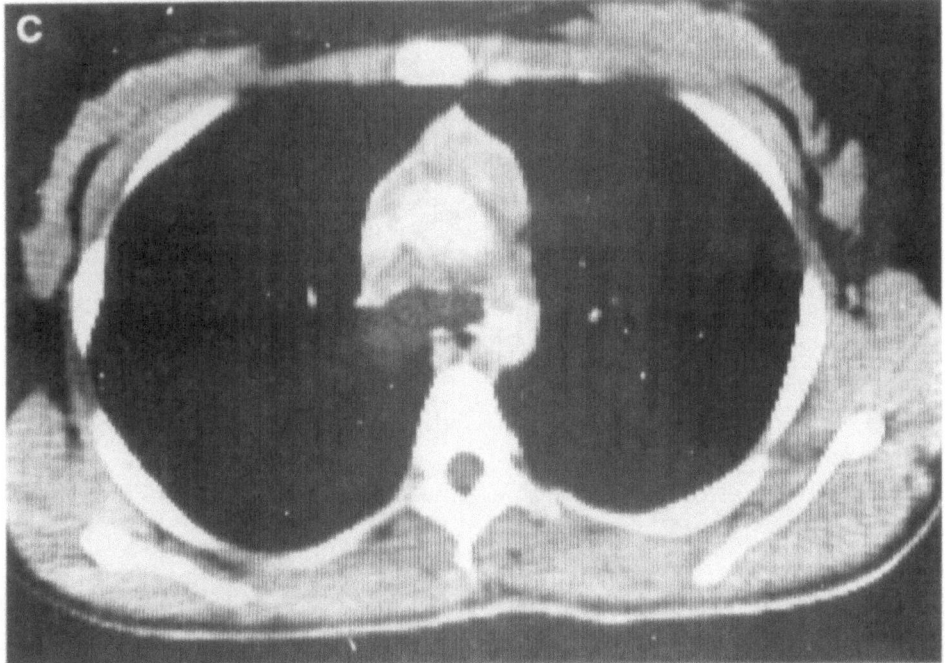

*Figure 14C.* CT section at the level of the carina reveals an unsuspected anterior mediastinal mass consistent with adenopathy in front of the contrast-filled aorta and superior vena cava.

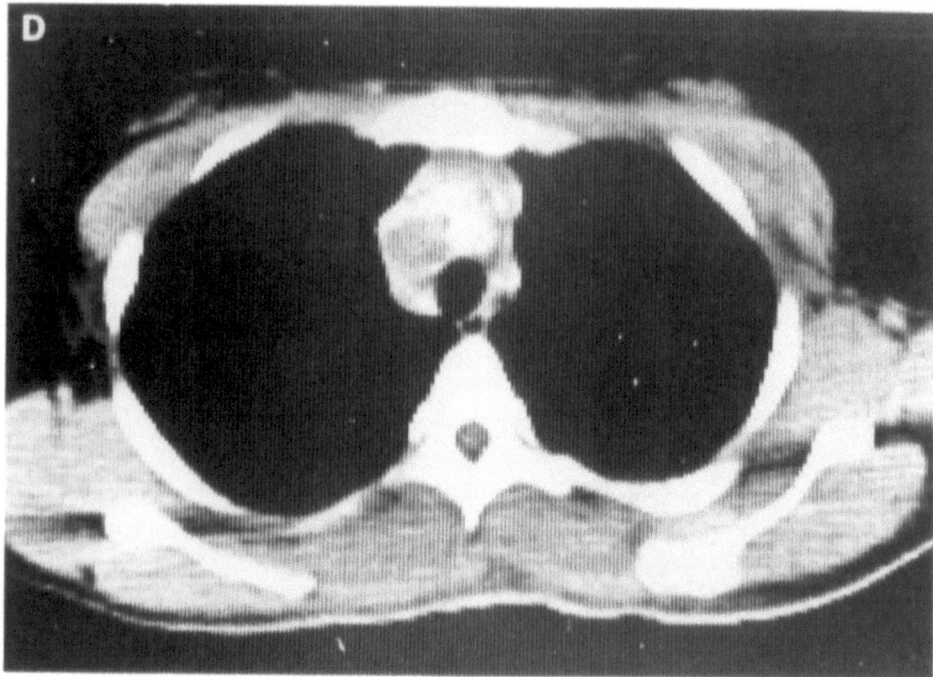

*Figure 14D.* CT section several centimeters higher shows a low-density right paratracheal lymph node mass corresponding to that seen in 14A.

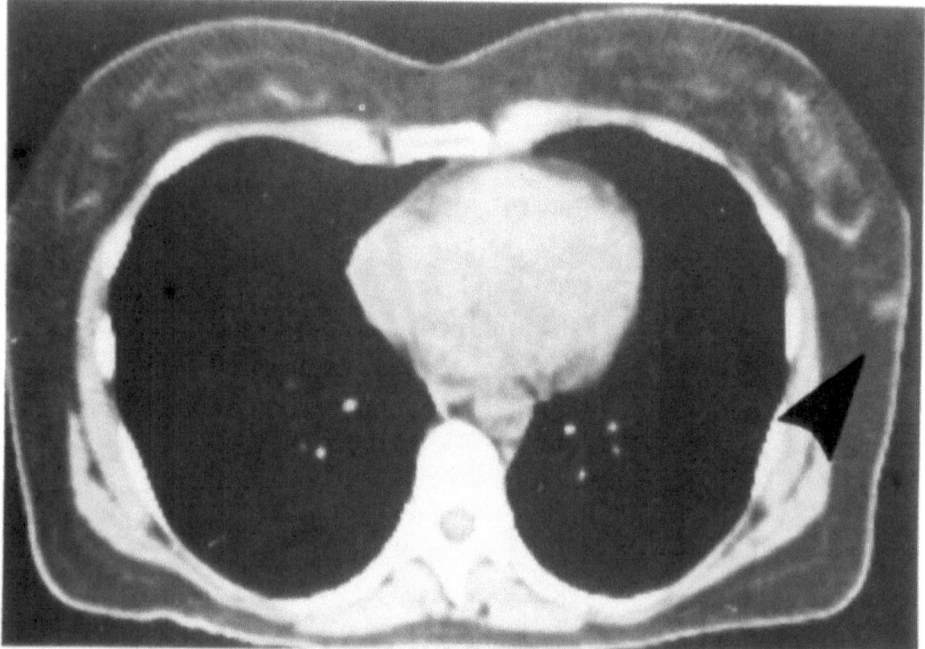

*Figure 15A.* Chest roentgenograms and conventional and computed tomograms all showed multiple bilateral pulmonary nodules in this 52-year-old woman, but only CT disclosed the metastatic deposits in the subcutaneous tissue of the lateral chest wall (arrowhead).

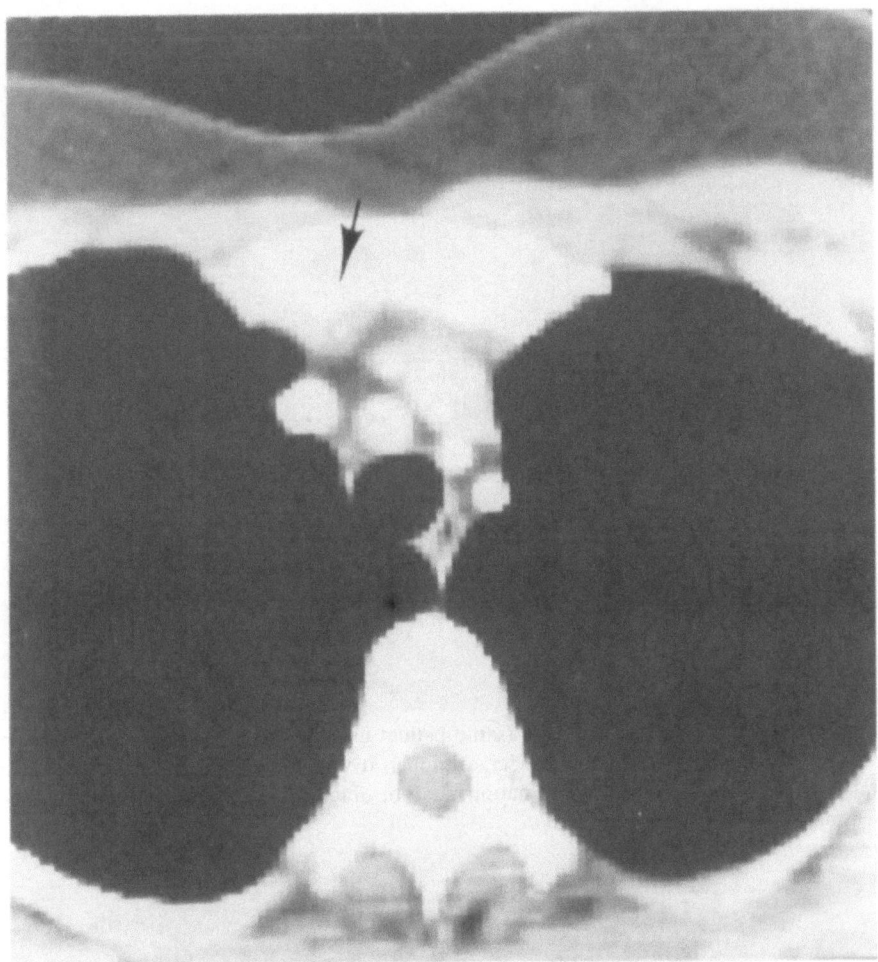

*Figure 15B.* The arrow points to a small square cursor which measures the average tissue density of a presumed retrosternal metastasis to allow it to be distinguished from the vascular structures behind which have been rendered quite dense with a bolus injection of iodinated contrast agent.

melanoma deposits. Well-controlled clinical studies would therefore seem to be beneficial in order to determine the relative importance and cost effectiveness of CT, conventional tomography and plain film radiography in routine follow-ups of melanoma patients at high risk for dissemination. Again, although the number of patients assigned to a high risk category in our prospective study is still too small for statistical analysis, it is interesting that both patients discovered only by CT to have systemic melanoma relapse had locally advanced disease (Clark Level IV) at initial diagnosis.

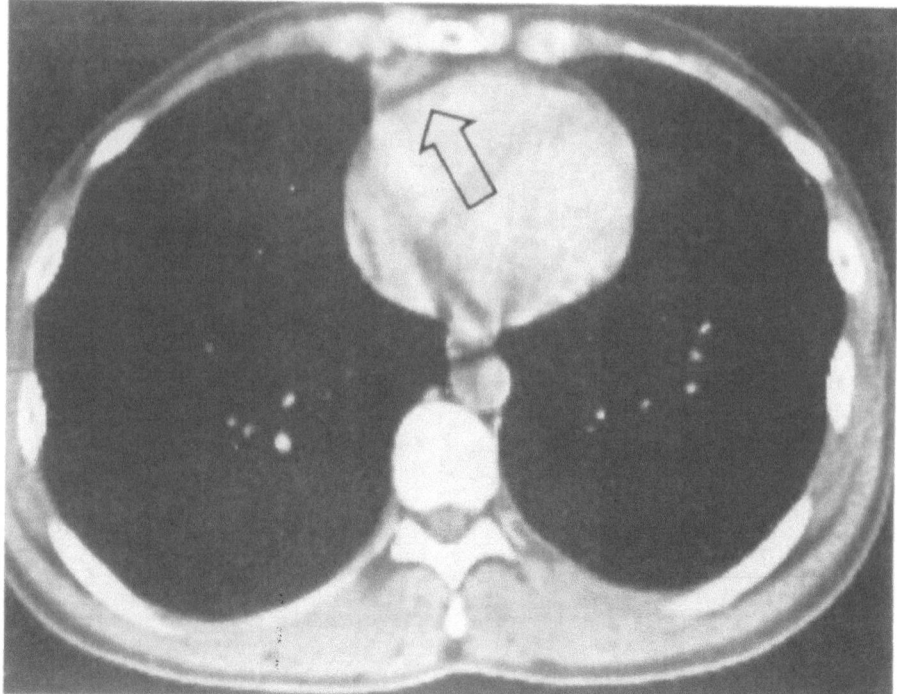

*Figure 16.* CT in this 32-year-old man (same patient as 10A and C) shows a soft tissue mass adjacent to the anterior right heart border. Although it was felt to most likely be a metastatic lymph node deposit, histologic confirmation was not obtained in view of the man's extensive disseminated disease.

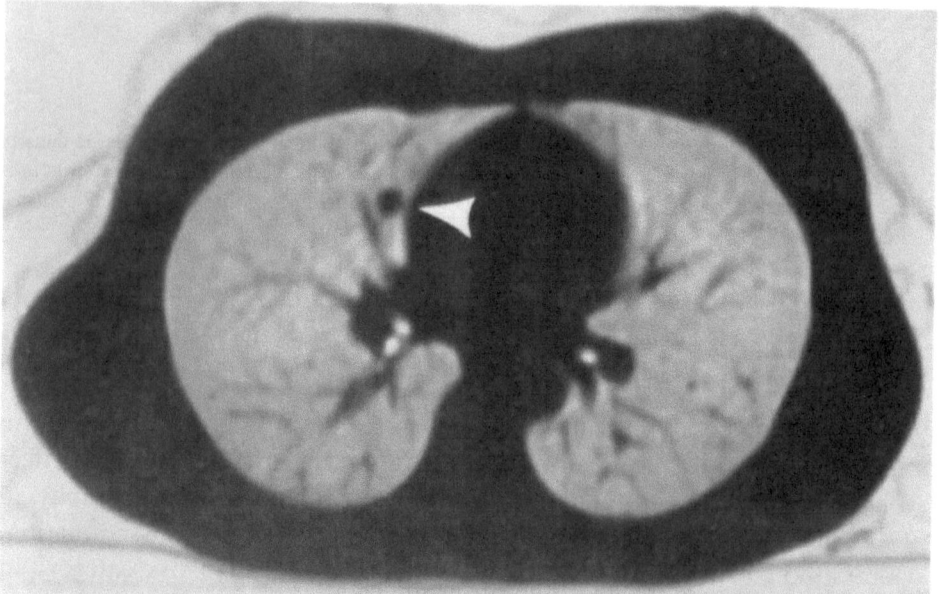

*Figure 17.* Even in retrospect the well-circumscribed 1 cm nodule defined here by CT between the right hilum and the heart border (arrowhead) was not apparent by high KVP chest radiographs or linear tomography.

*Thoracic radionuclide imaging*

The application of nuclear imaging to the routine staging and follow-up of malignant melanoma in general is described elsewhere (Chapter 11). In the specific evaluation of intrathoracic melanoma, the various radionuclides proven to have diagnostic efficacy assume only a minor role [34, 37, 92]. Gallium-67 for example localized correctly in 60% of 18 patients with melanoma lung metastases [86], but because of its nonspecificity in localizing radiotracer in sites of focal inflammation, a positive scan has tended to require confirmation [53]. An abnormal pulmonary accumulation of $^{67}$Ga-citrate for instance will follow recent oily contrast lymphangiography or BCG therapy [66, 59]. Based on these findings gallium-67 is currently employed as an adjunctive staging test, a method of monitoring treatment or a method of detecting occult recurrent disease [101]. No useful preoperative purpose has been found for gallium scanning which appears to be less sensitive than careful physical examination when assessing the primary melanoma site and its regional nodal drainage [108]. Evidence does suggest, however, that a negative $^{67}$Ga-citrate scintiscan is a reliable indicator of the disease-free state and that focal uptake in the lungs is highly suggestive of metastatic disease [13, 67].

It is not known whether newer "tumor specific" radionuclides will increase the specificity of nuclear medicine imaging of intrathoracic melanoma [68]. One recent report suggests a role for thallium-201 in the detection of cardiac metastatic tumors where technetium-99m stannous pyrophosphate has proven utility [71].

*Lymphangiography/angiography*

Although of proven value in the evaluation of inguinal, pelvic and abdominal nodal metastases, lymphangiography has a very limited usefulness in the staging of intrathoracic malignant melanoma [7, 26, 143]. At present its role is relegated to the confirmation of lymphatic as opposed to venous obstruction in the occasional patient with upper extremity edema or superior venal caval obstruction secondary to surgical dissection, radiation therapy or nodal metastases. Since most edema in surgically staged patients is a combination of lymphatic and venous occlusion, however, iodinated contrast injection into a hand or forearm vein, which is much more easily performed than lymphatic cannulation, is preferred [142].

When exact definition of the superior vena cava, its tributaries or collaterals, is desired, bilateral upper extremity injections or venous catheterization for superior and inferior cavography or azygography may be indicated. Venography demonstrates the venous morphology, possible compression,

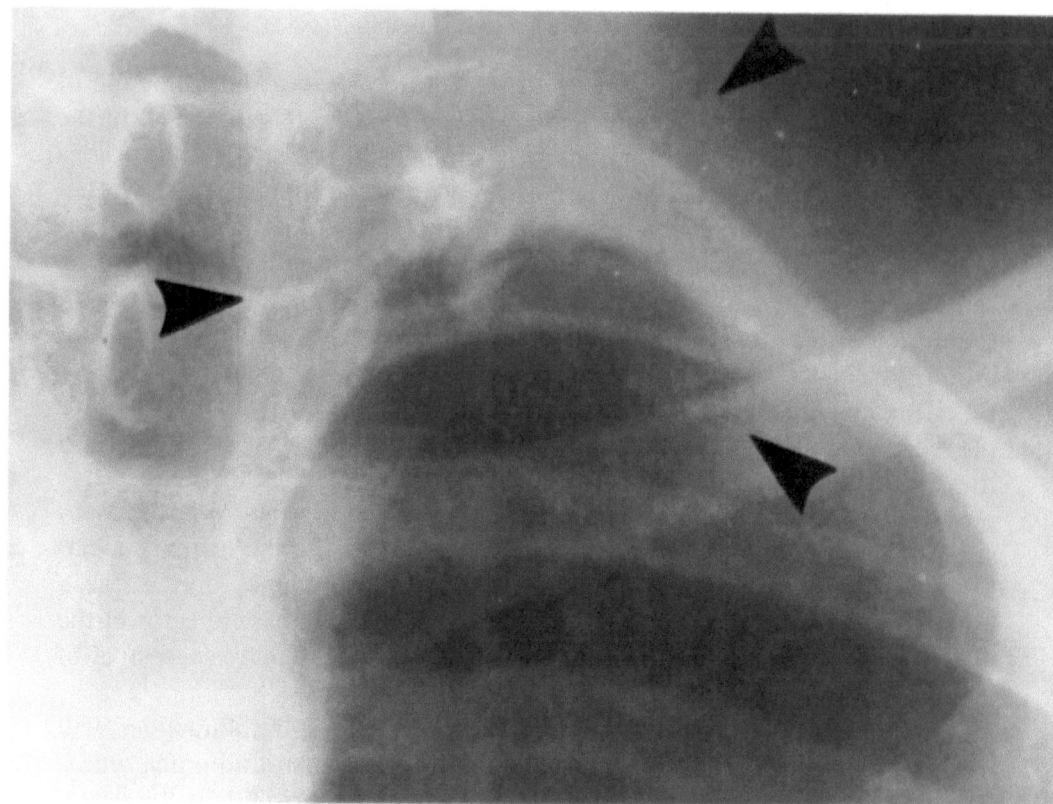

*Figure 18A.* Bipedal lymphangiography was performed in this young woman with locally advanced malignant melanoma to exclude distant disease prior to regional node dissection. Although pelvic and paraortic nodes were unremarkable, the nodal architecture in the left supraclavicular fossa is distorted, suggesting lymphadenopathy (arrows point to displaced, irregularly contoured nodes).

displacement or invasion and whether a thrombus is present. The exact histologic etiology of such venous occlusion may be determined by needle aspiration biopsy at the site of compression. Thin needle aspiration biopsy has proven to be of considerable value in evaluating superior vena caval syndromes secondary to mediastinal masses of various etiologies [109, 110].

The advent of chest CT has certainly complemented the more traditional approaches to mediastinal melanoma detection (plain films, conventional tomography, angiography) and has obviated the use of more experimental methods. One of these described in the literature involved opacification of the thoracic duct following surgical cannulation through a left supraclavicular fossa incision [47]. Water soluble and oily iodinated contrast material injected under high pressure allowed retrograde filling of the thoracic duct to the tenth or eleventh thoracic vertebral body in five of six patients, one of

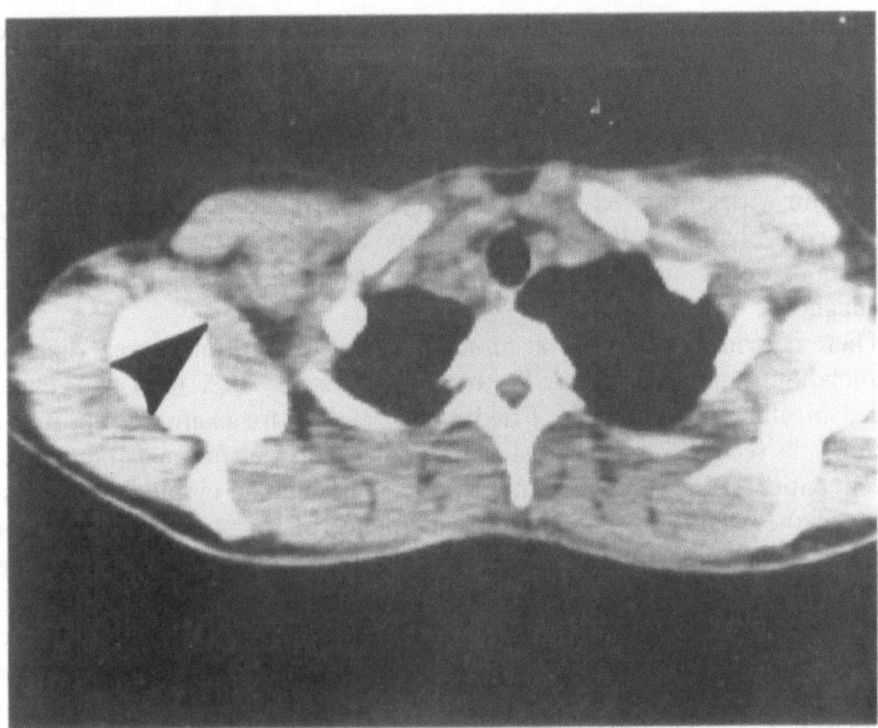

*Figure 18B.* CT and directed physical examination confirm the left supraclavicular mass.

whom had malignant melanoma. Despite the lack of serious complications of the procedure, it offered little diagnostic advantages, since no ductal pathologic processes were identified nor were lymph nodes visualized. It is known that bipedal contrast injections can opacify mediastinal, supraclavicular or axillary nodes either in normals or abnormals [10, 22]. Even though quite rare, one should be aware of the metastasis which can present on 24-hour chest follow-up films of such a bipedal lymphangiogram (Figure 18).

*Needle aspiration biopsy*

Any diagnostic modality may suffice in the occasional case to confirm the histopathologic presence of metastatic malignant melanoma to the chest. Thus, either rigid or flexible type bronchoscopy with endobronchial or transbronchial biopsy or brushing, thoracentesis, mediastinoscopy or even sputum cytology may yield a histologic diagnosis [135]. Short of open thoracotomy however, needle biopsy is the most effective means of obtaining tissue [51].

The method, precautions and contraindications of this procedure are adequately described in the literature [51]. The important distinction between thin needle aspiration for recovery of cytological material or small histological fragments and the use of large caliber cutting needles with their increased risk of complications has been emphasized [125]. Performance of aspiration with improved 22- to 18-gauge thin walled needles under fluoroscopic control and scrutiny of the recovered material by expert cytopathologists has made lesions throughout the chest safely accessible to this method of diagnosis.

There is evidence that the accuracy of needle aspiration biopsy diagnosis of melanoma metastases may be just as high as the 80% to 90+% experienced in other malignancies. Friedman et al. [42] for example reported on their 90/% recovery of diagnostic material in 74 melanoma patients. Only seven patients (9.5%) failed to provide a malignant cytologic diagnosis; three of these failed to show clinical evidence of malignancy in the lesion biopsied a year later. Air dried aspirates were obtained with 18-gauge needles and subjected to Wright-Giesma stains. Despite the wide diversity of cytologic patterns, with considerable variation in cell size, shape, nuclear changes, staining affinity and pigment distribution in the examined material, the authors felt that a high diagnostic success in malignant melanoma could be attributed to the recovery of rich cellular specimens. These were thought to be possible because of the nearly complete replacement of local tissue by tumor cells showing lack of cohesiveness and minimal necrotic change. The presence of melanin pigment was obviously the single most valuable morphologic marker. When not present, a differential diagnosis of multiple myeloma, soft tissue sarcoma or undifferentiated epithelial tumor was entertained, necessitating occasional electron microscopic studies or excisional biopsy. No complications were encountered in this series; however, no pulmonary biopsies were described.

The largest cytological series reporting high diagnostic accuracy of intrathoracic melanoma has come from evaluation of pleural effusions. Forty-three (78%) of the 55 specimens obtained from the pleural cavity in Hajdu and Savino's [50] series showed evidence of melanoma metastases. Bronchial spirates, on the other hand, allowed positive diagnosis in only 18% of their cases, while sputum cytology was diagnostic in 26% of 120 cases. In their description of the cytologic morphology, multinucleation was probably one of the more common findings as opposed to an almost total lack of intracellular cohesiveness and mitoses. All patients in the series died of their melanoma. The 17 showing positive pleural effusions lived an average of only three months following diagnosis, those with positive sputa lived five months.

A large series of percutaneous transthoracic needle aspiration biopsies of melanoma metastases has not yet been reported. In their significant mono-

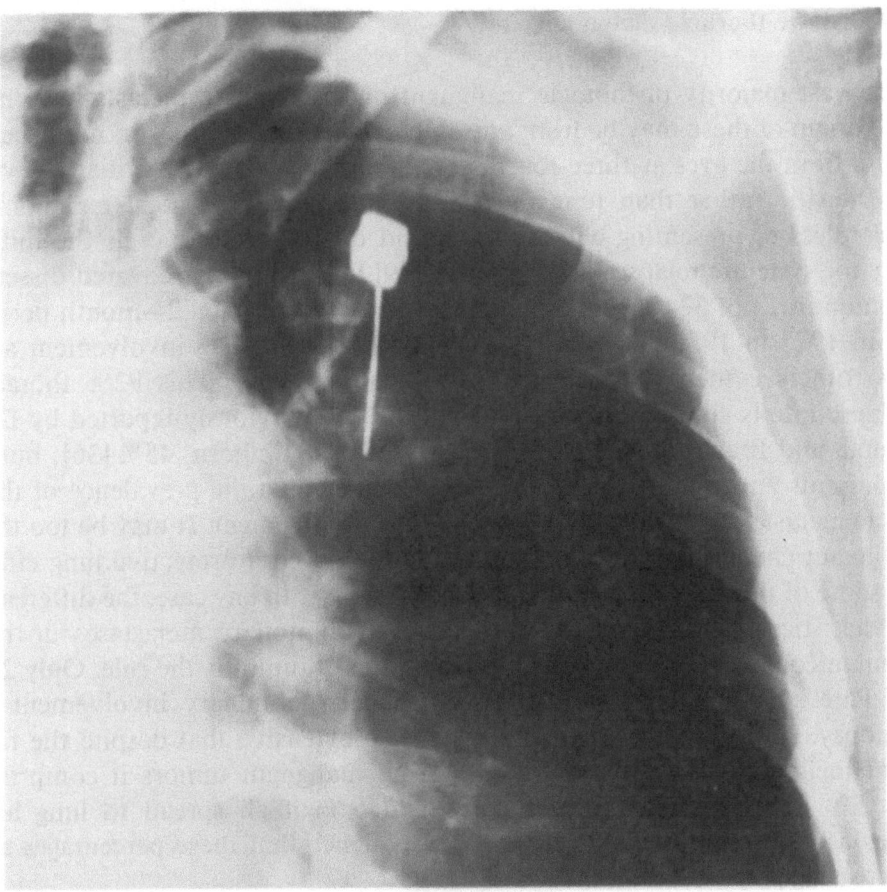

*Figure 19.* Percutaneous transthoracic needle aspiration biopsy to confirm suspected melanoma metastasis is performed as for any primary lung malignancy. Here a 22-gauge needle is aseptically passed into a left upper lobe nodular density from the preferred prone approach. The radiograph shows the needle tip within the lesion.

graph of 1966 Dahlgren and Nordenstrom [29] illustrate in situ electrocoagulation of a small left upper lobe melanoscarcoma metastasis following needle aspiration diagnosis. Interestingly, although the electrocoagulation procedure was an attempt to diminish possible tumor implantation along the needle track, it resulted in an apparent growth cessation of the metastasis during the patient's 13-month follow-up. Subsequent series have shown seeding of tumor cells from any malignancy to be vanishingly small following thin needle aspiration [125]. A case of melanoma implantation has yet to be reported to our knowledge.

Our personal experience with aspiration of intrathoracic metastatic melanoma is limited, although diagnostic material has been recovered in the few attempted (Figure 19). Our smears have been subjected to a modified rapid Papanicolaou method [51].

## Metastatic thoracic melanoma

The vast majority of thoracic malignant melanomas are metastatic. While the origin of these may be from any skin or visceral site, they do not usually arise from the eyes as three-fourths of all ocular melanomas initially develop hepatic rather than lung metastases [36]. Otherwise most melanomas regardless of presenting clinical stage tend toward the thorax as the initial site for systemic relapse. Gromet et al. [49] for example discovered dissemination in 13 of 324 melanoma patients followed during a 24-month period from 1975 to 1977. Ten of these 13 first presented lung involvement and two others evidenced mediastinal or pleural disease. This 92% thoracic relapse rate is considerably higher than the 7% previously reported by Das Gupta and Brasfield [31], Stehlin, 21% [132], or Einhorn, 45% [36], but it represents an initial incidence of relapse rather than the prevalence of thoracic metastases in those with other sites of involvement. It may be too that adjuvant chemotherapy or immunotherapy exerted a protective lung effect in some of those series as has been suggested [49]. In any case, the difference in statistics points to the observation that pulmonary metastases do not remain confined for long. True dissemination of tumor is the rule. Only 2% of Patel's [100] 216 patients showed isolated pulmonary involvement at autopsy. This degree of dissemination is so extensive that despite the fact that melanoma constitutes only 1% of all malignant tumors it comprises 5–15% of all pulmonary metastases and 5% of all spread to lung and mediastinum combined. There is even evidence that these percentages are increasing [17].

There is also evidence that the incidence of intrathoracic spread or the rapidity of metastasis to all stages may be related to initial tumor location [94]. Lesions of the head and neck for example consistently metastasize more rapidly than do extremity lesions [94]. Such metastases may likewise depend on primary tumor extent. Since it has been shown that overall mortality is directly related to Clark level of invason or Breslow tumor thickness [23, 63, 85] and cardiopulmonary metastases account for most deaths, one would postulate, therefore, a direct proportionality between extent of thoracic metastasis and microinvasion of the primary tumor. In actuality however the biologic behavior is unpredictable. Thoracic melanoma manifestations have been noted to vary with age, sex, heredity, geography, nationality, primary site, endocrine and immune status [1, 33, 99, 118]. They may also appear at any time after diagnosis, a case with metastatic changes 32 years after initial surgery having been reported [52]. The protean roentgenographic presentations of this fascinating tumor as influenced by these factors comprise the remainder of this chapter.

## Pulmonary parenchyma

Radiographic manifestations of metastatic thoracic melanoma are legion [82]. The most common presentation parallels that of metastases in general, consisting of one or more well-defined nodular lung masses with diameters of 3 mm to 6 cm or larger [40]. When multiple they are rarely the same size, reflecting their diversity of time of origin from the parent tumor and the growth milieu in which they come to rest (Figure 20). Lobulation, which also implies differential growth, (within parts of the lesion rather than in parts of the lung), is unusual. Only three of the 26 solitary nodules reviewed by Dahmash et al. [30] at Duke were not round or oval. One of these was umbilicated, one was fusiform, and the third was tear-drop shaped. Also, of those 26 lesions only one was not sharply demarcated (Figure 21). The same was true of multiple lesions which outnumber solitary

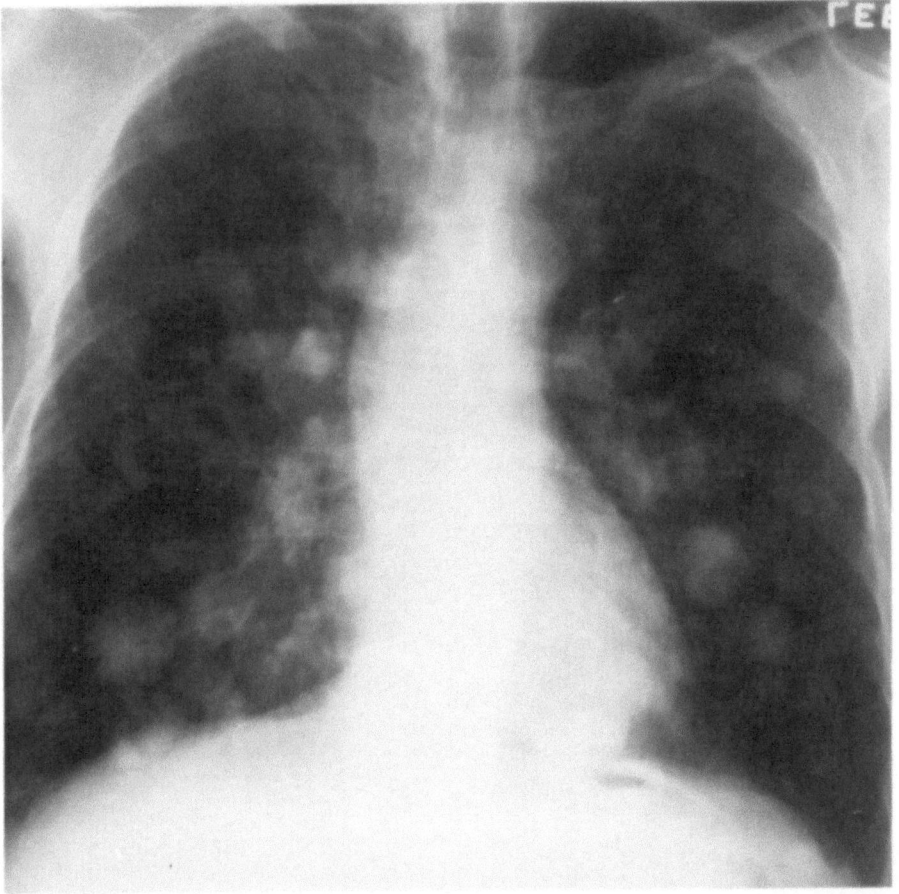

*Figure 20.* The PA chest view in this 61-year-old man obtained one month prior to his death from malignant melanoma shows the wide variation in diameter of the observable metastases, which range from a few millimeters to nearly four centimeters.

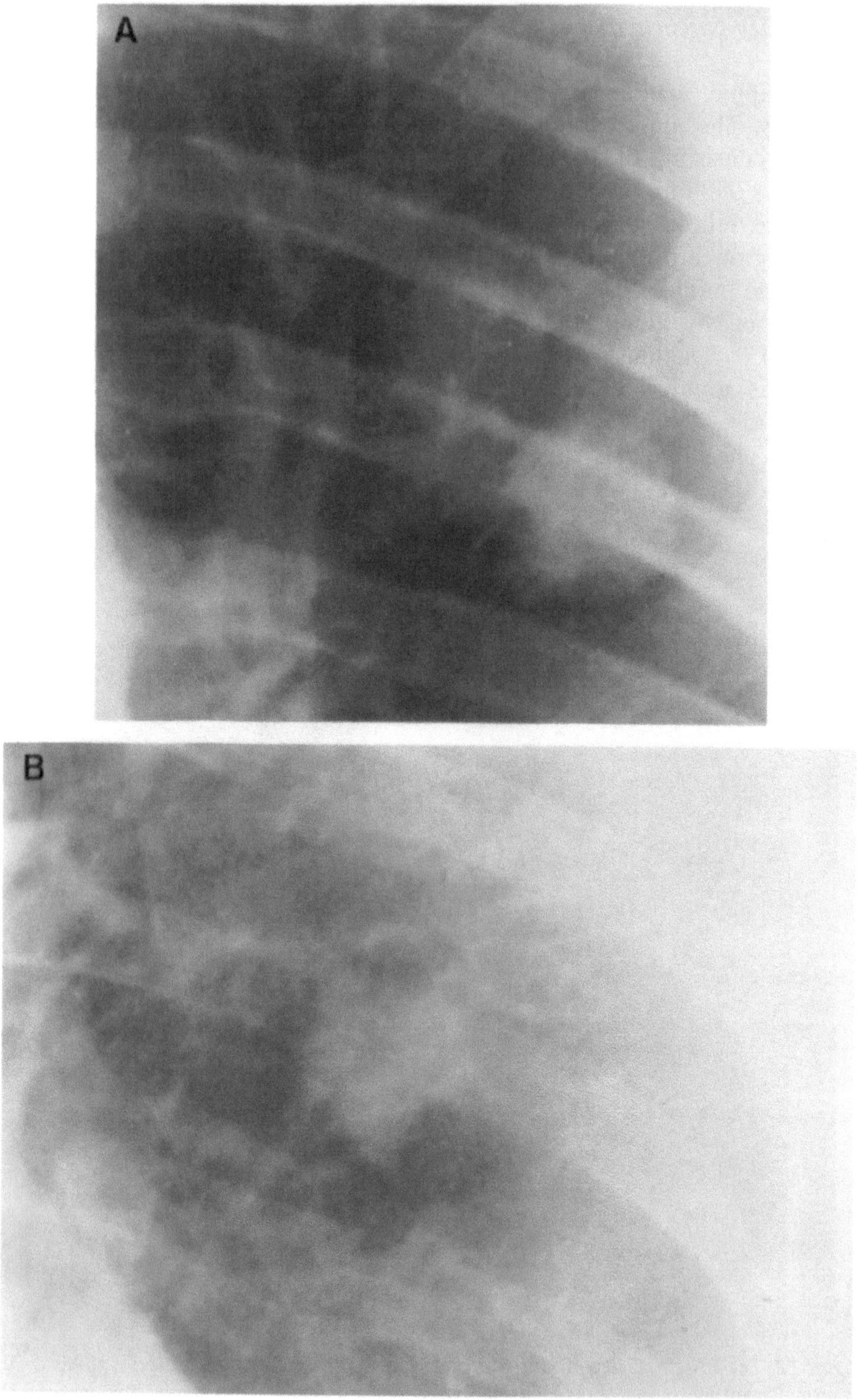

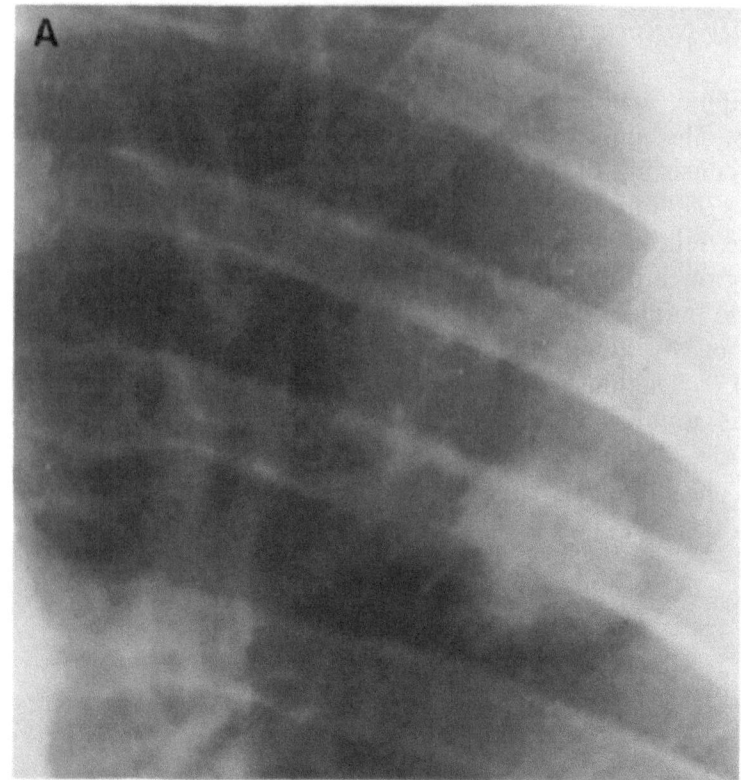

*Figures 21A, B.*

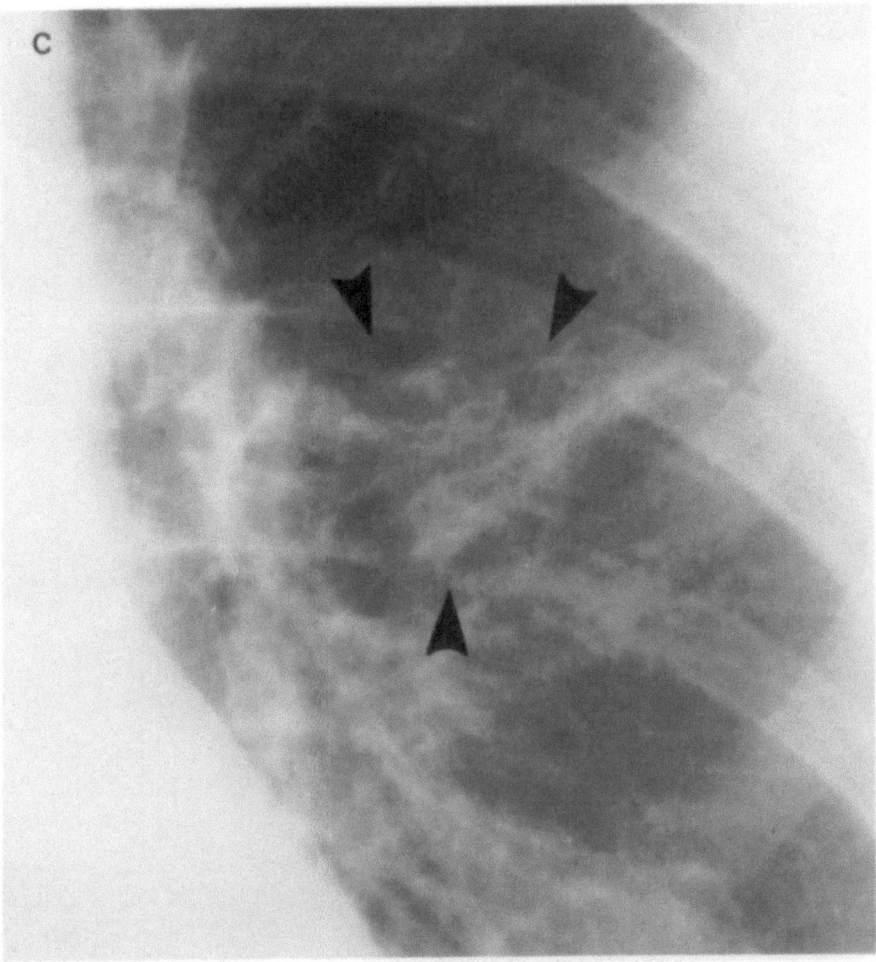

*Figure 21*. Coned views of PA chest films illustrate the typical and distinctly atypical appearances of several left midlung zone melanoma metastases; all measuring approximately 2 cm in diameter. (A, facing page) Two well-demarcated round nodules. (B, facing page) A solitary comet-shaped nodule with its tail pointing down. (C) An indistinct density of proven melanoma (outlined by arrow-heads).

nodules by 2 or 3 to 1 [30, 145]. Both solitary and multiple nodules tend toward an even distribution throughout the lung fields, from side to side and top to bottom [30]. Unilateral lung involvement however is not uncommon (Figure 22). Neifeld et al. [95] noted melanoma metastases limited to one lung on plain radiographs in seven of 19 patients, and in five unilateral disease was tomographically confirmed. Surgical confirmation was obtained in three of four patients manifesting a solitary nodule on both conventional studies. According to Webb's UCSF series [144, 145], 22 of 57 radiographically visible metastases had unilateral involvement.

Prognosis based on uniqueness or multiplicity of nodules varies in the

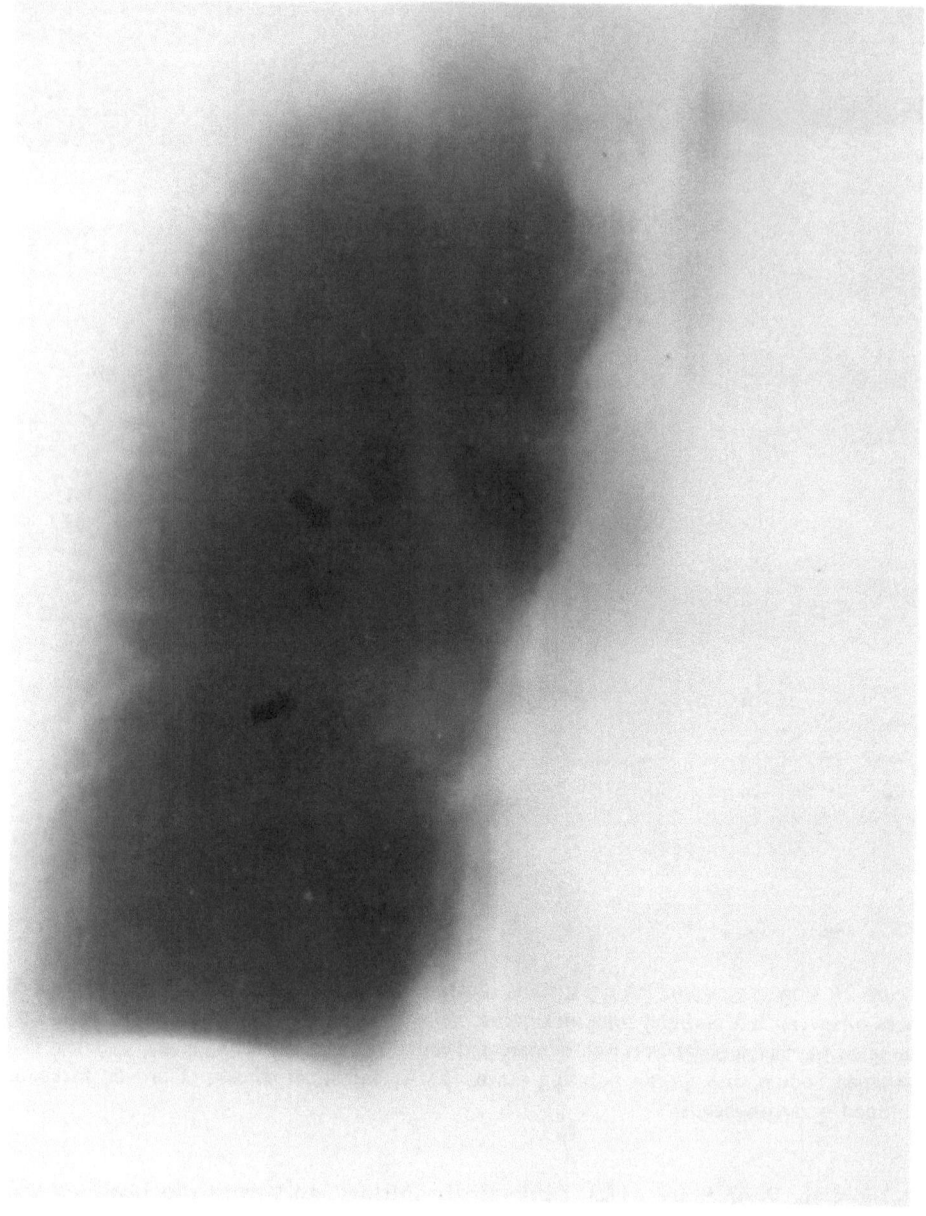

*Figure 22A.* This tomographic section shows the right perihilar mass (double arrows) of this 53-year-old man which was his only site of known malignant melanoma metastasis.

literature. Whereas survival after lesion detection averaged nine months and seven months for solitary or multiple nodules respectively in the UCSF series, in the Duke series a significant difference of 51 months for solitary and 31 months for multiple nodules was observed. Both series agree however in decrying the uniformly dismal outlook of those patients who mani-

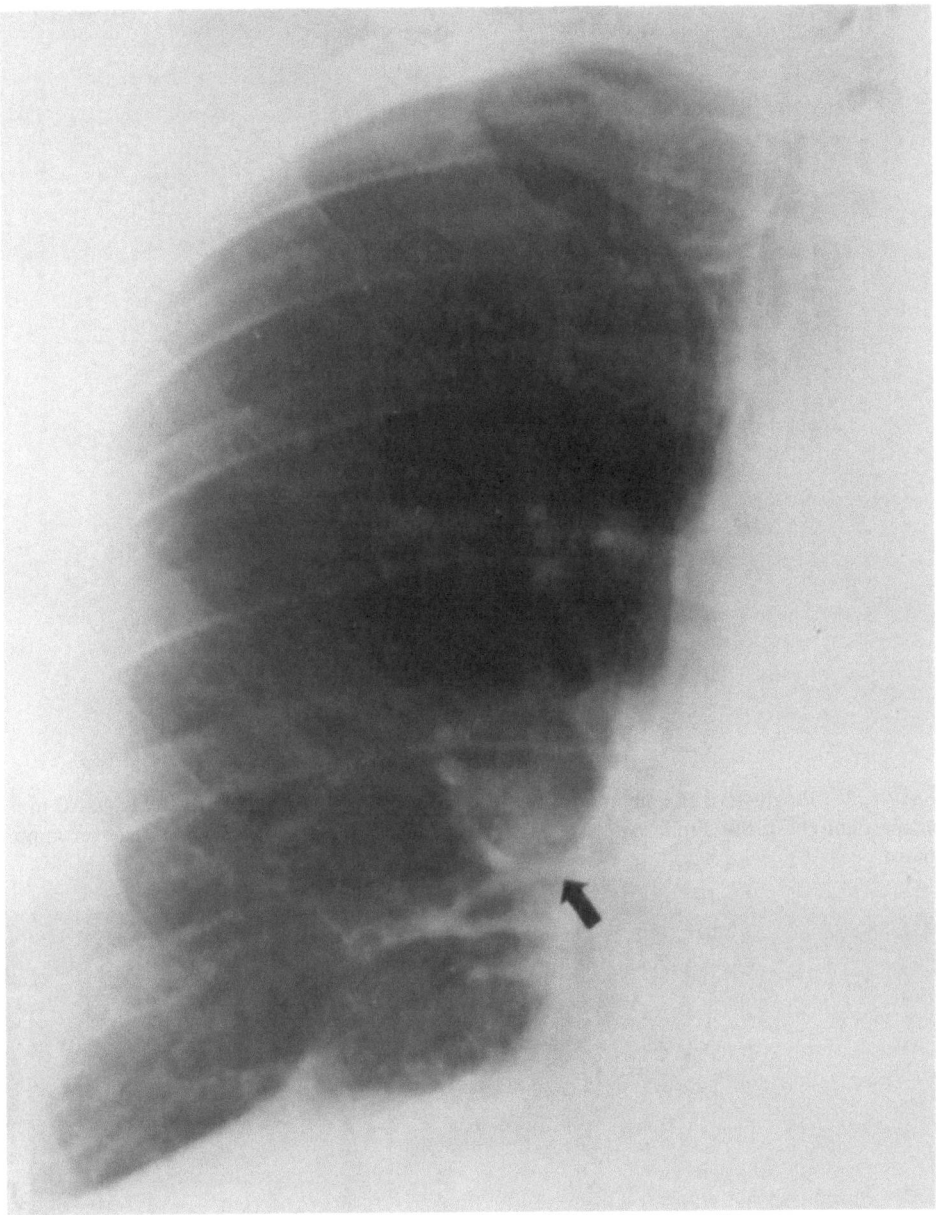

*Figure 22B.* Despite wedge resection of the mass, local recurrence was evident within four months (single arrow medial to surgical staples).

fest innumerable miliary (or snowstorm) metastases. Eight patients from UCSF and two from Duke died within an average span of five weeks to two months respectively, following the appearance of this pattern. Too few cases have been described to clearly separate the lymphangitic type appearance from this prognosis (Figure 23).

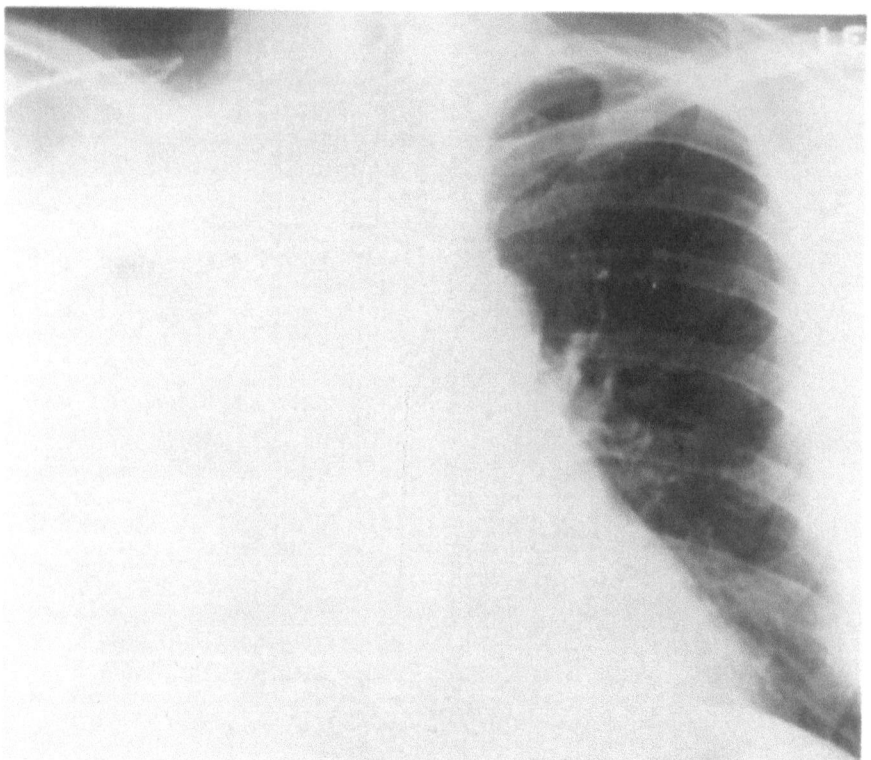

*Figure 22C.* Progressive enlargement of the locally recurrent metastasis gradually engulfed most of the right chest, but similar metastases to the left lung and pleural space were never appreciated.

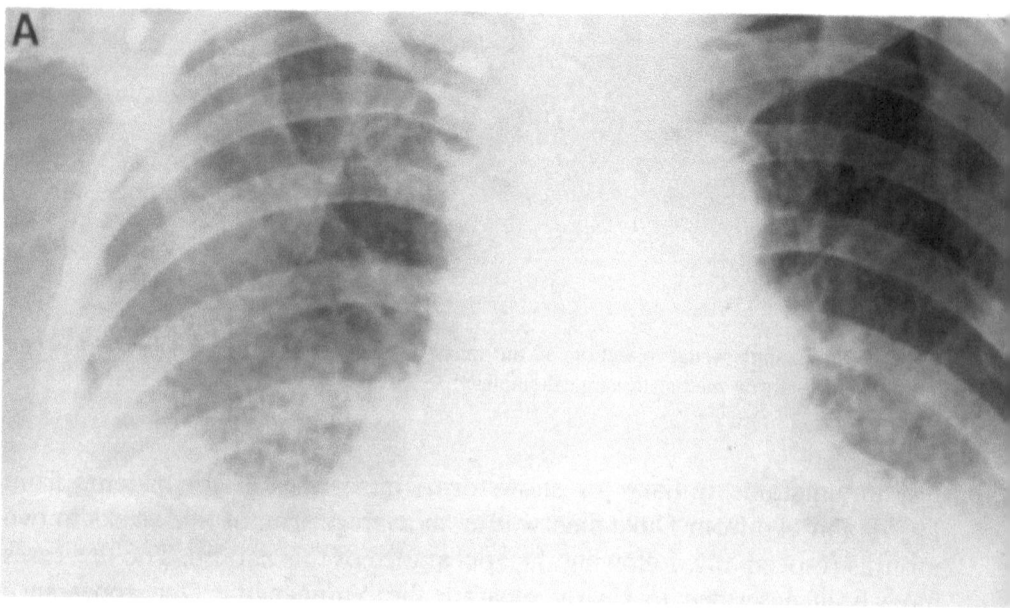

*Figure 23A.*

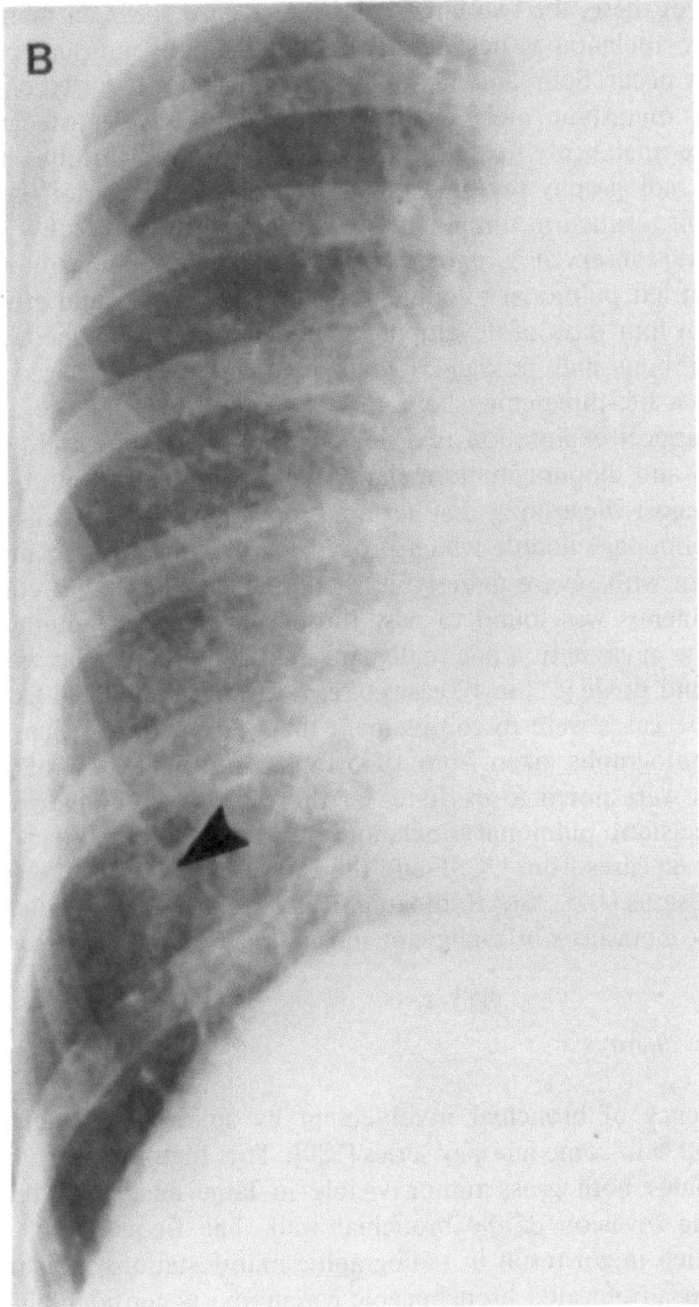

*Figure 23B.* AP (Figure A, bottom facing page) and oblique (Figure B) views of this 68-year-old woman with autopsy-proven pulmonary malignant melanoma show an ill-defined linear density pattern with Kerley's B lines (arrowhead points to the costophrenic angle where they are most apparent) characteristic of the lymphangitic tumor seen with certain tumors.

Neither of these, the two largest series to record roentgen manifestations of thoracic melanoma, has described the distinctly unusual phenomena which may occur. Sethi and Saxton [117] for instance reported on two cases of solitary metastatic melanoma associated with severe osteoarthropathy which were mistakenly treated for several months as arthridites before routine chest radiography revealed metastatic foci. Resection of the tumor in each patient resulted in immediate cessation of the arthropathy. Teung and Bonnet [149] observed a patient with widespread malignant melanoma, including a left pulmonary nodule and moderate left pleural effusion, who died within four days of developing a moderate left spontaneous pneumothorax. Gibbons and Devig [45] then described a middle-aged man who developed a life-threatening hemothorax as his first evidence of systemic relapse. Surgical exploration revealed blood oozing from multiple pleural, pericardial and diaphragmatic melanoma implants. Lahiri et al. [150] published a report illustrating distinct air bronchograms traversing a circumscribed pulmonary nodule which proved to be malignant melanoma in an elderly man with severe underlying rheumatoid arthritis. On cut section a patent bronchus was found to pass through the excised nodule. Finally a solitary case of cavitation in a malignant melanoma metastasis was collected by Dodd and Boyle [35] in 12 cases of cavitation accumulated from 1957 to 1961. These cases were to complement their earlier comprehensive review of chest radiographs taken from 1955 to 1957 in which 4% of pulmonary metastases were noted to cavitate. Of those 6729 earlier patients, 30 displayed metastatic pulmonary melanoma but none were cavitary. Likewise, among the 65 cases from UCSF and the 130 cases from Duke, there were no cavitary lesions [145, 30]. Radiographically identifiable calcification in a pulmonary metastasis of malignant melanoma is yet to be described.

*Pulmonary airways*

The frequency of bronchial involvement by solid tumor metastases approaches 50% in some autopsy series [109]. This high incidence of involvement includes both gross tumor visible in large and small bronchi and microscopic invasion of the bronchial wall. The frequency of metastatic disease which might result in radiographic manifestations indistinguishable from a centrally located bronchogenic carcinoma is considerably less. This was placed at 2% in a retrospective review of 1359 autopsies at Walter Reed General Hospital [15], 21 of which involved melanoma patients. It was thought to represent approximately 5% of the cases described by King and Castleman [62]. One of their 11 cases displayed "melanosarcoma" thought to arise from the meninges. This tumor presented as a 4 mm nodule protruding into the lumen of a bronchus 9 mm in diameter.

Metastatic melanoma may involve a bronchus in three ways: 1) by direct metastasis to the bronchial wall, 2) by invasion from a pulmonary parenchymal metastasis and 3) by direct extension from a mediastinal lesion [114]. All three are usually late manifestations, since even in hematogenous spread to the bronchus, hilar or mediastinal lymphadenopathy is frequently present at postmortem examination. This necessitates a careful search for such nodal metastases before definitive resection of the bronchus is attempted.

Radiologic as well as clinical symptoms of patients with melanoma which involve bronchi simulate those with bronchogenic carcinoma. Cough, hemoptysis and, less frequently, shortness of breath and wheezing, lead to the radiologic examination. This in itself may be quite variable. Segmental, lobar or whole lung atelectasis is the most commonly observed finding on plain chest films (Figure 24). In Webb and Gamsu's series [145] eight of 65 patients showed segmental or lobal atelectasis. Five of these demonstrated ipsilateral hilar lymph node enlargement, while visible bronchial narrowing was present in two. One of those showing radiographic atelectasis was found to have a bronchial metastasis at autopsy. In another a fungating intratracheal mass measuring 1 cm in diameter was discovered just above the carina. Occasionally the lesion may be so small that bronchography or bronchoscopy, or even sputum cytology [106] may be the only means of implicating an otherwise negative chest film. Bronchoscopy with biopsy is certainly the most reliable means of obtaining histological verification of a suspected endobronchial metastasis. An unusual case showing the palliative utility of repeated bronchoscopic resections of endobronchial melanoma producing whole lung collapse has been published [24]. Another case showing diffuse melanosis of the airways diagnosed bronchoscopically has been reported [135]. Postbronchoscopy expectoration of a melanoma mass has even occurred [135].

As the endobronchial metastasis enlarges, it may engulf bronchial cartilages and invade pulmonary parenchyma creating a visible plain film mass, usually in hilar areas. Or it may produce a dumbbell-shaped mass by growth between cartilaginous rings [114]. The subepithelial location of some melanomas within bronchi also allows distal bronchiectasis when obstruction is incomplete; or distal pneumonia or air entrapment when relatively more complete. Such a case of air trapping involving a right middle and lower lobe was shown by Fraser and Pare [40]. In their thinking malignant melanoma shows an unusual propensity for metastasis to bronchial walls.

It is important to realize that a bronchial malignancy in a patient with melanoma may be either a metastasis or a second primary tumor originating in the lung. Histologically different primary cancers have been observed in 7.4% of the 216 autopsies performed on melanoma patients from Roswell Park [100]. This concurs with the incidence of approximately 6%

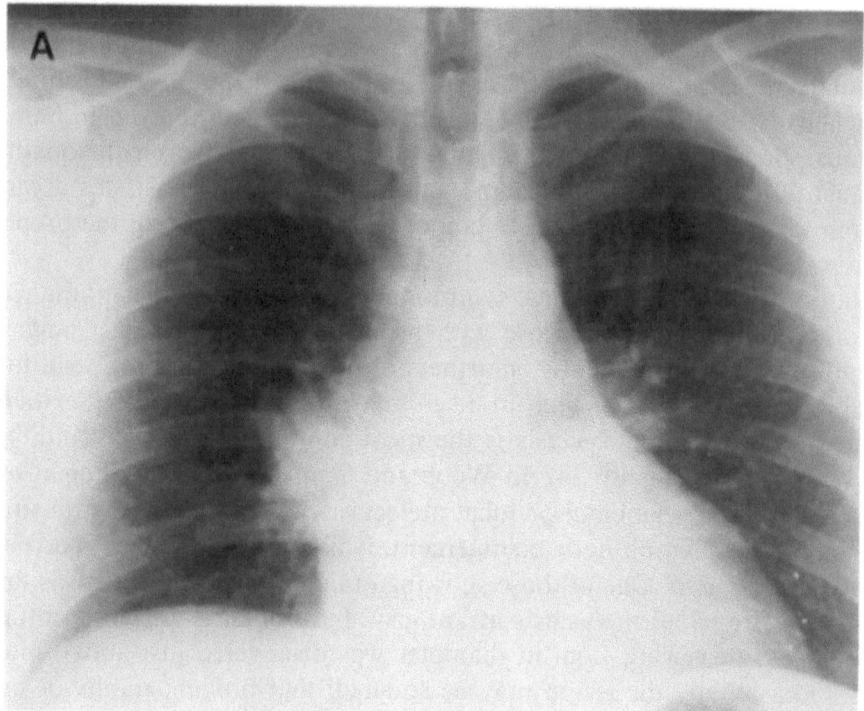

*Figure 24.* Although occasionally due to endobronchial metastases, most major atelectasis on melanoma chest films is due to extrinsic compression by lymphadenopathy. Figure A shows modest bilateral hilar and mediastinal lymph node enlargement without volume loss in a 45-year-old man. Figure B (next page) obtained four months later shows marked interval growth of the hilar masses and resultant right lower lobe atelectasis (open arrows).

(range 2.7–10.6%) gathered from the literature by Baldwin and Wisner [9] and that reported by Budman et al. [17]. Updates during the last decade suggest that this incidence is increasing, the reason probably being multifactorial. When a lung cancer is involved it usually follows the diagnosis of the associated malignancy [107]. There are exceptions such as in the 14-year-old girl who developed a posterior thoracic wall melanoma 13 years following encleation for a retinoblastoma [137]. Five reported melanoma patients who subsequently developed bronchogenic carcinomas 1, 1, 9, 10, and 12 years later show this trend [19]. At least two patients described in the literature developed synchronous primaries, the lung cancer being discovered on preoperative evaluation of the melanoma [19]. One of these showed anaplastic epidermoid carcinoma and the other adenocarcinoma. Interestingly two others were oat cell carcinomas [107]. A natural association of oat cell carcinoma and melanoma has been suggested on the basis of their similar embryologic origin as manifested in the multiple-endocrine-adenomatosis syndromes [96, 127].

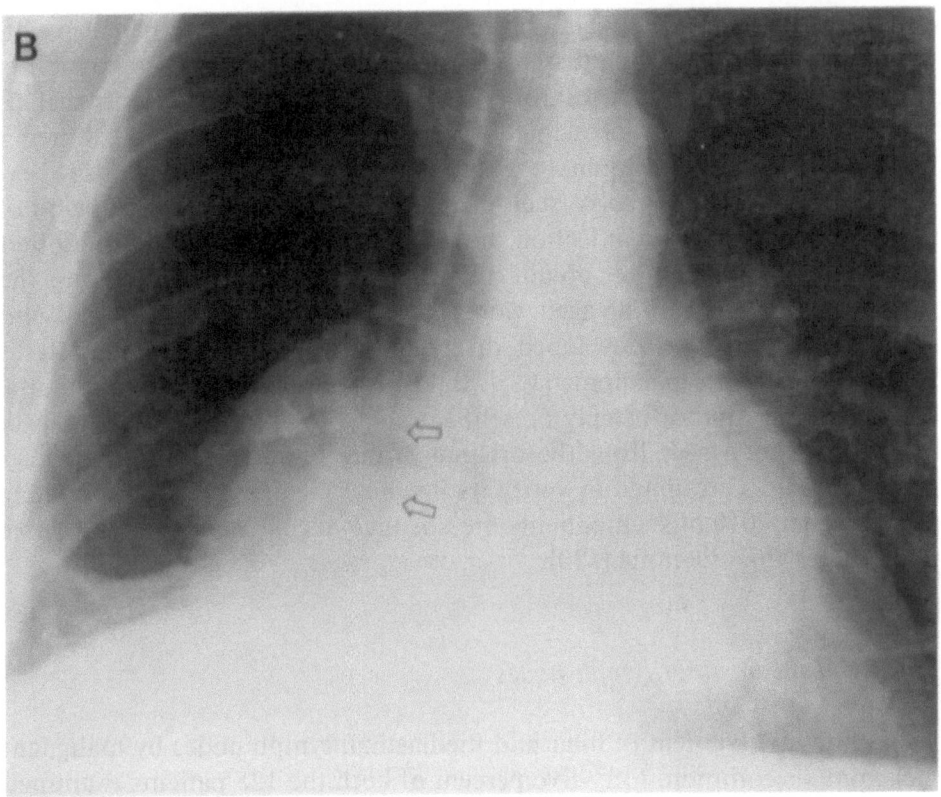

*Figure 24B.*

An association of a malignant melanoma and chronic lymphocytic leukemia (CLL) has also been noted [48]. Of 4869 patients with CLL, second primaries subsequently appeared in 234. Besides lung cancer and soft-tissue sarcomas, the risk was significantly elevated for malignant melanoma. Among those with untreated CLL, a three-fold increase of melanoma was found. In view of the proclivity of both diseases to form roentgenographically observable thoracic lymphadenopathy, this association is important. Ipsilateral intrathoracic lymphadenopathy associated with a solitary lung nodule is likewise typical of bronchogenic carcinoma but can certainly be seen with melanoma as evidenced by the three cases of Webb and Gamsu [145].

When lung nodules are multiple and unilateral, it has been suggested that ipsilateral thoracic lymph node enlargement should bring an infectious process such as tuberculosis or fungal pneumonia to mind [144]. At least two surveys, however, have indicated the rarity with which melanoma patients are afflicted with active tuberculosis, suggesting the possibility of an immunological cross-reactivity between tubercle bacilli and melanoma cells. Only one of all patients (179) treated at the National Cancer Institute (NCI) and none of 2131 melanoma patients at risk at another larger cancer center contracted active TB [98]. That one NCI patient developed apparent reactivation of old TB following dissemination of his melanoma. The possibility of pulmonary abnormality resulting from various therapeutic agents such as the infiltrative process occasionally seen with BCG (Bacillus Calmette-Guerin) and its methanol extraction residue (MER) also exists [73, 129, 141]. To resolve such diagnostic dilemmas as the suspicion of a second malignancy or infection, needle aspiration biopsy or some other diagnostic mechanism to obtain tissue may be needed. Such was the reported case of a middle-aged woman with preexisting endometrial and colon carcinoma who developed discrete nodular pulmonary metastases from her malignant melanoma [135]. Baldwin and Wisner [9] stress that the second primary tumor usually presents at about the time one would expect to uncover metastases from the original primary and, unless further diagnostic measures are made to verify its histology, it may be inappropriately treated. That 70% of such patients died of their second cancer in one series underscores this dilemma [130].

*Hilar and mediastinal lymph nodes*

Metastatic involvement of hilar and mediastinal lymph nodes by malignant melanoma is common. Fifty-five percent of both the 125 patients examined at autopsy by Das Gupta and Brasfield [31] and the 216 patients reviewed by Patel et al. [100] evidenced intrathoracic lymphadenopathy. A similar percentage was found radiographically by Webb and Gamsu [145] in 65 patients with known (31 autopsies) or clinically suspected (34 cases) hilar and mediastinal melanoma. The strong correlation of lung metastases and nodal metastases was shown, since only three of those 65 had isolated lymphadenopathy. Similar statistics were seen in other series where two patients out of 52 [76] and nine of 130 [30] (Figure 25) showed radiographic lymph node enlargement without pleural or parenchymal disease. Of course all of these studies are subject to the foibles of plain chest film diagnosis, as previously discussed. Despite these limitations a synopsis of obvious radiographic lymph node melanoma is instructive.

Hilar lymphadenopathy is larger and more frequently seen than mediastinal lymph node enlargement. Mediastinal lymphadenopathy involving either azygous, ductus or paratracheal nodes can occur singly but is uncommon without concommitant hilar involvement (Figure 26). Two-thirds of patients display unilateral lymph node enlargement. Bilateral enlargement may be symmetric [44] or asymmetric [30] (Figure 24). Symmetrical adenopathy mimicking sarcoidosis occurred in two of 30 Duke patients and five of 28 UCSF patients. Subcarinal or posterior mediastinal lymphadenopathy is uncommon; isolated anterior mediastinal involvement is rare. Every

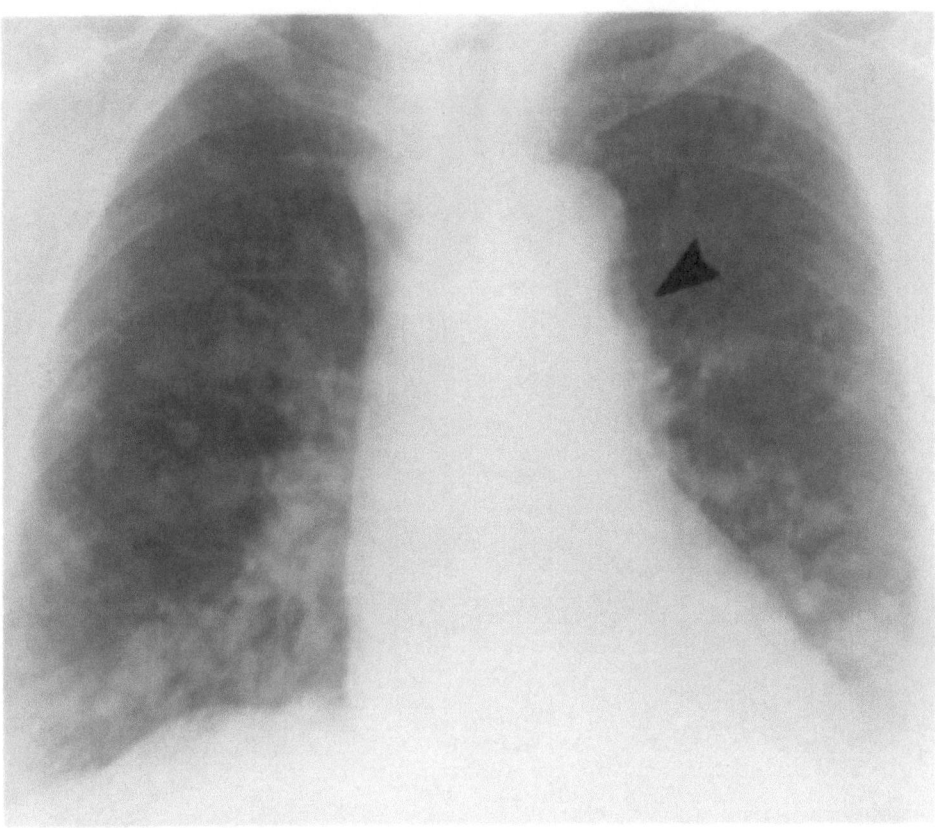

*Figure 25.* The typical association of pulmonary parenchymal and nodal melanoma metastases is shown in the PA chest film of this 66-year-old woman who displays bilateral paratracheal, ductus (arrowhead) and right hilar lymphadenopathy.

combination of metastatic adenopathy and pulmonary nodule(s) has occurred except for their simultaneous appearance in contralateral chest cavities. The same may be said for pleural effusions appearing with adenopathy.

In all probability two mechanisms allowing malignant cells into thoracic lymph nodes are operant in melanoma: direct and indirect. Direct lymphatic spread such as might result from capture of melanoma cells by the lymph system would involve the predictable progression of tumor up through existing lymphatics into the thoracic duct. Once cells from the head, arms or lower body approached the thoracic duct, they might reflux into bronchopulmonary or mediastinal lymph nodes due to lymphatic valvular incompetence. They might even pass to these nodes via existing aberrant or antegrade intercommunications [10]. One argument for this direct seeding of intrathoracic nodes is the finding by Webb [144] that hilar and mediastinal lymphadenopathy was more often than not preceded by regional metastases, which had appeared months to years earlier.

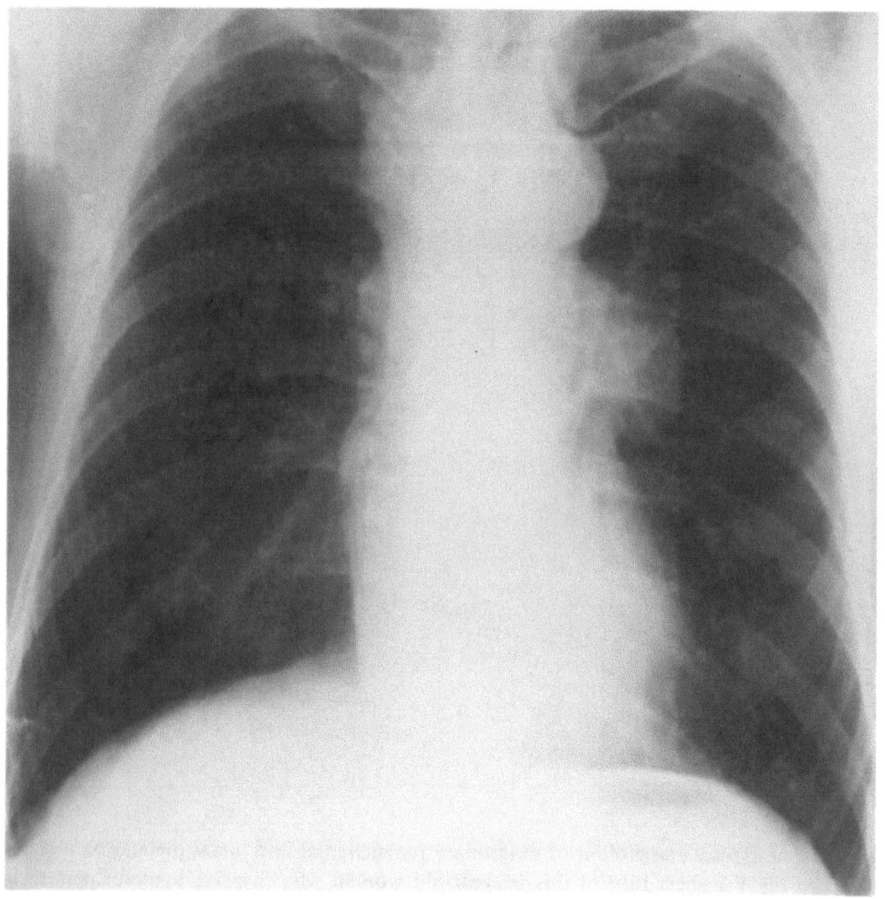

*Figure 26.* This 53-year-old man without demonstrable pulmonary parenchymal nodules manifests metastases to the right paratracheal and left hilar lymph nodes.

Good arguments likewise exist for an indirect or secondary route of melanoma spread to intrathoracic nodes once metastases have been hematogenously implanted in the lung. Certainly the natural history of lymphatic spread of bronchogenic carcinoma has set this precedent. The percentage of known hematogenous pulmonary metastases coincides favorably with known lymphadenopathy. Furthermore tumor invasion of pulmonary lymphatics occurred in one third of the autopsied patients with node metastases in Webb's series [144] and was recognized in at least nine of 29 patients in Cahan's [19]. Occurrence of this indirect route of node metastasis would also help explain the association of lymphadenopathy and pulmonary nodules and the large intrathoracic nodal metastases occasionally seen in the absence of extrathoracic adenopathy.

*Mediastinum*

That mediastinal involvement by metastatic melanoma is common has been shown by the frequency of late mediastinal lymphadenopathy already discussed. Direct extension into organs surrounding these lymph nodes (e.g., superior vena caval obstruction) or direct hematogenous metastasis to those organs is considerably less common. We could find only one description of secondary melanoma to the thymus for instance [31] as opposed to the high incidence of thyroid metastases [5]. When thymic metastases from other carcinomas occur, as they did in 7% of Middleton's 102 cases [84], they are almost always the expression of generalized disease. As such, they are more likely to be found at autopsy than surgically. A primary thymic melanoma has not been documented. Esophageal melanomas are described elsewhere (see Chapter 5).

*Heart and pericardium*

Secondary neoplasms of the heart and pericardium are 20 to 40 times more common than primary cardiac tumors, having been reported in 1–5% of all autopsies and in 10–25% of patients succumbing to malignancy [12, 14, 64]. In absolute numbers lung and breast carcinoma lead that list of metastases. In total percentage of cardiac involvement, however, malignant melanoma predominates [12]. Glancy and Roberts [44] of the National Heart Institute (NHI) found 64% of their 70 autopsy cases to contain melanoma. Others have reported the incidence of heart involvement from 40% to 55% and of pericardial involvement from 10% to 24% [65]. Subdividing the NHI series one finds 73% of the cardiac metastases affecting the endocardium, 78% involving the epicardium and 98%, or 44 of the 45 patients, having myocardial metastases. Tumor invasion was usually nodular rather than interstitial; therefore few, if any, myocardial fibers remained within most of the larger nodules. Extension through the entire wall of one or more cardiac chambers, usually on the right, occurred in a third of the cases. The most common pathway for initial tumor to reach the heart, however, is not by direct extension but rather appears to be either by retrograde extension of mediastinal metastases through subepicardial lymphatic vessels [64] or hematogenous spread from distant sites [126]. This tendency toward formation of nodules in melanoma is probably what allows the high diagnostic accuracy of echocardiography, cardiac catheterization and angiocardiography, which approach 100% detection [14]. An antemortem diagnosis of the extremely rare valvular metastasis, however, is yet to be made. The NHI series described two such cases involving the tricuspid valve and Thomas et al. [139] added another which had produced tricuspid stenosis. A fourth was

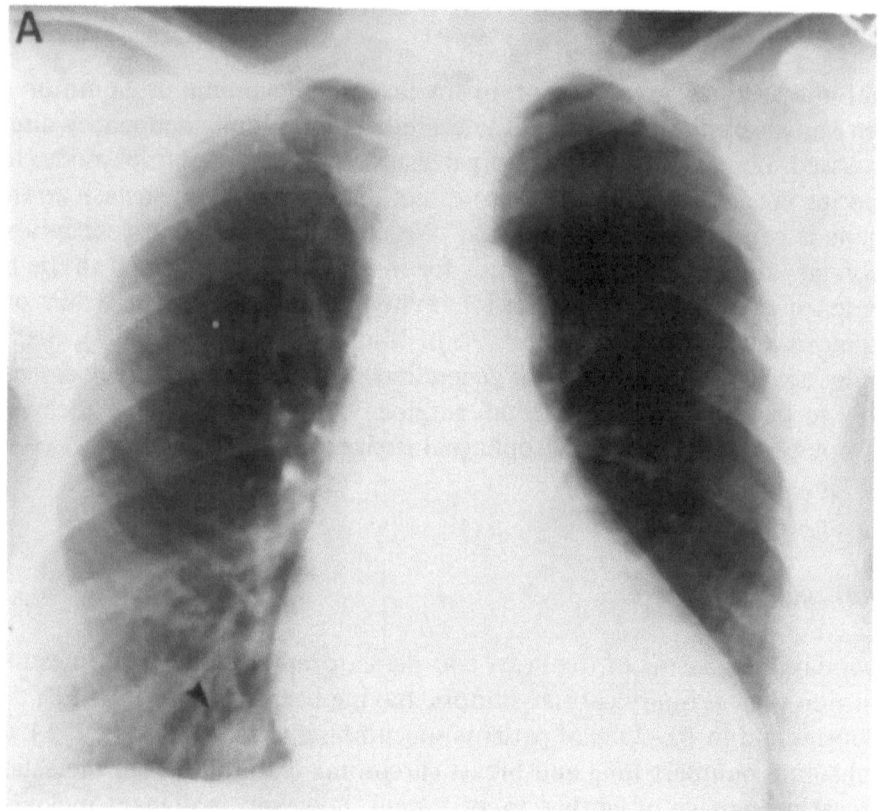

*Figure 27A.* Initial PA (A) and lateral (B, next page) chest views of this 74-year-old woman with cutaneous malignant melanoma disclosed an enlarged cardiac silhouette as well as a right lower lobe pulmonary metastasis (arrowhead). Her age, clinical course and radiographic follow-up suggested an atherosclerotic basis for the cardiomegaly.

reported by Bryant and Vuckovic [18] which caused inflow obstruction of the right heart resulting in a murmur, conduction abnormalities and chronic congestive heart failure.

In the NHI cases, the gross extent of cardiac involvement was divided into three equal categories: slight, moderate or extensive. On the average, patients with extensive tumor had larger hearts, which could be reflected roentgenographically. The nonspecificity of chest film cardiomegaly, however, has been underscored by the postmortem finding of concomitant atherosclerotic myocardial disease and melanoma metastases [145] (Figure 27). Despite this nonspecificity and its infrequency of appearance, rapid cardiac enlargement has been reported as the most significant radiologic sign of melanoma metastasis to the heart [14] and the most ominous [64]. Based on

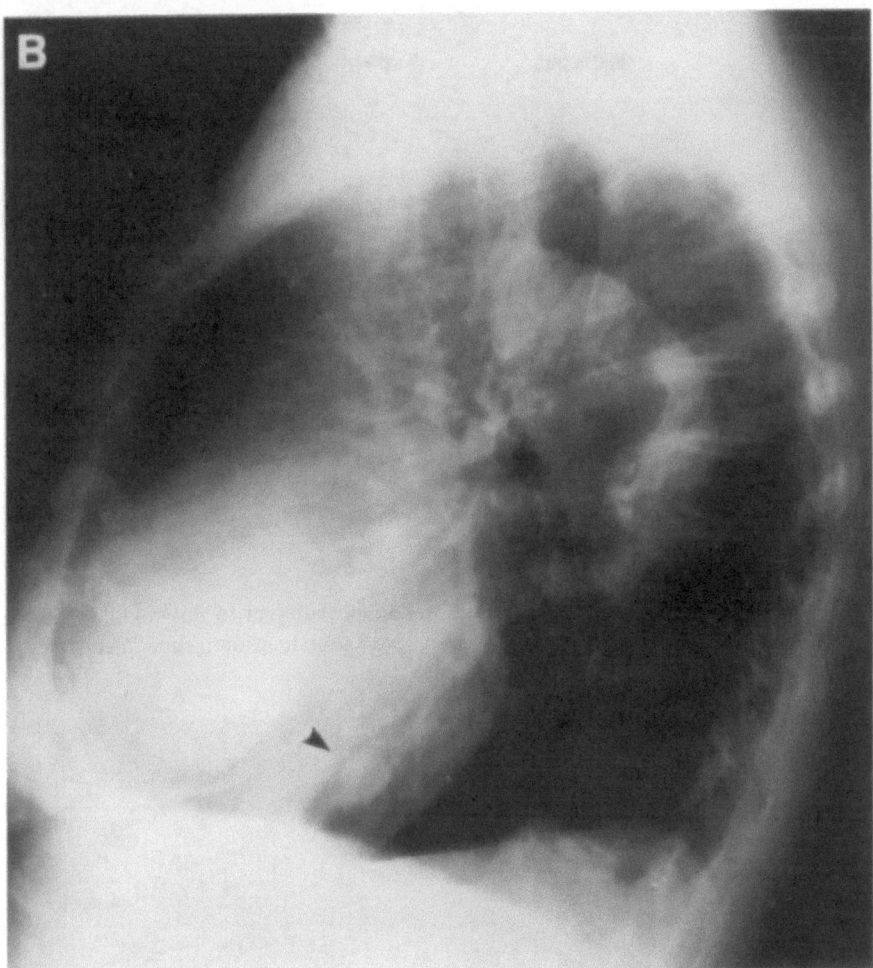

*Figure 27B.*

their data Glancy and Roberts [44] also list one or more of the following as strongly suggestive: 1) acute pericarditis, 2) cardiac constriction or tamponade, 3) onset of ectopic tachycardia, 4) development of second- or third-degree atrioventricular block and 5) onset of definite cardiac failure. Since these may be a manifestation of other organ failure produced by the tumor's propensity to metastasize widely before causing death, they are likewise nonspecific. Melanoma metastases to other organs almost always accompany heart metastases. Remarkably 80% of 62 Memorial patients [31] with cardiac metastases also had multiple cutaneous and subcutaneous metastases. Therefore despite a high frequency of myocardial involvement by melanoma, the clinical import is usually small [146].

Detection of pericardial effusion, especially tamponade, is of clinical importance however. Most cases with significant cardiac metastatic impairment have pericardial involvement with resultant effusion and tamponade.

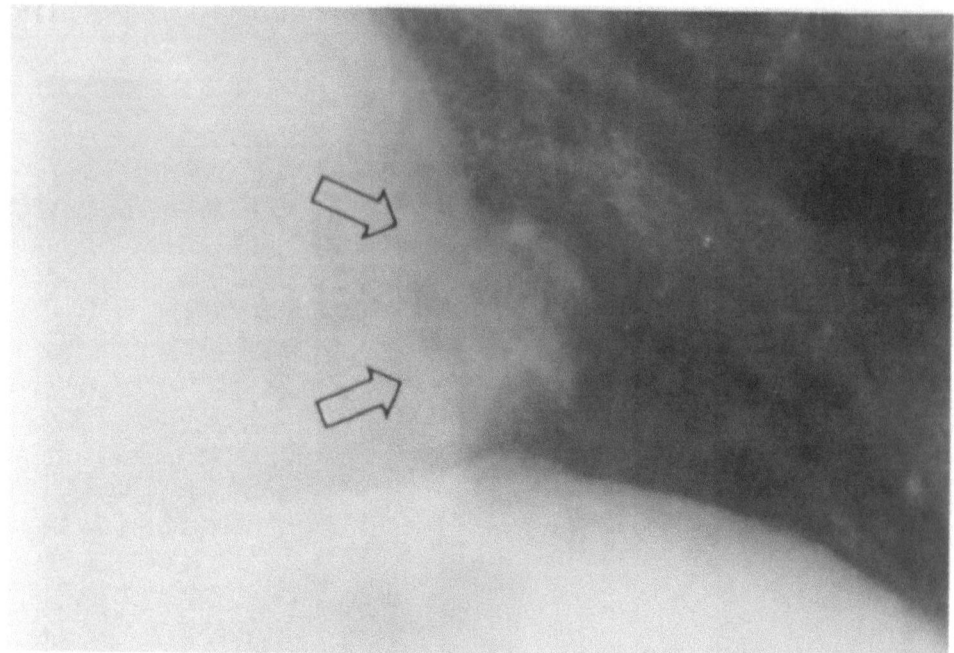

*Figure 28A.* This unique pleural based nodule was found adjacent to this middle-aged man's cardiac apex simulating an epicardial metastasis. No other lung or pleural metastases were identified.

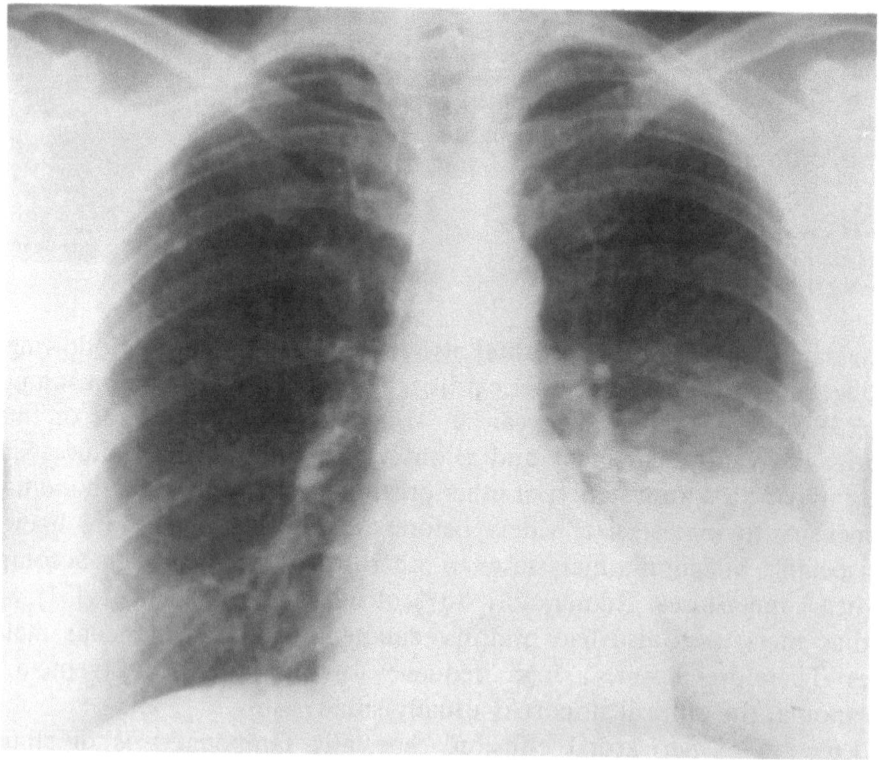

*Figure 28B.* Pa chest radiograph in a 51-year-old man with a large pleural-based melanoma mass representing his only known thoracic disease.

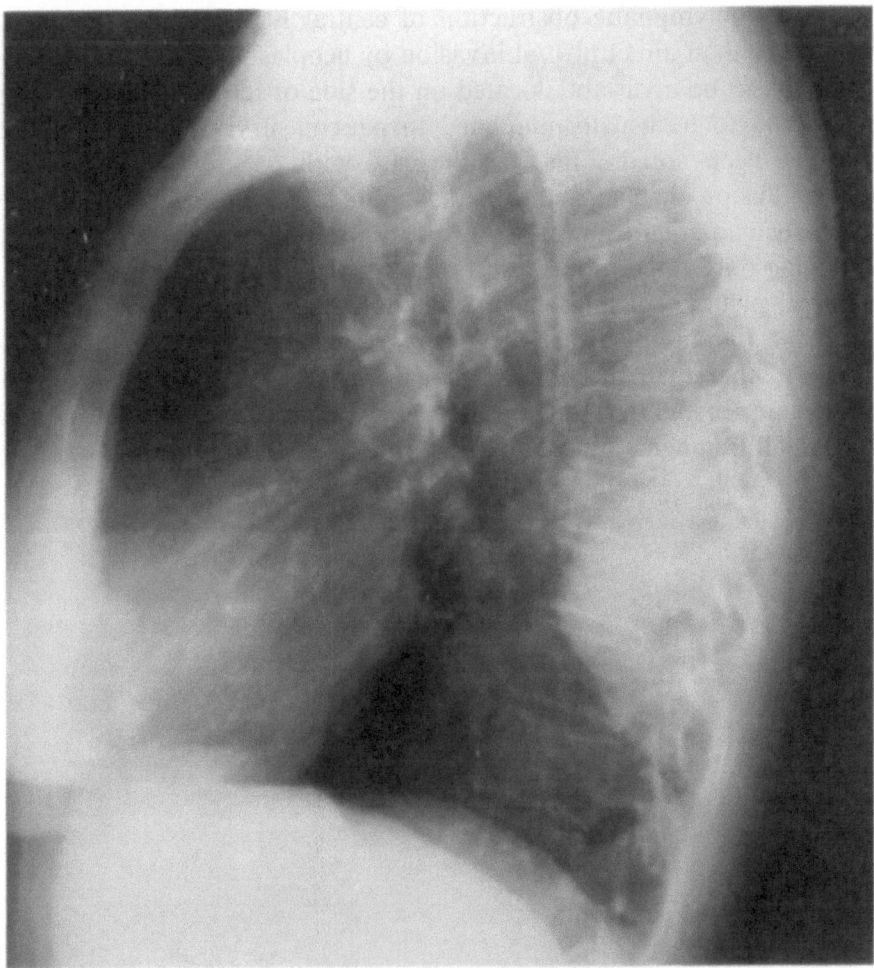

*Figure 28C.* Lateral view positions the mass posteriorly. Adjacent ribs are uninvolved.

Direct constriction by the malignancy may also occur, although isolated pericardial melanoma is exceedingly rare [77, 124]. These problems usually result in distressing symptoms to the patient and, since they are readily diagnosable by echography, attempted palliation may be beneficial [20, 70, 72].

*Pleural space and diaphragm*

The association of pleural effusion with hilar and mediastinal lymph node metastases has already been mentioned. Such serous effusions are thought to result from lymphatic obstruction of central lymph nodes replaced by tumor rather than direct pleural invasion by neoplastic cells [83]. They tend to be small, to be invariably located on the side of radiographic lymphadenopathy and to be usually unrelated to patient survival [58, 145]. Exceptions have been noted. This was the case with one Duke patient whose massive effusion displaced the mediastinum [30]. Respiratory embarrassment in such a patient can markedly affect longevity, the average life expectancy being only three months according to Das Gupta [31].

Bilateral pleural effusions have been noted to relate to the presence of hepatic melanoma metastases [83]. In actuality most pleural metastases from sites other than the lung are considered to represent tertiary spread from hepatic secondaries [40]. In rare cases hematogenous spread by embolism of small fragments of tumor into pulmonary arteries has occurred [83].

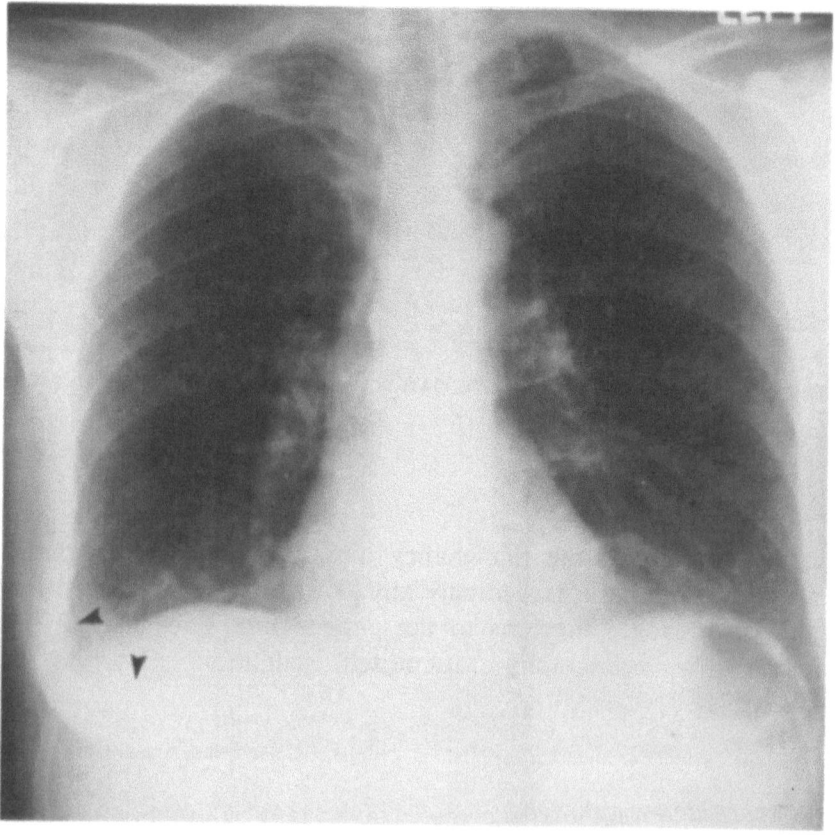

*Figure 29A.* PA chest roentgenogram shows a small right pleural effusion in a young woman with malignant melanoma. Although lymphadenopathy is not apparent, CT may be necessary to detect subtle node enlargement not appreciated on conventional studies.

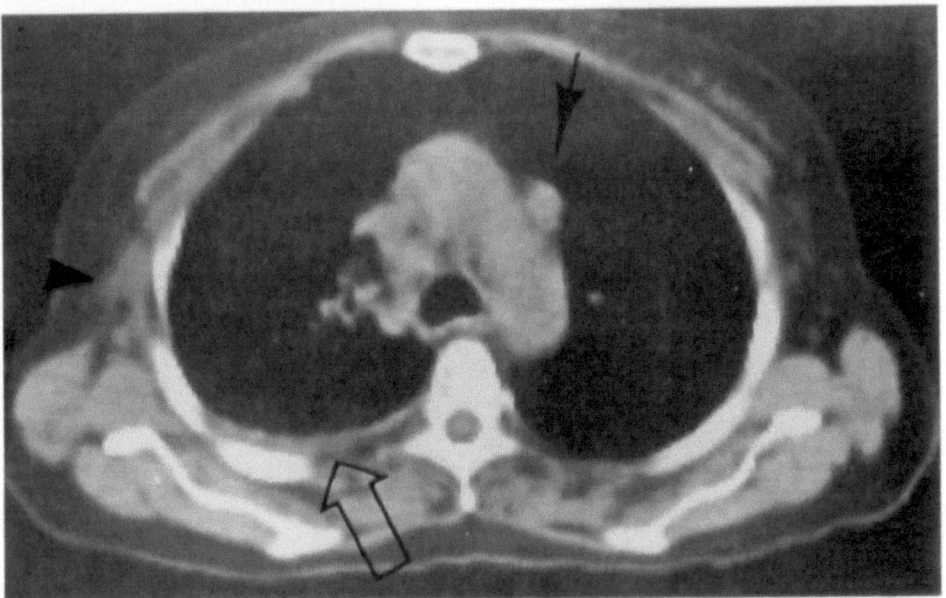

*Figure 29B.* Only CT demonstrated the mediastinal adenopathy (solid arrow) present in this elderly woman with metastatic melanoma involving the right axilla (arrowhead). Bilateral hilar adenopathy (not shown) was associated with a right pleural effusion (open arrow).

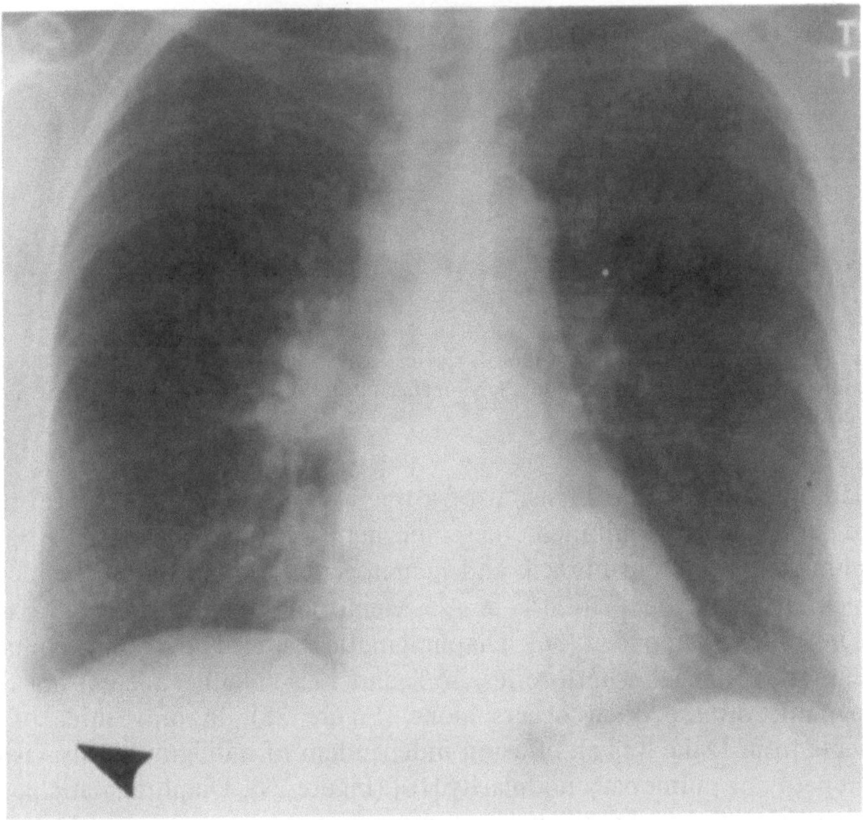

*Figure 29C.* Typical small pleural effusion accompanying unilateral hilar enlargement (arrowhead).

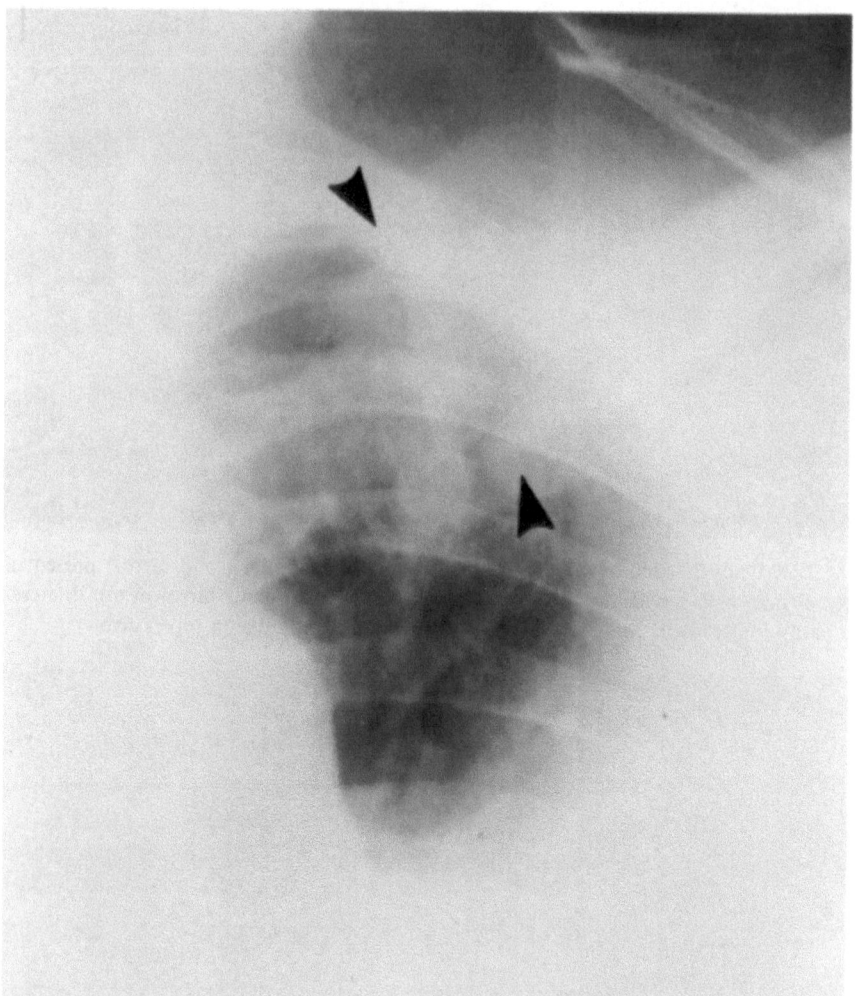

*Figure 30A.* Metastatic expansion of the left clavicular head (between arrowheads) visible with difficulty on the PA chest view due to a large malignant pleural effusion and the normal apical lung densities.

Theoretically chest wall invasion of a massive melanoma could also provoke an effusion. Combined, these mechanisms (i.e., obstructive, transdiaphragmatic or transthoracic and hematogenous) produced an incidence of pleural involvement of 24% in 125 Memorial patients [31] and 15% of M. D. Anderson autopsies [36]. Diaphragmatic disease had an approximately similar incidence in both series, 15% and 17%. Neither pleural nor diaphragmatic disease often occurs alone (Figure 28). In only three of 20 patients from Duke was an effusion independent of radiographically visible adenopathy or pulmonary nodularity [10] (Figure 29). Diaphragmatic paralysis resulting from phrenic nerve compression or invasion has been described with other findings such as a mediastinal mass [52].

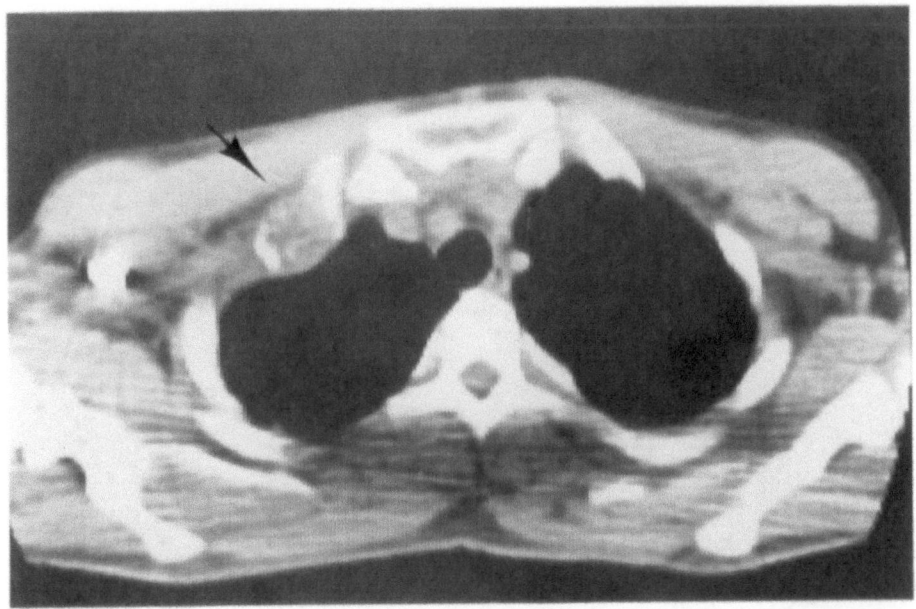

*Figure 30B.* CT demonstration of lytic melanoma metastasis (arrow) involving the opposite clavicle in a 23-year-old man with lung and mediastinal involvement.

*Extrapleural space.* An extrapleural mass was evident in 15 of the 130 available chest roentegenograms reviewed by Dahmash et al. [30]. One of these had an apical mass without the rib destruction that was displayed in all of the others. The majority were characterized by random combinations of pleural effusion, adenopathy and pulmonary nodules (Figure 30). Since skeletal melanoma in general is described elsewhere (Chapter 15), those findings which are reflected on routine chest radiography will be only briefly mentioned here.

In their review of the 1677 patients treated for melanoma at Duke from 1956 to 1976, Stewart et al. found osseous metastases in 6.9% [133]. Three-fourths of the diagnoses were established by conventional radiography, the remainder by radionuclide bone scan, biopsy, etc. Under ideal circumstances chest films might have shown metastases in the clavicle (seven cases), scapula (four), humerus (five), ribs (32) and thoracic spine (36) or in 84 of the 190 lesions, 44%. When Dahmash et al. [30] reviewed a similar number of cases from the same institution, (albeit the cases were somewhat different because of a different time interval) 17 bone metastases were identified. These lytic lesions were localized to ribs in all but one patient who had involvement of the thoracic spine, ribs and scapula [116]. Since only half of the chest films of the 260 with thoracic metastases were available for this study, one could reasonably double the data to get a rough idea of the accuracy of chest films in detecting these skeletal abnormalities. This would

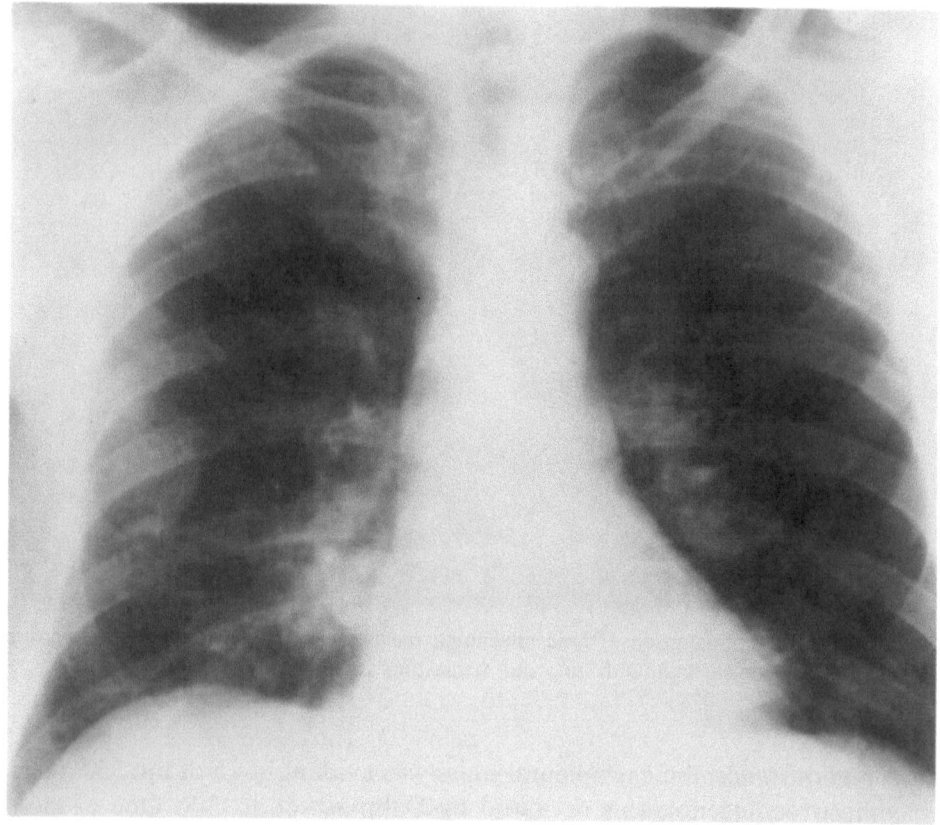

*Figure 31.* The PA chest film in this man with pulmonary metastases for three years shows the typical soft tissue density associated with rib destruction by melanoma. He expired shortly thereafter.

suggest that routine PA and lateral chest views are reasonable for detecting melanoma rib metastases but are poor for spine detection [39]. Probably the association of extrapleural masses with adjacent bone destruction serves to call rib metastases to the radiologist's attention (Figure 31).

The high frequency of osseous metastases presenting in the chest field of vision should alert the examining physician to a careful scrutiny of the skeleton. Of course when the patient is symptomatic, detailed views or bone scans of the area of interest are warranted.

## Primary thoracic melanoma

Primary visceral melanomas are distinctly uncommon [41]. Some continue to debate the existence of even one case [8]. Given the proclivity of malignant melanoma to metastasize to virtually everywhere in the body, the difficulty of identifying an occult ocular or cutaneous primary lesion and the known spontaneous regression rate of melanoma, this reluctance is understandable. Based on similarities of survival between melanomas with known primaries and those 4% of 2446 patients from the M.D. Anderson Hospital without a known primary, Baab and McBride [8] concluded that spontaneous regression of the original melanoma and subsequent discovery of the metastasis, whether in a lymph node or visceral site, was the probable explanation. That such tumors metastasize in toto has even been postulated [8].

On the other hand, primary visceral melanomas may be real. As Das Gupta [32] pointed out, it is impossible to prove a negative hypothesis and too tenaciously adhering to the above reasoning may exclude the unusual primary melanoma from being what it really might be. With this in mind the following reported cases of "primary" intrathoracic melanomas are presented.

## Lung parenchyma

In 1967 Jensen and Egedorf [60] proposed clinical criteria to suggest the primary lung occurrence of a melanoma: 1) no previous removal of pigmented skin tumors; preferably no removal of any skin tumors, 2) no ocular tumors, 3) only a solitary lung tumor in the surgical specimen, 4) tumor morphology consistent with a primary tumor, 5) no other surgically demonstrable melanomas and 6) careful autopsy exclusion of another possible primary, particularly in the skin and eyes. While the authors accepted two earlier cases as fulfilling these criteria, in actuality one originated in a bronchus [112] and the other patient had not come to autopsy, being alive ten years following left lower lobectomy for his solitary melanoma [105]. Their description of a 61-year-old woman, who underwent resection of a 6–10 cm left upper local recurrence, was the first case to satisfy all the criteria. One other lung melanoma verified by autopsy [136] has been reported. Both presented radiographic appearances identical to those of bronchogenic carcinoma in general. Four patients living at the time of their case publication have fulfilled the other clinical criteria suggested by Jensen and Egedorf. To obviate the need for autopsy in these, Allen and Drash [3] have revived a previously suggested pathologic standard consisting of the following: 1) junctional change with "nesting" of melanoma cells just beneath the bronchial epithelium, 2) bronchial epithelial invasion by melanoma cells in an area of intact epithelium and 3) the presence of an obvious melanoma beneath. It has been postulated that such tumors may arise from melanocytes which have migrated with the downward extension of the primordial tubular respiratory tract during fetal life [80]. Others have speculated that these tumors may arise from areas of respiratory squamous metaplasia [4].

*Tracheobronchial tree*

The first well-documented instance of possible primary bronchial melanoma appeared in a 45-year-old man who presented with sudden severe hemoptysis [112]. Bronchoscopy showed a large polypoidal tumor arising from the left lower lobe which largely blocked the upper lobe bronchus orifice. Pneumonectomy was performed. Two months later a large right apical pulmonary metastasis was demonstrated roentgenographically and by the sixth postoperative month the patient had expired. Autopsy disclosed multiple metastatic pulmonary nodules but failed to reveal an alternate site of primary melanoma. Other possible, but not completely proven, surgical cases have been described by Allen and Spitz [4] and Hsu et al. [55]. A recent possible primary bronchial melanoma in a Nigerian woman was presented [2]. Chest radiographs in her case, as in the others, matched those of any large centrally located bronchogenic carcinoma with perihilar mass and obstructive atelectasis. Microscopic sections show pleomorphic tumor cells and many multinucleated cells often arranged in whorls. Scattered cells reacted positively to Fontana's melanin stain. In the intact bronchial epithelium, beyond the site of primary growth, junctional nevus changes were found lending credence to the origin of the tumor from bronchial epithelial melanoblasts.

At least two melanomas have been said to arise from the trachea. The first presented by x-ray and bronchoscopy as a 2 cm mass partially obstructing the lower tracheal lumen [106]. Surgical resection of the tumor in this 35-year-old man and subsequent postmortem examination fulfilled the clinical criteria of a primary melanoma. The second was seen in a middle-aged woman who presented with shortness of breath from a radiographic right parahilar mass [89]. A bluish flat lesion on the posterior wall of the trachea was seen bronchoscopically. A primary tracheal melanoma with lymph node metastases was presumed on histological examination of the resected specimen. The flat configuration of the tumor appeared unique as did the absence of surrounding squamous metaplasia, suggesting an origin of the melanoma directly from nonsquamous mucosa. This corroborates findings in the upper respiratory tract, where melanomas probably arise from melanocytes in the respiratory mucosa and do not necessarily need a milieu of squamous epithelium [80].

*Pleura*

Primary pleural melanoma has been postulated only once to our knowledge [128]. This occurred in a 49-year-old black man suffering from recent marked weight loss. Chest radiographs and fluoroscopy demonstrated opacification of the entire lower right lung with coexistent right-sided pleural effusion and a posterolateral extrapleural mass. Thoracentesis, cope needle biopsy and percutaneous transthoracic needle biopsy were nondiagnostic. Open lung biopsy, however, revealed a large bulky mass adhèrent to the pleura. Histological interpretation of the specimen was initially equivocal but subsequent review by the Armed Forces Institute of Pathology confirmed a diagnosis of melanoma. Despite the patient's initial response to chemotherapy, he later died of pulmonary thromboemboli. Autopsy failed to show tumor other than that confined to the original surgical site. Seemingly, then, this case also meets the primary criteria set forth by Jensen and Egedorf [60].

## Mediastinum

Few reported cases of apparent malignant melanoma presenting as mediastinal masses exist. One was associated with weight loss, malaise and fever in a 31-year-old man whose chest radiograph demonstrated a left superior mediastinal mass displacing the trachea slightly to the right [38]. Mediastinoscopy and subsequent biopsy produced clumps of large cells containing prominent eosinophilic nucleoli and cystoplasm showing brown melanin pigment characteristic of malignant melanoma. Standard radioisotope scans were normal but a bone marrow biopsy also revealed melanoma. Despite treatment with DTIC (dacarbazine) the patient died six months later.

The finding of marrow melanoma at the time of original diagnosis and lack of subsequent autopsy confirmation to exclude an occult ocular or mucosal lesion place this case at variance with the criteria established by Jensen and Egedorf [60].

An earlier report described the appearance of calcification in a thoracic posterior mediastinal mass of the 12-year-old girl previously discussed [131]. Cutaneous melanotic lesions are common in adolescents [134] but malignant melanoma is decidedly uncommon. An incidence of 0.3–0.4% of a tumor, which in itself only accounts for 1–2% of all cancers in the United States, has been attributed to pediatric melanoma. Metastases from such tumors, excluding the very aggressive melanomas associated with giant nevi, are also the exception [97]. Stromberg [134] describes only 47 documented cases of metastatic melanoma in prepubertal children, although once a metastasis does occur it behaves in an adult fashion. Obviously then primary malignant melanomas in children must be rare. To have such a tumor occur in a mediastinal location and with calcification certainly exhausts the odds of duplication of the case reported by Stanley et al. [131]. These authors felt that it was probable that their tumor arose from the paravertebral sympathetic ganglia, sites of known origin and calcification of other neuroectodermal neoplasms [28]. Autopsy in their patient was limited to the thorax, excluding the possibility of defining other skin, mucosal, retinal or leptomeningeal primary sites.

In all probability this tumor was not unlike primary malignant melanocytic tumors of the sympathetic chain described in Millar's 1932 original case [87] and updated by Fu et al. in 1975 [43]. Together those authors presented four patients. In two, tumor arose from thoracic sympathetic ganglia, while cervical or lumbar sites accounted for the other two. The original description was that of a 34-year-old man in whom an approximately 6 cm left paravertebral mass invading the lung, pleura and chest wall was found at autopsy. Metastatic melanomatous nodules involved the contralateral lung, liver, adrenal gland and skull base. A well-demarcated 4 cm mass, also in the left posterior mediastinum, was discovered on routine chest radiography in the other patient with apparent melanoma of sympathetic ganglion origin. Although the mass did not appreciably change during the next year, the 34-year-old hypertensive man in whom it occurred died of postoperative complications following its removal. Both of the other two patients with suspected primary sympathetic chain melanoma died of disseminated intrathoracic tumor, which on electron microscopic examination was indistinguishable from malignant melanoma of the skin [43]. The detailed ultrastructural studies of Fu et al. [43], Mishima [88] and others [28, 127] have indicated a close kinship of melanoma and the multiple tumors originating in tissue of the sympathetic nervous system. In view of their probable common origin from the same primordial neural crest cells, this is more readily understandable.

# References

1. Ackerman LV and Del Regato JA: Cancer: Diagnosis, Treatment and Prognosis. CV Mosby, St. Louis, 1962.
2. Adebonojo SA, Grillo IA and Durodola JI: Primary malignant melanoma of the bronchus. J Natl Med Assoc 71 (6):579–581, 1979.
3. Allen MS, Jr and Drash EC: Primary melanoma of the lung. Cancer 21:154–158, 1968.
4. Allen AC and Spitz S: Malignant melanoma: a clinicopathological analysis of the criteria for diagnosis and prognosis. Cancer 6:1–45, 1953.
5. Amer EH, Al-Shrraf M and Viatkevicius VK: Clinical presentation, natural history and prognostic factors in advanced malignant melanoma. Surg Gynecol Obstet 149:687–692, 1979.
6. Aranha GV, Simmons RL, Gunnarsson A, Grage TB and McKhann CF: The value of preoperative screening procedures in Stage I and II malignant melanoma. J Surg Oncol 11:1–6, 1979.
7. Ariel IM: The use of lymphangiography in melanoma. Surgery 76:654–655, 1974.
8. Baab GH and McBride CM: Malignant melanoma — the patient with an unknown site of primary origin. Arch Surg 110:896–900, 1975.

9. Baldwin JN and Wisner R: Multiple primary neoplasms. Am J Surg 111:230–233, 1966.

10. Baltaxe HA and Constable WC: Mediastinal lymph node visualization in the absence of intrathoracic disease. Radiology 90:94–98, 1968.

11. Bein ME, Greenberg M, Liu P, Ohara J, Bassett LW, Schaefer CJ and Steckel RJ: Pulmonary nodules: detection in 1 and 2 cm full lung linear tomography. Am J Roentgenol 135:513–520, 1980.

12. Berge T and Sievers J: Myocardial metastases: a pathological and electrocardiographic study. Br Heart J 30:383–390, 1968.

13. Bilgi C, Brown NE, McPherson TA and Lentle B: Pulmonary manifestations in patients with malignant melanoma during BCG immunotherapy. Chest 75 (6):685–687, 1979.

14. Borgren HG, DeMaria AN and Mason DT: Imaging procedures in the detection of cardiac tumors with emphasis on echocardiography: a review. Cardiovasc Intervent Radiol 3:107–125, 1980.

15. Braman SS and Whitcomb ME: Endobronchial metastasis. Arch Intern Med 135:543–547, 1975.

16. Breslow A: Thickness, cross-sectional areas and depth of invasion in the prognosis of cutaneous melanoma. Ann Surg 172:902–908, 1979.

17. Budman DR, Camacho E and Wittes RE: The current causes of death in patients with malignant melanoma. Eur J Cancer 14:327–330, 1977.

18. Bryant J and Vuckovic G: Metastatic tumors of the endocardium. Arch Pathol Lab Med 102:206–208, 1978.

19. Cahan WG: Excision of melanoma metastases to lung: problems in diagnosis and management. Ann Surg 178 (6):703–709, 1973.

20. Cham WC, Freiman AH, Carstens PHB and Chu FCH: Radiation therapy of cardiac and pericardial metastases. Radiology 114:701–704, 1975.

21. Chang AE, Schaner EG, Conkle DM, Flye MW, Doppman JL and Rosenberg SA: Evaluation of computed tomography in the detection of pulmonary metastases. Cancer 43:913–916, 1979.

22. Clark RA and Colley DP: Pulmonary lymphatics visualized during pedal lymphangiography. Radiology 136:29–32, 1980.

23. Clark WH, Jr, From L, Bernardino EA and Mihm MC: The histogenesis and biologic behavior of primary human malignant melanoma. Cancer Res 29:705–727, 1969.

24. Clerf LH: Melanoma of bronchus: metastasis simulating bronchogenic neoplasm. Ann Otol Rhinol Laryngol 43:887–891, 1934.

25. Conrad FG: Cures achieved in patients with metastatic malignant melanoma of the skin. Cancer 30:144–147, 1972.

26. Cox KR, Hare WSC and Bruce PR: Lymphography in melanoma: correlation of radiology with pathology. Cancer 19:637–647, 1966.

27. Curtis AM, Ravin CE, Collier PE, Putman CE, McLoud T and Greenspan RH: Detection of metastatic disease from carcinoma of the breast: limited value of full lung tomography. Am J Roentgenol 134:253–255, 1980.

28. D'Abrera VS and Burfitt-Williams W: A melanotic neuroectodermal neoplasm of the posterior mediastinum. J Pathol 111:165–172, 1973.

29. Dahlgren S and Nordenstrom B: Transthoracic Needle Biopsy. Year Book Publ, Chicago, 1966.

30. Dahmash NS, Chen JTT, Ravin CE, Putman CE, Seigler HF and Reed JC: Metastatic melanoma to the thorax — a report of 130 patients (submitted for publication).

31. Das Gupta T and Brasfield RD: Metastatic melanoma — a clinicopathological study. Cancer 17:1323–1339, 1964.

32. Das Gupta T, Brasfield RD and Paglia MA: Primary melanomas in unusual sites. Surg Gynecol Obstet 128:841–847, 1969.

33. Del Regato JA and Spjut JH: Malignant melanomas. In: Del Regato and Spjut JA (eds) Cancer, pp 208–223. CV Mosby, St. Louis, 1977.

34. Devereux D, Johnston G, Blei L, Head G, Makuch R and Burt M: The role of bone scans in assessing malignant melanoma in patients with Stage III disease. Surg Gynecol Obstet 151:45–58, 1980.

35. Dodd GD and Boyle JJ: Excavating pulmonary metastases. Am J Roentgenol 85:277–293, 1961.

36. Einhorn LH, Burgess MA, Vallejos C, Bodey GP, Sr et al: Diagnostic correlations and response to treatment in advanced metastatic malignant melanoma. Cancer Res 34:1995–2004, 1974.

37. Evans RA, Bland KI, McMurtrey MJ and Ballantyne AJ: Radionuclide scans not indicated for clinical Stage I melanoma. Surg Gynecol Obstet 150:532–534, 1980.

38. Feldman L and Kricun ME: Malignant melanoma presenting as a mediastinal mass. J Am Med Assoc 241 (4):396–397, 1979.

39. Fornasier VL and Horne JG: Metastases to the vertebral column. Cancer 36:590–594, 1975.

40. Fraser RG and Pare JAP: Diagnosis of diseases of the chest. In: Fraser RG and Pare JAP (eds) Metastatic Neoplasms, Chap 8, pp 1117–1134. WB Saunders, 1979.

41. Fraser RG and Pare JAP: Diagnosis of diseases of the chest. In: Fraser RG and Pare JAP (eds) Primary Melanoma of the Lung, p 1000. WB Saunders, Philadelphia, 1979.

42. Friedman M, Forgione H and Shanbhag V: Needle aspiration of metastatic melanoma. Acta Cytol 24 (1):7–15, 1980.

43. Fu YS, Kaye GI and Lattes R: Primary malignant melanocytic tumors of the sympathetic ganglia, with an ultrastructural study of one. Cancer 36:2029–2041, 1975.

44. Glancy DL and Roberts WC: The heart in malignant melanoma. Am J Cardiol 21:555–571, 1968.

45. Gibbons JA and Devig PM: Massive hemothorax due to metastatic malignant melanoma. Chest 73:123, 1978.

46. Goldsmith HS: Melanoma: an overview. CA-A Cancer J Clin 29 (4):194–279, 1979.

47. Gothlin J, Dahlback O, Dencker H, Hakansson GH and Lunderquist A: Retrograde angiography of the human thoracic duct. Am J Roentgenol 124:472–476, 1975.

48. Greene MH, Hoover RN and Fraumeni JF: Subsequent cancer in patients with chronic lymphocytic leukemia — a possible immunologic mechanism. J Natl Cancer Inst 61 (2):337–340, 1978.

49. Gromet MA, Ominsky SH, Epstein WL and Blois MS: The thorax as the initial site for systemic relapse in malignant melanoma. Cancer 44:776–784, 1979.

50. Hajdu SI and Savino A: Cytologic diagnosis of malignant melanoma. Acta Cytol 17:320–327, 1973.

51. Heaston DK, Mills SR, Moore AV and Johnston WW: Percutaneous thoracic needle biopsy. In: Putman C (ed) Diagnostic Imaging in Pulmonary Disease. Appleton-Century-Crofts, New York, 1981.

52. Hilbish TF: Roentgen manifestations of malignant melanoma. Am J Roentgenol 78:769–779, 1957.

53. Hoffer PB: The utility of gallium-67 in tumor imaging: a comment on the final reports of the cooperative study group. J Nucl Med 19:1082–1083, 1978.

54. Holmes EC, Ramming KP, Eilber FR and Morton DL: The surgical management of pulmonary metastases. Semin Oncol 4 (1):65–69, 1977.

55. Hsu C, Wu S and Chen C: Melanoma of the lung. Chin Med J 81:263–266, 1962.

56. Huffman TA and Sterin WK: Ten-year survival with multiple metastatic malignant melanoma. Arch Surg 106:234–235, 1973.

57. Ishihara T, Kikuchi K, Ikeda T, and Yamazaki S: Metastatic pulmonary disease: biologic factors and modes of treatment. Chest 63:227–232, 1973.

58. Izbicki R, Weyhing BT, Baker L, Caoili EM and Vaitkevivius VK: Pleural effusion in cancer patients. Cancer 36:1511–1518, 1975.
59. Jackson FI, McPherson TA and Lentle BC: Gallium-67 scintigraphy in multisystem malignant melanoma. Radiology 122:163–167, 1977.
60. Jensen OA and Egedorf J: Primary malignant melanoma of the lung. Scand J Respir Dis 48:127–135, 1967.
61. Jost RG, Sagel SS, Stanley RJ and Levitt RG: Computed tomography of the thorax. Radiology 126:125–136, 1978.
62. King DS and Castleman B: Bronchial involvement in metastatic pulmonary malignancy. J Thorac Surg 12:305–315, 1943.
63. Kirkwood JM, Tonkonow B, Nordlund JJ, Ariyan S, Forget B and Lerner A: Melanoma: a multidisciplinary overview of current concepts and management. Conn Med 44 (1):21–26, 1980.
64. Kline IK: Cardiac lymphatic involvement by metastatic tumor. Cancer 29:779–808, 1972.
65. Lee YN: Malignant melanoma: pattern of metastasis. CA-A Cancer J Clin 30:137–142, 1980.
66. Lentle BC, Scott JR, Noujaim AA and Jackson FI: Iatrogenic alterations in radionuclide biodistributions. Semin Nucl Med 9:131–143, 1979.
67. Licata G, Bongiorno A and Scaffidi A: Diagnostica L'oncoscintigrafia polmonare con $^{67}$Ga. Minerva Med 69:357–368, 1978.
68. Lilien DL, Jones SE, O'Mara RE, Salmon SE and Durie BGM: A clinical evaluation of indium-111 bleomycin as a tumor-imaging agent. Cancer 35:1036–1049, 1975.
69. Littleton JT, Durizch ML and Callahan WP: Linear vs pluridirectional tomography of the chest: correlative radiographic anatomic study. Am J Roentgenol 134:241–248, 1980.
70. Lokich JJ: The management of malignant pericardial effusions. J Am Med Assoc 224:1401–1404, 1973.
71. Lubell DL and Goldfarb CR: Metastatic cardiac tumor demonstrated by $^{201}$Thallium scan. Chest 79:98–99, 1980.
72. Luce JK: Chemotherapy of melanoma. Semin Oncol 2:179–185, 1975.
73. Lundy J, Damjanov I, Ballow M, Henken M and Mitchell MS: Pulmonary granulomas in a patient on MER therapy. Yale J Biol Med 50:665–668, 1977.
74. McCarthy WH, Shaw HM and Milton GW: Spontaneous regression of metastatic malignant melanoma. Clin Oncol 4:203–207, 1978.
75. McCormack PM, Bains MS, Beattie EJ and Martini N: Pulmonary resection in metastatic carcinoma. Chest 73:163–166, 1978.
76. McLoud TC, Kalisher L, Stark P and Greene R: Intrathoracic lymph node metastases from extrathoracic neoplasms. Am J Roentgenol 131:403–407, 1978.
77. Mann T, Brodie BR, Grossman W and McLaurin L: Effusive-constrictive hemodynamic pattern due to neoplastic involvement of the pericardium. Am J Cardiol 41:781–786, 1978.
78. Mathisen DJ, Flye MW and Peabody J: The role of thoracotomy in the management of pulmonary metastases from malignant melanoma. Ann Thorac Surg 27:295–299, 1979.
79. Mastrangelo MJ, Bellet RE, Berkelhammer J and Clark WH, Jr: Regression of pulmonary metastatic disease associated with intralesional BCG therapy of intracutaneous melanoma metastases. Cancer 36:1305–1308, 1975.
80. Mesara BW and Burton WD: Primary malignant melanoma of the upper respiratory tract. Cancer 5:217–255, 1968.
81. Meyer JE and Stolbach L: Pretreatment radiographic evaluation of patients with malignant melanoma. Cancer 42:125b–126, 1978.
82. Meyer JE: Radiographic evaluation of metastatic melanoma. Cancer 42:127–132, 1978.
83. Meyer PC: Metastatic carcinoma of the pleura. Thorax 21:437–443, 1966.

84. Middleton G: Involvement of the thymus by metastatic neoplasms. Br J Cancer 20:41–46, 1966.

85. Mihm MC, Clark WH, Jr and Reed RJ: The clinical diagnosis of malignant melanoma. Semin Oncol 2 (2):105–118, 1975.

86. Milder MS, Frankel RS, Bulkley GB, Ketcham AS and Johnston GS: Gallium-67 scintigraphy in malignant melanoma. Cancer 32:1350–1356, 1973.

87. Millar GW: A malignant melanotic tumor of ganglion cells arising from a thoracic sympathetic ganglion. J Pathol 35:351–357, 1932.

88. Mishima Y: Melanotic tumors. In: Zelickson AS (ed) Ultrastructure of Normal and Abnormal Skin, pp 388–424. Lea & Febiger, 1967.

89. Mori K, Cho H and Som M: Primary "flat" melanoma of the Trachea. J Pathol 121:101–105, 1977.

90. Morton DL, Joseph WL, Ketcham AS et al: Surgical resection and adjuvantive immunotherapy for selected patients with pulmonary metastases. Ann Surg 178:360–366, 1973.

91. Muhm JR, Brown LR and Crowe JK: Use of computed tomography in detection of pulmonary nodules. Mayo Clin Proc 52:345–348, 1977.

92. Muss HB, Richards IF, Barnes PL, Willard VV and Cowan RJ: Radionuclide scanning in patients with advanced malignant melanoma. Clin Nucl Med 4:516–518, 1979.

93. Nathanson L: Spontaneous regression of malignant melanoma: a review of the literature on incidence, clinical features and possible mechanisms. Natl Cancer Inst Monogr 44:67–76, 1976.

94. Nathanson L, Hall TC and Farber S: Biological aspects of human malignant melanoma. Cancer 20:650–655, 1967.

95. Neifeld JP, Michaelis LL and Doppman JL: Suspected pulmonary metastases, correlation of chest x-ray, whole lung tomograms and operative findings. Cancer 39:383–387, 1977.

96. Nissenblatt MJ and Wu HV: Malignant melanoma and small-cell carcinoma of the lung. N Engl J Med 302:636, 1967.

97. Olbourne NA and Harrison SH: Malignant melanoma in childhood. Br J Plast Surg 27:305–307, 1974.

98. Oster MW: Tuberculosis in malignant melanoma. Med Pediatr Oncol 2:439–440, 1976.

99. Pack GT, Gerber DM and Scharnagel IM: End results in the treatment of malignant melanoma. Ann Surg 136:905–911, 1952.

100. Patel JK, Didolkar MS, Pickren JW and Moore RH: Metastatic pattern of malignant melanoma – a study of 216 autopsy cases. Am J Surg 135:807–810, 1978.

101. Pinsky SM and Henkin RE: Gallium-67 tumor scanning. Semin Nucl Med 6:397–409, 1976.

102. Plesnicar S, Klanjscek G and Modic S: Actual doubling time values of pulmonary metastases from malignant melanoma. Aust N Z J Surg 48:23–26, 1978.

103. Raptopoulos V, Schellinger D and Katz S: Computed tomography of solitary pulmonary nodules: experience with scanning times longer than breath-holding. J Comput Assisted Tomography 2:55–60, 1978.

104. Ravin CE, Wallin K and Sorenson J: Chest tomography – a practical approach. Appl Radiol, 1977.

105. Reed RJ, III and Kent EM: Solitary pulmonary melanomas. J Thorac Cardiovasc Surg 48:226–231, 1964.

106. Reid JD and Mehta VT: Melanoma of the lower respiratory tract. Cancer 12:627–631, 1966.

107. Reynolds RD, Pajak TF, Greenberg BR, Shirley JH et al: Lung cancer as a second primary. Cancer 42:2887–2893, 1978.

108. Romolo JL and Fisher SG: Gallium-67 scanning compared with physical examination in the preoperative staging of malignant melanoma. Cancer 44:468–472, 1979.

109. Rosenberger A and Adler O: Fine needle aspiration biopsy in the diagnosis of mediastinal lesions. Am J Roentgenol 131:239–242, 1978.

110. Resenberger A and Adler O: Superior vena cava syndrome — a new radiologic approach to diagnosis. Cardiovasc Intervent Radiol 3:127–130, 1980.

111. Rosenberger MB, Lisa JR and Trinidad S: Pitfalls in the clinical and histological diagnosis of bronchogenic carcinoma. Dis Chest 49:396–404, 1966.

112. Salm R: A primary malignant melanoma of the bronchus. J Pathol Bacterial 85:121–126, 1963.

113. Schaner EG, Chang AE, Doppman JL, Conkle DM, Flye MW and Rosenberg SA: Comparison of computed and conventional whole lung tomography in detecting pulmonary nodules — a prospective radiologic-pathologic study. Am J Roentgenol 131:51–54, 1978.

114. Schoenbaum S and Viamonte M: Subepithelial endobronchial metastases. Radiology 101:63–69, 1971.

115. Seigler HF and Fetter BF: Current management of melanoma. Ann Surg 186:1–12, 1977.

116. Selby HM, Sherman RS and Pack GT: A roentgen study of bone metastases from melanoma. Radiology 67:224–228, 1956.

117. Sethi SM and Saxton GD: Osteoarthropathy associated with solitary pulmonary metastasis from melanoma. Can J Surg 17:221–224, 1974.

118. Shaw HM, Milton GW, McCarthy WH, Farago GA and Dilworth P: Effect of smoking on the recurrence of malignant melanoma. Med J Aust 1:208–209, 1979.

119. Shirakawa S, Luce JK, Tannock I and Frei E, III: Cell proliferation in human melanoma. J Clin Invest 49:1188, 1970.

120. Siegelman SS: Computed tomography. In: Siegelman SS, Stitik FP and Summer WR (eds) Pulmonary System: Practical Approaches to Pulmonary Diagnosis, Vol 1, p 818. Grune & Straton, New York, 1979.

121. Siegelman SS, Zerhouni EA, Leo FP, Khouri NF and Stitik FP: CT of the solitary pulmonary nodule. Am J Roentgenol 135:1–13, 1980.

122. Silverberg E: Cancer statistics, 1980. CA-A Cancer J Clin 30:23–38, 1980.

123. Simeone JF, Putman CE and Greenspan RH: Detection of metastatic malignant melanoma by chest roentgenography. Cancer 39:1993–1996, 1977.

124. Singh A and Krishan I: Cardiac tamponade following secondary pericardial carcinosis in malignant melanoma. Indian Heart J 394–396, 1967.

125. Sinner WN: Complications of percutaneous transthoracic needle aspiration biopsy. Acta Radiol Diagn 17:813, 1976.

126. Smith LH: Secondary tumors of the heart. Rev Surg 33:223–231, 1976.

127. Smith LH: Thoracic neurolophomas. Ann Surg 23:586–592, 1977.

128. Smith S and Opipari MI: Primary pleural melanoma — first reported case and literature review. J Thorac Cardiovasc Surg 75:827–831, 1978.

129. Sparks FC: Hazards and complications of BCG immunotherapy. Med Clin North Am 60:499–509, 1976.

130. Stalker LK, Phillips RB and Pemberton JJ: Multiple primary malignant lesions. Surg Gynecol Obstet 68:595, 1939.

131. Stanley P, Seigel SE and Isaacs H: Calcification in a paraspinal malignant melanoma in a child. Am J Roentgenol 129:143–145, 1977.

132. Stehlin JJ, Hills WJ and Rufino C: Disseminated melanoma: biologic behavior and treatment. Arch Surg 94:495–501, 1967.

133. Stewart WR, Gelberman RH, Harrelson JM and Seigler HF: Skeletal metastases of melanoma. J Bone J Surg 60-A:645–649, 1978.

134. Stromberg BV: Malignant melanoma in children. J Pediatr Surg 14:465–467, 1979.

132

135. Sutton FD, Vestal RE and Creagh CE: Varied presentations of metastatic pulmonary melanoma. Chest 64:415–419, 1974.
136. Taboada CF, McMurray JD, Jordan RA and Seybold WD: Primary melanoma of the lung. Chest 62:629–631, 1972.
137. Tefft M, Vawter GF and Mitus A: Second primary neoplasms in children. Am J Roentgenol 103:800–822, 1968.
138. Theros EG: Varying manifestations of peripheral pulmonary neoplasms: a radiologic-pathologic correlative study. Am J Roentgenol 128:893–914, 1977.
139. Thomas JH, Panoussopoulos DG, Jewell WR and Pierce GE: Tricuspid stenosis secondary to metastatic melanoma. Cancer 39:1732–1737, 1977.
140. Twersky J and Levin DC: Metastatic melanoma of the adrenal. Radiology 119:627–628, 1975.
141. Voith MA, Lichtenfeld KM, Schimpff SC and Wiernik PH: Systemic complications of MER immunotherapy of cancer, pulmonary granulomatosis and rash. Cancer 43:500–504, 1979.
142. Wallace S, Jackson L, Dodd GD and Greening RR: Lymphatic dynamics in certain abnormal states. Am J Roentgenol 91:1187–1206, 1964.
143. Wallace S and Jing BS: Carcinoma. In: Clouse ME (ed) Clinical Lymphography, Sec 7, pp 185–273. Williams and Wilkins, Baltimore, 1977.
144. Webb WR: Hilar and mediastinal lymph node metastases in malignant melanoma. Am J Roentgenol 133:805–810, 1979.
145. Webb WR and Gamsu G: Thoracic metastasis in malignant melanoma: a radiographic survey of 65 patients. Chest 71:176–181, 1977.
146. Wenger NK: Cardiac tumors. In: Hurst JW and Logue BB (eds) Diseases of the Heart and Pericardium, pp 1668–1681.McGraw-Hill, New York, 1978.
147. Wilkins EW, Jr, Head JM and Burke JF: Pulmonary resection for metastatic neoplasms in the lung. Experience at the Massachusetts General Hospital. Am J Surg 135 (4):480–483, 1978.
148. Wolfe S and Popp RL: Diagnosis of atrial tumors by ultrasound. Circulation 39:615–622, 1969.
149. Yeung K and Bonnet JD: Spontaneous pneumothorax with metastatic malignant melanoma. Chest 71:435–436, 1977.
150. ZuWallack RL, Urman JD and Lahiri B: Metastatic melanoma: another cause of a solitary pulmonary nodule with an air bronchogram. Radiology 123:286, 1977.

# 5. Radiographic manifestations of metastatic melanoma to the gastrointestinal tract, hepatobiliary system, pancreas, spleen and mesentery

WILLIAM M. THOMPSON

Malignant melanoma metastasizes widely and involves most organs in the body [1–19]. In particular, gastrointestinal metastases, although commonly found at autopsy, have not been generally well recognized premortem. Das Gupta and Brasfield [6] found only a 9% incidence of gastrointestinal metastatic melanoma in patients premortem compared to a 60% incidence in their autopsy series [6, 7]. Melanoma is probably the most common malignancy to metastasize in the gastrointestinal tract and other intra-abdominal organs [11]. Many reports illustrating the radiographic features of metastatic melanoma to the stomach and small bowel have been published [20–46]. Although the occurrence of primary melanoma of the gastrointestinal tract has been reported, the majority of lesions found are metastatic. The two exceptions are esophagus and anus [47–67]. Melanocytes are present at these two sites.

The two most common sites of metastasis to the gastrointestinal tract and abdomen are the small bowel and liver (Table 1). In most series, these two sites are involved in over half of the patients. The esophagus, stomach, colon, pancreas, spleen, gallbladder and mesentery may also be involved (Table 1). At Duke only 90 of approximately 2000 patients have had proven metastatic malignancy to the gastrointestinal tract and abdomen. This is a lower incidence than in most reported series (Table 1). Although our series extended over 15 years, most metastases have been diagnosed in the past five years as our awareness of metastatic disease has increased. Many of our patients who expired did not have an autopsy. Most of the 90 patients had more than one metastatic site with multiple metastases found in the liver, small bowel and stomach. The interval between initial discovery of the primary melanoma and the radiographic demonstration of metastatic disease ranged from three months to thirteen years (average five years). A small number of patients presented with a gastrointestinal and/or abdominal metastatic lesion without a primary ever being discovered and a few patients had evidence of abdominal and/or gastrointestinal metastases when the primary lesion was discovered.

In addition to disseminating widely, no tumor is more unpredictable than melanoma. Melanoma has a relatively high rate of spontaneous regression. There may also be long intervals between removal of the primary and

*Seigler, H. F. (ed.), Clinical Management of Melanoma. ISBN 978-94-009-7495-1*
© *1982, Martinus Nijhoff Publishers, The Hague/Boston/London.*

*Table 1.* Incidence of metastatic melanoma—autopsy (A) † and clinical (C) series.

| Series ( ) | Total patients | Esophagus | Stomach | Duodenum | Small intestine | Colon | Liver | Gall-bladder | Pancreas | Spleen | Mesentery |
|---|---|---|---|---|---|---|---|---|---|---|---|
| Das Gupt and Brasfield (A) [6] | 125 | 4% | 26% | 12% | 58% | 22; | 68% | 15% | 53% | 36% | — |
| Einhorn et al. (A) [72] | 96 | 3% | 7% | — | 26% | 14% | 76% | 4% | 38% | 43% | — |
| Mayer (A) [15] | 74 | — | 26% | — | 34% | 24% | 54% | 20% | 32% | 27% | — |
| Nathanson et al. (A) [16] | 22 | 36% | 36% | 36% | 36% | 77% | | 41% | 36% | — | — |
| Patel et al. (A) [17] | 216 | 9% | 23% | — | 36% | 28% | 58% | 9% | 38% | 31% | — |
| Goldstein et al. (C) [11] | 67 | 7% | 24% | 19% | 48% | 4% | 24% | 4% | — | — | 32% |
| Potchen et al. (C) [28] | 46 | — | 24% | — | 31% | 20% | 52% | 20% | 37% | 20% | — |
| Duke (C & A) * | 90 | 2% | 7% | 3% | 50% | 16% | 29% | 3% | 10% | 13% | 14% |

† Most patients had more than one metastatic lesion.
* Incomplete data from 2000 patients. Only 90 have been identified with metastasis.

appearance of metastases [71–76]. For instance, ten to 15 years may pass between removal of a choroidal melanoma and the development of hepatic metastases. Recent advances in immuno- and chemo-therapy have extended the survival of patients with melanoma [71–76]. Melanoma patients with small bowel metastases have improved survival following resection of solitary as well as multiple lesions [76]. Thus, full knowledge of the potential spread of melanoma, its radiographic appearance, and accurate and timely clinical and radiologic evaluation should further contribute to improved survival.

This chapter summarizes the radiologic features of metastatic melanoma to the abdomen excluding the retroperitoneum and genitourinary tract. The radiographic features are discussed by anatomic location. In each section the relative incidence, clinical features, radiographic appearance and differential diagnosis are presented. The final section summarizes an overall approach for the radiographic evaluation in patients with suspected metastatic melanoma to the abdomen. Although experience is limited, the potential impact of ultrasound and computed body tomography (CT) in patients with metastatic melanoma is discussed [77–83].

**Esophagus**

Malignant melanoma of the esophagus is rare. It can occur as either a metastatic or primary lesion [47–58]. The esophagus is the least commonly affected hollow viscus (Table 1). Das Gupta and Brasfield reported a 4% incidence of esophageal metastasis in their autopsy series [7]. Goldstein et al. had five of 67 (7%) patients with metastatic lesions in the esophagus [11]. However, two of these were adjacent metastatic lesions in the mediastinum. Only three were primary intrinsic esophageal lesions.

Primary esophageal melanoma has been reported [47–58]. The diagnosis of a primary esophageal melanoma should be based on the following criteria: 1) the tumor should have a characteristic structure of a melanoma and contain demonstrable melanin, 2) it should arise from an area of junctional change in the squamous epithelium and 3) the adjacent epithelium should also show junction changes with the presence of cells containing melanin pigment [56]. Raven and Dawson indicated that in many cases the epithelium over the tumor is often ulcerated and a direct origin from junctional epithelium may not be detectable [56]. Therefore, they felt that if either the second or third criterion is fulfilled, the tumor may then be considered a primary lesion. The lesion is still rare enough that it continues to be reported. In our series of over 1000 patients with carcinoma of the esophagus, we have not observed a primary melanoma of the esophagus. Our files also fail to show any definite intrinsic metastatic melanoma to the esopha-

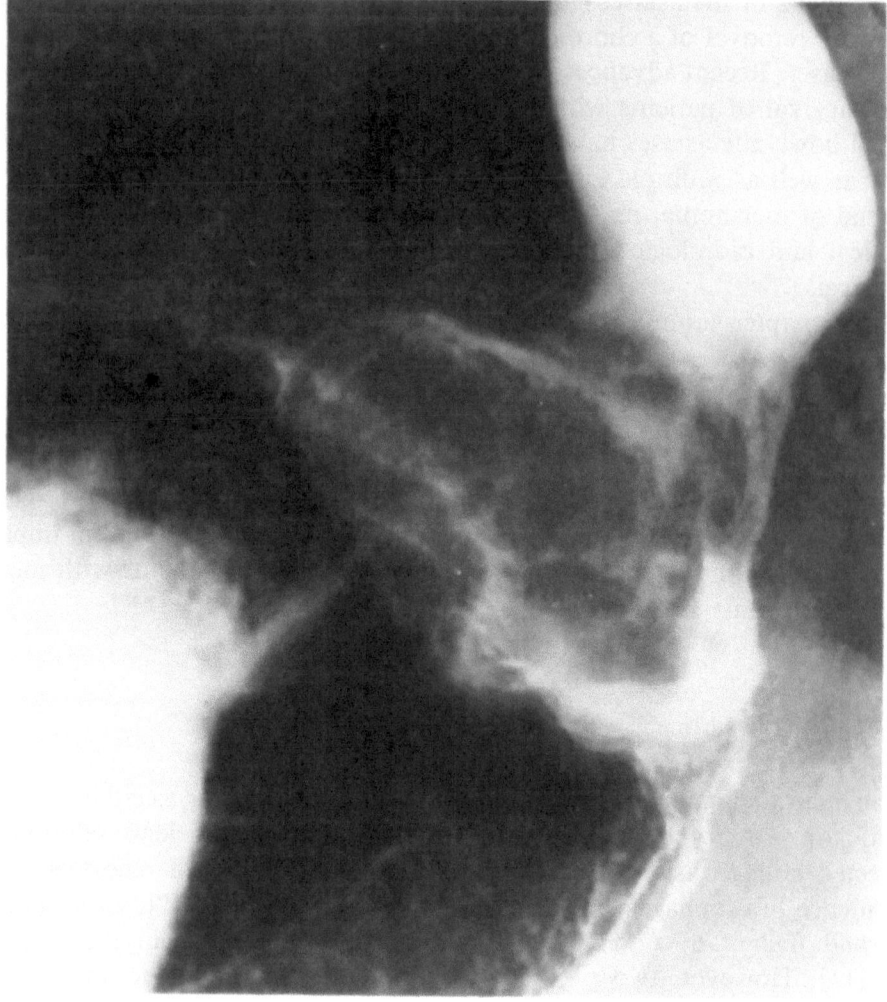

*Figure 1.* Large polypoid mass at gastroesophageal junction without evidence of obstruction in more proximal esophagus.

gus; however we have seen a few patients with extrinsic metastatic lesions in the mediastinum compressing the esophagus.

Patients with either primary or secondary melanoma of the esophagus will usually present with dysphagia or bleeding or both. The symptoms may be mild and inconstant consisting of epigastric fulness, substernal pressure and precordial burning [47–58]. Endoscopically the tumor may be difficult to differentiate from other lobulated tumors such as leiomyoma, fibroma, carcinosarcoma and leiomyosarcoma. In most reported cases of primary melanoma of the esophagus, the tumor grew to considerable size within the esophageal lumen before symptoms were apparent. Dysphagia is probably

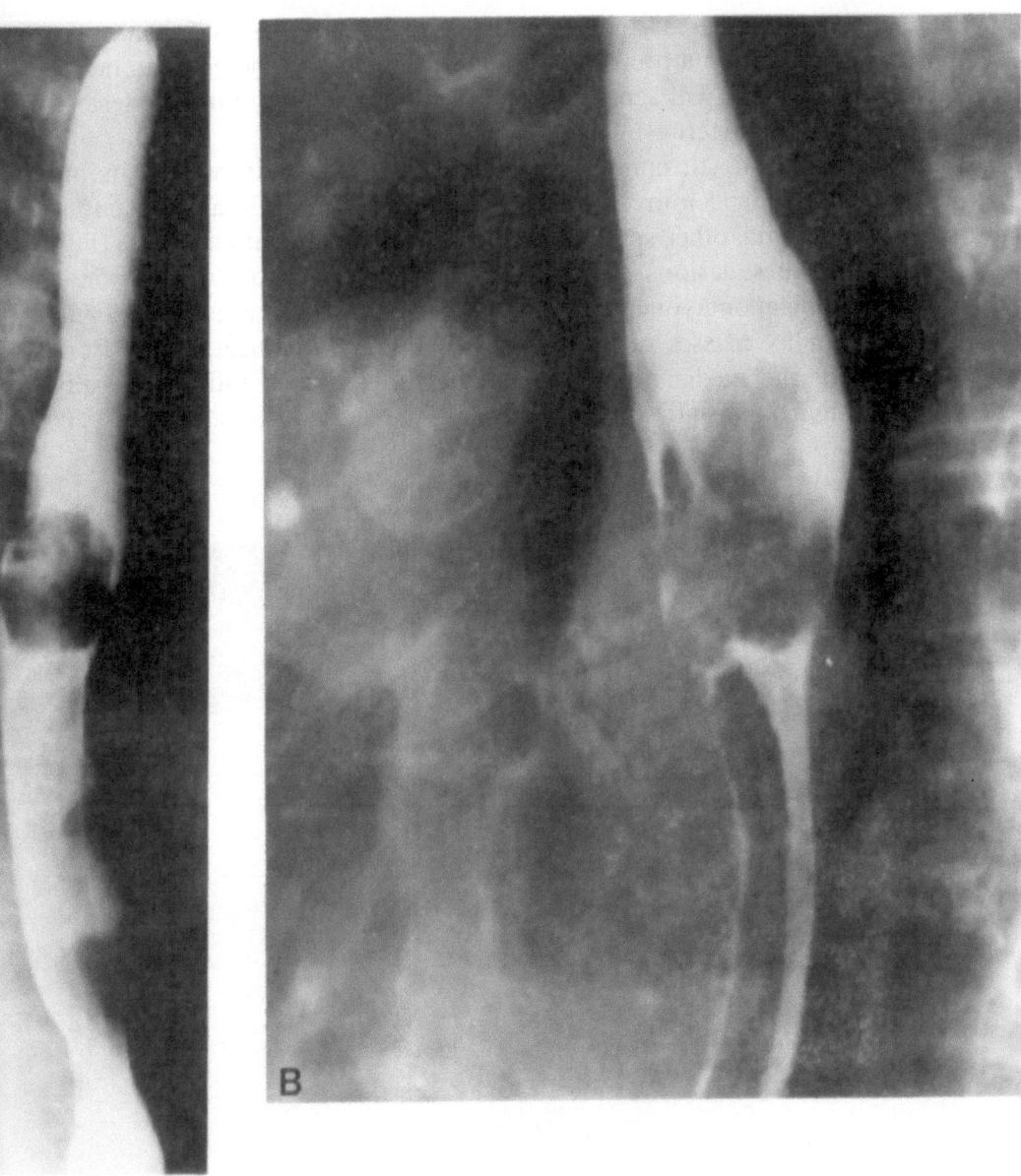

*Figure 2.* Large bulky polypoid mass in midesophagus due to carcinosarcoma (A, B).

related to ulcerated mucosa rather than to the mass itself, because in most cases there is little dilatation above the large lobulated mass.

With extrinsic lesions, there will be radiographic evidence of extrinsic impression on the esophagus by a large adjacent mass. If the large mass invades the wall, large ulcerated areas may be present [11]. Intrinsic lesions, either primary or secondary, will present as a large bulky polypoid mass with little dilatation or evidence of obstruction above the mass (Figure 1).

There may be large areas of ulceration and, at times, the lesion may be indistinguishable from a primary esophageal carcinoma. There are no radiographic features that will separate primary from secondary intrinsic lesions in the esophagus (Figure 2).

Differential diagnostic considerations in the absence of known melanoma include leiomyoma, leiomyosarcoma, carcinosarcoma, primary squamous or adenocarcinoma, other spindle cell tumors and adenomatous polyps (Figure 2). All of these lesions are rare and, without the history of a previous diagnosis of melanoma, one could not distinguish between a melanoma and other large bulky masses in the esophagus. Finally, extrinsic lesions from melanoma of the mediastinum can not be differentiated radiographically from any other metastatic mediastinal lesion invading the esophagus.

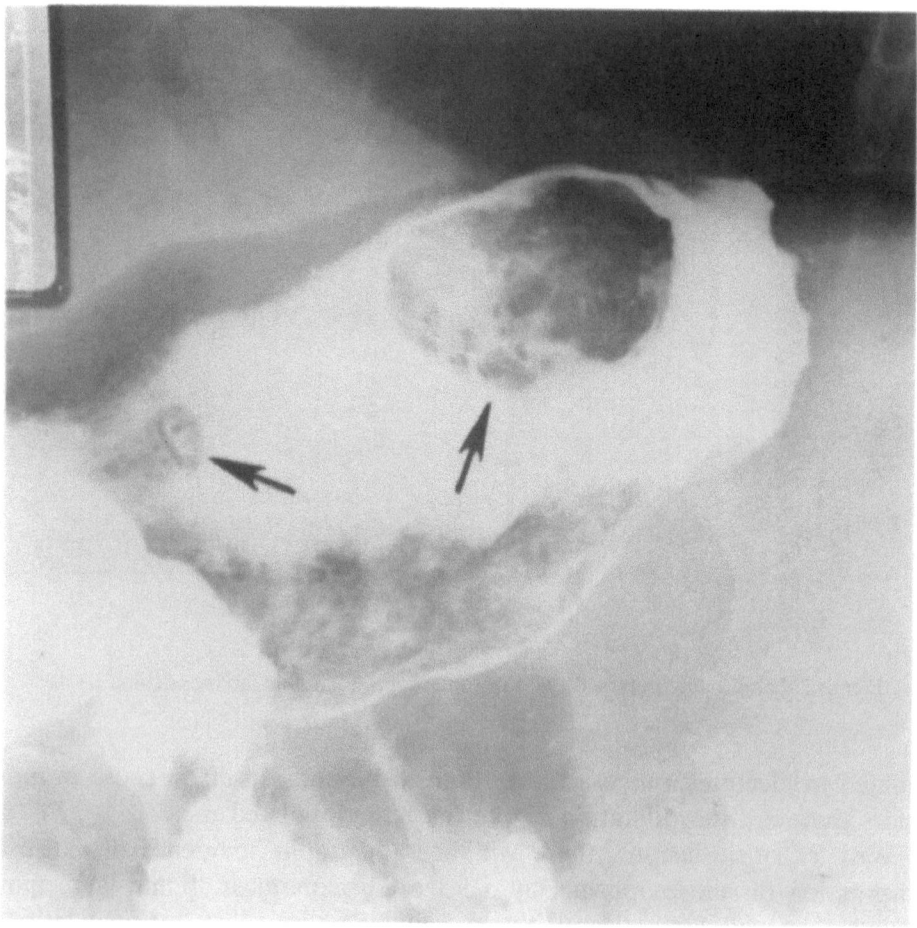

*Figure 3A.* Single contrast view of two polypoid lesions in proximal stomach due to metastatic melanoma (arrows).

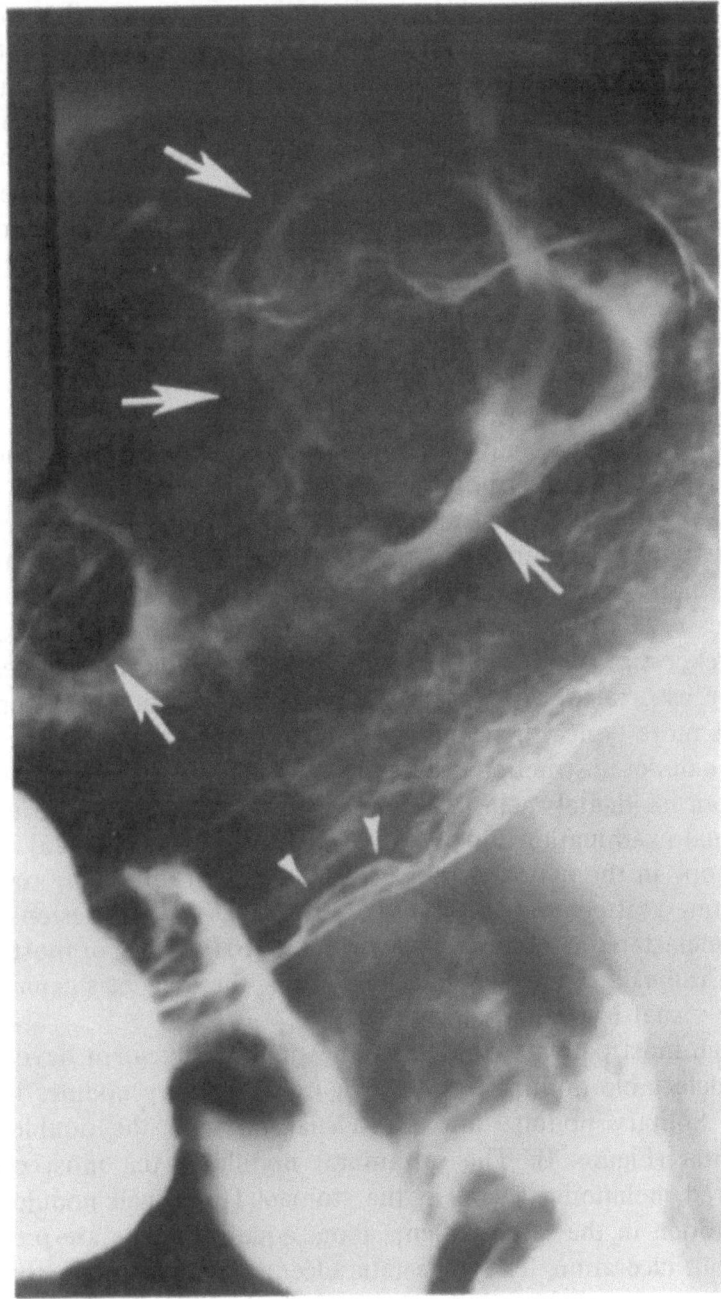

*Figure 3B*. Double contrast view of proximal stomach shows two metastatic lesions (arrows) as well as small lesion (arrowheads) not shown on single contrast study.

The double contrast esophogram is more sensitive for detecting subtle lesions of the esophagus than the routine barium swallow [84]. With a large, bulky metastatic lesion from melanoma, the double contrast exam does not aid in lesion detection but it can more clearly show the extend of a lesion and the surface characteristics [84]. Thus, for any large bulky lesion, such as a metastatic or primary melanoma of the esophagus, a double contrast examination is recommended to determine the extent of the lesion and to detect subtle areas of ulceration.

## Stomach

The stomach is the second most common site for metastatic melanomas (Table 1) [6, 11]. Furthermore, melanoma is one of the most common lesions to ppoduce metastatic lesions in the stomach [27].

Patients with melanoma of the stomach usually present with nausea or vomiting, nonspecific abdominal discomfort and pain suggestive of peptic ulcer disease. General features of malignancy such as weight loss, malaise and anorexia may also be present [20–29]. Ulcerative mucosal lesions are frequently associated with enteric blood loss. A gradual development of anemia is more typical than massive hemorrhage. Annular lesions are rare but gastric outlet obstruction occurs in some patients with melanoma. Occasionally, an incidental metastatic lesion is discovered during an upper gastrointestinal examination for peptic ulcer disease (Figure 4) [25].

Endoscopy in the patient with gastrointestinal bleeding may reveal polypoid lesions scattered throughout the stomach. If these lesions are pigmented, metastatic melanoma is likely [31, 32]. However, in most cases the polypoid lesions are not pigmented and, thus, the diagnosis cannot be suggested by visual inspection alone.

Although most patients with gastrointestinal involvement have radiographically detectable multiple lesions (Figure 3), solitary nodules have been reported. Solitary nodules are best visualized with the double contrast examination (Figure 4). The intramural nodule is the most commonly encountered melanoma lesion in the stomach [11]. Such nodules vary in size and, often in the same patient, about equal numbers are present with and without ulceration. The metastatic ulcerating mass in the stomach originating from the mucosa has been described as the bull's eye or target lesion (Figure 4). These are seen in other metastatic lesions but are more common with melanoma. This lesion is more common in the stomach than elsewhere in the gastrointestinal tract [11, 30]. However, the bull's eye lesion is less common than polypoid masses.

Since most patients with polypoid and ulcerative lesions in the stomach are also known to have melanoma, the numerous differential diagnostic

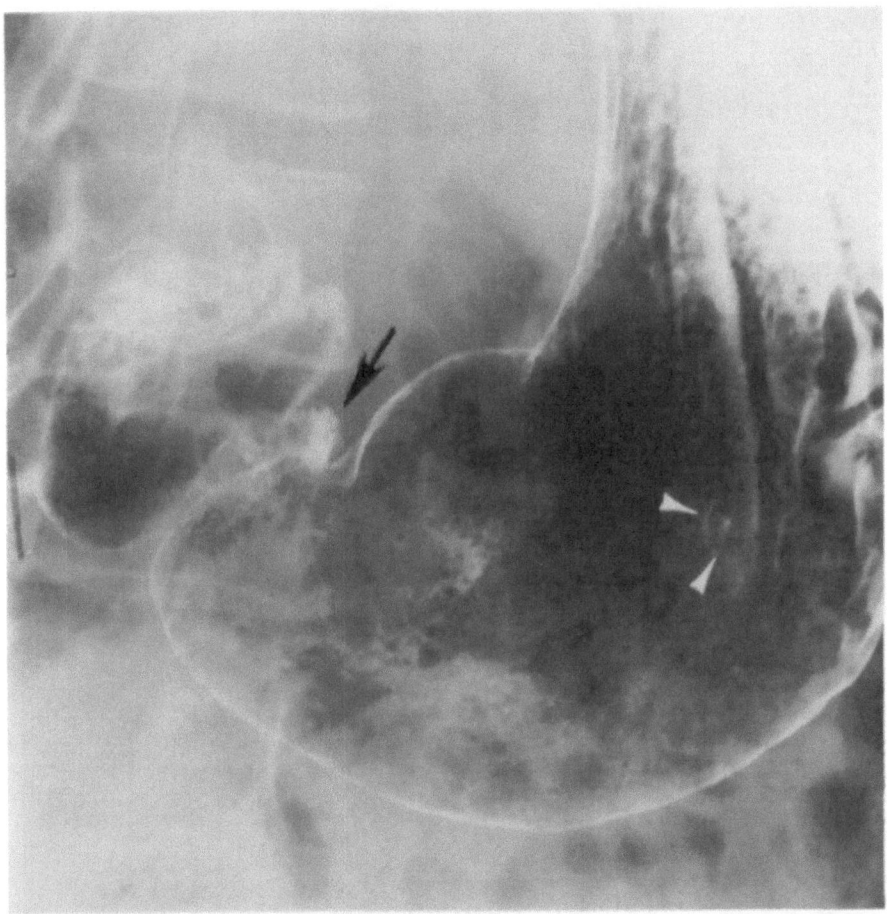

*Figure 4A.* Double contrast view of distal stomach showing pyloric ulcer (arrow). Small bull's eye lesion (arrowheads) in more proximal stomach.

possibilities are of little practical importance [11]. In the absence of known history of melanoma, the ulcerative lesion can be seen with both benign and malignant spindle cell lesions, with metastatic lesions (most commonly from breast and lung), ectopic pancreas, carcinoid tumors, primary carcinoma and lymphoma. The polypoid lesions may represent adenomatous polyps and may reflect the spectrum of multiple polyposis of the gastrointestinal tract or inflammatory gastric polyposis.

Goldstein et al. [11] and Laufer [84] showed that the double contrast examination is more sensitive than the routine examination for detecting small lesions (less than 1 cm in diameter) in the stomach, especially for detecting the small submucosal nodules that may occur in patients with metastatic melanoma (Figure 3). Thus, the double contrast examination is

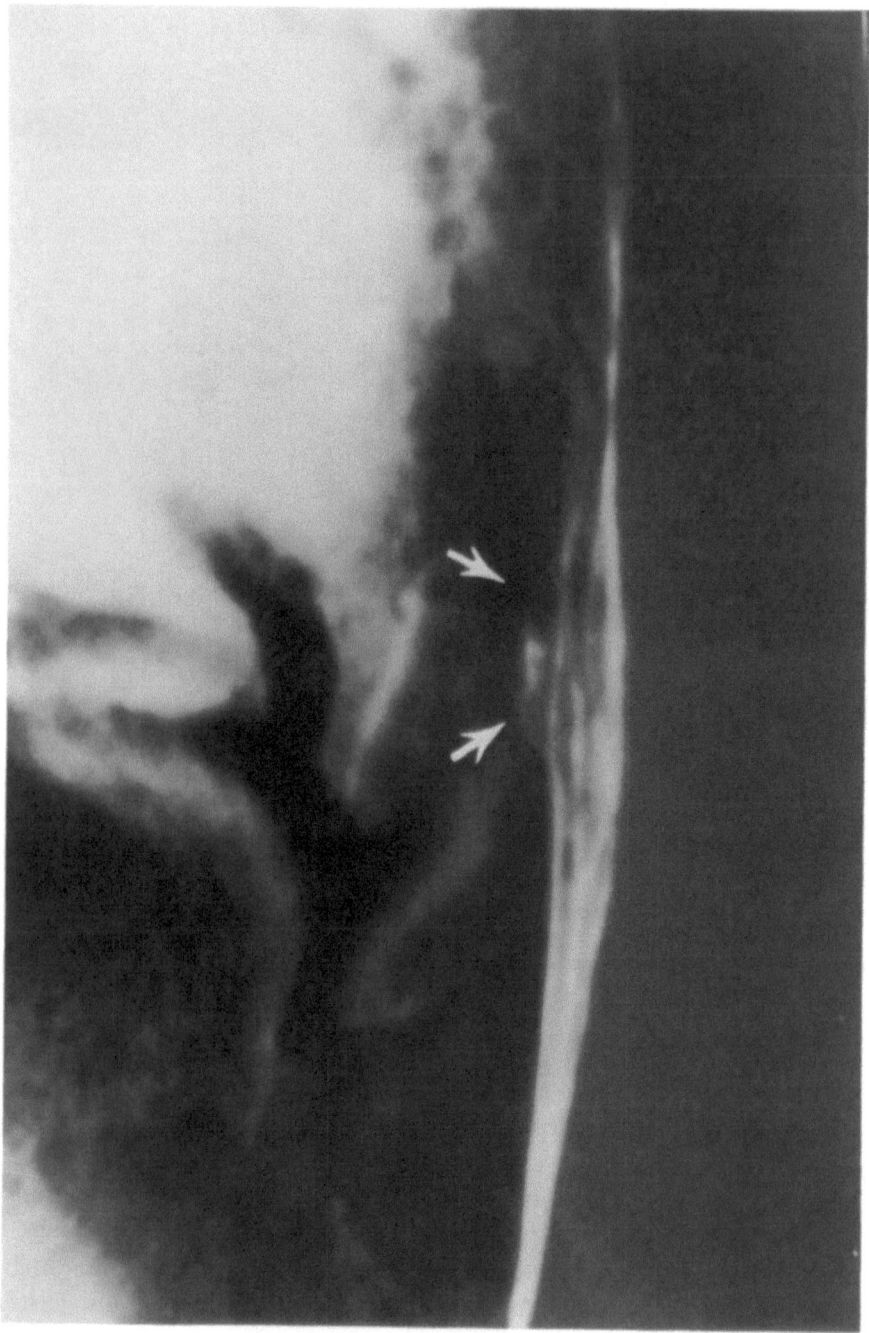

*Figure 4B.* Coned down tangential view of umbilicated bull's eye lesion originating from the gastric wall (arrows).

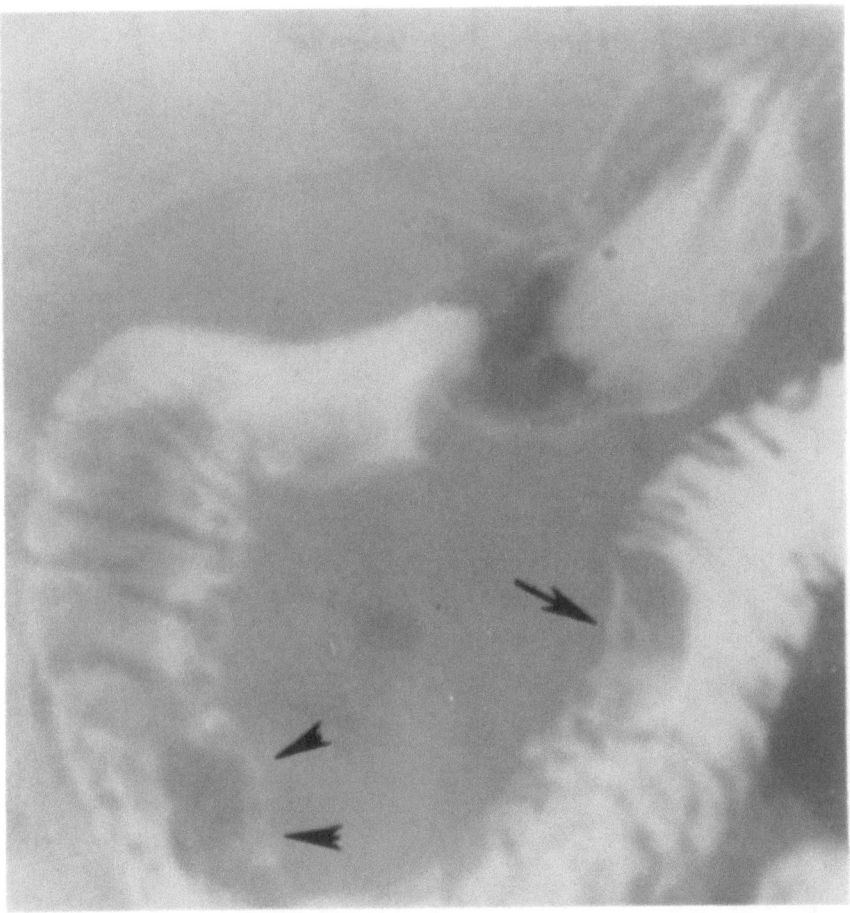

*Figure 5.* Spot film from a gastrointestinal series showing the normal ampulla of Vater (arrowheads), and an intramural polypoid metastatic lesion from melanoma in the fourth portion of the duodenum (arrow).

recommended for any patient with a known melanoma who also has gastrointestinal symptoms suggesting peptic ulcer disease or gastrointestinal bleeding, or both.


## Duodenum

Among the hollow viscus, the duodenum is the third most common site for metastatic melanoma (Table 1). Most cases of metastatic disease of the upper gastrointestinal tract involve lesions in both the stomach and duodenum. Occasionally, however, solitary lesions of either the stomach or duodenum are encountered [11].

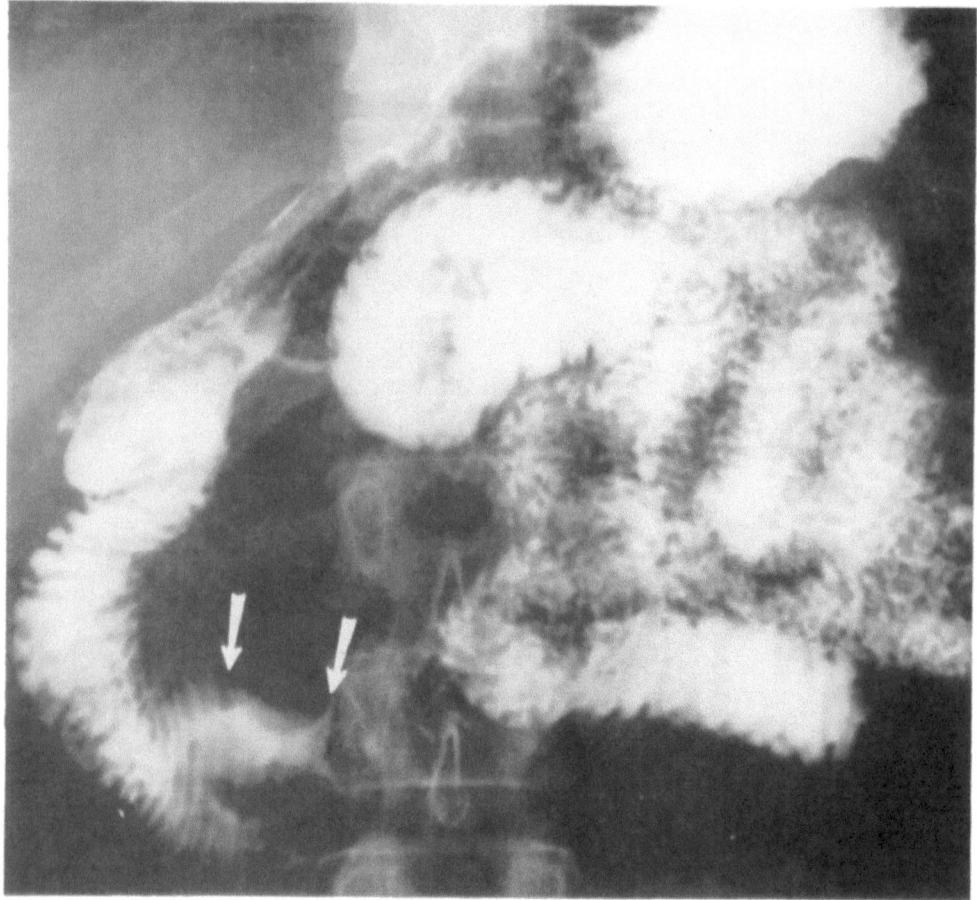

*Figure 6A.* Large intussuscepting polypoid mass in third portion of duodenum (arrows) due to metastatic melanoma.

Since patients with duodenal involvement also usually have either gastric or small bowel metastases, they will present with gastrointestinal bleeding or pain, or both. Like stomach lesions, duodenal lesions can also be identified endoscopically [29]. Furthermore, a specific diagnosis can be made for pigmented lesions. In many cases, however, the lesions are ulcerated without definite pigment. These require endoscopic biopsy for tissue diagnosis.

Radiographically, the most common duodenal lesion is the polypoid mass with or without central ulceration (Figures 5, 6). Usually, many similar lesions are present in both the stomach and small bowel [11]. Goldstein et al. [11] concluded that about equal numbers of patients have either ulcerated or nonulcerated nodules and, in some cases, both types of nodules can occur in the same patient. Large exophytic masses, either in the duodenal

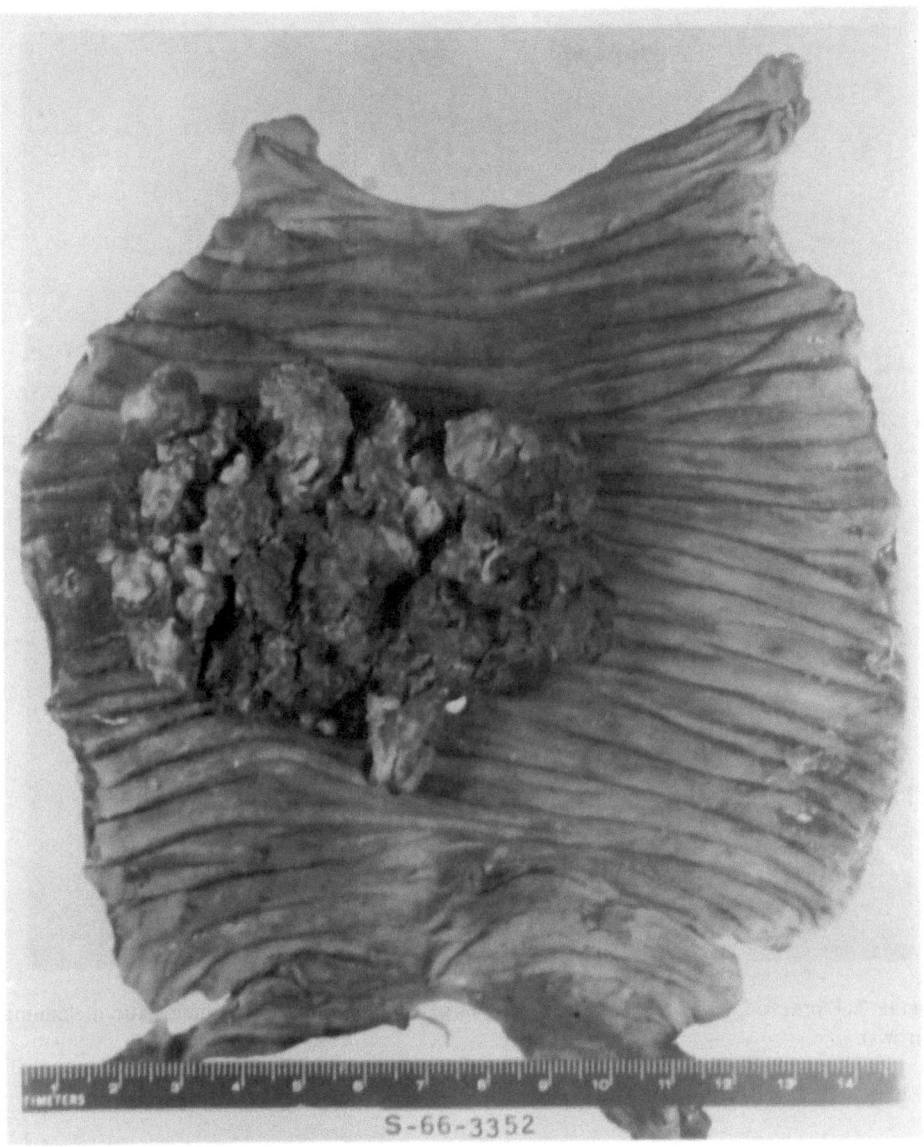

*Figure 6B.* Gross resected section of duodenum showing large irregular polypoid metastatic melanoma.

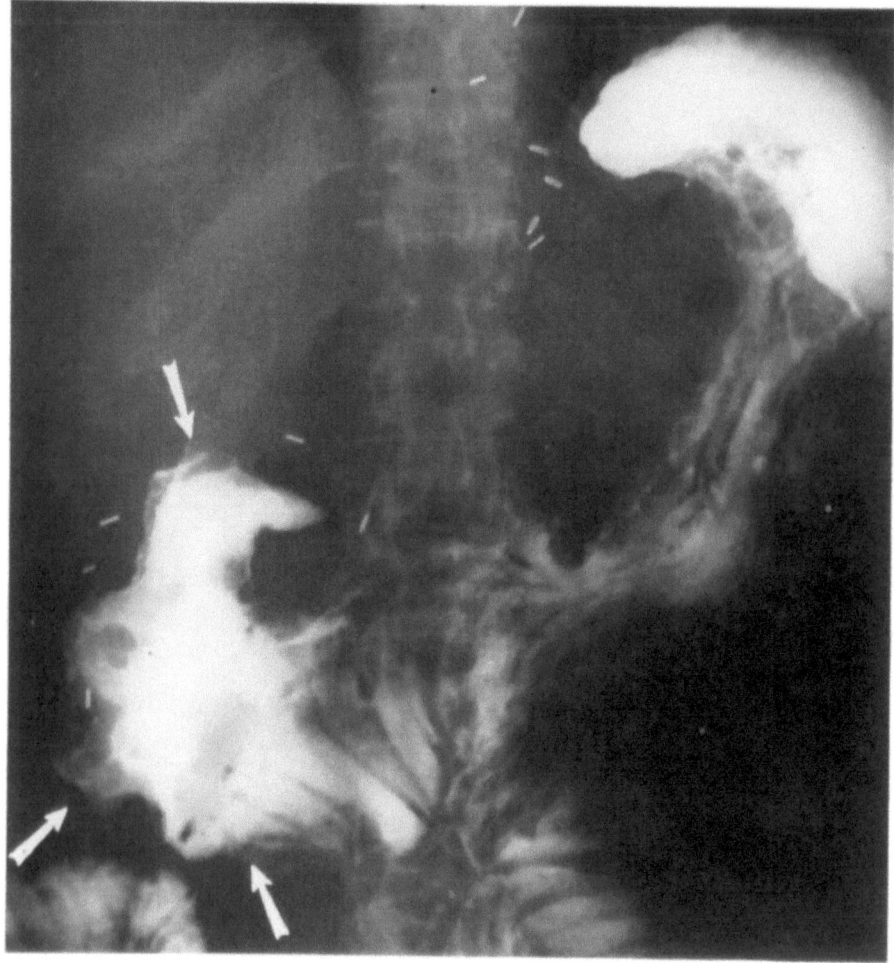

*Figure 7.* Upper GI series in patient showing large exophytic ulcerating metastatic melanoma (arrows).

wall or in the paraduodenal area, may produce large areas of ulceration or mass effect, or both (Figure 7).

The radiographic approach and the differential diagnosis of metastatic lesions of the duodenum are similar to those in the stomach. Double contrast views are important for detecting small subtle lesions [84].

## Small bowel

Following the liver, the small intestine is the most common site of metastatic disease to the abdomen. It is also the most common intestinal site to

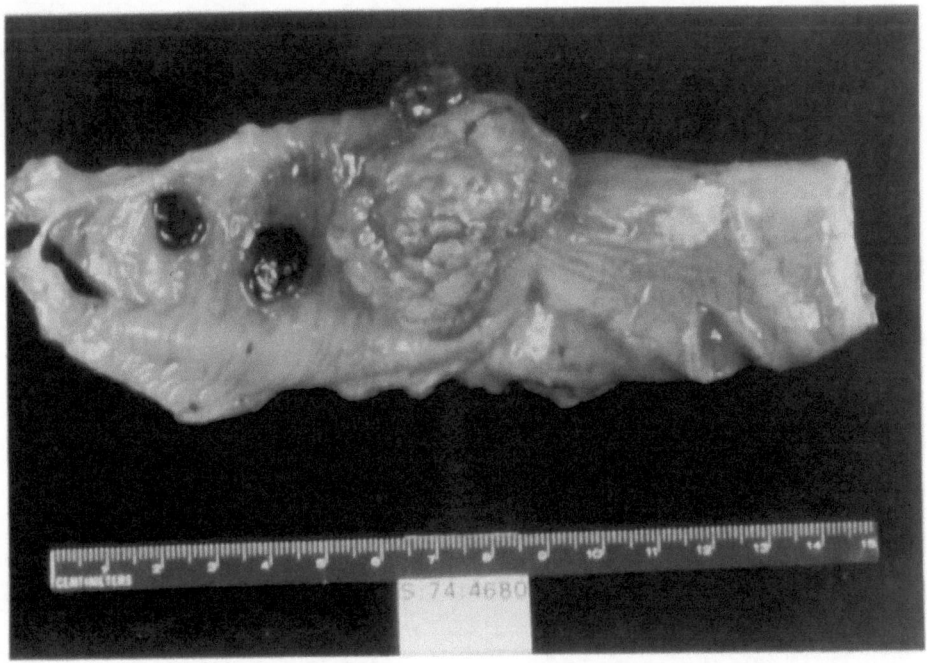

*Figure 8.* Gross pathological specimen from small bowel showing three pigmented and one larger nonpigmented metastatic lesion. Note the marked difference in size between the largest and smallest lesion.

be affected by metastatic melanoma (Table 1) [34–46]. This is probably because it receives the majority of the mesenteric blood supply. Embolic metastases usually implant in the submucosa and grow rapidly to various sizes (Figure 8). However, these tumor deposits generally do not stimulate a fibrotic reaction. Thus, there is little propensity to produce bowel obstruction unless the lesions are associated with intussusception. These characteristics suggest that melanoma in the small bowel behaves more like lymphosarcoma than other forms of metastatic disease.

Patients with metastatic melanoma to the small bowel generally present with manifestations of blood loss or abdominal pain, or both. The pain is usually due to bowel obstruction. The blood loss from the metastatic lesions is usually occult [42]; however, massive gastrointestinal bleeding can occur from metastatic melanoma to the small bowel [39, 42]. Often, patients with gastrointestinal bleeding have large excavating metastases but some may have multiple intramural nodular lesions. Patients with bowel obstruction usually present with abdominal pain and, in most cases, the obstruction is due to an intussuscepting metastatic deposit. These deposits may be either solitary or multiple. Malabsorption from diffuse metastatic small bowel melanoma can also occur [34].

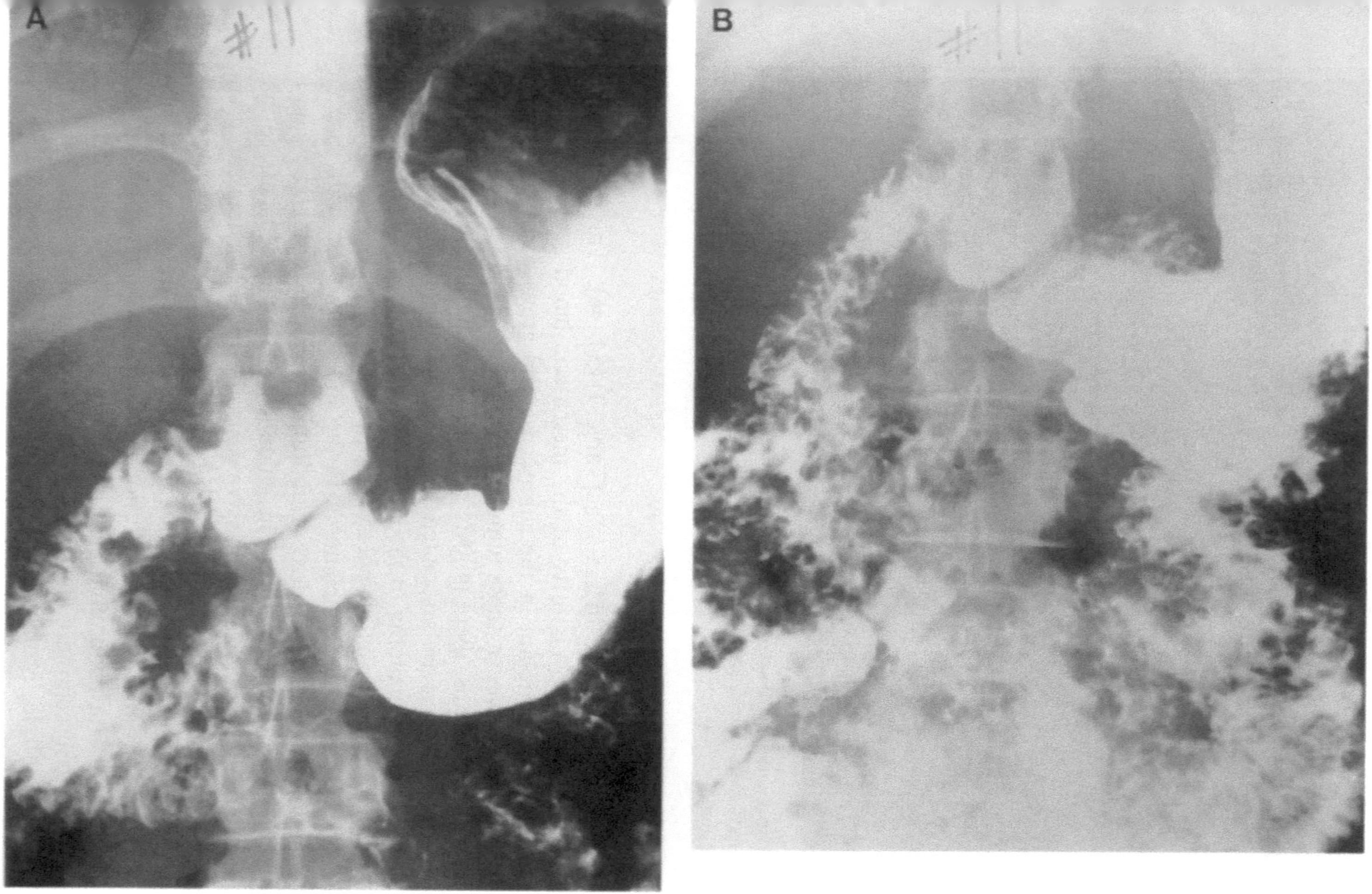

148

*Figure 9.* Two films (A, B) from an upper gastrointestinal examination and small bowel follow through showing diffuse nodularity of the duodenum and small bowel from metastatic melanoma (case courtesy of Dr. George Norton. Little Rock. Arkansas).

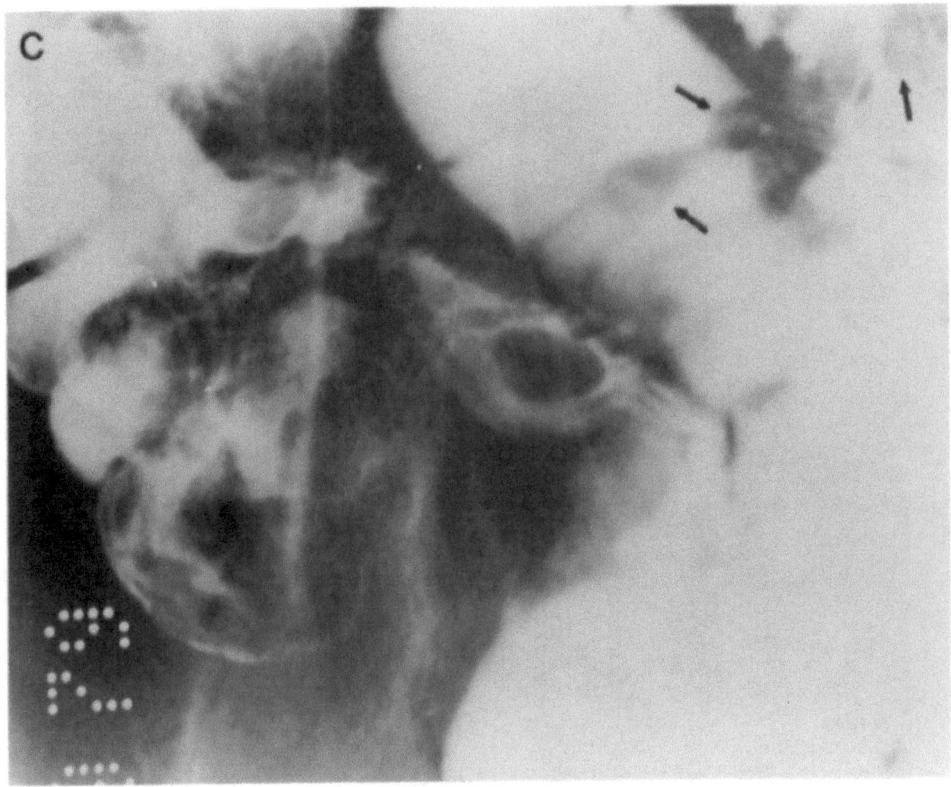

*Figure 9C.* Spot film from terminal ileum (arrows) showing numerous small metastatic lesions (arrows).

There is a wide spectrum of the radiographic manifestations of metastatic melanoma to the small bowel [11, 42]. A frequent manifestation is the presence of one or more intramural nodules (Figures 9-11). These may vary from a few millimeters up to 5-6 cm. In many instances, a definite intussusception due to submucosal lesion can be demonstrated (Figures 11-13). However, many patients have evidence of small bowel obstruction by plain film radiography but the barium studies only confirm the presence of the obstruction without identifying the exact site and cause (Figures 12, 13).

In the Duke experience, about one-half the patients had polypoid lesions and, in many of these, multiple lesions were demonstrated radiographically (Figures 8-12). In some patients, solitary lesions were demonstrated radiographically; however, multiple lesions were found during surgical exploration. The lesions vary from 3 to 4 mm up to 5 to 6 cm in diameter. While areas of necrosis were found in many lesions at surgery (Figures 14-16), we observed only one instance of a necrotic lesion producing the so-called target or bull's eye lesion (Figure 16). This lesion appears as a large, centrally

150

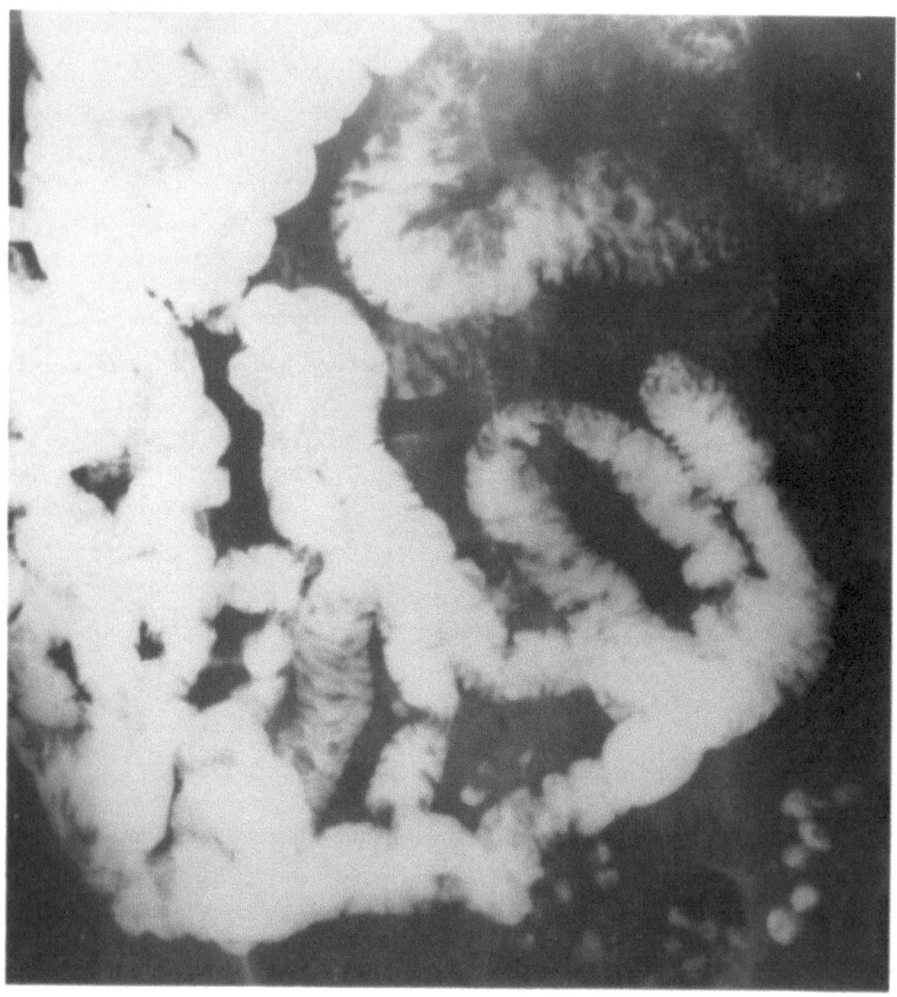

*Figure 10.* A single film from small bowel follow through examination showing multiple nodular lesions due to metastatic melanoma.

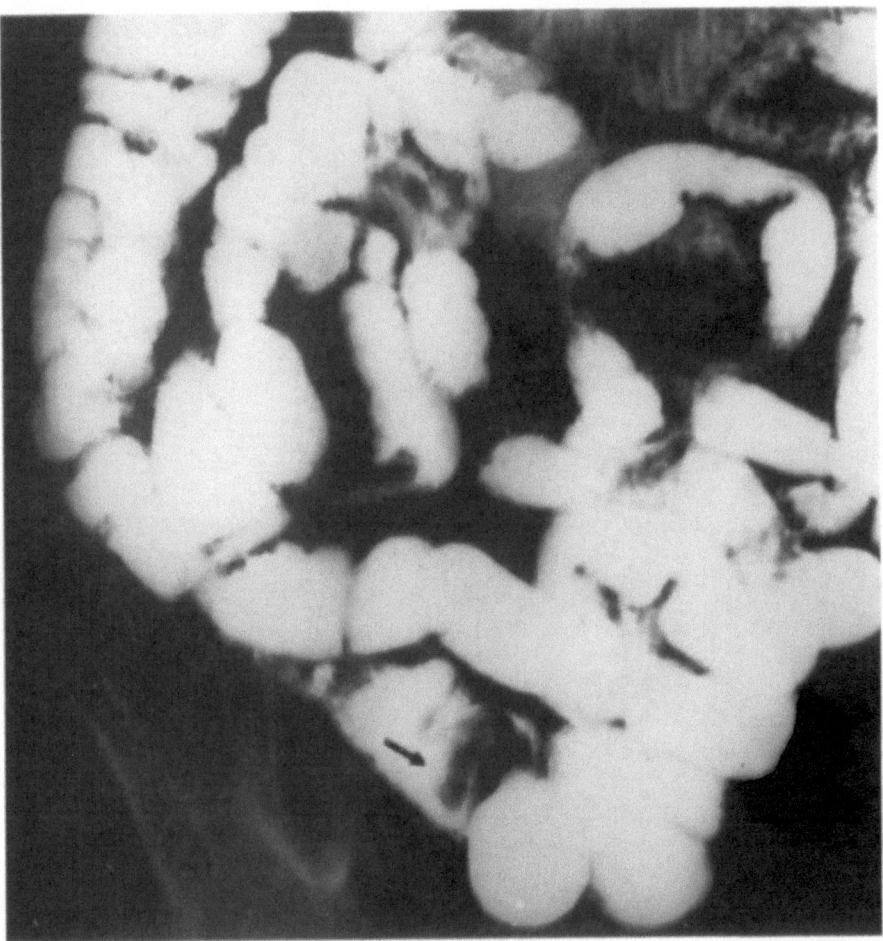

*Figure 11A.* A single film from small bowel follow through examination showing large polypoid defect in distal ileum (arrow) due to metastatic melanoma.

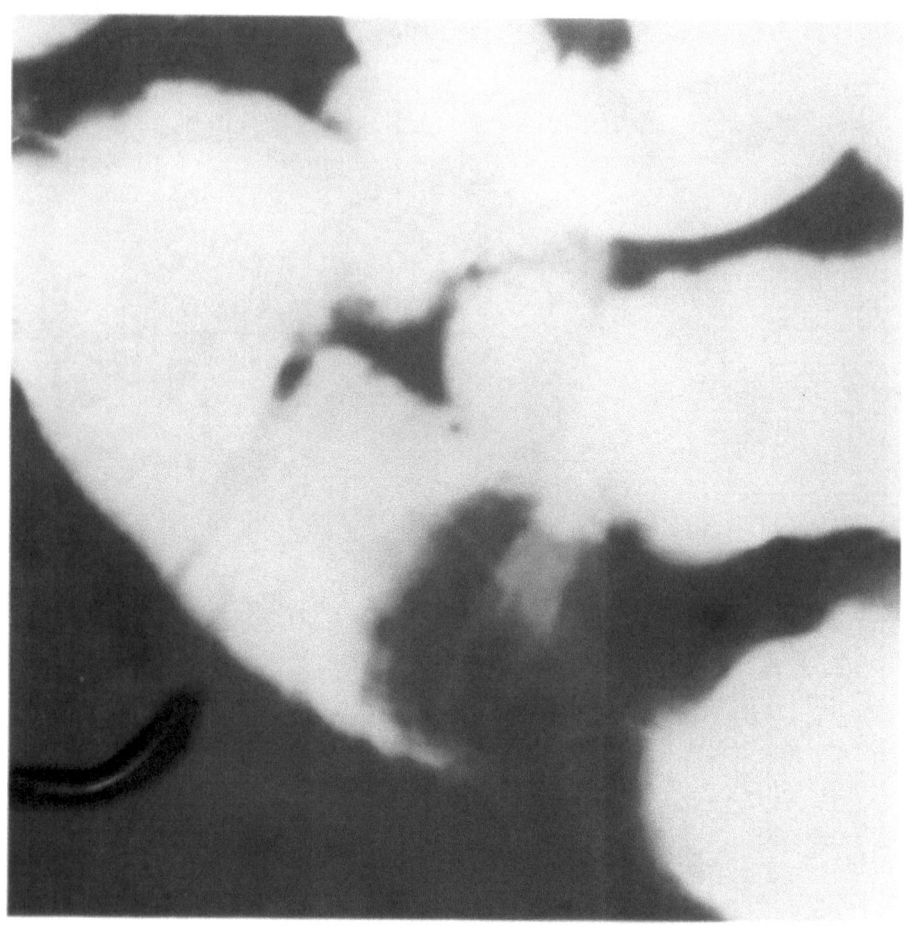

*Figure 11B.* Spot film showing distal ileum containing intussuscepting polypoid metastatic melanoma.

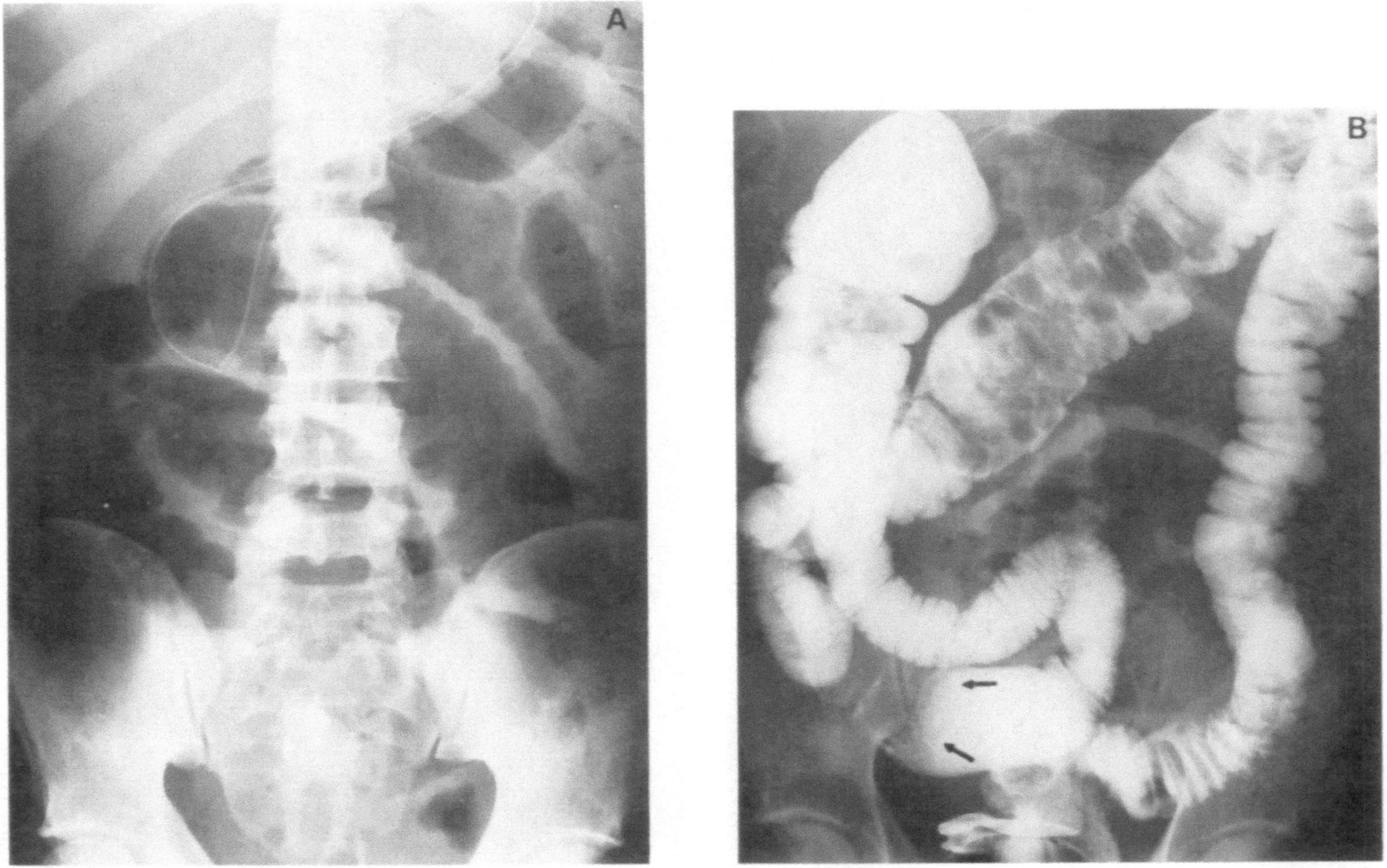

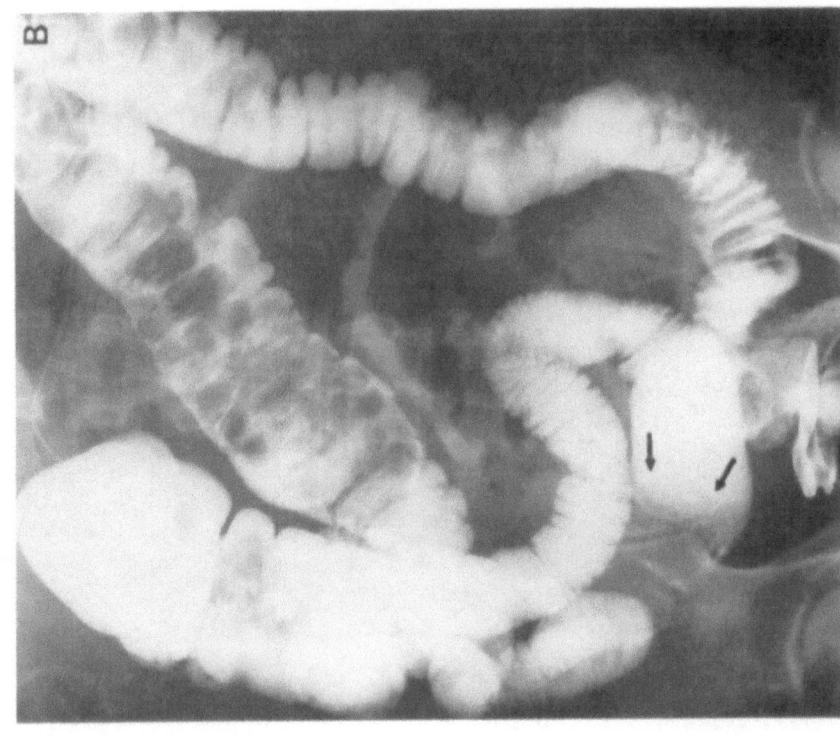

*Figure 12A.* Supine film of abdomen showing multiple dilated loops of small bowel due to small bowel obstruction. (B) Barium enema on same day showing intussuscepting polypoid mass due to melanoma in distal ileum (arrows). Intussuscepting lesion was producing the small bowel obstruction.

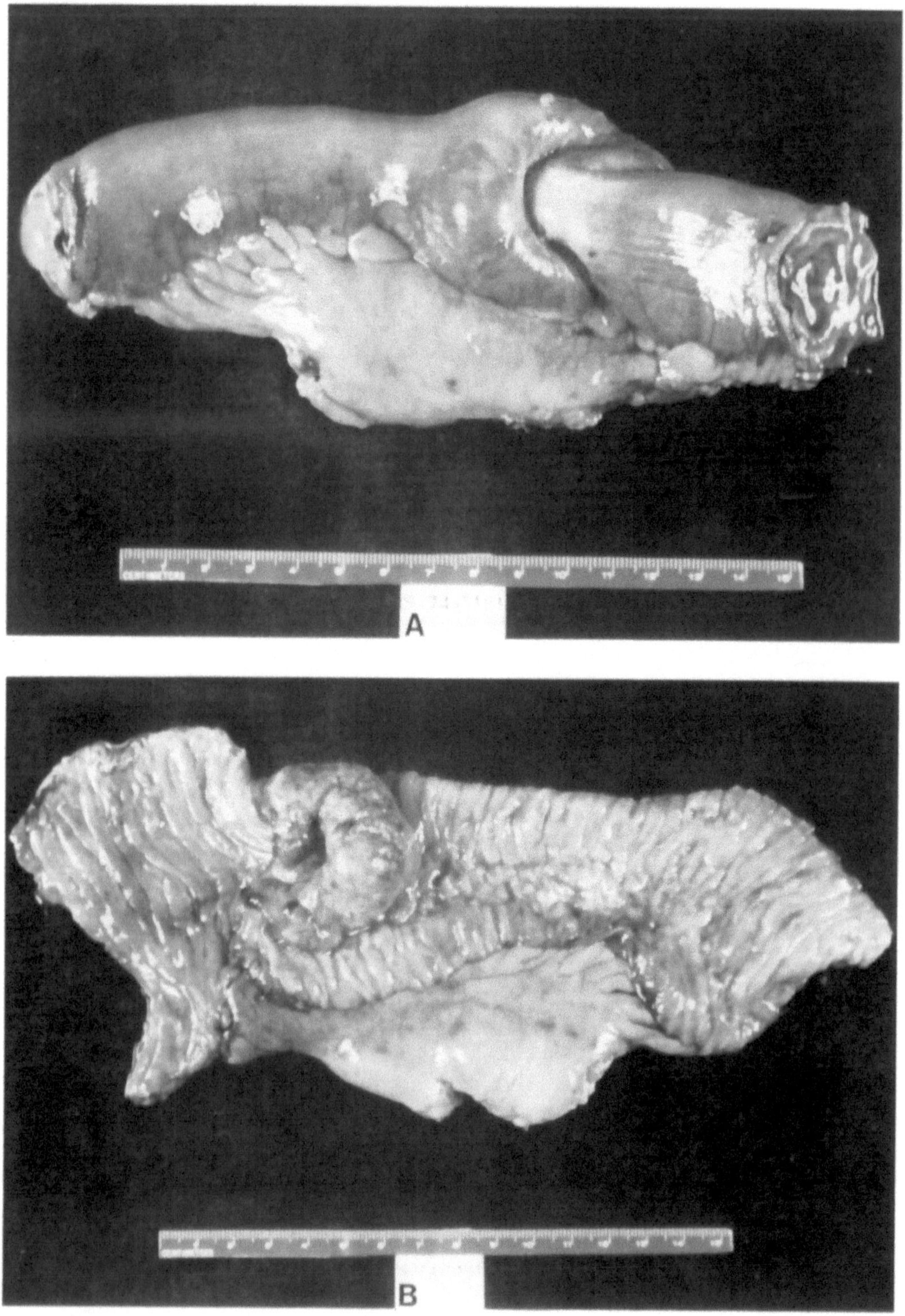

154

*Figures 13A, B.*

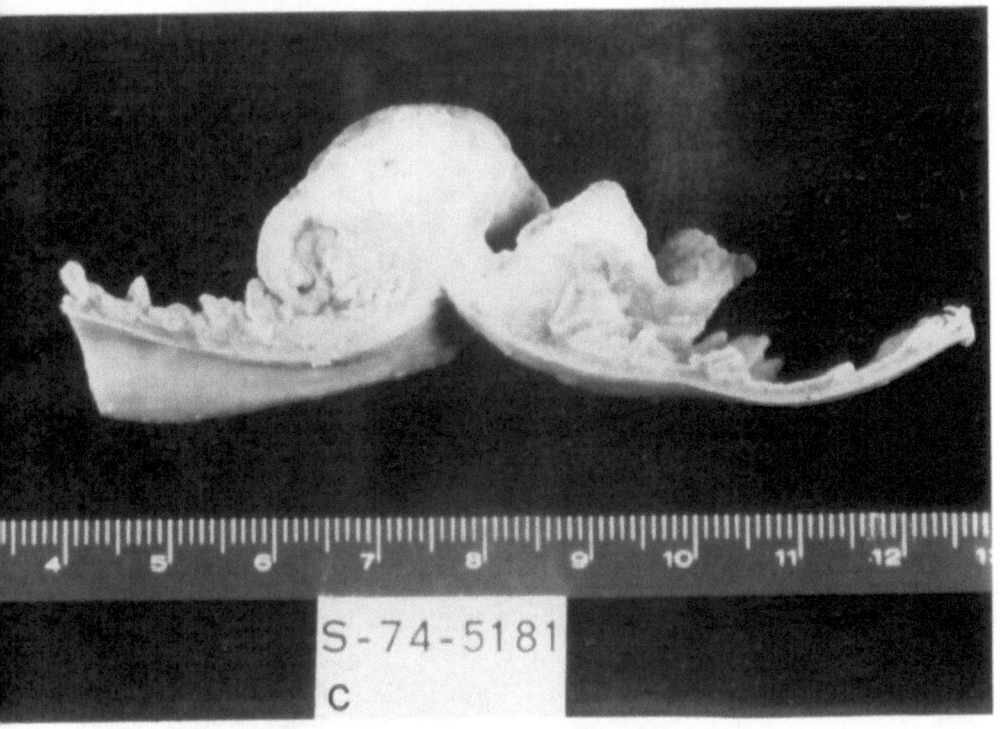

S-74-5181

C

*Figure 13.* (A, facing page) Serosal view of resected small bowel segment showing intussuscepting lesion due to metastatic melanoma. (B, facing page) Mucosal surface of resected specimen showing the intussuscepting submucosal metastatic lesion producing the intussusception. (C) Cross-section of metastatic lesion in small bowel showing the intussuscepting submucosal lesion.

located accumulation of barium within an ulceration or depression of the mural nodule. Radiographic detection of numerous bull's eye lesions of various sizes strongly suggests metastatic melanoma especially where there is a history of a previous excision of a melanoma; however, bull's eye lesions are not commonly demonstrated in the small bowel [11, 42].

The other broad category of metastatic melanoma to the small bowel is the ulcerating lesion (Figures 17–19). In our experience, the frequency of ulcerating lesions was equal to that of polypoid masses. These ulcerating lesions represent large excavating masses and vary from 5 to 6 cm up to as much as 10–12 cm in diameter (Figures 17–19). These lesions rarely produce obstruction but are very commonly associated with gastrointestinal bleeding. In one instance, massive gastrointestinal bleeding occurred from a large excavating metastatic deposit [42]. While metastatic lesions are well known to occur throughout the small intestine in patients with leiomyosarcoma and lymphoma, it has only been recently emphasized to occur with metastatic disease particularly with metastatic melanoma [46]. Many of

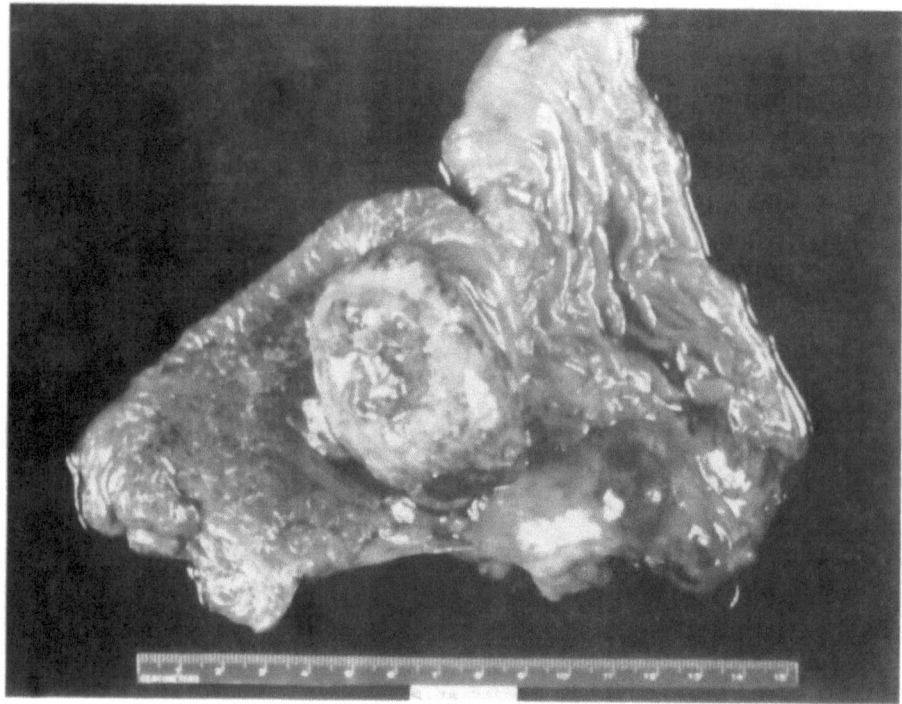

*Figure 14.* Resected specimen of large solitary ulcerating metastatic melanoma deposit in small bowel.

these lesions may mimic primary carcinoma but they are usually much larger than primary carcinoma. They rarely produce a desmoplastic reaction and narrowing of the bowel, a common manifestation of small bowel adenocarcinoma. Mesenteric metastases are discussed in a separate section.

In 1961, McNeer and Das Gupta reported that 99% of stage three melanoma patients die within one year after staging [14]. Since then surgical treatment complimented by adjuvant therapy and immunotherapy have become available. Now many patients with stage three melanoma live more than a year following therapy [42, 72–76]. In one series the average survival was three years following treatment [75]. However, malignant melanoma is an unpredictable disease because of a relatively high rate of spontaneous regression. This has led some authors to suggest that improved survival rate is due to greater clinical awareness of the disease, aggressive radiographic examination in addition to more effective therapeutic regimens [71–76]. Because of the increased chances for survival, we believe that patients with malignant melanoma who present with abdominal signs or symptoms (pain, palpable mass or gastrointestinal blood loss) should be examined by small bowel enteroclysis [42, 75]. This technique produces a continuous column

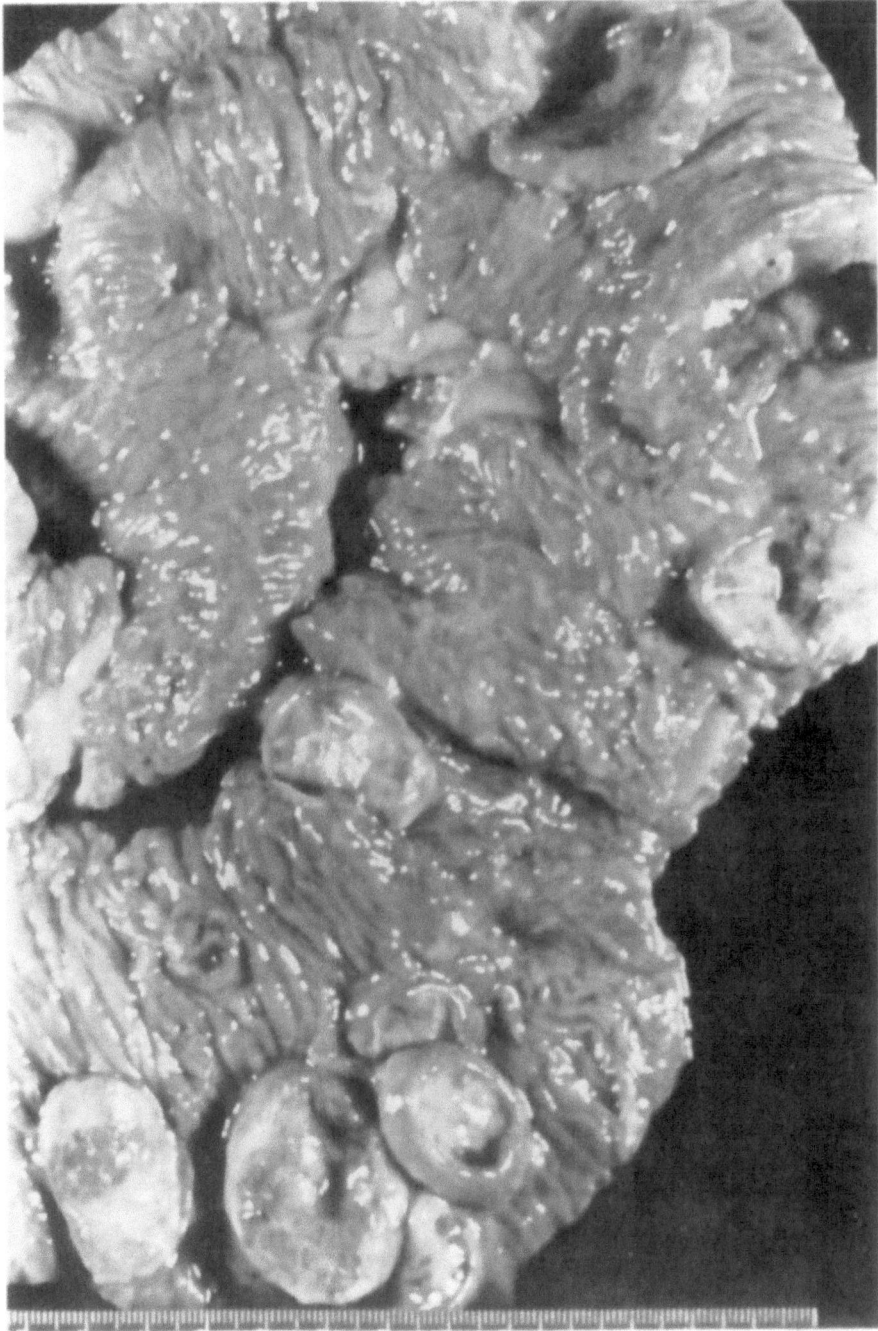

*Figure 15.* Close-up view of resected small bowel segment showing multiple submucosal nodules containing central areas of ulceration.

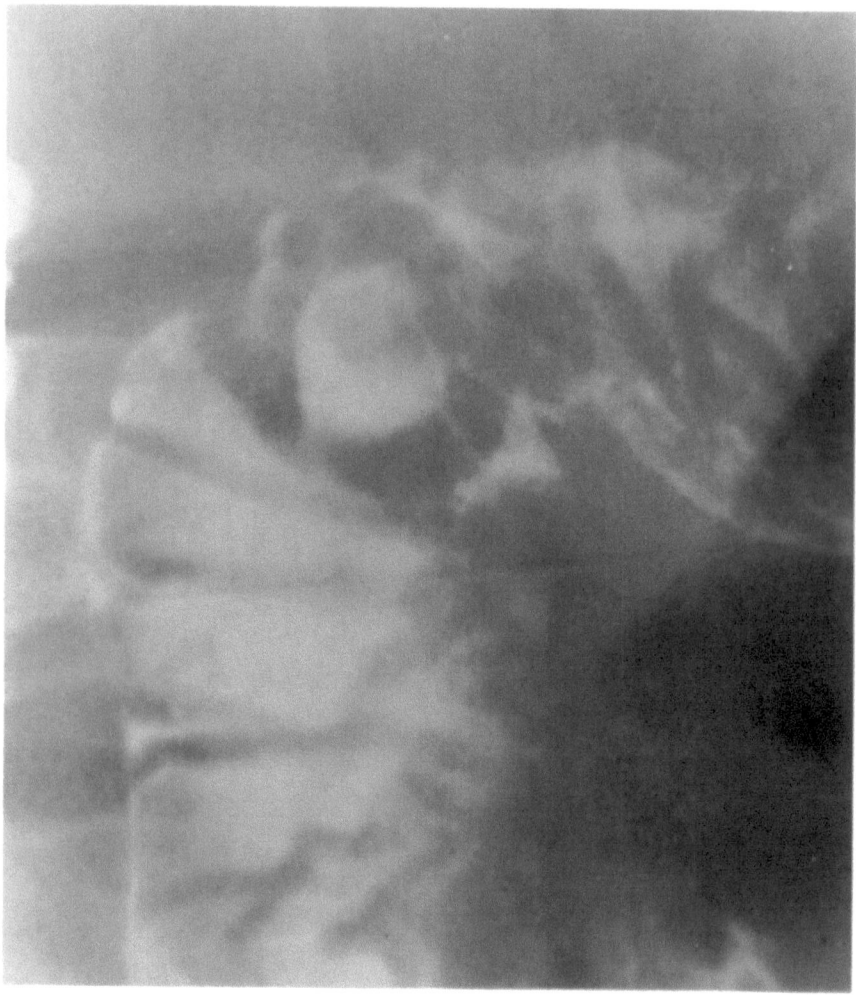

*Figure 16.* Coned down spot film from small bowel series showing the classic bull's eye lesion due to metastatic melanoma.

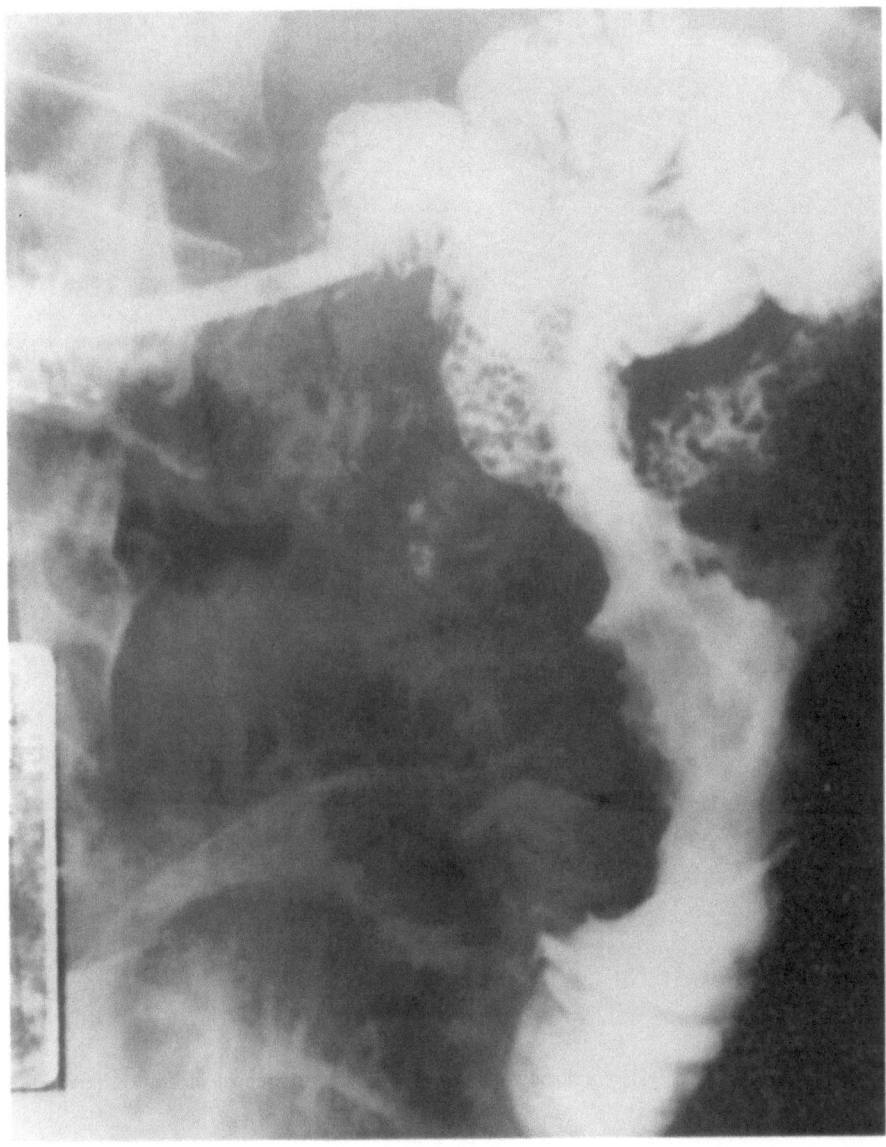

*Figure 17.* Close-up view from small bowel enteroclysis showing a large ulcerating polypoid mass in proximal jejunum due to metastatic melanoma.

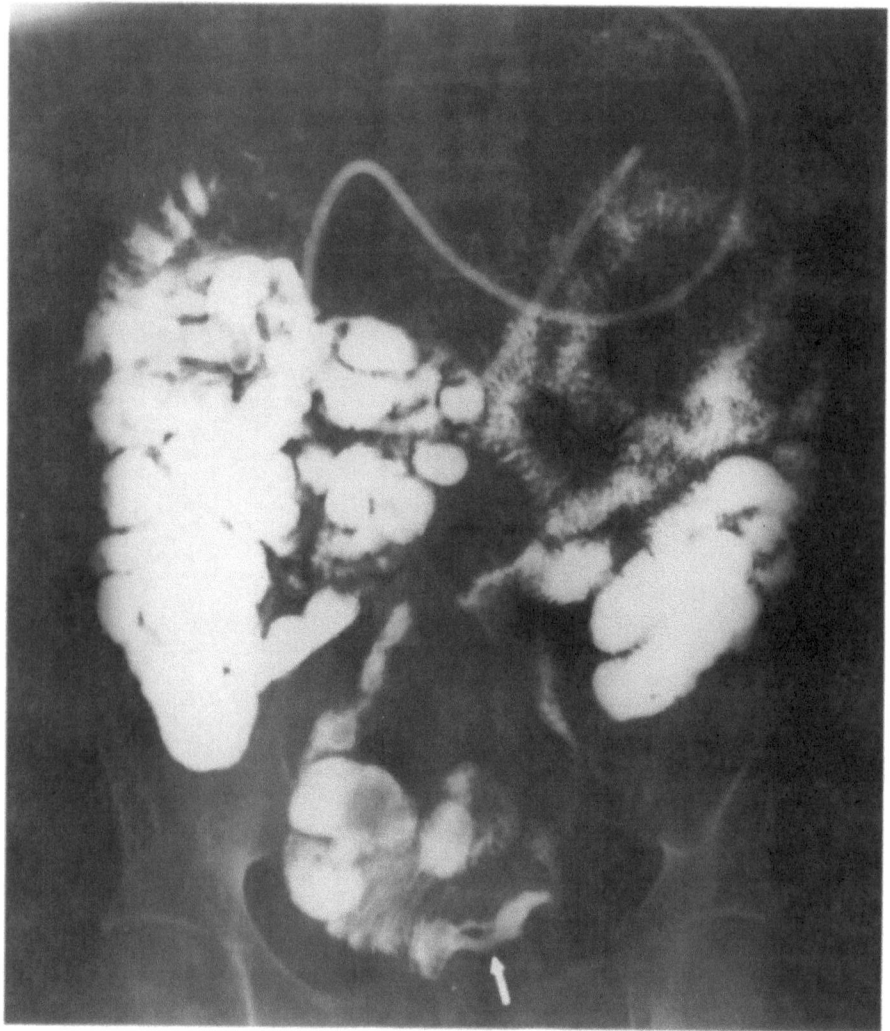

*Figure 18A.* Enteroclysis small bowel exam showing long area of ulceration (arrow).

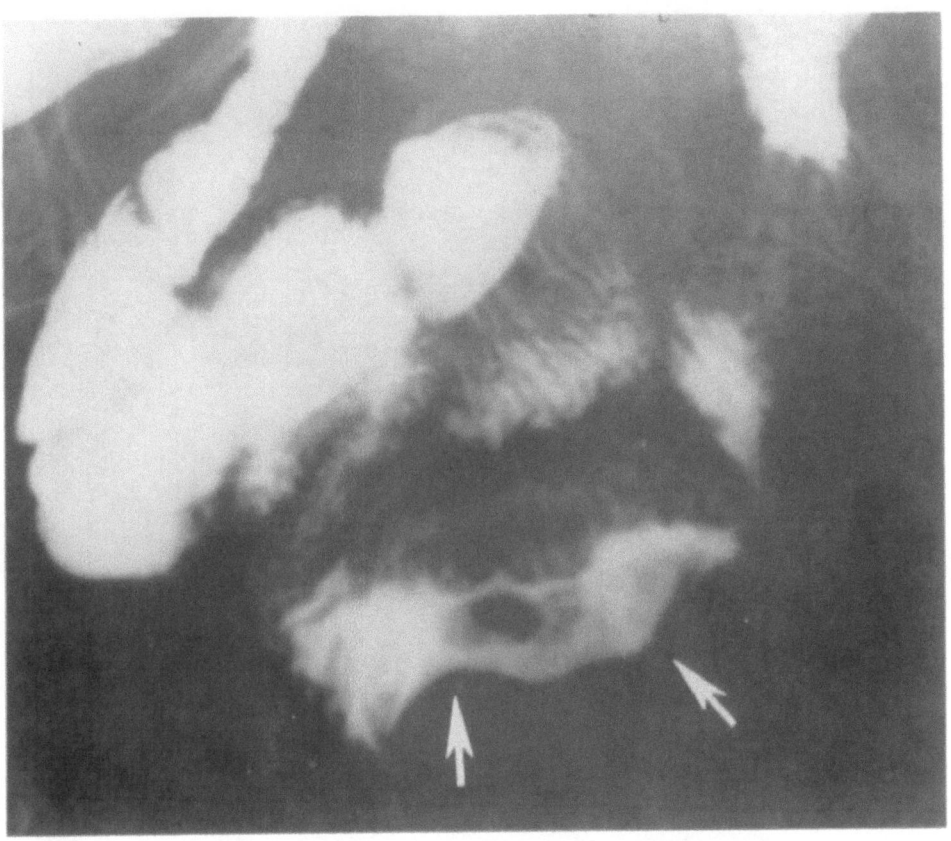

*Figure 18B.* Spot film showing the ulcerated metastatic lesion (arrows).

of barium in the small bowel and the distention of the wall of the small bowel facilitates the recognition of the polypoid lesions or contour defects (Figure 18). Enteroclysis affords sufficient advantages over the conventional small bowel follow-through examination. The applications and benefits of this approach have been thoroughly described [85–87]. However, if the clinical or plain film radiographic indications suggest any extremely distal ideal lesion, we would begin the radiographic workup with a retrograde small bowel examination using the technique described by Miller [88] (Figure 12B).

The differential diagnostic considerations of patients with either nodular lesions or large excavating lesions in the small bowel usually are limited, since most of these patients have a history of melanoma. However, without such a history, a large excavating lesion could represent a primary lymphoma or lymphosarcoma as well as a metastatic lesion from the lung, retroperitoneum or colon. The polypoid lesions could also represent hematogenous metastases. The polyposis syndromes are also a consideration. Solitary

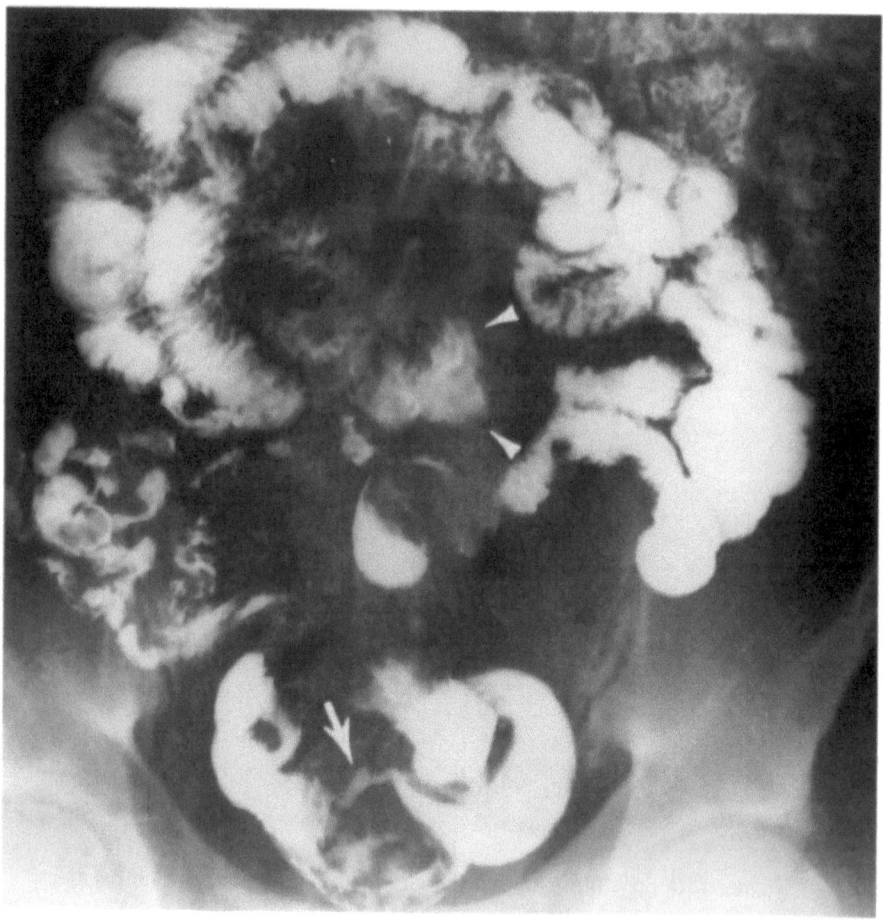

*Figure 19A.* A single film from small bowel follow through examination showing ulcerative lesion (arrowheads) as well as polypoid lesion (arrow). Both lesions due to metastatic melanoma.

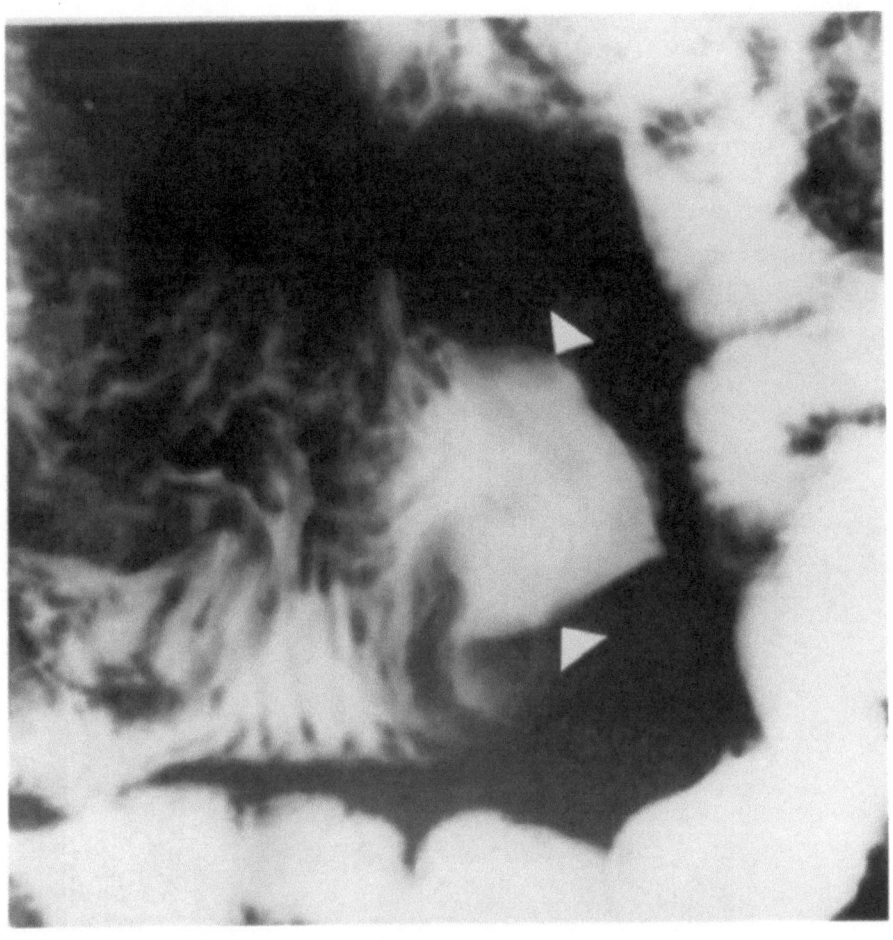

*Figure 19B.* Spot film of ulcerative lesion (arrows) in mid small bowel.

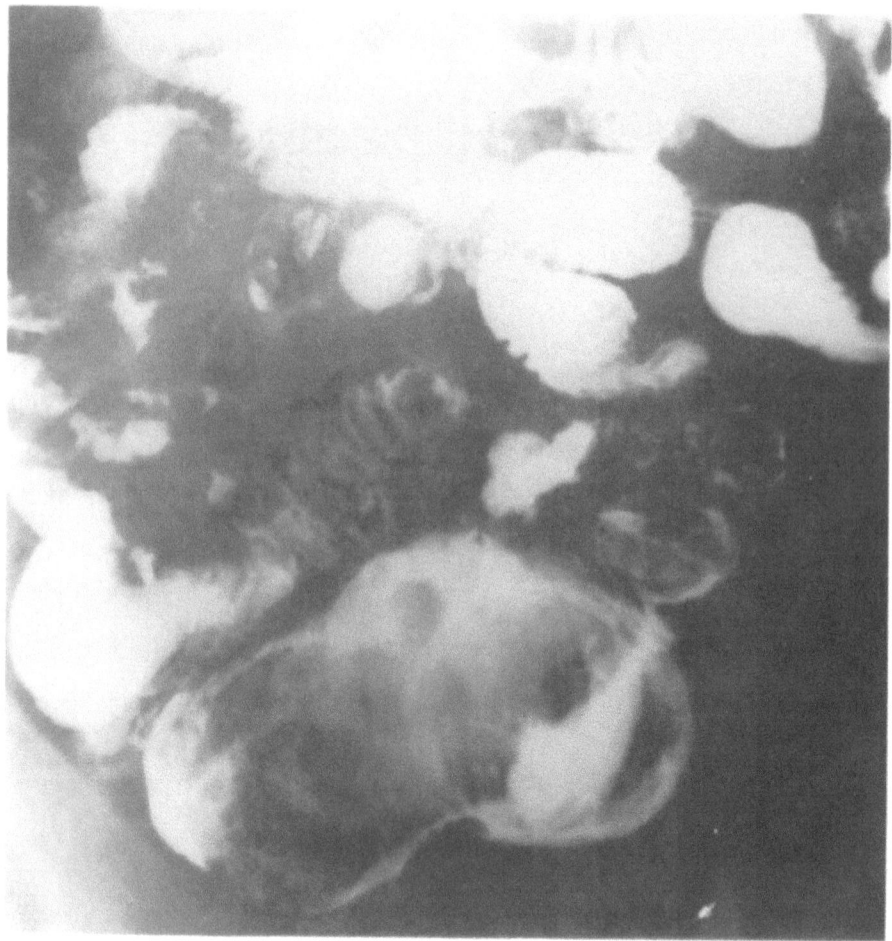

*Figure 19C.* Spot film of small bowel loops in pelvis showing larger intussuscepting polypoid lesion.

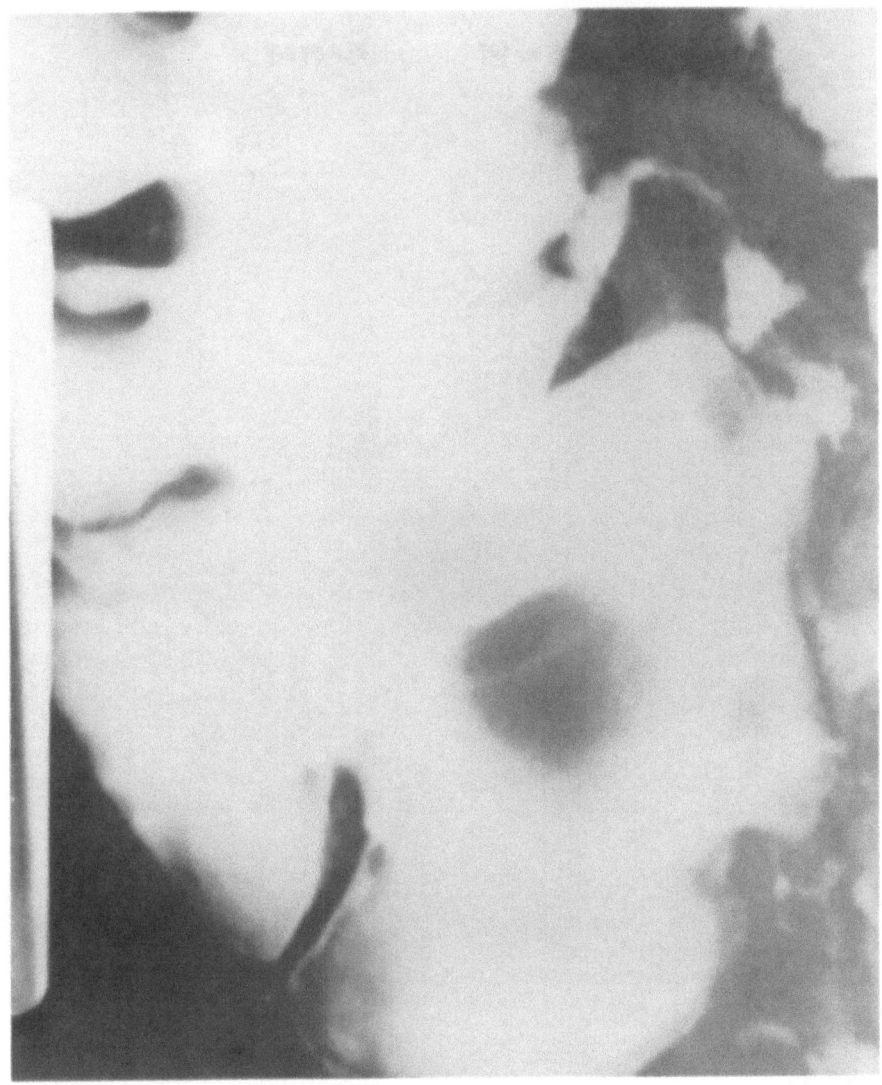

*Figure 20A*. Solitary polypoid lesion in cecum due to metastatic melanoma.

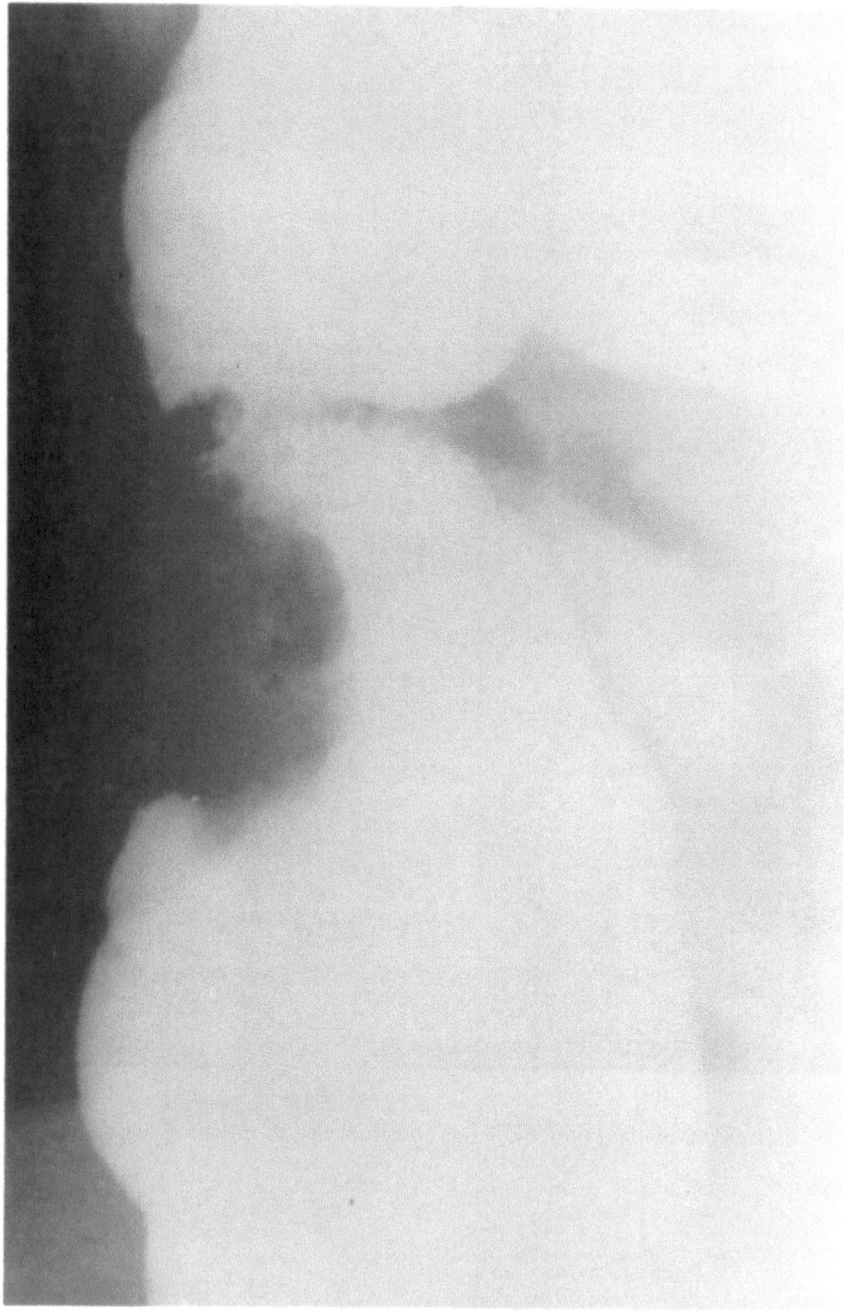

*Figure 20B.* Large exophytic metastasis invading right colon in same patient.

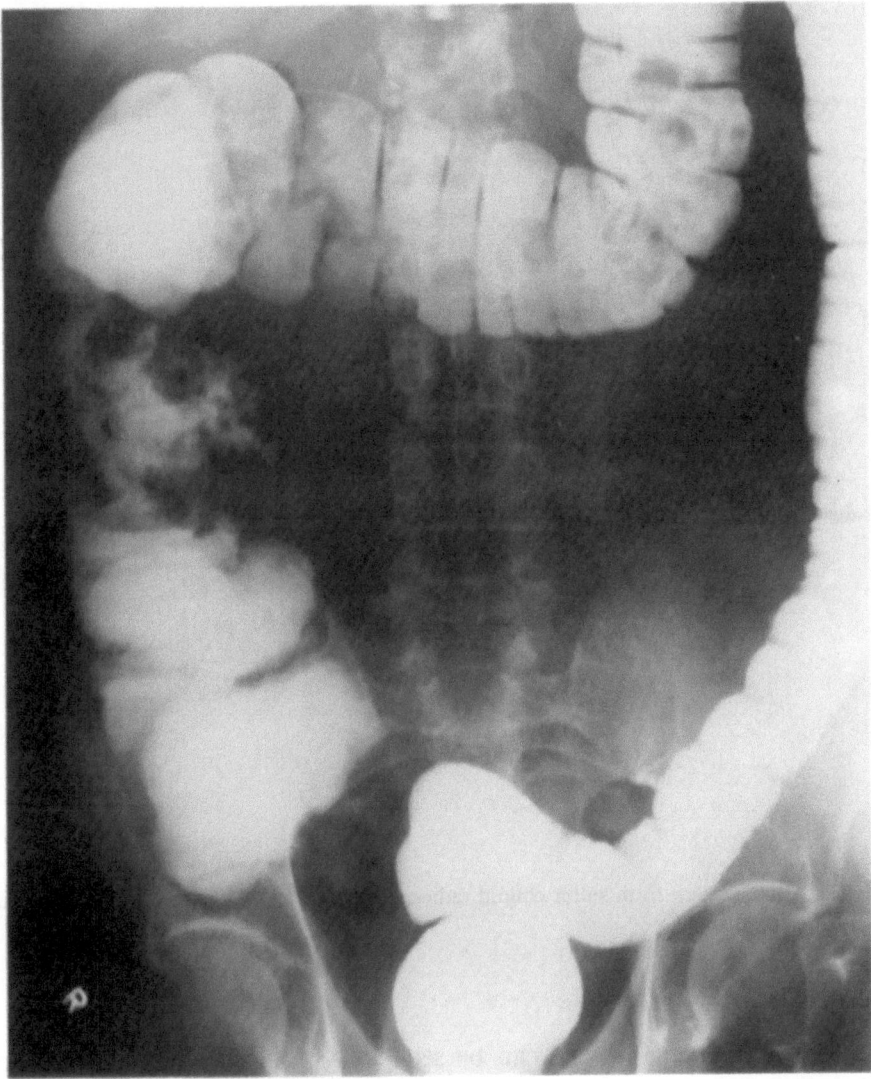

*Figure 21.* Full column barium enema showing large ulcerative excavating mass in ascending colon due to metastatic melanoma.

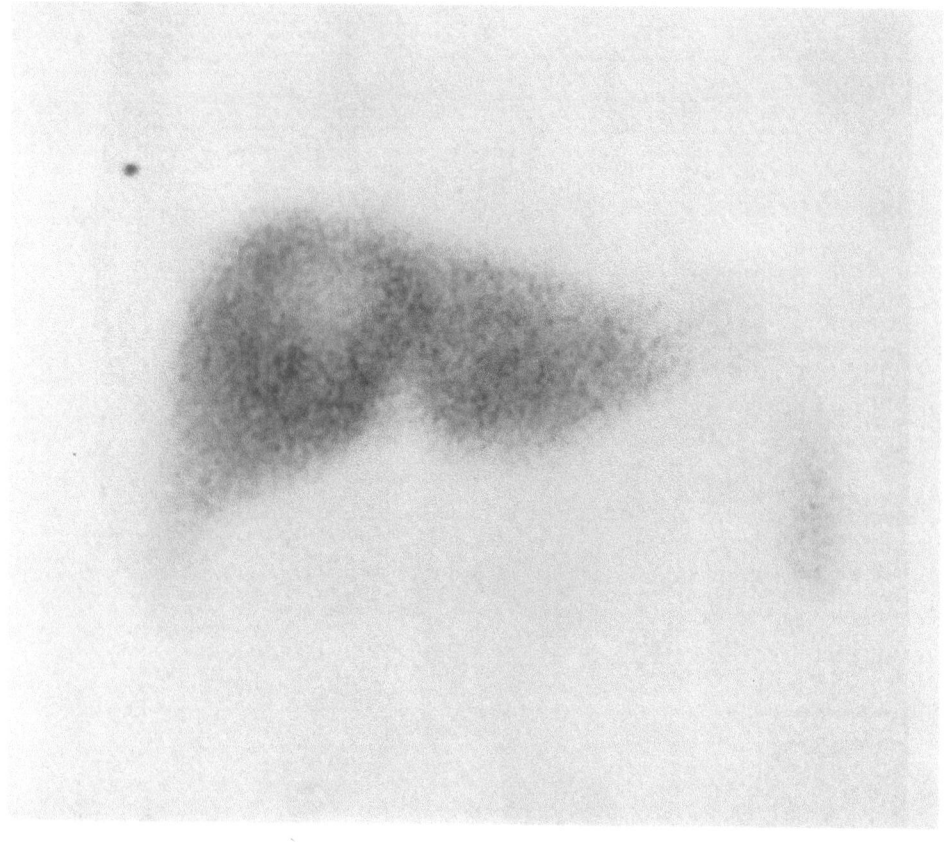

*Figure 22.* Anterior view from sulfur colloid radionuclide scan of liver showing large metastatic deposit in right lobe.

or multiple bull's eye lesions can be seen in lymphoma, leiomyomas, neurofibromas or their sarcoma counterparts [30]. Lesions which may produce a target lesion are aberrant pancreas, carcinoid tumor, carcinoma, eosinophilic grannuloma, Kaposi's sarcoma as well as metastatic lesions.

## Colon

Few colonic metastases from melanoma are discovered clinically or radiographically. Probably in part due to the infrequent examination of the colon in melanoma patients. Reports indicating the colon to be a fairly common site of metastasis in patients with metastatic melanoma are usually based on autopsy series (Table 1). On postmortem examination colon metastases occur with equal frequency to those in the stomach (Table 1). Only three of

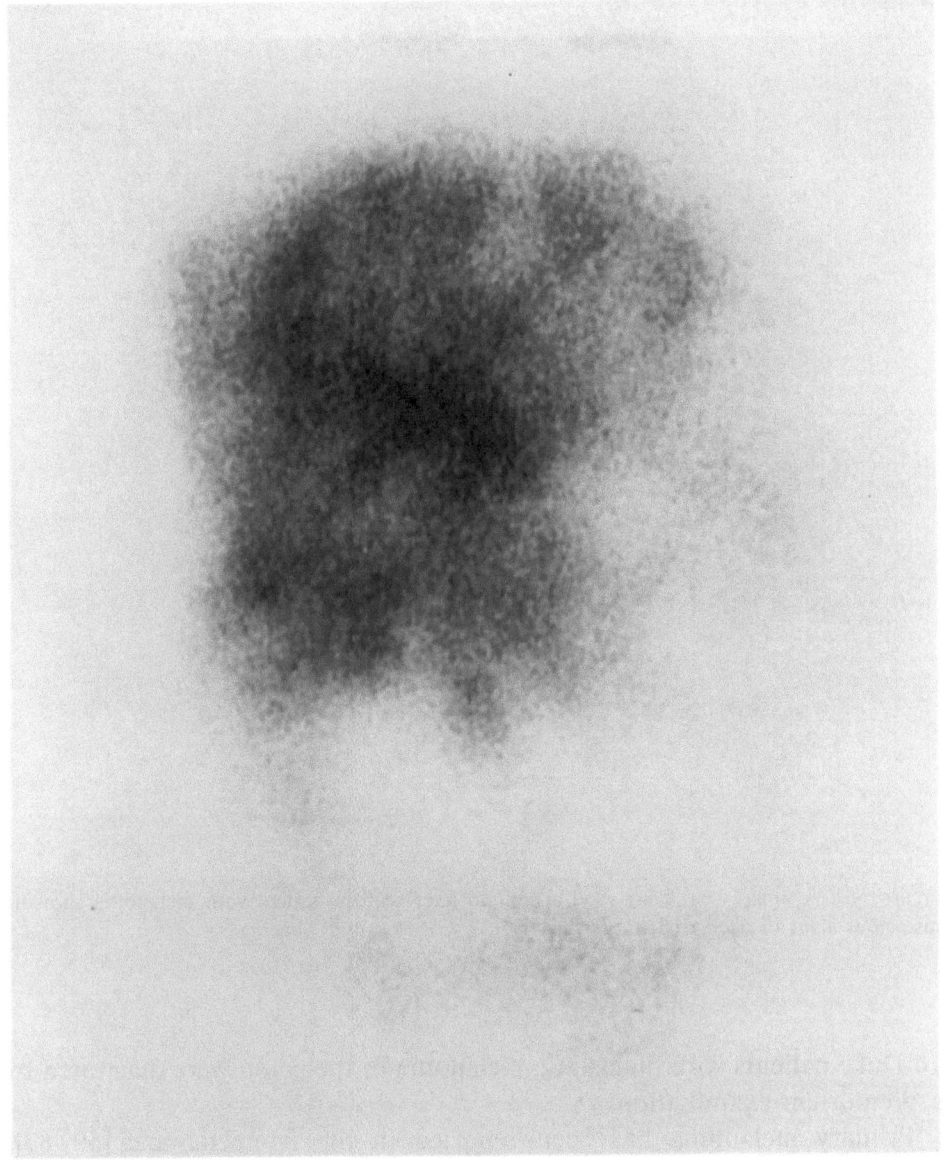

*Figure 23.* AP view of sulfur colloid liver scan showing diffuse enlargement of liver with numerous areas of decreased tracer concentration due to metastatic melanoma.

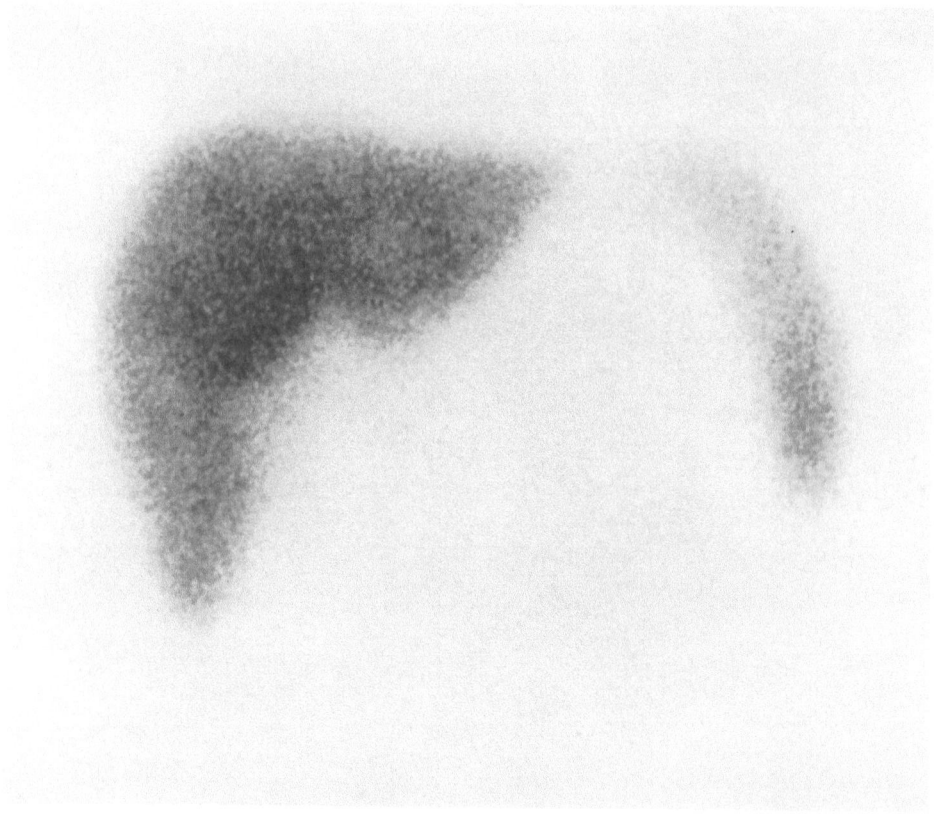

*Figure 24A.* A single view from a sulfur colloid liver scan in patient with melanoma showing suspicious areas of decreased tracer activity.

14 Duke patients with metastatic melanoma of the colon were diagnosed by a premortem examination.

Primary melanoma has been reported in the anorectal area [59–67]. These lesions may be especially difficult to diagnose when they lack melanin. Usually these melanoma patients present with symptoms similar to those of adenocarcinoma of the rectum. They will have gastrointestinal bleeding and, if the lesion becomes large enough, obstruction can occur. The anal lesions may be either intra- or extra-rectal. If they are intra-rectal, they can be identified both by physical exam and proctoscopy. Since most of the anorectal melanomas are situated at or near the anorectal line, the majority do not penetrate past the anal sphincter [59–67]. Thus, many lesions initially may be mistaken for an adenocarcinoma of the rectum. There have also been case reports of patients who had large intussuscepting metastases from anal melanoma which produced bowel obstruction [61].

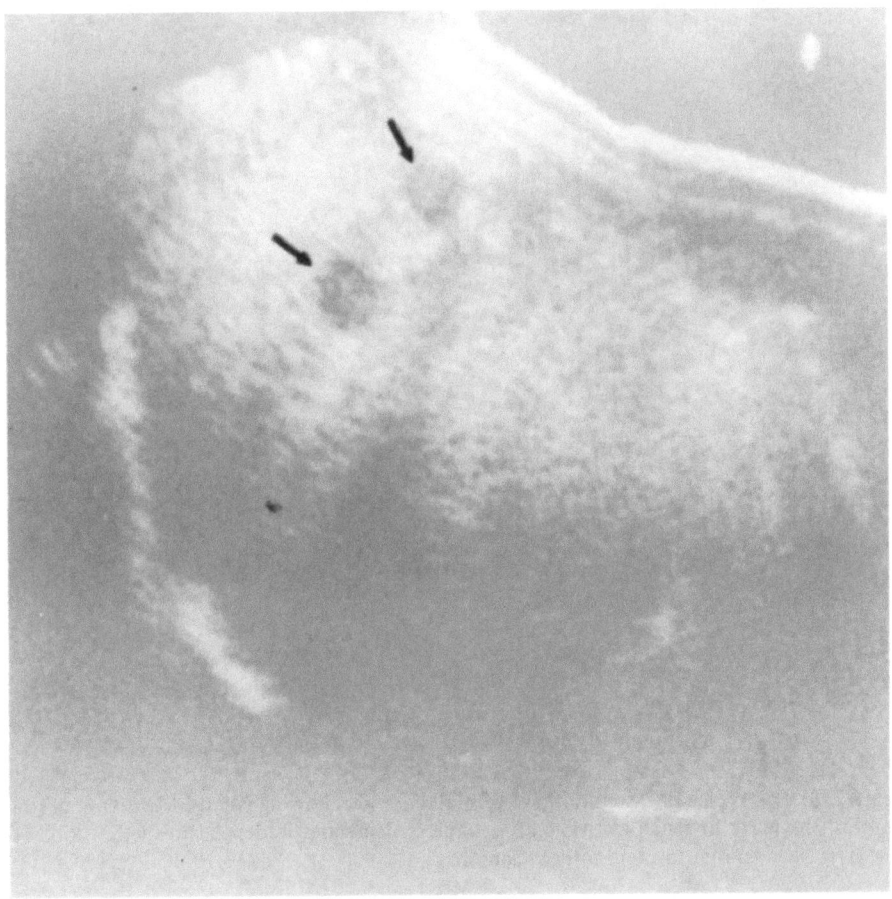

*Figure 24B.* Ultrasound confirms the presence of metastatic melanoma in the liver (arrows).

Metastatic melanoma in the colon may present as multiple polyps [89], solitary polyps (Figure 20A), intussusception, submucosal nodules, large ulcerative lesions in the anorectal region and extrinsic masses ulcerating the colon (Figure 20B) [11]. They also may present as large, bulky excavating ulcerative masses (Figure 21). A distal polypoid lesion in the ileum may intussuscept and produce ileal-colonic intussusception. This entity may be difficult to separate from a primary cecal-colonic intussusception. Large mesentery or intraperitoneal masses may also produce significant displacement of the colon, particularly in the rectosigmoid area.

In most cases there is little to consider in terms of differential diagnosis, since the patient will have a history of melanoma. Without a history of melanoma the differential diagnosis would be determined by the radiographic findings and could include primary colon carcinoma, lymphoma, metastatic lesions, cloacogenic carcinoma, villous adenoma, polyposis syndromes

172

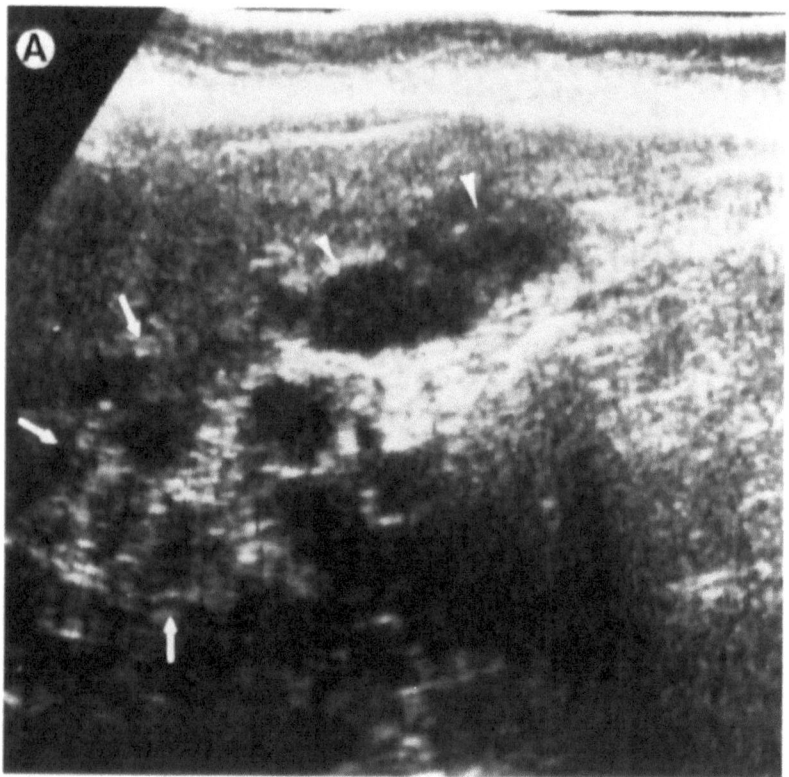

*Figure 25A.* Transverse ultrasound image of midabdomen showing enlarged lymph nodes in the region of the porta hepatis (arrows) and a sonolucent metastatic deposit in the left lobe of the liver (arrowheads) due to metastatic melanoma.

and, rarely, inflammatory bowel disease. The radiographic approach will vary depending upon the specific signs and symptoms produced by the metastatic lesion. If the patient has only intestinal bleeding, a double contrast enema may reveal lesions that appear very similar to those of primary carcinoma or multiple polyposis. If there are physical findings of bowel obstruction, then a routine contrast enema may show a stenotic, ulcerating or an intussuscepting metastatic lesion. Lesions in the anorectal area are extremely difficult to evaluate radiographically. Unless there is a significant obstructing component, we prefer to perform a double contrast enema to define the rest of the colon.

## Liver

The liver is the most common site for metastatic melanoma in the abdomen (Table 1). In one autopsy series, as many as one-half of the patients had

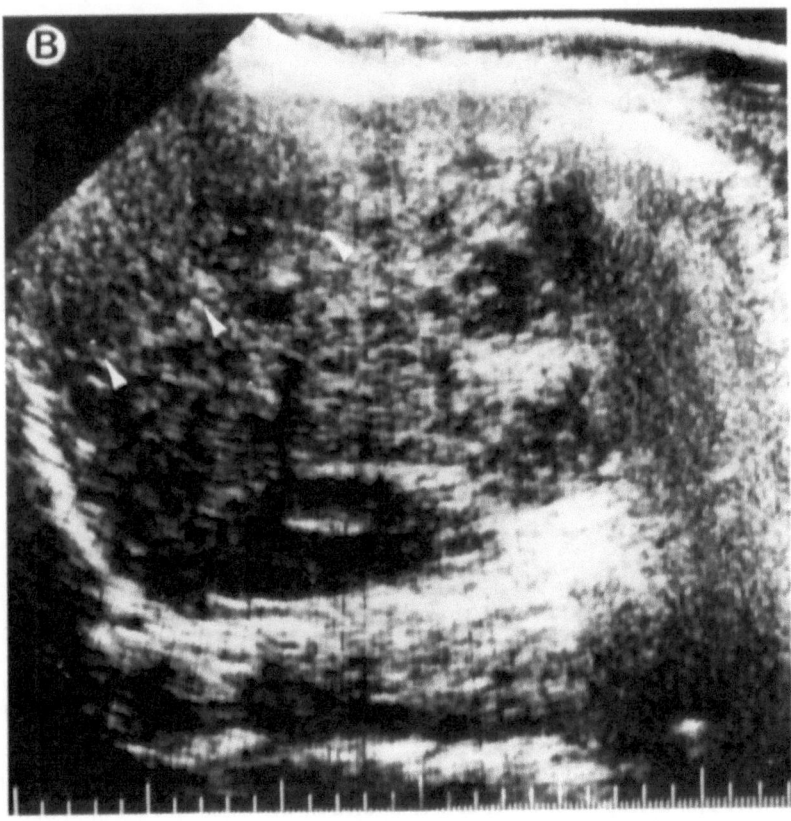

*Figure 25B.* Longitudinal scan in same patient through liver and right kidney showing diffuse increased echogenecity in a large metastatic deposit in the right lobe of the liver. Normal liver outlined by arrowheads.

metastatic disease to the liver [6]. Based on premortem examination, Goldstein et al. found 16 of the 67 patients had metastatic lesions in the liver [11]. Amer et al. reported that 14% of their patients had hepatic metastases at the time the initial melanotic lesion was discovered. In this group of patients 52% developed liver metastases prior to death. Another 24% were found to have metastatic deposits at autopsy. Thus, 76% of the patients in this study were found to have metastatic melanoma of liver at autopsy [1]. In the Duke series, about 25% of the patients who had widespread metastatic disease also had evidence of liver metastases (Table 1).

When liver-spleen scans were performed in the absence of documented metastatic disease, they were only helpful in 2% of 700 patients [75]. A liver-spleen scan may demonstrate a shift of tracer activity from the liver to the spleen which reflects either the reticuloendothelial stimulation of the tumor itself or the effect of chemotherapeutic or immunotherapeutic regim-

A

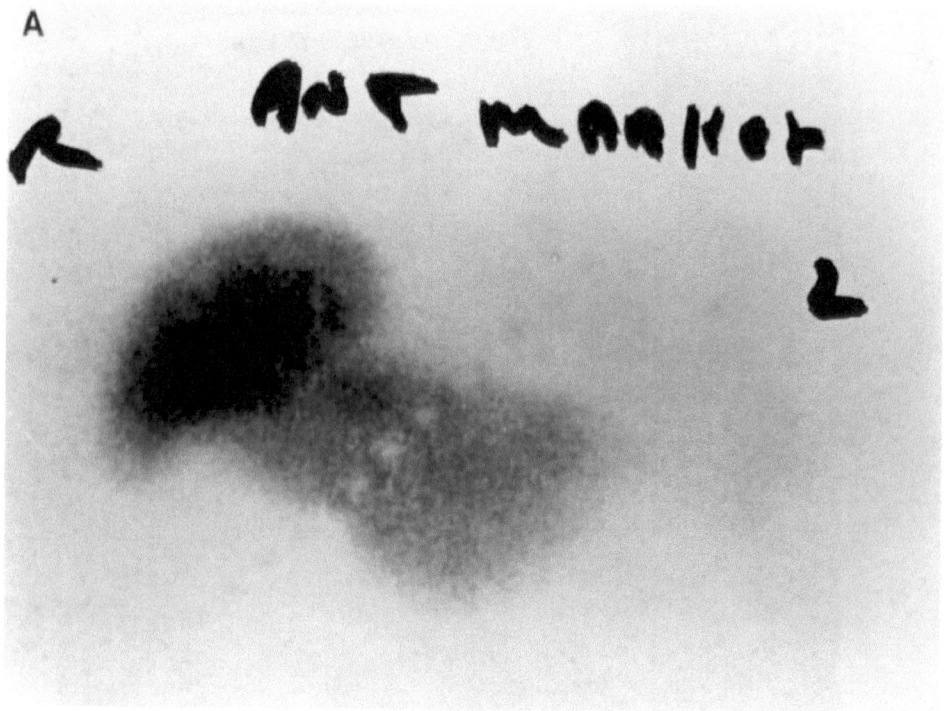

*Figure 26A.* Sulfur colloid liver scan in patient with suspected melanoma showing enlarged left lobe of liver and a suggestion of an abnormal area of decreased tracer concentration in right lobe. Findings suggest possibility of metastatic disease.

ens [75]. This type of pattern is easily differentiated from focal metastatic defects.

Unless there is massive replacement of the liver by a metastatic lesion, patients with metastatic disease may exhibit little clinical evidence of metastatic spread. For example, in one series one-half of the patients with hepatic metastases have had normal sized livers, while only one-third of patients without proven liver metastases had hepatomegaly [1]. Chemical studies measuring serum glutamic-oxalacetic transaminase and serum glutamic-pyruvic transaminase were only helpful in about 50 % of the patients and the alkaline phosphatase levels were only helpful in 77 % [1]. However, all patients with abnormal results on all three tests were found to have metastatic disease at operation or autopsy even when some of the patients had had normal liver scans [1]. Negative percutaneous biopsies of the liver do not rule out the possibility of an underlying metastasis to the liver. It is well recognized that percutaneous biopsies of the liver failed to detect hepatic metastases in about 30 % of patients with proven metastases [1].

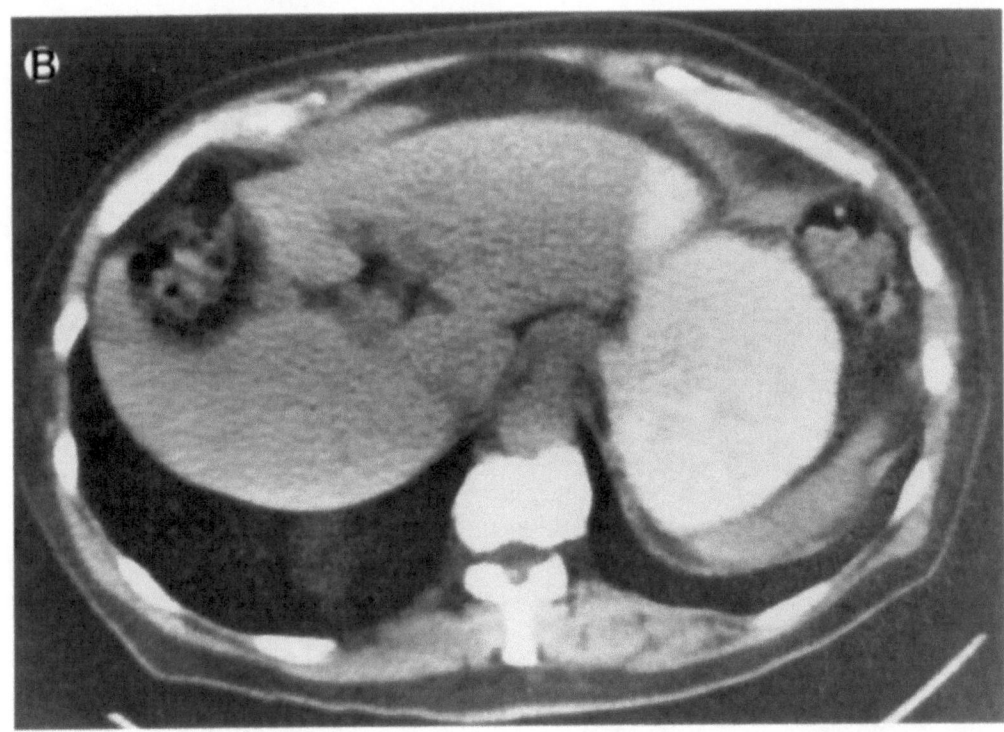

*Figure 26B.* CT scan showing the area of decreased attenuation in the liver on the liver scan due to colonic interposition. There is no evidence of metastatic disease to the liver.

Most patients with liver metastases will be suspected on the basis of widespread metastases and, thus, they will undergo a liver scan. Multiple, solitary (Figure 22) and diffuse metastatic deposits (Figure 23) may be detected by a liver scan. However, as previously mentioned a shift of tracer material from the liver to the spleen may not reflect metastatic disease but may be the result of therapy [75]. Thus, further evaluation of the liver by either ultrasound or CT may be necessary to confirm the presence or absence of metastatic disease (Figure 24).

There are a number of different echogenic appearances produced by metastatic disease in the liver [78, 82]. Unfortunately, there is no correlation between the echogenic characteristics of the lesion and its predominant tissue type [77]. There may be a well-defined, sonolucent area surrounded by normal liver parenchyma (Figures 24, 25A). Typically, fine lower level echos are noted within these lesions indicating their solid nature (Figure 25B). The so called bull's eye lesion has a dense central focus surrounded by a more lucent periphery. The periphery is, in turn, readily separable from the adjacent liver. This lesion is caused by many types of metastatic lesions. The most common metastatic appearance in the liver is the single or multiple

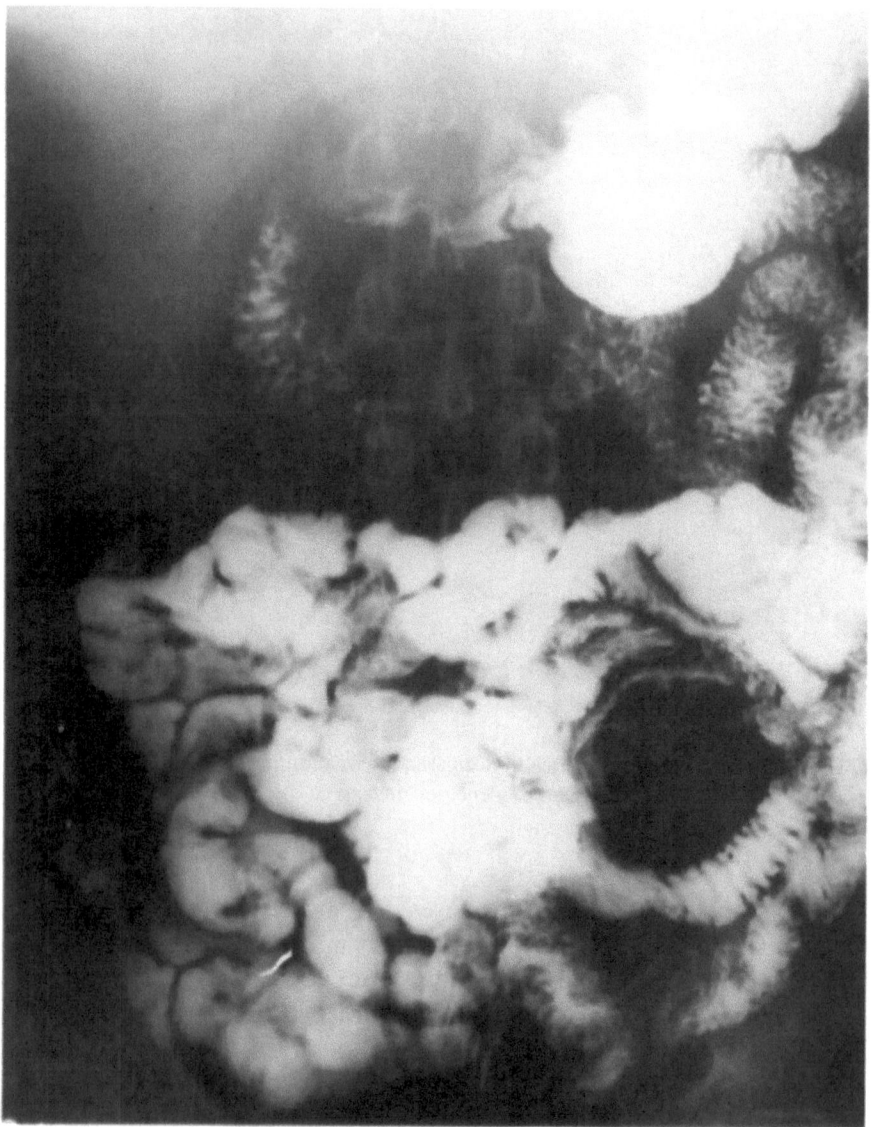

*Figure 27A.* Film from a small bowel follow through examination in a patient with a metastatic deposit to the mesentery. Note displaced loops of small bowel.

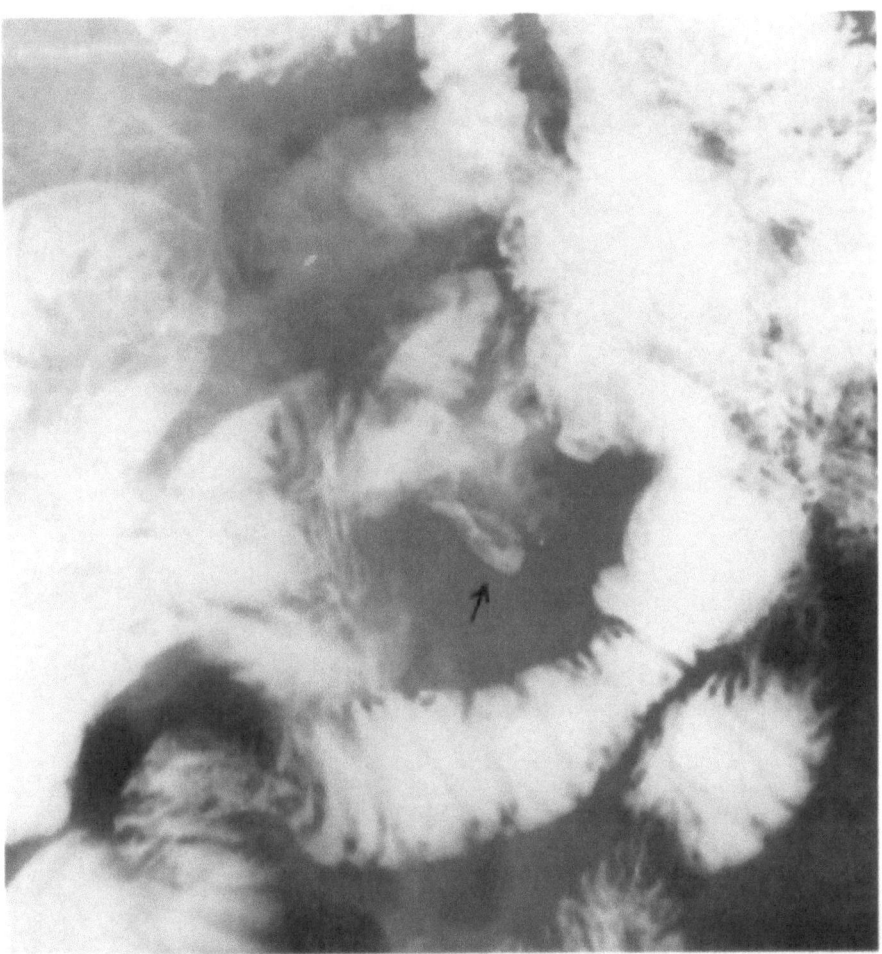

*Figure 27B.* Coned down view further along in the small bowel follow through examination of the left lower quadrant shows an area of ulceration (arrow) in the mesenteric deposit due to metastatic melanoma.

dense mass [78, 82]. These lesions can be differentiated from less echogenic surrounding parenchyma. Whether single or multiple, these lesions tend to be large, usually over 5 to 6 cm in diameter. This type of lesion is common in patients with adenocarcinoma and, although not specifically reported in melanoma, melanotic metastases could show this type of pattern. Another type of hepatic lesions is a totally echo-free mass which may simulate a cyst on the ultrasonogram [78, 82].

In addition to ultrasound, computed tomography (CT) of the liver has been used to confirm the presence or absence of metastatic lesions suggested by a liver radionuclide scan. Occasionally, congenital abnormalities have been confused with metastatic lesions in the liver and the CT scan has been

178

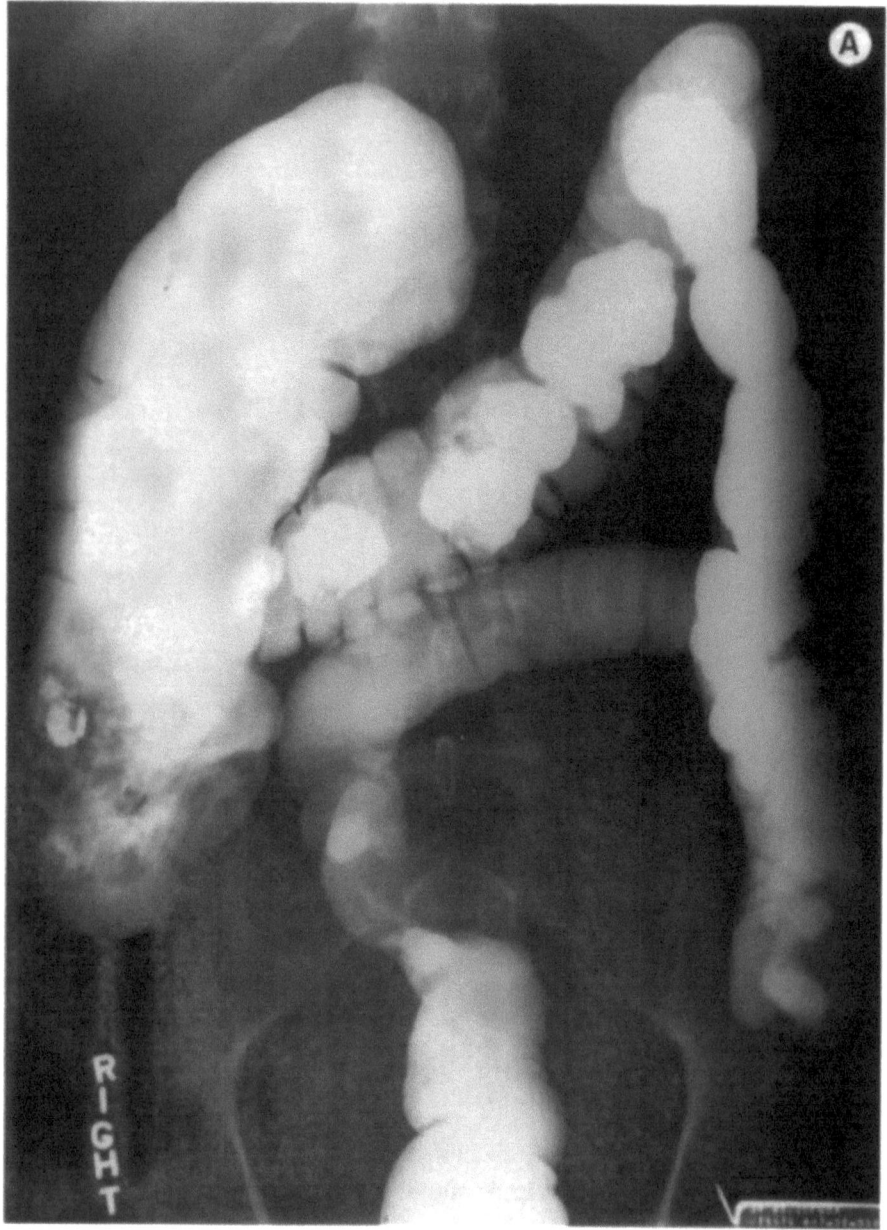

*Figure 28.* AP (A) and lateral views (B, next page) from barium enema shows large mesenteric pelvic mass displacing retosigmoid colon due to metastatic melanoma.

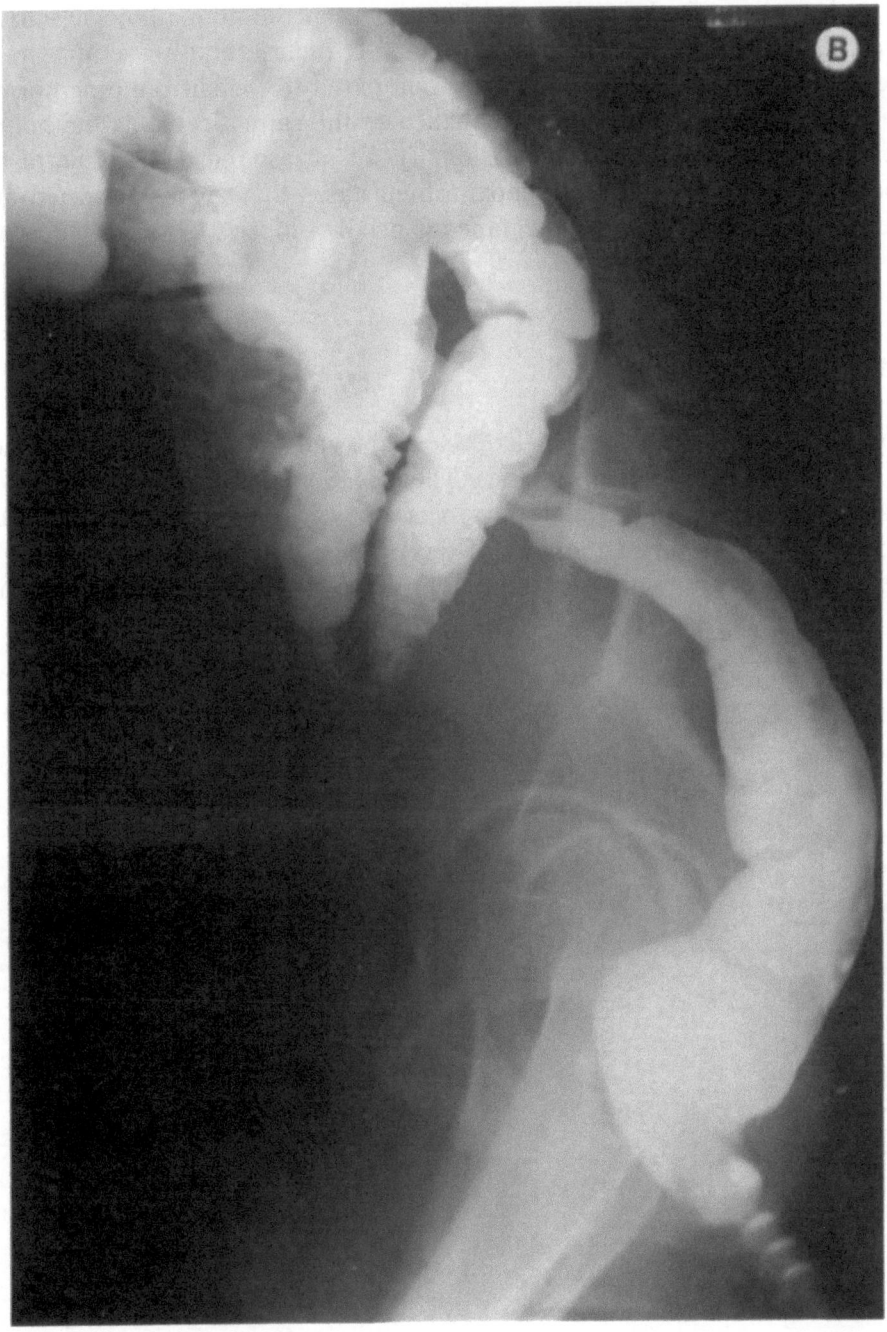

*Figure 28B.*

the principal method for distinguishing between the nonpathologic variant and metastatic disease (Figure 26). With CT, metastatic disease appears as areas of decreased radiodensity when compared to the surrounding normal liver. Also, these lesions do not enhance to the same degree as the noninvolved liver [77, 79, 81, 83]. Occasionally, an ultrasound or CT scan of the abdomen might demonstrate hepatic metastases that are unsuspected and they can be used to direct percutaneous needle biopsies of suspected metastatic lesions to the liver.

## Gallbladder

The incidence of metastatic melanoma to the gallbladder has been reported to be as high as 15 % in some series (Table 1). Some reports suggest primary melanoma of the gallbladder may occur [68–70], but since melanocytes have not been found in the wall of the normal gallbladder, melanomas of the gallbladder are metastatic lesions [11, 87–91]. Autopsy series show that

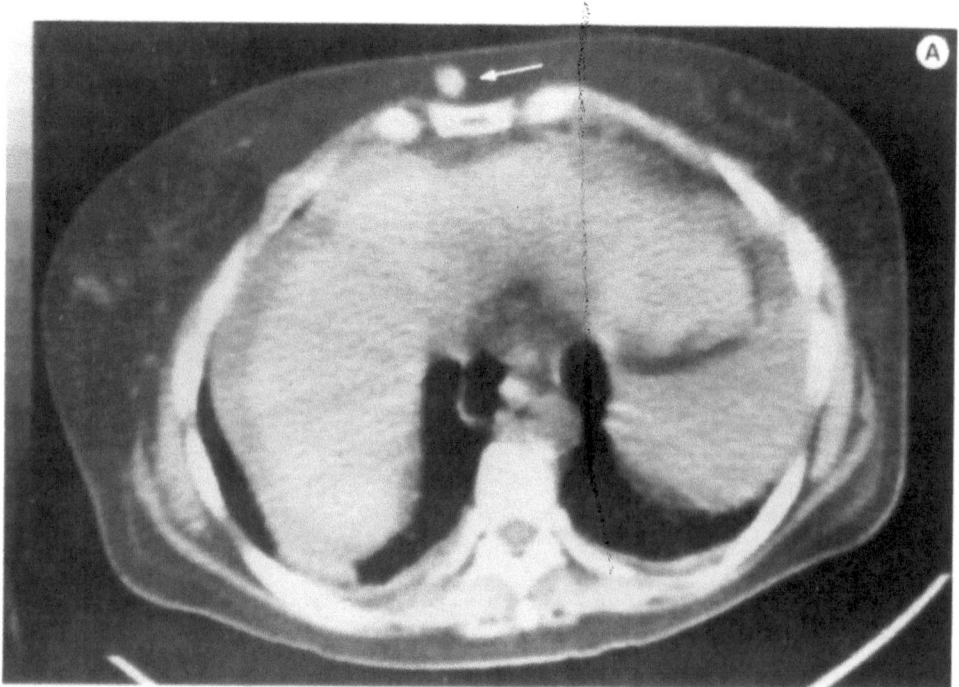

*Figure 29A.* CT scans through the upper abdomen at three different levels showing multiple subcutaneous metastatic lesions (small arrows). Ascites is present around the liver on all three scans and Figure 29C (next page) shows a large intrapancreatic metastatic lesion. There are also numerous metastatic nodular lesions in the retroperitoneum, in the region of the adrenal and kidneys, felt to be due to metastatic disease.

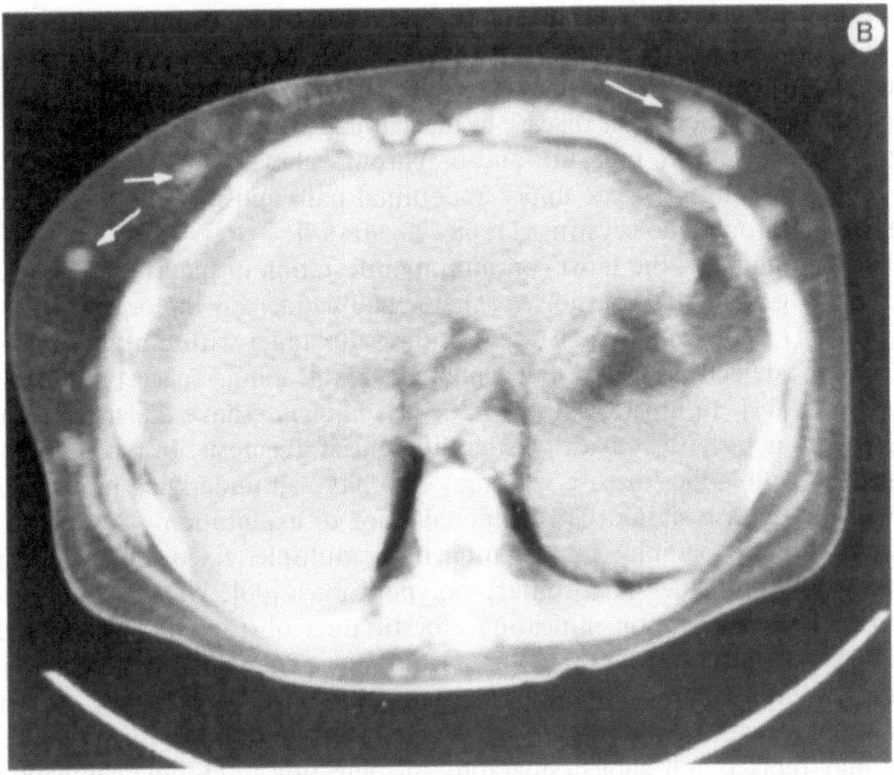

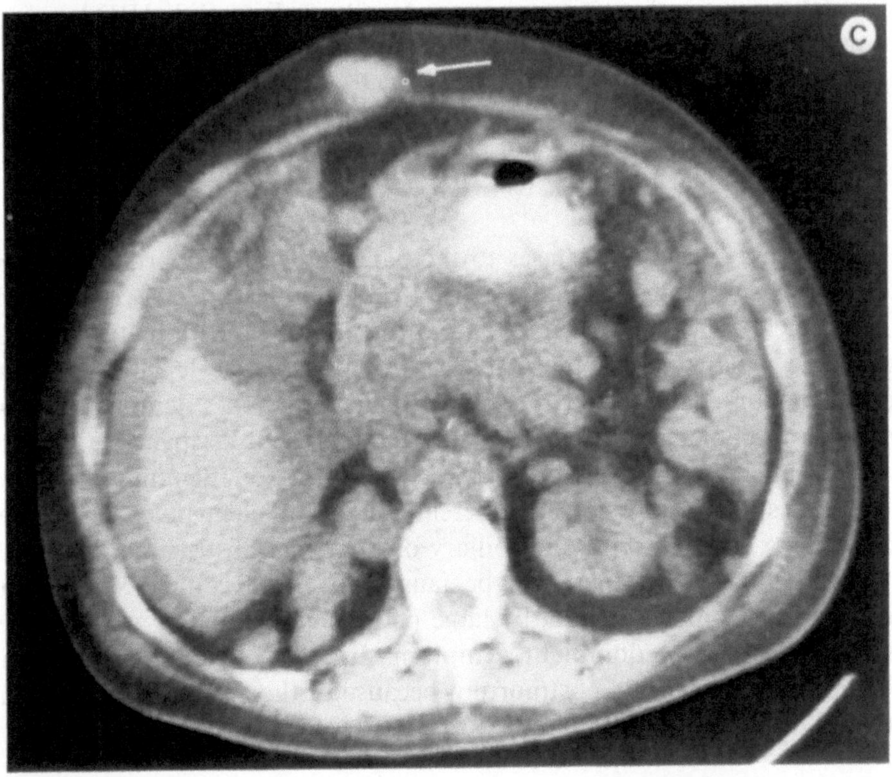

*Figures 29B, C.*

metastatic disease to the gallbladder occurs more frequently than is clinically detected (Table 1). In most cases where metastatic disease is discovered premortum, it usually is associated with acute cholecystitis [11, 90–94].

Patients with metastatic disease to the gallbladder usually present with the signs and symptoms of acute and/or chronic cholecystitis. Occasionally, patients complain of vague upper abdominal pain and undergo surgery for suspected chronic cholecystitis [11, 68–70, 90–94].

Radiographically, the most common manifestation of metastatic melanoma to the gallbladder is a nonvisualizing gallbladder on the oral cholecystogram [11]. However, visualization of the gallbladder with multiple or solitary filling defects attached to the gallbladder wall should suggest metastatic melanoma [11]. In most cases, the patient is known to have melanoma and, thus, there is little to consider in the differential diagnosis. In patients with suspected gallbladder disease who may also have an underlying melanoma, metastatic disease should be considered prior to exploration.

Oral cholecystography may demonstrate multiple, fixed filling defects within the gallbladder or a solitary polypoid mass [90]. Usually, however, there is nonvisualization indicating a cystic duct obstruction. Intravenous cholangiography is not usually used in these patients. In patients with chronic symptoms, oral cholecystography remains the mainstay for the diagnosis of gallbladder disease. However, ultrasound is rapidly changing and may replace oral cholecystography for detection of chronic gallbladder disease. If the patient's symptoms are acute, the radionuclide HIDA scan is the most appropriate initial examination to exclude acute cholecystitis [95].

## Pancreas

In one autopsy series, metastases to the pancreas and periportal area were found with a surprisingly high frequency (53%) (Table 1). However in Goldstein's clinical series there were only four (6%) patients with metastatic disease in the region of the biliary tree and/or pancreas [11]. These patients had obstruction of the biliary tree by peripancreatic nodes demonstrated by percutaneous cholangiography [11, 96]. Pancreatic and peripancreatic nodal involvement may also produce compression on the duodenum.

The metastatic lesions to the pancreatic area are silent unless the nodes become large enough to produce biliary or duodenal obstruction. With biliary obstruction, the patient will be jaundiced. With compression of the duodenum or stomach or both by large peripancreatic nodes, gastric outlet obstruction is the predominant symptom. In most series, peripancreatic involvement is diagnosed postmortem because of the absence of symptoms (Table 1).

If the metastatic mass is large, the upper gastrointestinal exam may show extrinsic compression of the antrum and/or duodenal loop by the large pancreatic mass or nodes. If the patient is jaundiced, CT and ultrasound may show evidence of dilated bile ducts and a mass in the region of the pancreas. A percutaneous cholangiogram can be used to demonstrate the location of the lesion and percutaneous biopsy may help establish a diagnosis. Percutaneous drainage of the biliary system should be considered in any jaundiced patient who also has evidence of metastatic melanoma [97–99].

The patient with metastasis to the pancreatic region would likely be known to have widespread melanoma. Thus, there is little to consider in the differential diagnosis. Metastatic lesions in the head of the pancreas and peripancreatic lymph nodes are usually impossible to differentiate from primary pancreatic neoplasm.

## Spleen

Metastatic disease to the spleen is almost always silent and usually discovered at autopsy (Table 1). Melanoma is one of the few primary tumors that

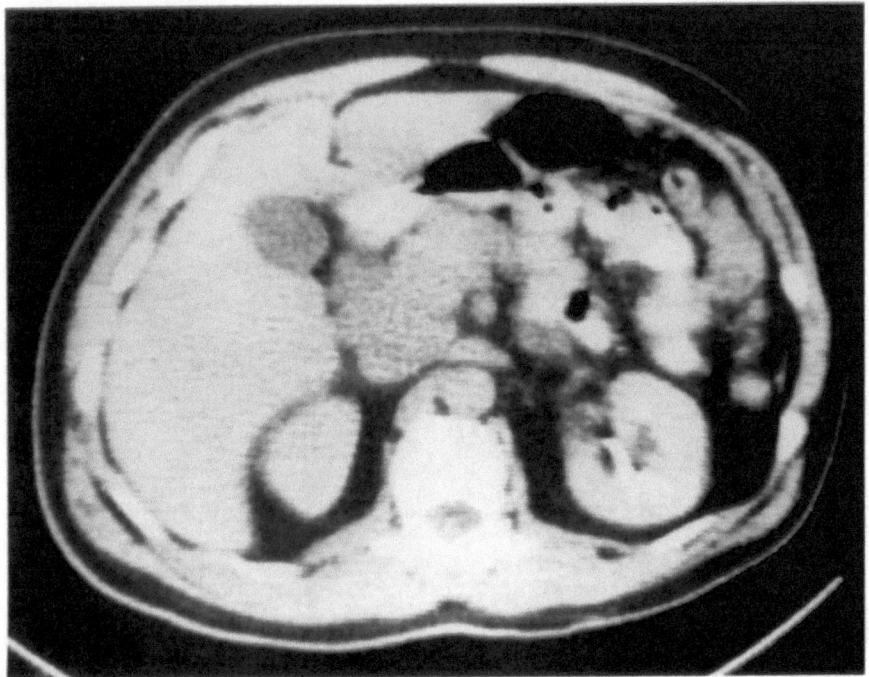

*Figure 30.* CT scan through the midabdomen in a patient with known melanoma demonstrating a large metastatic lesion in the head of the pancreas.

will metastasize to the spleen but rarely produces symptoms related to the metastasis. In most patients splenic metastasis would be an incidental finding on a nuclear medicine scan, ultrasound or CT.

### Mesentery

The mesentery and omentum can also be sites for metastatic melanoma (Table 1) [100]. In Goldstein's series eight of 67 patients had metastatic masses in the mesentery in one report and one patient had an omental metastasis [11]. We found 13 patients in the Duke series with metastatic deposits in the mesentery, primarily affecting the small bowel. Such masses are almost purely extrinsic, causing impression or displacement or both of the loops of bowel (Figures 27, 28). Goldstein et al. [11] reported several patients had invasion of the small bowel. They concluded that it is not possible to be certain if such masses originate in the bowel wall with subsequent exoenteric extension or arise in the mesentery [11]. We have had

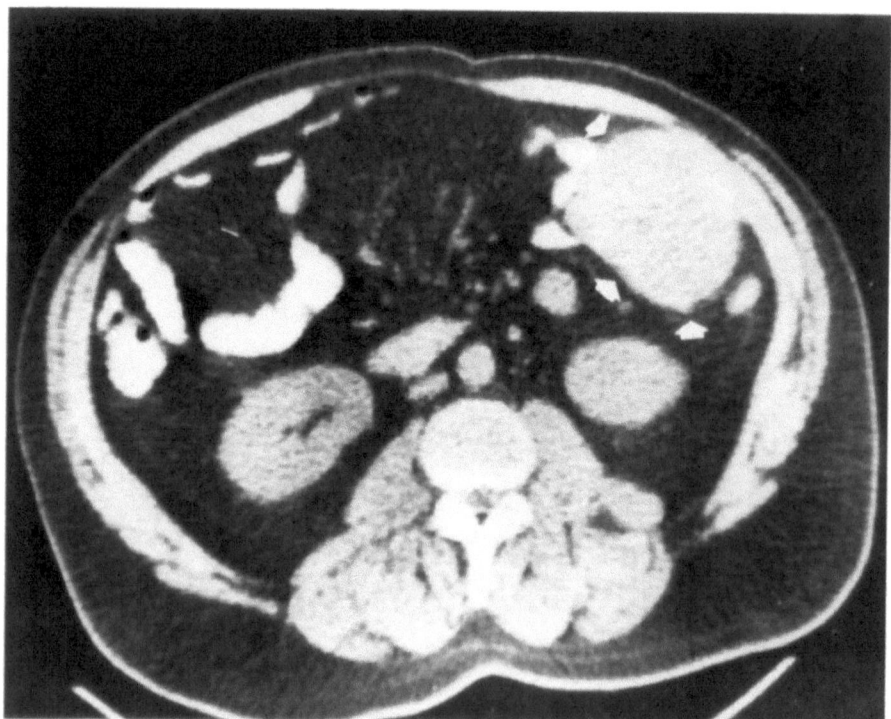

*Figure 31.* CT scan through the abdomen in apatient with a palpable mass in the left abdomen. A large metastatic lesion is demonstrated (arrows). Evaluation of CT numbers showed the mass to contain calcium which is an extremely rare occurrence in metastatic melanoma.

one similar patient (Figure 27). These metastases may invade omental and mesenteric arteries and produce significant intra-abdominal bleeding (Figure 28). Except for patients bleeding and evidence of extrinsic compression and associated with bowel obstruction, the mesenteric metastases are silent in most patients. In our study most of these types of mesenteric lesions were found at autopsy.

## Future of ultrasound and CT

Most of the 2000 patients in our study were not evaluated by ultrasound or CT. However, both of these modalities were used effectively in a few patients to prove or disprove the presence of intrahepatic disease (Figures 24, 26). CT was also extremely helpful for evaluating intra-abdominal masses and mediastinal disease (Figure 29A). A number of subcutaneous metastases were detected with CT (Figures 29A–C). Both CT and ultrasound were extremely valuable for evaluating the liver as well as the peripancreatic region (Figure 30), mesentery (Figure 31) and retroperitoneal area (Figure 32). Both these modalities have been used by others to stage lymphoma and,

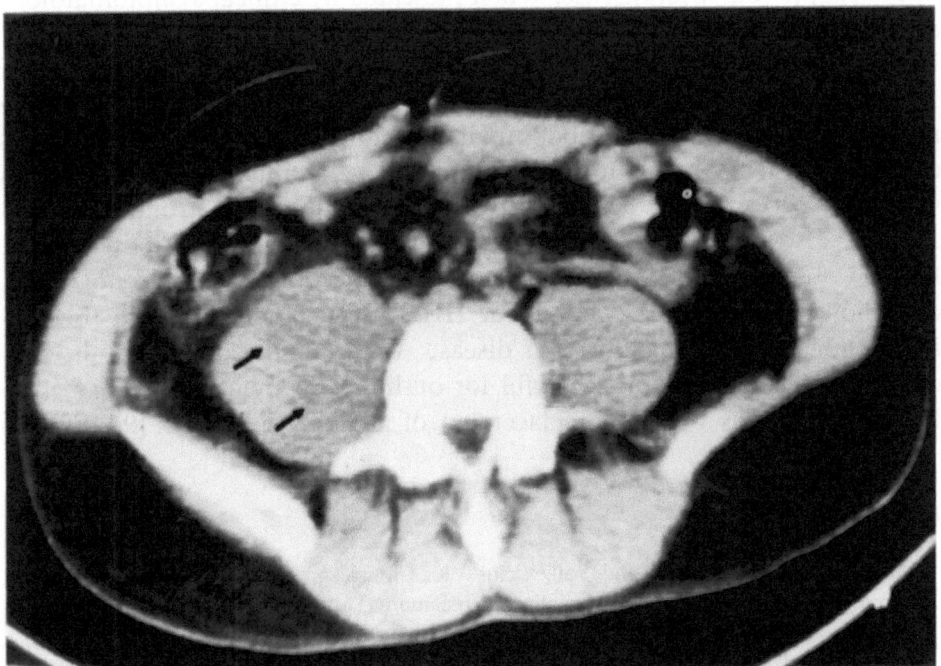

*Figure 32.* CT scan through the lower abdomen showing a low-density metastatic deposit involving the medial aspect of the right ileopsoas muscle (arrows).

186

therefore, they also could be used for the overall staging of melanoma. However, the overall accuracy of ultrasound and CT in staging melanoma is not known.

## Summary

In the past, metastatic involvement of the gastrointestinal tract indicated widespread disease and a poor prognosis. In 1965, one study reported that 99% of the patients died within one year of the first clinical evidence of visceral metastasis. The prognosis with metastasis to other abdominal sites was similarly poor [14]. Recently, new chemotherapeutic agents and combined chemotherapy and immunotherapy with disseminated melanoma have improved the prognosis for these patients [75]. Because many patients with small bowel metastases can now be treated to prolong survival, the search for metastatic disease within the gastrointestinal tract should be aggressive to permit early treatment.

It is only through the aggressive use of radiographic procedures in attempting to diagnose metastatic disease as soon as possible that one may improve the overall survival rate from this devastating disease. Patients with melanoma should undergo a screening chest examination as described in the chapter on chest disease. When indicated by clinical symptomatology or signs of chemical abnormalities, liver-spleen, bone, and brain scans may be helpful for staging the disease. Confirmation of an abnormal liver-spleen scan by either ultrasound or CT, and percutaneous needle biopsy may be necessary in many cases. If abdominal symptomatology suggests blood loss or if intermittent obstruction occurs, we believe a small bowel enteroclysis should be performed. Double-contrast colon and upper gastrointestinal exams are also important for evaluating anyone with gastrointestinal blood loss. Evaluation of the biliary system should be done by ultrasonography, oral cholecystograms, or radionuclide HIDA in melanoma patients presenting with symptoms of gallbladder disease. With jaundiced patients the percutaneous cholangiogram is helpful for outlining a potential site for percutaneous biopsy as well as for placement of a drainage catheter [97–99].

## References

1. Amer MH, Al-Saraaf M and Vaikevicius VK: Clinical presentation, natural history and prognostic factors in advanced malignant melanoma. Surg Gynecol Obstet 149:687–692, 1979.
2. Backman H: Metastasis of malignant melanoma in the gastrointestinal tract. Geriatrics 24:112–120, 1969.
3. Beckley D: Alimentary tract metastases from malignant melanoma. Clin Radiol 25:385–389, 1974.

4. Byrd BF and Morton CE: Malignant melanoma metastatic to the gastrointestinal tract from an occult primary tumor. South Med J 71:1306–1308, 1978.

5. Chandler AB and Jones FG: Malignant melanoma of the gastrointestinal tract. Am Surg 17:719–721, 1951.

6. Das Gupta TK and Brasfield R: Metastatic melanoma: a clinicopathological study. Cancer 17:1323–1339, 1964.

7. Das Gupta TK and Brasfield RD: Metastatic melanoma of the gastrointestinal tract. Arch Surg 88:969–973, 1964.

8. Das Gupta TK, Brasfield RD and Paglia MA: Primary melanomas in unusual sites. Surg Gynecol Obstet 128:841–848, 1969.

9. Frasen-Moodie A, Heghas RG, Jones SM, Shorley BA and Snape L: Malignant melanoma metastases to the alimentary tract. Gut 17:206–209, 1976.

10. Giler S, Kott J and Urca I: Malignant melanoma metastatic to the gastrointestinal tract. World J Surg 3:375–379, 1979.

11. Goldstein HM, Talal Beydoun M and Dodd GD: Radiologic spectrum of melanoma metastatic to the gastrointestinal tract. Am J Roentgenol 129:605–612, 1977.

12. Halbish TF: Roentgen manifestations of malignant melanoma. Am J Roengental 78:769–779, 1957.

13. Lee Y-TN: Malignant melanoma: pattern of metastasis. CA-A Cancer J Clin 30:137–142, 1980.

14. McNeer G and Das Gupta TK: Life history of melanoma. Am J Roengental 93:686–694, 1965.

15. Meyer JE: Radiographic evaluation of metastatic melanoma. Cancer 42:127–132, 1978.

16. Nathanson L, Hall TC and Farber S: Biological aspects of human malignant melanoma. Cancer 20:650–655, 1967.

17. Patel JK, Didolkar MP and Pickren JW: Metastatic pattern of malignant melanoma: a study of 216 autopsy cases. Am J Surg 135:807–810, 1978.

18. Pomerantz H and Margolin HN: Metastases to the gastrointestinal tract from malignant melanoma. Am J Roengentol 88:712–717, 1962.

19. Willbanks OL and Fogleman MJ: Gastrointestinal melanosarcoma. Am J Surg 120:602–606, 1970.

20. Baxkman H and Davidson L: Metastases of malignant melanoma in the stomach and small intestine. Acta Med Scand 178:329–335, 1965.

21. Booth JB: Malignant melanoma of the stomach. Br J Surg 52:262–269, 1962.

22. Calderon R, Ceballos J and McGraw JP: Metastatic melanoma of the stomach. Am J Roengentol 74:242–245, 1955.

23. Davis GH and Zollinger RW: Metastatic melanoma of the stomach. Am J Surg 99:94–96, 1960.

24. Dutta SK and Costa BS: Umbilicated gastric polyposis: an indicator of metastatic gastric tumor. Am J Gastrol 71:598–604, 1979.

25. Goldman SL, Pollak EW and Wolfman EF: Gastric ulcer, an unusual presentation of malignant melanoma. J Am Med Assoc 237:52, 1977.

26. Karparov M and Koyundjiev I: The roentgen image of metastatic melanoma in the upper gastrointestinal tract. Radiol Diagn 6:761–S, 1965.

27. Menuck LS and Amberg JR: Metastatic disease involving the stomach. Am J Dig Dis 20:903–913, 1975.

28. Potchen EJ, Khung CL and Yatsuhashi M: X-ray diagnosis of gastric melanoma. N Engl J Med 271:131–136, 1964.

29. Reed PI, Raskin HF and Graff PW: Malignant melanoma of the stomach. J Am Med Assoc 182:298–299, 1962.

30. Reeder MM and Cavanagh RC: "Bull's eye" lesions: solitary on multiple nodules in the

gastrointestinal tract with larger central ulceration. J Am Med Assoc 229:825–826, 1974.

31. Richte R, Panish J and Berel G: Endoscopic findings in melanoma metastatic to the stomach. Gastrointest Endosc 18:172–173, 1972.

32. Stalder GA: Malignant melanoma of the stomach. Gastrointest Endosc 16:30–32, 1969.

33. Sivak MV and Sullivan BH: Endoscopic diagnosis of malignant melanoma metastatic to the duodenum. Gastrointest Endosc 22:36–38, 1975.

34. Benisch BM, Abramson S and Present DH: Malabsorption and metastatic melanoma. Mt Sinai J Med N Y 39:474–477, 1972.

35. Bierne MF: Malignant melanoma of the small intestine. Radiology 65:749–754, 1955.

36. Cavanagh RC, Buchignani JC and Rulon DB: Metastatic melanoma of the small intestine: radiological pathological conference of the month from the Armed Forces Institute of Pathology. Radiology 101:195–200, 1971.

37. Harris MN: Massive gastrointestinal hemorrhage. Arch Surg 88:1049–1051, 1964.

38. Helidonis ES, Meyers EN and Barnes EL, Jr: Metastasis of malignant melanoma of the nasal mucosa to the small intestine. Laryngoscope 86:1734–1737, 1976.

39. Karakousis C, Holyoke ED and Douglass HO: Intussusception as a complication of malignant neoplasm. Arch Surg 109:515–518, 1974.

40. Macbeth WAAG, Gwynne JF and Jamieson MG: Metastatic melanoma in the small bowel. Aust N Z J Surg 38:309–315, 1969.

41. Meyers MA and McSweeney J: Secondary neoplasms of the bowel. Radiology 105:1–11, 1972.

42. Oddson RA, Rice RP, Seigler HF, Thompson WM, Kelvin FM and Clark WC: The spectrum of small bowel melanoma. Gastrointest Radiol 3:419–423, 1978.

43. Paglia MA and Exclby PY: Recurrent intussusception from metastatic melanoma. N Y State J Med 68:3061–3062, 1968.

44. Richie RE, Reynolds OH and Sawyers JL: Tumors metastatic to the small bowel from extra-abdominal sites. South Med J 66:1383–1387, 1973.

45. Smith SJ, Carlson HC and Gisvold JJ: Secondary neoplasms of the small bowel. Radiology 125:29–33, 1977.

46. Zornoza J and Goldstein HM: Cavitating metastasis of the small intestine. Am J Roengentol 129:613–615, 1977.

47. Bingham DLC, Chadsey LC, Ramchand S et al: Primary melanocarcinoma of the esophagus. Can Med Assoc J 105:607–610, 1974.

48. Brodenick PA, Allegra SR and Corvese CT: Primary malignant melanoma of the esophagus: a case report. Acta Cytol 16:159–164, 1972.

49. Fowler M and Sutherland HD'A: Malignant melanoma of the esophagus. J Pathol Bacterol 64:473–477, 1952.

50. Garfinkle MJ and Cahan Wa: Primary melanocarcinoma of the esophagus: first histologically proven case. Cancer 5:921–926, 1952.

51. Hendricks GL, Jr, Barnes WT and Suter HJ: Primary malignant melanoma of the esophagus. Am J Surg 40:468–473, 1974.

52. Hosoda S, Minakami I and Murakami M: An autopsy case of primary malignant melanoma of the esophagus. Tap J Cancer Clin 15:752–759, 1969.

53. Musher DR and Linder AE: Primary melanoma of the esophagus. Am J Dig Dis 19:855–859, 1974.

54. Picconi VA, Klopstock R, LeVeen HJ et alb: Primary malignant melanoma of the esophagus associated with melanosis of the esophagus. J Thorac Surg 59:864–870, 1970.

55. Raven RW: Rare tumors of the pharynx and esophagus. Ann N Y Acad Sci 114:1061–1079, 1971.

56. Raven RW and Dawson I: Malignant melanoma of the esophagus. Br J Surg 51:551–555, 1964.

57. Sakornpant P, Barlow P and Bevar CM: Two cases of primary malignant melanoma of the esophagus. Br J Surg 51:386–388, 1964.
58. Waken JK and Bullock WK: Primary melanocarcinoma of the esophagus. Am J Clin Pathol 38:415–421, 1962.
59. Balthazar EJ and Javors B: Anorectal melanoma. Am J Gastroenterol 63:79–83, 1975.
60. Garnick M and Lokich JJ: Primary malignant melanoma of the rectum: rationale for conservative surgical management. J Surg Oncol 10:529–531, 1978.
61. Gupta S and Rastogi BE: Metastatic anal melanoma presenting as double intussusception of the small bowel. Am J Proctol 28:49–57, 1977.
62. Husa A and Hockerstedt K: Anorectal malignant melanoma: a report of fourteen cases. Acta Clin Scand 140:68–72, 1974.
63. Mason JK and Holwig FB: Ano-rectal melanoma. Cancer 19:39–50, 1966.
64. Moroson BC and Volkstadt H: Malignant melanoma of the anal canal. J Clin Pathol 16:126–132, 1963.
65. Nyquist A and Tillander H: Malignant melanoma of the anal canal. Acta Clin Scand 135:730–732, 1969.
66. Pack GT and Oropeza R: A comparative study of melanoma and epidermoid carcinoma of the anal canal. Dis Colon Rectum 10:161–176, 1967.
67. Sinclair DM, Hannah G, McLaughlin JS et al: Malignant melanoma of the anal canal. Br J Surg 57:808–811, 1970.
68. Rafrensperger EC, Brason FW and Triano G: Primary melanoma of the gallbladder. Am J Dig Dis 8:356–363, 1973.
69. Rosenthal SR: Primary melanocarcinoma of the gallbladder. Am J Cancer 15:2288–2300, 1931.
70. Zemlyn S: Metastatic melanoma of the gallbladder. Radiology 87:744–745, 1966.
71. Cohen DM, Greenspan EM, Weiner MJ et al: Triple combination therapy of disseminated melanoma. Cancer 29:1489–1495, 1972.
72. Einhorn LH, Burgess MA, Vallegos C, Bodey GP, Sr, Gutterman A, Mauligit G, Hersh EM, Luce JK, Frei E, III, Freirech AJ and Gottlieb JA: Prognostic correlations and response to treatment in advanced metastatic malignant melanoma. Cancer Res 34:1995–2004, 1974.
73. Maurer LH, McIntyre OR and Rueckent F: Spontaneous regression of malignant melanoma. Am J Surg 127:397–403, 1974.
74. McCarthy WH, Shaw HM and Milton GW: Spontaneous regression of metastatic malignant melanoma. Clin Oncol 4:203–207, 1978.
75. Seigler HF and Fetter BF: Current management of melanoma. Ann Surg 186:1–12, 1977.
76. Storm FK and Morton DL: Treatment of metastatic disease. Adv Surg 13:33–68, 1979.
77. Frick MP, Knight LC, Feinberg SB, Loken MK and Gedgaudas E: Computed tomography, radionuclide imaging and ultrasonography in hepatic mass lesions. Comput Tomogr 3:49–55, 1979.
78. Green B, Bree RL, Goldstein HM et al: Gray scale ultrasound evaluation of hepatic neoplasms: patterns and correlations. Radiology 203–208, 1977.
79. Kreel L: Computerized tomography and the liver. Clin Radiol 28:571–581, 1977.
80. Marchal GJ, Baert Al and Wilms GE: CT of noncystic liver lesions: bolus enhancement. Am J Roengentol 135:57–65, 1980.
81. Moss AA, Schrump FT, Schnyder P, Korobkin M and Shimshak RR: Computed tomography of focal hepatic lesions: a blind clinical evaluation of the effect of contrast enhancement. Radiology 131:427–430, 1979.
82. Scheible W, Gosink BB and Leopold GR: Gray scale echographic patterns of hepatic metastatic disease. Am J Roengentol 129:983–987, 1977.

83. Wooten WB, Bernardino ME and Goldstein HM: Computed tomography of necrotic hepatic metastases. Am J Roengentol 131:839–842, 1978.

84. Laufer I: Double Contrast Gastrointestinal Radiology with Endoscopic Correlation. WB Saunders, Philadelphia, 1979.

85. Ekberg O: Double contrast examination of the small bowel gastrointestine. Radiology 1:349–352, 1977.

86. Sanders DE and Ho CS: The small bowel enema: experience with 150 examinations. Am J Roengentol 127:743–751, 1976.

87. Sellink JL: Radiologic examination of the small bowel by a duodenal intubation. Acta Radiol 15:318–332, 1974.

88. Miller RE: Reflux examination of the small bowel. Radiol Clin North Am 7:175–184, 1969.

89. Sacks BA, Joffe N and Antonioli DA: Metastatic melanoma presenting clinically as multiple colonic polyps. Am J Roengentol 129:511–513, 1977.

90. Herrington JL, Jr: Metastatic malignant melanoma of the gallbladder masquerading as cholelithiasis. Am J Surg 109:676–678, 1965.

91. Jones CH: Malignant melanoma of the gallbladder. J Pathol 81:423–430, 1961.

92. Peison B and Rabin L: Malignant melanoma of the gallbladder: report of 3 cases and review of the literature. Cancer 37:2448–2454, 1976.

93. Ronca PC: Benign and malignant disease: metastatic malignant melanoma, cholecystitis and cholelithiasis. Am J Gastroenterol 50:307–314, 1968.

94. Shimkin PM, Solowax MS and Jaffe E: Metastatic melanoma of the gallbladder. Am J Roengentol 116:393–395, 1972.

95. Rosenthall L, Shaffer EA and Lesbona R: Diagnoses of hepatobiliary disease by $^{99m}$Tc-HIDA cholescintigraphy. Radiology 26:467–474, 1978.

96. Cole HS and Freston JW: Recurrent melanoma presenting with obstructive jaundice: report of two cases. Rocky Mount Med J 70:42–46, 1973.

97. Ferrucci JT, Jr, Wittenberg J, Sarno RA and Dreyfuss JR: Fine needle transhepatic cholangiography: a new approach to obstructive jaundice. Am J Roengentol 127:403–407, 1976.

98. Harbin WP and Ferrucci JT, Jr: Nonoperative management of malignant biliary obstruction: a radiologic alternative. Am J Roengentol 135:103–107, 1980.

99. Hoevels J, Lunderquist A and Ihse I: Percutaneous transhepatic intubation of bile ducts of combined internal-external drainage in preoperative and palliative treatment of obstructive jaundice. Gastrointest Radiol 3:23–31, 1978.

100. Zboralske FF and Bessolo RJ: Metastatic carcinoma to the mesentery and gut. Radiology 88:302–310, 1967.

# 6. Malignant melanoma of the eye

ARTHUR C. CHANDLER, Jr.

## Introduction

From the time they begin training, most ophthalmologists are taught and believe that any pigmented lesion about the eye or its adnexa, including the conjunctiva and the skin of the lids, is suspect and should be observed frequently. Although these lesions may represent nevi, melanocytomas or other benign pigment disturbances, the ophthalmologist is all too aware of the potential malignancy of these lesions and their consequences. Exactly what mechanisms cause the alteration of normal pigment-producing cells to become malignant is poorly understood at best, and what causes some normal cells to become more malignant in their activity than others is suspect. Furth [1], in 1961, outlined the possible etiologic factors as being: A) genetic factors, B) hormones and C) carcinogens, agents that initiate modifications of nucleic acid causing loss of proper response to homeostatic regulators. Many investigators believe that viruses may be among the most potent of the carcinogens.

Heredity does not seem to be very important in the genesis of pigmented tumors [2]. It is of interest, however, that the rare occurrence of ocular pigmented tumors of a malignant type in the black race may well suggest factors that are determined genetically. Conjunctival pigmentation in the members of the black race seems to remain benign; whereas in the nonblack races, these lesions all too frequently progress toward or are transformed into less benign and more malignant lesions.

The histology and pathogenesis of melanin-containing cells are discussed elsewhere in this book by Dr. Klintworth.

Malignant melanomas of the eye can occur primarily in any area that contains melanin-producing cells, including the skin, conjunctiva and uveal tract. They also can occur in the orbit as primary lesions, but these are frequently secondary to extensions from primary lesions within the eye or as a metastasis from a lesion elsewhere in the body. Uveal melanomas can also occur as a result of a metastasis from elsewhere or, of course, can be the primary site giving metastatic lesions elsewhere in the body.

The ophthalmologist's dilemma with melanomas of the choroid concerns a reasonable certainty in the differential diagnosis and decision upon the

*Seigler, H. F. (ed.), Clinical Management of Melanoma. ISBN 978-94-009-7495-1*
© *1982, Martinus Nijhoff Publishers, The Hague/Boston/London.*

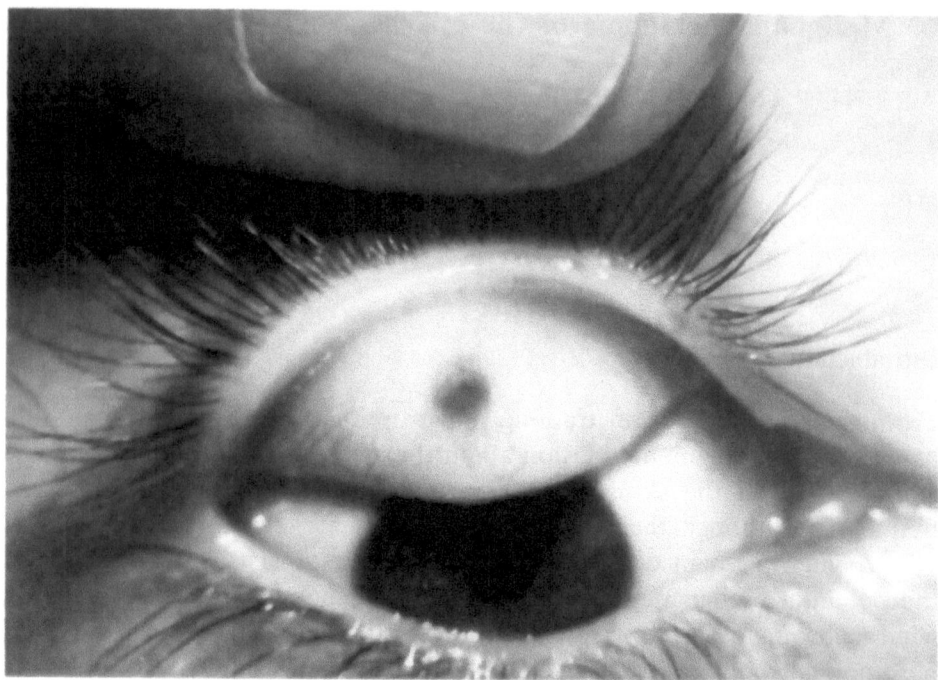

*Figure 1.* Metastatic malignant melanoma to the tarsal conjunctiva. Primary site was a cutaneous lesion of the hip area.

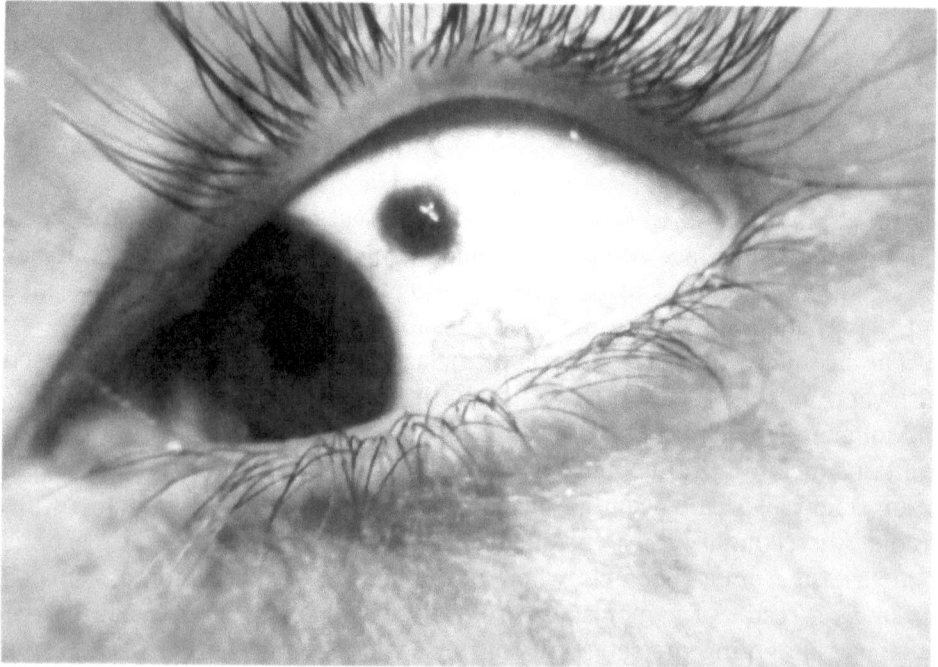

*Figure 2.* Metastatic malignant melanoma to the sclera of the left eye. Primary site was a cutaneous malignant melanoma of the left hip.

type of therapy. Until very recently, the ability to obtain a tissue diagnosis of choroidal lesions to histologically confirm the diagnosis of a malignancy did not exist and many ancillary diagnostic tests have been devised to supplement the clinical observation and impression.

## Skin and conjunctival melanomas

Melanomas in the skin of the lids or in the periocular area are treated by excisional biopsy and wide margins with pathologic confirmation and any adjunctive therapy as would be carried out with a primary melanoma malignancy elsewhere in the body. Metastatic lesions to the skin of the lids (Figure 1) and the conjunctiva or sclera (Figure 2) from primary lesions elsewhere in the body are treated in a palliative manner, the agressiveness being determined by the general effect of widespread dissemination of the disease.

The diagnosis of the myriad of pigmented lesions about the lid and conjunctiva can be determined histologically without compromising the appearance or function of the structure. Spencer [3] has suggested in his classification for hyperpigmented melanocytic lesions that the conjunctiva pigmentation of the focal type would either be diagnosed as a nevus (Figure 3) or a

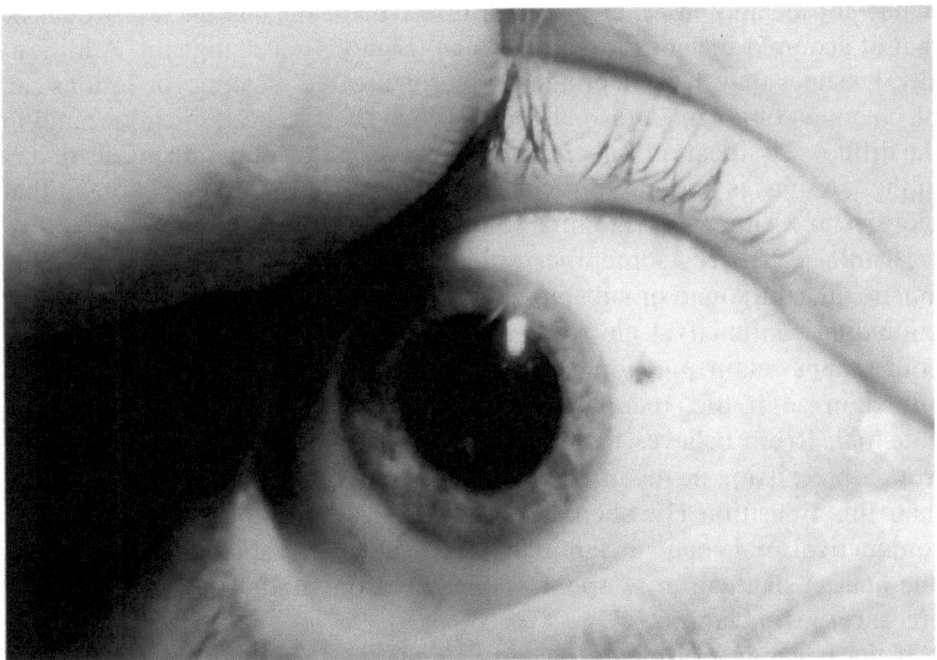

*Figure 3*. Small pigmented nevus of the conjunctiva.

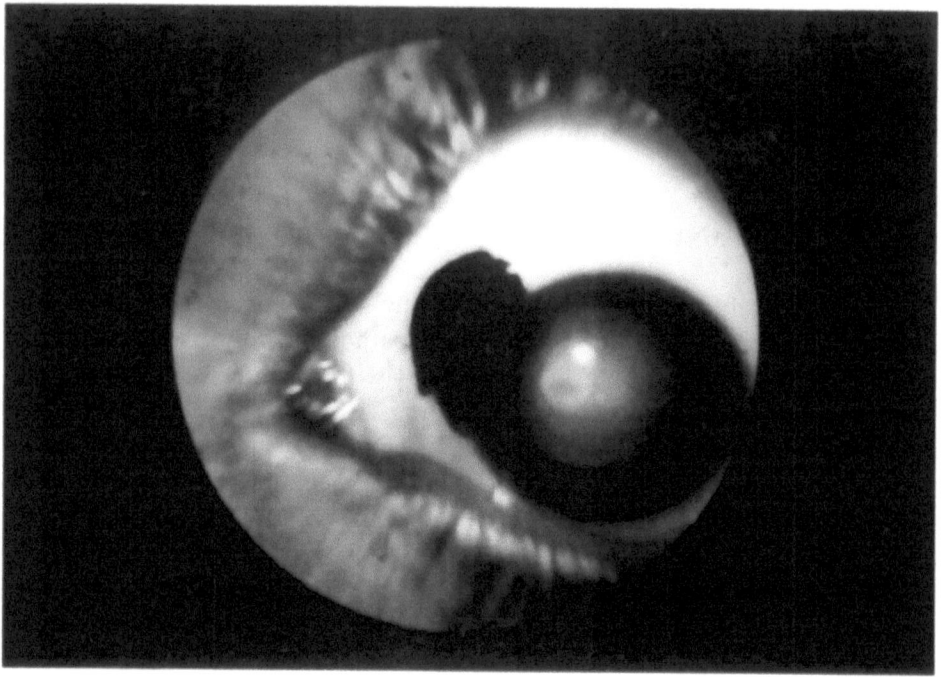

*Figure 4.* Large acquired area of benign melanosis of the conjunctiva.

malignant melanoma, whereas the diffuse type of the conjunctiva would be that of acquired melanosis, either benign (Figure 4) or malignant. Additionally, he states that the subepithelial hyperpigmented melanocytic lesions can be blue nevi of a benign or malignant type in the focal classification; and in the diffuse classification, subepithelial melanosis. Again the diagnosis of any of these lesions is no more difficult than superficial lesions elsewhere in that biopsies and laboratory examination can be carried out.

Histologically, it is sometimes difficult to determine whether a nevus is junctional, compound or subepithelial. Reese has reported in analyzing over a hundred conjunctival nevi and nevi of the skin of the lids that 95% of both groups retain junctional activity. If these junctional changes are acquired in adult life, there seems to be a higher incidence of malignant potential. Reese believes that the instance of malignant melanoma arising from a preexisting nevus in the skin of the lids or the conjunctiva is higher than this transition elsewhere in the body. He feels about one-quarter of conjunctival malignant melanomas arise from preexisting congenital nevi, one-quarter of them arise spontaneously and one-half arise from acquired precancerous melanosis [4].

If the nevus is considered by the patient to be unsightly, the only indicated treatment would be excision. It is not generally felt that a partial excision of a nevus excites active growth. Since nevi about the lids or the conjunctiva are more apt to undergo malignant change, removal of these, particularly when small, reduces that risk and does not reduce the function of the eye or the lids.

## Melanomas of the iris

Malignant melanomas of the iris (Figure 5) comprise only about 6% of the melanomas of the uveal tract [2]. These lesions, however, do create some problems in absolute diagnosis in that any excisional biopsy requires intraocular surgery with removal of a part of the iris, leaving a defect that may not seriously involve vision, but may well create a cosmetic defect and frequently some degree of photophobia or even monocular diplopia.

Iris freckles are observed in a large proportion of the population and are quite anterior in their location. They are congenital and only rarely change in size or number. Freckles are not seen before the sixth year of life and seldomly are noted before the twelfth year. Reese states that 48% of all adults have unilateral or bilateral iris freckles [4]. A melanoma of the iris is more extensive than a freckle and clinically appears to be more elevated,

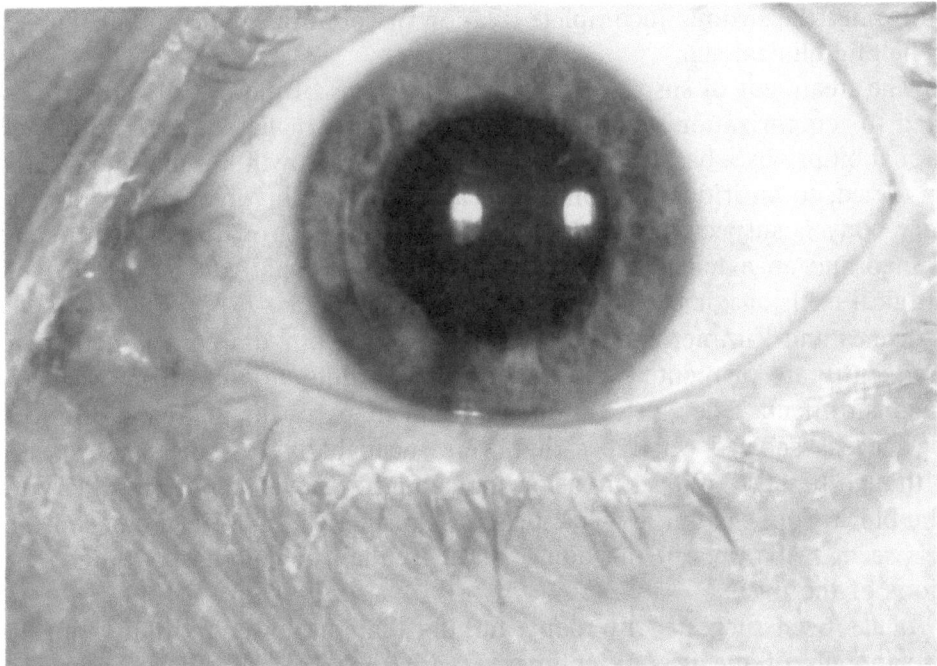

*Figure 5.* Biopsy proven malignant melanoma of the iris.

occasionally increasing the iris thickness. A shortening of the anterior stroma causing an ectropion of the pupillary margin with the pigment epithelium being pulled toward the periphery by stromal shortening is occasionally seen. Most investigators believe that malignant melanomas of the iris develop from benign melanomas. Therefore, it would seem prudent that any elevated pigmented lesion of the iris be carefully observed for growth. The iris melanoma, be it benign or malignant, is asymptomatic in most cases, but occasionally the tumor can extend into the angle and/or ciliary body causing glaucoma with resultant reductions of vision and/or pain. The inferior and inferiotemporal quadrants in the periphery is the location at which these tumors are most often seen [5].

A biopsy of this lesion, unless it is a total excisional biopsy, is thought to be contraindicated because of the possibility of seeding. The $^{32}$P (radioactive phosphorus) test had not been shown to be helpful for suspected lesions confined to the iris. Fluorescein angiography of the iris may be helpful in distinguishing between nevi and melanomas but frequently is not too helpful in determining the malignancy of the lesion. There is an absolute rarity of metastases from an isolated iris lesion and this would dictate no treatment in the absence of confirmed growth of the lesion.

When the melanoma is in the far periphery of the iris, it is frequently difficult to determine whether or not the ciliary body is involved. It is felt by many that the appearance of blood vessels in the tumor or coursing to it may well be significant regarding the activity of the lesion. If the tumor infiltrates the stroma, incomplete dilation or splinting of the pupil becomes a helpful clinical sign.

The treatment of suspicious pigmented lesions of the iris should be limited to temporization when no documented growth has occurred, to excisional biopsy by a basal iridectomy when there is growth but the angle is not involved, to an iridocyclectomy if local nondiffuse involvement of the ciliary body is suspected, or finally, to enucleation if growth has been determined and an extension of the tumor is beyond what can be handled by surgical excision, or because of secondary glaucoma.

Rones and Zimmerman [5] have stated that lyomyosarcomas of the iris frequently are pigmented and, therefore, the differentiation from melanomas is difficult. They also commented that many of the pigmented tumors of the iris showed cell types that were incapable of distance metastases, although because of local invasion they could cause glaucoma secondary to the blocking of the outflow channels. It is of interest that melanomas of the iris seem to be present in younger patients than melanomas of other portions of the uvea.

It has been suggested by many authors that the lower mortality rate in melanomas of the iris, as compared with those of the ciliary body and choroid, is probably secondary to their being seen more easily and followed with more concern. Cleasby [6] reported in 1958 that 13 patients followed five years or longer with confirmed diagnoses of malignant melanomas of the iris survived. Of his series of 23 patients, the other eight had been followed for a shorter period but they were still living and there were no signs of metastases. It is of interest that 17 of the 21 cases had epithelioid or spindle cell-type disease, the former type having a high metastatic potential from the choroidal malignant lesion.

**Malignant melanomas of the ciliary body**

Approximately 9% of uveal malignant melanomas occur in the ciliary body [8, 9]. It would appear that the age of onset of melanomas of the ciliary body is approximately that of melanomas of the choroid, both showing the highest occurrence in the fifth decade. Bilateral melanomas of either the ciliary body or the choroid appear to be extremely rare. Ciliary body melanomas are extremely difficult to diagnose unless they are large enough to be visible with indirect ophthalmoscopy or the gonioscope or have displaced the iris anteriorly or the lens toward the opposite side (Figure 6). At times, the only indication of such a growth may be an invasion into the angle of the anterior chamber, which can be visualized. Change in vision is noted,

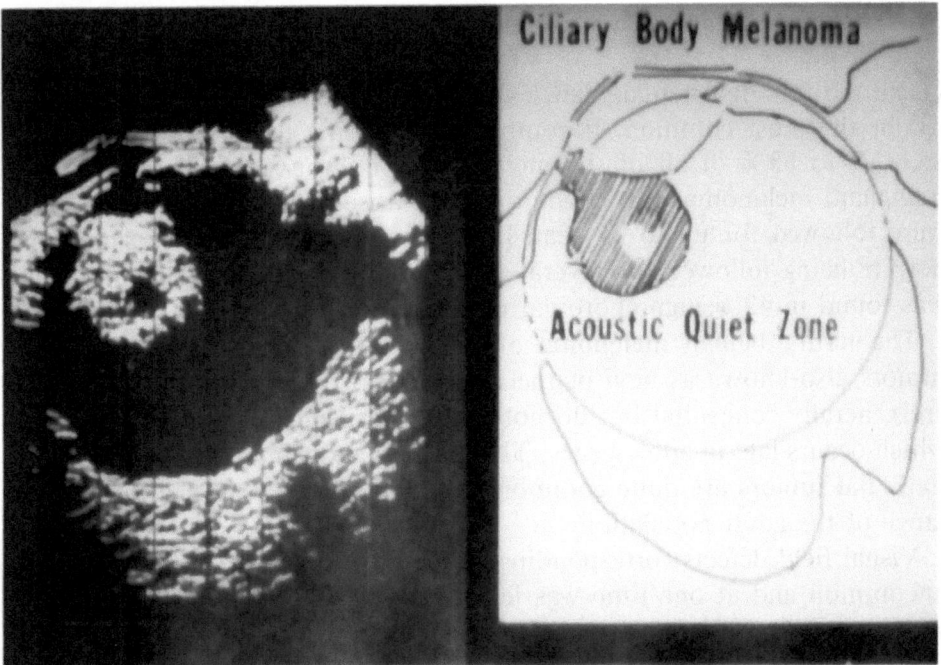

*Figure 6.* Ultrasonographic view of large malignant melanoma of the ciliary body.

perhaps because of the shift of the lens. Pain, secondary to increased intraocular pressure, and inflammation of the iris are common complaints with patients who have ciliary body melanomas.

Transillumination is occasionally of help in a large mass to differentiate it from a ciliary body cyst, but generally transillumination is not of help, particularly in small tumors. Once the solid lesion has been initially observed, any increase in size can be considered ominous. Radioactive phosphorus studies may be of a great deal of value if the lesion is sufficiently large. If there is activity in the anterior chamber, a paracentesis can be performed and the aqueous can be studied cytologically [9].

Enucleation may be the operation of choice when the diagnosis is fairly certain unless the patient is one eyed. Excision of the neoplasm, if small enough, could be considered as well as radiation therapy as alternative therapeutic methods. Because the overall mortality rate of patients with tumors of the ciliary body and choroid is approximately 29% within the first five years and 40% within the first ten years [10], older patients, particularly those with only one eye, can be observed. In the case of ciliary body malignant melanomas alone, there is apparently a 60% survival rate through the first decade [11]. Reese [4] reports a 50% survival rate after five years but only a 35% survival rate after ten or more years. He also states that such lesions arising elsewhere have a mortality rate of 80–90%.

## Malignant melanomas of the choroid

Of all the intraocular malignancies, malignant melanoma of the choroid is by far the most common. It comprises, according to various series, from 85% [2] to 88% of all of the melanomas of the uveal tract [4]. Verified malignant melanomas of the choroid have arisen from suspected nevi that were followed for up to 25 years [2]. However, another series states that despite being followed for several years, no evidence of malignant change was found in 42 benign choroidal melanomas [12].

The term "benign melanoma of the uvea" refers to those pigmented tumors also known as nevi or melanocytomas. It is felt that these tumors are generally congenital but do not appear until pigmentation is acquired, which occurs late in adolescence. These round and smooth bordered, essentially flat tumors are quite common, probably being present in the 6–10% range of the adult population.

Visual field defects corresponding to the position of the benign tumor is uncommon and at one time was felt not to exist at all. However, Tamler and Maumenee [13] found that field defects did exist if small targets were used.

It would appear that, since it is felt that malignant melanomas only rarely are the result of conversion from a benign nevus, the malignant melanoma may arise from pigment-bearing cells that are not predisposed to form nevi. Calender [14] described a cell classification due to cell type in 1931. These cell types have to do with the prognosis for survival and are discussed elsewhere in this book. It is well known in ophthalmology that the least malignant of the melanomas of the choroid is that of the spindle-A type makeup. But this is not the most common type with spindle cell B and a combination of spindle cell and epithelioid cell type comprising approximately 75% of all intraocular melanomas. Prognosis seems also to be dependent upon the size of the tumor at the time of diagnosis and treatment [15]. A more recent report [16] suggests that not only the size of the lesion, but the cell type, the amount of pigmentation, scleral extension, mitotic activity, location of the anterior margin of the tumor and optic nerve extension are good prognostic indicators for survival. The four worst factors for prognosis seem to be a combination of cell type, largest dimensions, scleral extension and mitotic activities.

The malignant melanoma of the choroid is not infrequently first observed through routine funduscopy. These are generally of the small type and other symptoms are rare unless the tumor is quite large or located near the posterior pole where changes in visual acuity can be expected with tumors of relatively small size. Invariably, visual field defects do arise, secondary to

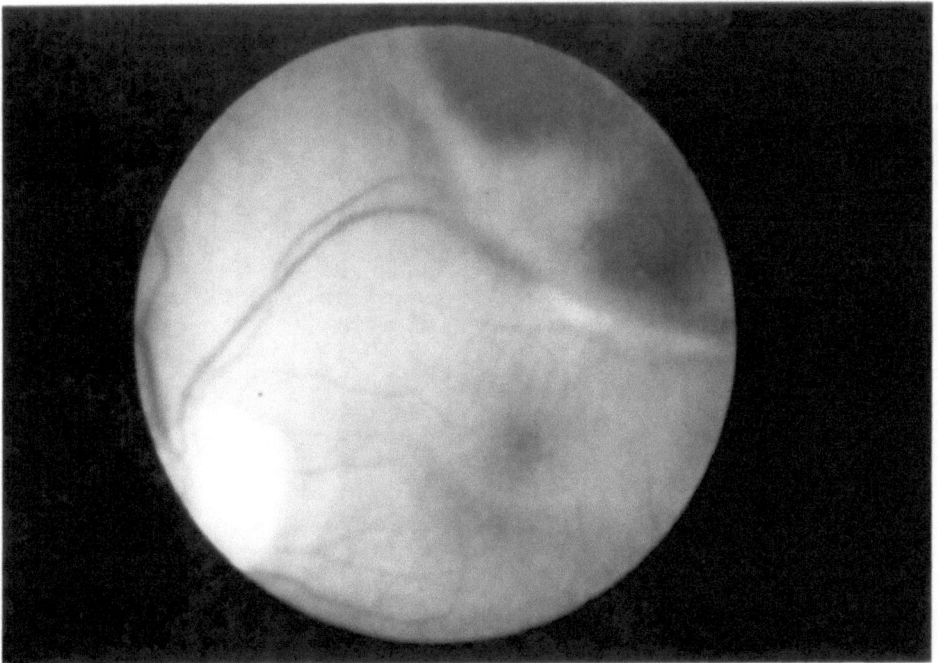

*Figure 7.* Large peripherial malignant melanoma at the equator of the left eye showing retinal folds or stria toward the macula.

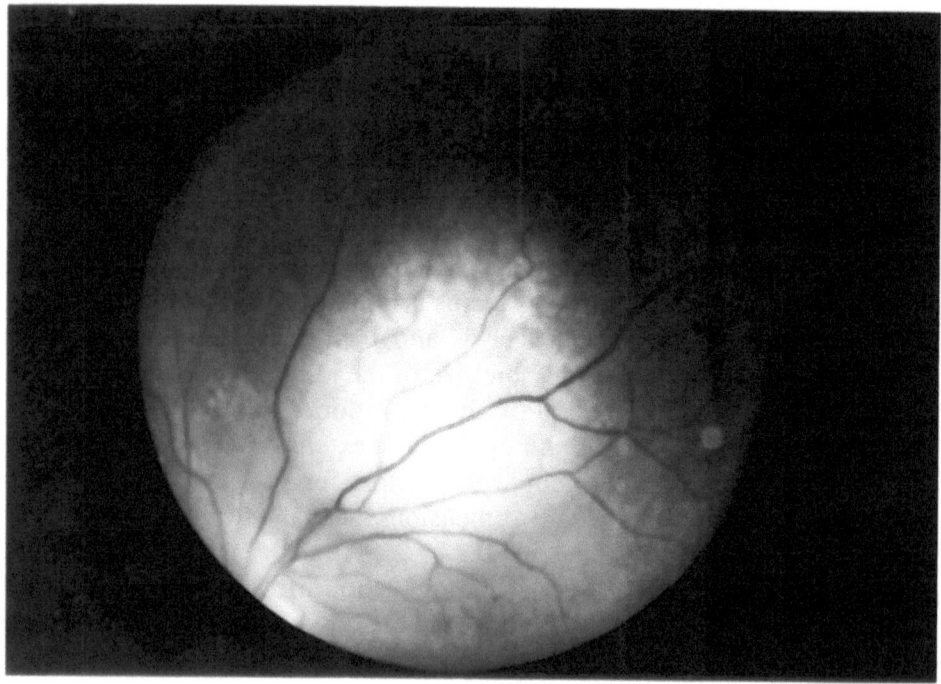

*Figure 8.* A melanotic malignant melanoma in the superior temporal region of a left eye.

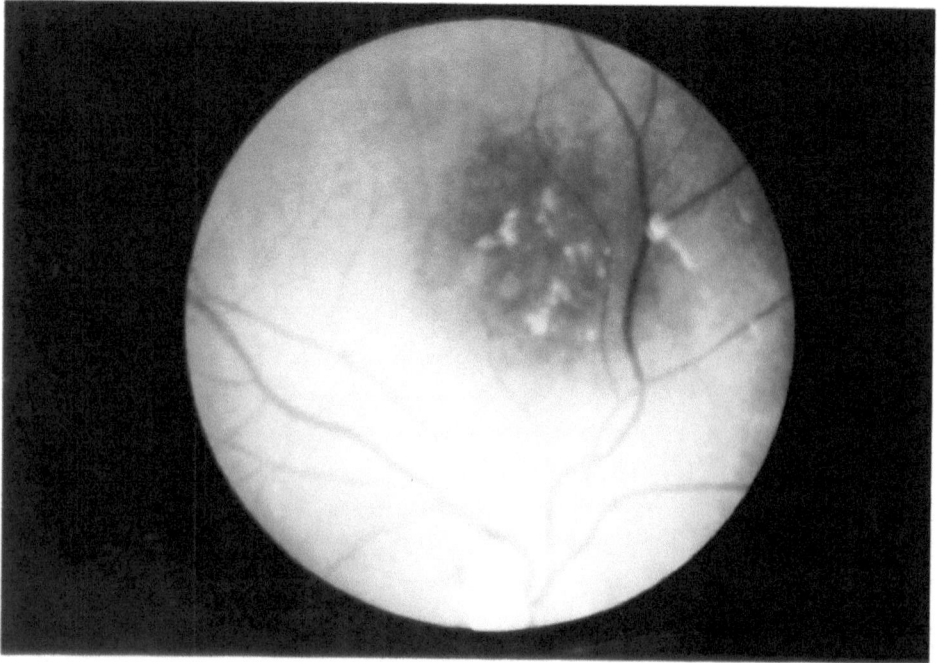

*Figure 9.* Scattered orange pigment overlying the surface of an elevated pigmented lesion of the choroid.

retinal involvement in the area overlying the malignant melanoma. The clinical appearance of the melanoma may be that of a moderately dark lesion which is somewhat elevated (Figure 7) to one in which there is essentially no pigmentation at all (Figure 8). Characteristically, there is a druse-like disturbance on the surface and a development of an orange pigment deposit in the superficial area over the tumor [17] (Figure 9). As long as the media is clear, observation of the tumor with its feathery edges and its growth along with absence of transillumination (particularly if the tumor is located anterior to the equator) helps considerably in the clinical diagnosis. However, as the tumor increases in size, there is produced an exudation which creates a retinal detachment which, if high enough, may obscure the visualization of the tumor itself.

Visual changes in image size or configuration (metamorphopsia) may also be an initial complaint if the tumor is located in the paramacula area. If the tumor is anterior enough or large enough, secondary glaucoma may be produced and pain becomes one of the initial symptoms.

At one time, bleeding was not believed to be part of the melanoma process, but is is now universally recognized that hemorrhage can occur if the tumor becomes large enough and necrotic enough. With necrosis, an inflammatory response also may occur, producing ocular congestion.

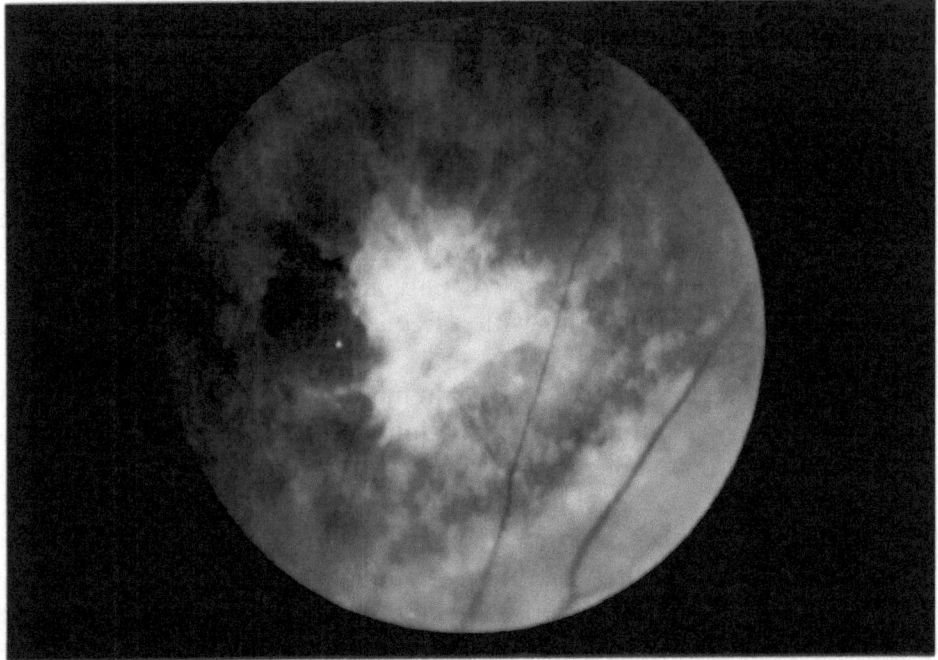

*Figure 10.* Malignant melanoma of the choroid, which resembled an inflammatory process and remained stable under observation for approximately 12 years. On enucleation, a spindle cell B type malignant melanoma was diagnosed histologically.

Visual field defects in melanomas, particularly those with serous attachments, although shallow, will invariably give larger defects than the scotomas demonstrated from benign melanomas. The latter shows scotomas that are of the same or less size than the defect seen by the ophthalmoscope or indeed may not exist at all.

With careful observation, a malignant melanoma will show clumps of pigment if the neoplasm is close to the retina. It may resemble old inflammatory lesions or scars (Figure 10). As the tumor extends through Bruch's membrane, retinal detachments invariably occur.

In general, when the medium is reasonably clear, the clinical findings will allow the examining physician to establish the diagnosis of a choroidal melanoma. However, when the medium is not clear, false positive diagnoses are frequently made [18]. The reverse is also true in that out of 212 eyes with opaque medium, which were studied at the Armed Forces Institute of Pathology, 113 showed unsuspected melanomas [19].

Newer techniques have further added to the diagnostic certainty of these lesions, particularly in the face of a hazy medium. Radioactive phosphorus or $^{32}$P has been used since 1952 in an attempt to differentiate malignant melanomas of the uvea from other lesions [20]. $^{32}$P uptake simply is the measurement of the radioactive phosphate ion incorporated into newly formed nucleic acids in cell nuclei. Since malignant cells are more rapidly growing as reflected by tumor growth, $^{32}$P uptake should be higher in neoplastic cells than in normal cells. It is also known that $^{32}$P enters hemorrhagic and inflammatory tissues at a higher rate than normal.

Beta-emitting agents show poor tissue penetration and radioactive phosphorus is a Beta emitter. The average tissue penetrance is only 2–3 mm and therefore the detector must be placed very close to the tumor. An increase in uptake of greater than 50% over the involved area as compared with a similar, noninvolved area is considered suspicious. It should be emphasized, however, that a positive test is only an adjunct to the clinical diagnosis. False positive tests occur with a frequency of 1% to 4% and are due to a vast array of variables [21].

Ultrasonography has proven to be extremely helpful, but again not 100% reliable in the detection and differentiation of intraocular tumors. Ossoinig [22] has stated that malignant melanomas of the choroid and ciliary body can be detected if their elevation from the sclera is 0.75 mm or 1.5 mm in the ciliary body. He feels that melanomas can be differentiated from other similar lesions with an accuracy of greater than 95% if their elevation is at least 1.5 mm in the choroid and 3 mm in the ciliary body from the sclera (Figures 11, 12). With A scan ultrasonography, scleral infiltration or extension can be detected and, with the aid of the B scan, orbital involvement can be demonstrated. This technique is particularly helpful when retinal detachment obscures the visualization of the suspected underlying mass.

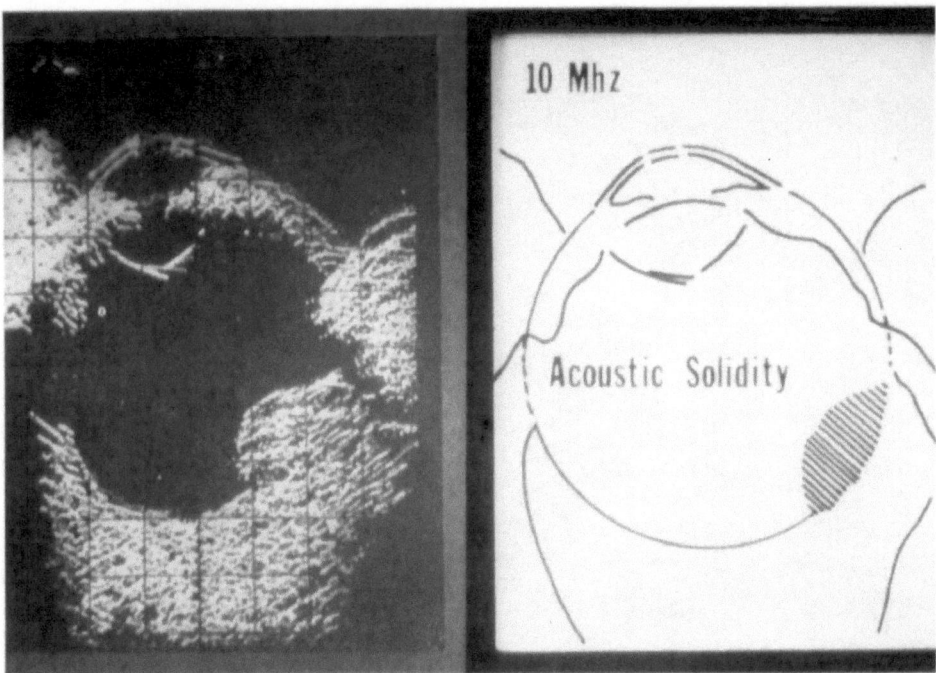

*Figure 11.* Malignant melanoma of the choroid showing acoutic solidity with 10 MHz transmission on B scan.

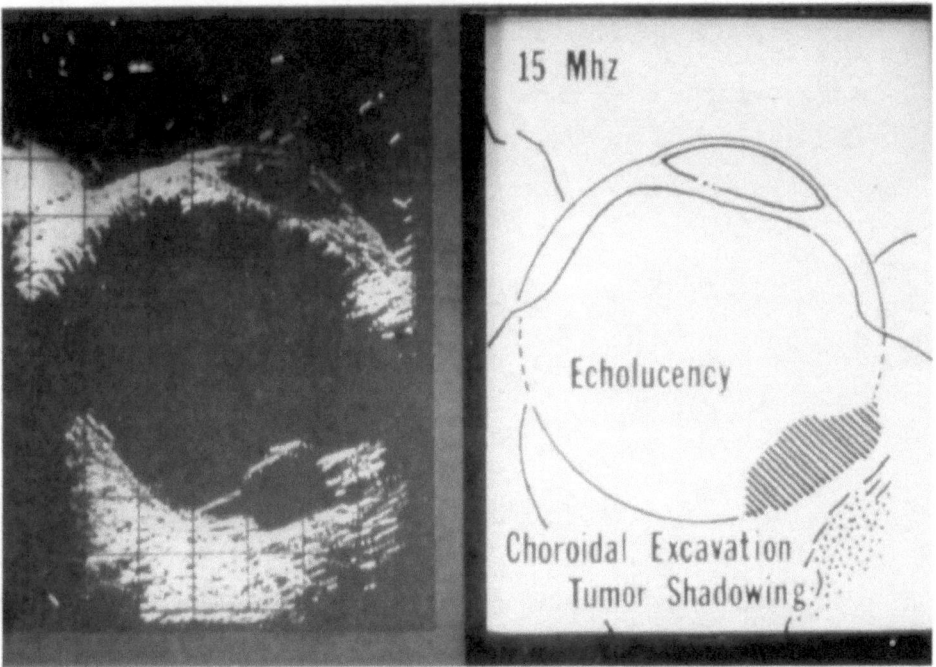

*Figure 12.* Same melanoma as in Figure 11 showing echolucency using the 15 MHz transmission.

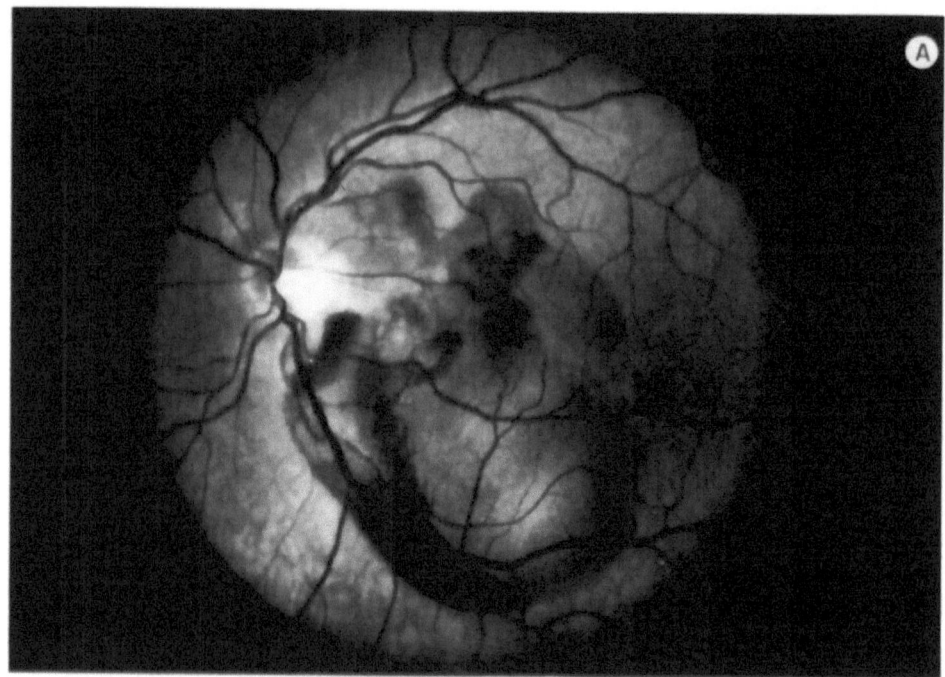

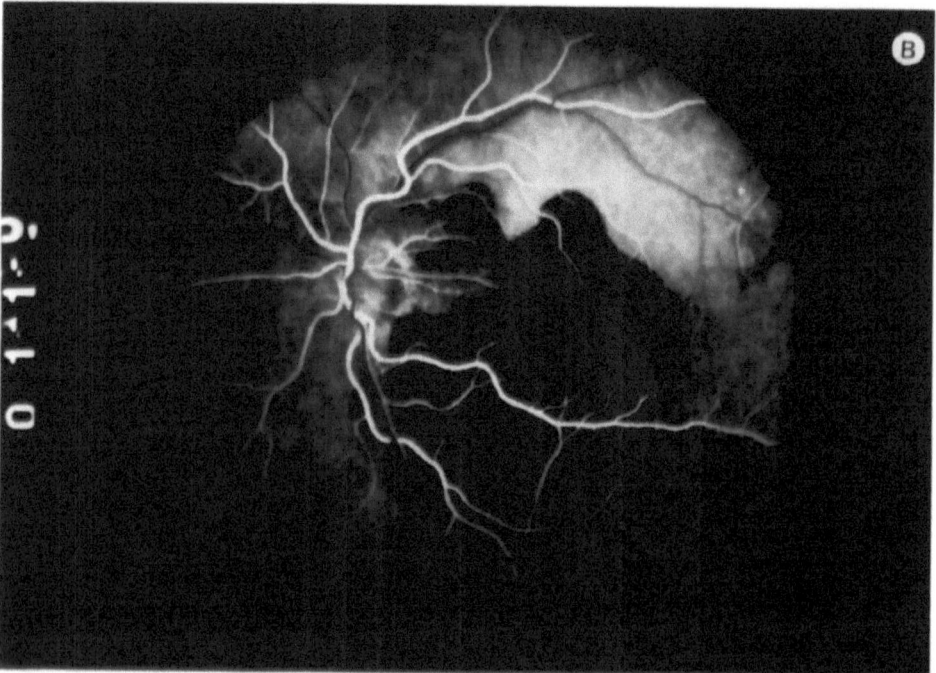

*Figure 13.* (A) Large subretinal hemorrhage in the inferior temporal quadrant of the left eye. (B) Fluorescein angiography confirming the diagnosis of subretinal hemorrhage shown in Figure 13A.

Fluorescein angiography is also extremely helpful in the differentiation of lesions simulating choroidal melanomas and iris melanomas. In the case of choroidal nevi or subretinal hemorrhage, the choroidal fluorescein pattern is obliterated (Figure 13A, B). If drusen do exist on the surface of the nevus, these may show typical window defects.

Fluorescein angiograms will, in the case of malignant melanoma, reveal irregular fluorescence, which is thought to be caused by loss of pigment from the pigment epithelium, leakage from the surface of the tumor and areas of hypofluorescence in the area of the orange pigmentation previously discussed (Figure 14). The leakage of fluorescein is independent of the location of the drusen [23].

The combination of clinical impression of a pigmented mass, including the feathery edge, the appearance of an orange pigment on the surface, changes in the visual fields or metamorphopsia, combined with a positive [32]P uptake, suggestive angiography and ultrasonography all aid in the increased certainty of positive diagnosis. No amount of testing, however, will negate the clinical impression from firsthand examination and observation, particularly with small tumors that show definite growth (Figure 15).

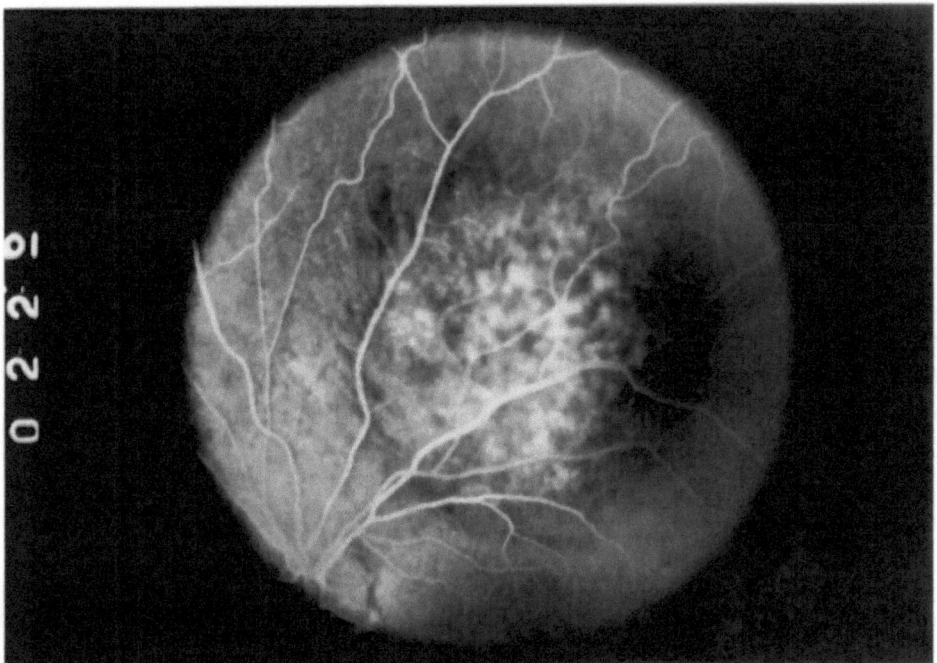

*Figure 14.* Fluorescein angiography of confirmed malignant melanoma showing the irregular fluorescence.

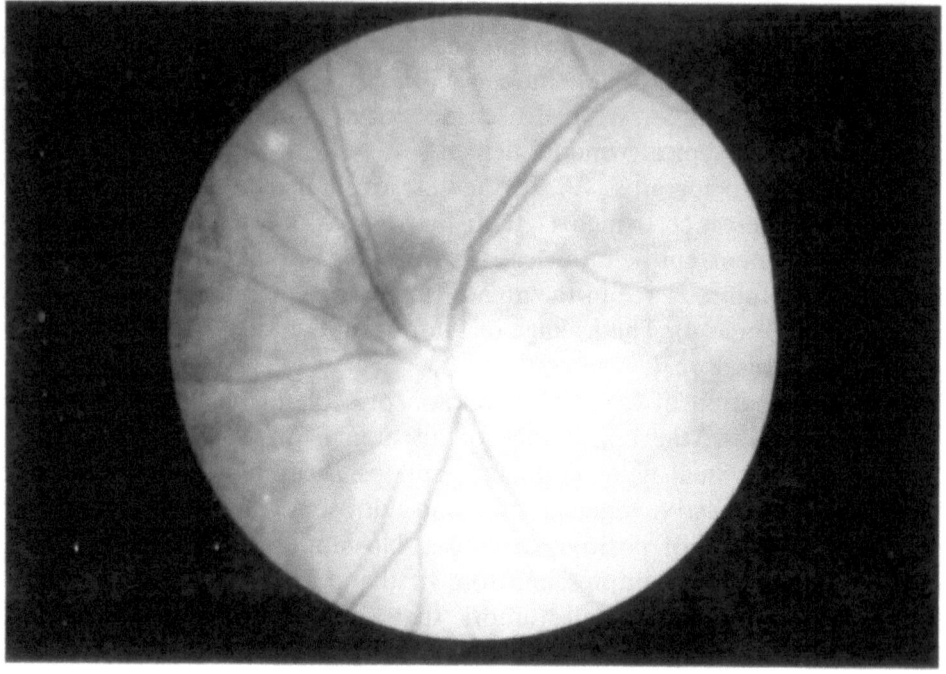

*Figure 15.* Elevated pigmented lesion at the border of the optic disc in a left eye.


## Treatment

In the past, a diagnosis of malignant melanoma, regardless of its size, of the choroid and ciliary body demanded enucleation as the only treatment of choice. Although some disagreement may well exist, it would seem that large tumors which show evidence of activity, are causing inflammation and reduction of vision, particularly when the fellow eye is normal, should have enucleation. Since untreated uveal melanomas have been said to rarely metastasize unless showing the above finding, one is faced with the dilemma of whether to treat small melanomas (less than 1400 mm$^3$ in size) or whether to just observe the patient. Much of the recent controversy has come from a report by Zimmerman and his co-workers [24] in which they reiterated that uveal melanomas rarely metastasize before the patient is referred for treatment. This group showed in their paper a remarkable increase in the death rate of patients with posterior uveal melanomas after enucleation when compared with those not treated.

It is suggested that although blood borne metastases are known to occur from uveal melanomas, they frequently cause no immediate problems because of the immune reaction of the body to these cells. Elsewhere in this book, a discussion upon the delay of clinical findings with metastases from cutaneous melanomas has been discussed, and it may well be that we are sitting on a time bomb from early metastases from uveal melanomas, but they frequently do not become evident for some time.

Fraunfelder and associates [25] in 1977 advocated a no-touch type of enucleation which allows reduction of manipulation of the extraocular muscles and increase of intraocular pressure which supposedly reduces the amount of blood borne metastases from the choroidal pressure which supposedly reduces the amount of blood borne metastases from the choroidal circulation.

Apple and Blodi [26], however, have shown that there is a slow and rapid growth phase of intraocular melanomas. They feel that during the period of rapid growth, metastasis, as well as other complications, are more apt to occur as well as cellular type change, perhaps from spindle A to epithelial, etc. It is during this time that decisions are frequently made to enucleate because of change in growth and appearance, and it may also be within this time span that metastasis to distance organs is also at its peak. Hence, the increased incidence of metastatic disease and death after enucleation may well be part of the natural history of the disease rather than on the basis of enucleation itself.

If one then agrees that either the natural history or standard enucleation does increase the chance for death from ocular melanoma, what course should one take, particularly when the tumor is small? If the clinician waits until there is evidence of activity and rapid growth, then perhaps a great disservice is done to the patient. However, is enucleation necessary to treat these small melanomas that show evidence that they are melanomas, malignant or with malignant potential, or should more conservative tumor eradication be carried out? This type of question becomes very important in patients whose only remaining eye is affected by the tumor or who are advanced in age. It may well be that this question applies to all patients.

As an alternative to enucleation, therapy with photocoagulation, radiotherapy, diathermy and cryotherapy have all been advocated. One should remember that observation is acceptable if there is some question in the observer's mind after using his diagnostic tests that the lesion is not unequivocally a melanoma. We have seen lesions that have been suspicious and followed for many years before a definite diagnosis could be made (Figure 10). Vogel [27], in 1972, has shown that a lesion being no greater than 10 mm in its greatest diameter and 2 mm in elevation will respond well to Xenon arc photocoagulation. Of course, these lesions should be in areas far enough from the macula or disc that the surrounding photocoagulation will not affect central vision. The $^{32}P$ test has been converted to a negative result after properly applied Xenon photocoagulation [28].

Stallard [29], in 1968, showed that cobalt-60 in an applicator using large doses of ionizing radiation can be curative with malignant melanomas of

208

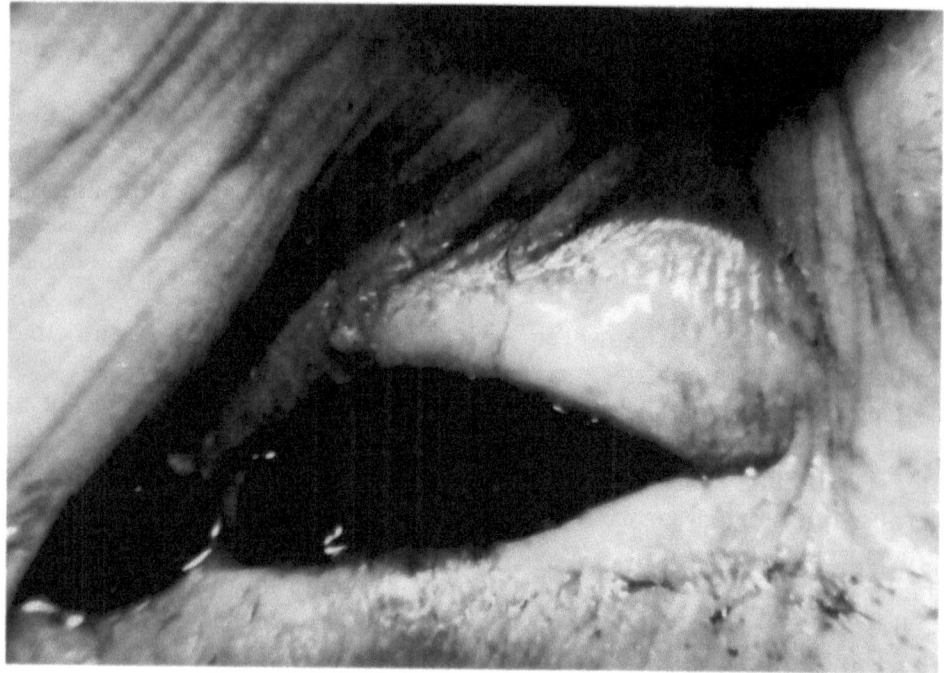

*Figure 16.* Recurrence of orbital malignant melanoma one year after enucleation of a left eye.

the choroid. More recently, proton radiation has shown potential [30]. [123]Iodine shows great potential in that construction of metal eye placques can be used so the tumor can be treated sparing the rest of the eye [31].

Transcleral diathermy may be effective, but it is generally felt that because of the damage to the sclera, the malignant cells may be able to escape into the periocular tissues more readily.

Cryotherapy has generally not been found to be completely satisfactory.

Until now the intraocular or transcleral removal of the tumor by surgical means has had only limited success.

Orbital recurrences after enucleation (Figure 16) can be treated by exenteration, radiotherapy or by palliative means.

## Summary

With astute clinical observation and the proper use of the newer diagnostic tools, the diagnosis of malignant melanoma of the eye should be accurate 99% of the time. Since iris lesions do not frequently metastasize, one should attempt surgical removal of these only if activity and growth are observed to prevent glaucoma and inflammatory complications as well as large extensions into the ciliary body. Small tumors of the ciliary body can also be removed surgically and large posterior uveal tumors will probably require enucleation although the older techniques may have to be modified in the light of statistical evidence that metastatic problems are accentuated with increase in intraocular pressure. Small lesions that are showing only early activity and are not involving central vision may well respond favorably to conservative methods other than observation. Larger lesions may also do well when the conservative treatment is decided upon in the cases of elderly patients or one eyed individuals.

There are no absolute answers and only nonemotional scientific observation on this tumor because of its ubiquitousness, and its frequent response to the body's immune system may perhaps give us the answers.

## References

1. Furth J: Vistas in the etiology and pathogenesis of tumors. Fed Proc Fed Am Soc Exp 20:865–873, 1961.
2. Hogan MJ: Clinical aspects management, and prognosis of melanomas of the uvea and optic nerve. In: Boniuk B (ed) Ocular and Adnexal Tumors. CV Mosby, St.Louis, 1964.
3. Spencer WH: Discussion in Reese AB: congenital melanomas. Trans Am Ophthalmol Soc 71:186–192, 1973.
4. Reese A: Tumors of the Eye, 3rd ed. Harper & Row, Hagerstown, 1976.
5. Rones B and Zimmerman LE: The prognosis of primary tumors of the iris treated by iridectomy. Arch Ophthalmol 60:193–205, 1958.
6. Cleasby G: Malignant melanomas of the iris. Arch Ophthalmol 60:403–417, 1958.
7. Martin-Jones JD: Uveal sarcomata. Br J Ophthalmol (Supp II):1–94, 1946.
8. Reese AB: The association of uveal nevi and skin nevi. Trans Am Ophthalmol Soc 49:47–57, 1952.
9. Bruckner R and Ludin H: Cytodiagnosis of tumors in ophthalmology. Ophthalmologica 133:169–175, 1957.
10. Paul EV, Parnell BL and Fraker M: Prognosis of malignant melanoma of the choroid and ciliary body. Int Ophthalmol Clin 2:387–402, 1962.
11. Hopkins RE and Carriker RR: Malignant melanoma of the ciliary body. Am J Ophthalmol 45:835–843, 1958.
12. Tamler E: A clinical study of choroidal nevi: a follow-up report. Arch Ophthalmol 84:29–32, 1970.
13. Tamler E and Maumenee AE: A clinical study of choroidal nevi. Arch Ophthalmol 62:196–202, 1959.
14. Callender GR: Malignant melanotic tumors of the eye: study of histologic type in 111 cases. Trans Am Acad Ophthalmol Otolaryngol 36:131–142, 1931.
15. Flocks M, Gerende JH and Zimmerman LF: The size and shape of malignant melanomas of the choroid and ciliary body in relation to prognosis and histologic characteristics. Trans Am Acad Ophthalmol Otolaryngol 59:740–758, 1955.
16. McLean IW and Foster WD: Prognostic factors in small malignant melanomas of choroid and ciliary body 95:48–58, 1977.
17. Smith LT and Irvine AR: Diagnostic significance of orange pigment accumulation over choroidal tumors. Am J Ophthalmol 76:212–216, 1973.

18. Kirk H and Petty R: Malignant malanoma of the choroid: a correlation of clinical and histological findings. Arch Ophthalmol 56:843–860, 1956.

19. Makley T and Teed R: Unsuspected intraocular malignant melanomas. Arch Ophthalmol 60:475–478, 1958.

20. Thomas C, Krohmer M and Storaasli J: Detection of intraocular tumors with radioactive phosphorus. Arch Ophthalmol 47:276, 1952.

21. Zakov ZN, Cook SA, Albert DM and Weichselbaum RR: False-positive phosphorus-32 uptake tests in the diagnosis of ocular melanoma, In: Albert and Weichselbaum (eds) International Ophthalmology Clinics (advances regarding the pathogenesis and treatment of ocular tumors), pp 117–121. Little, Brown, Boston, 1980.

22. Ossoinig K: Standardized echography: Basic principles, clinical applications and results. In: Albert and Weichselbaum (eds) International Ophthalmology Clinics (Advances regarding the pathogenesis and treatment of ocular tumors), pp 127–210. Little, Brown, Boston, 1980.

23. Gass JDM: Differential Diagnosis of Intraocular Tumors. CV Mosby, St. Louis, 1974.

24. Zimmerman LE, McLean IW and Foster WD: Does enucleation of the eye containing a malignant melanoma prevent or accelerate the dissemination of tumor cells? Br J Ophthalmol 62:420–425, 1978.

25. Fraunfelder FT, Boozman FW, Wilson RS and Thomas AH: No-touch technique for intraocular malignant melanomas. Arch Ophthalmol 95: 1616–1620, 1977.

26. Apple DJ and Blodi FC: Uveal melanocytic tumors: a grouping according to phases of growth and prognosis with comments on current theories of nonenucleation treatment. In: Albert and Weichselbaum (eds) International Ophthalmology Clinics (Advances regarding the pathogenesis and treatment of ocular tumors), pp 33–61. Little, Brown, Boston, 1980.

27. Vogel MH: Treatment of malignant choroidal melanomas with photocoagulation. Evaluation of ten year follow-up data. Am J Ophthalmol 74:1, 1972.

28. Shields JA, Annesley WH, Jr, Federman JL et al: Fluoroscrein and $^{32}$P studies in photocoagulated melanomas. Presented at First International Photocoagulation Congress, New York, September, 1975. CV Mosby, St. Louis, 1976.

29. Stallard HB: Malignant melanoblastoma of the choroid. Mod Probl Ophthalmol 7:16, 1968.

30. Constable I: Proton irradiation for small malignant melanomas of the choroid. In: Brockhurst, Boruchoff, Hutchinson and Lessell (eds) Controversy in Ophthalmology, pp 626–634. WB Saunders, Philadelphia, 1977.

31. Packer S and Rothman M: Radiotherapy of choroidal melanoma with iodine 125, In: Albert and Weichselbaum (eds) International Ophthalmology Clinics (Advances regarding the pathogenesis and treatment of ocular tumors), pp 135–142. Little, Brown, Boston, 1980.

# 7. Central nervous system melanoma

S. CLIFFORD SCHOLD, Jr., DENNIS E. BULLARD and
WESLEY A. COOK

## Introduction

Malignant melanomas arise from neural crest-derived melanocytes, which
are found in the skin, mucous membranes, uveal tract and in the pia-
arachnoid of the central nervous system (CNS). Theoretically, primary malignant melanomas can arise in any of these sites. However, the vast majority of melanomas arise in the skin, so that tumors found in other locations
are generally the result of metastasis. This chapter will review involvement
of the CNS by metastatic melanoma and will describe briefly the melanomas which originate in the brain and spinal cord.

## Parenchymal metastases

### Incidence

Melanoma is the third most common form of parenchymal CNS metastasis.
Only lung and breast cancer are found more commonly in the brain, in large
part because of their greater overall frequency. Vieth and Odom reported
that in 49 of 313 patients (16%) with clinically diagnosed brain metastases
the primary tumor was melanoma [1]. In a series of 426 patients with metastatic brain tumors referred to M.D. Anderson Hospital for chemotherapy,
Einhorn et al. found that 47 (11%) had melanoma [2]. Posner and Chernik
reported that 50 of 225 cases (22%) of intracerebral metastasis seen at
autopsy at Memorial Sloan-Kettering Cancer Center (MSKCC) between
1970 and 1976 were melanoma [3]. In other autopsy series the incidence of
melanoma has ranged from 4% to 10% of all metastatic brain tumors [4–6]
(Table 1).

Brain metastases are also found in a large percentage of patients dying
from melanoma. Posner reported that 50 of 125 melanoma patients (40%)
studied at autopsy had intracerebral metastasis [3]. The incidence has
ranged from 39% to 91% in other autopsy series [2, 5–10] (Table 2). Multiple metastatic lesions were present in the nervous system in 62–95% of
cases in three of these studies. Thus, roughly $\frac{1}{2}$ of patients dying from

*Seigler, H. F. (ed.), Clinical Management of Melanoma. ISBN 978-94-009-7495-1*
© *1982, Martinus Nijhoff Publishers, The Hague/Boston/London.*

*Table 1.* The Incidence of melanoma in autopsy series of brain metastases

| Reference | $\dfrac{\text{\# of cases of melanoma}}{\text{\# of cases of brain metastases}}$(%) |
|---|---|
| Posner [3] | 50/225  (22) |
| Markesbury [4] | 19/187  (10) |
| Aronson [5] | 13/358  (4) |
| Chason [6] | 10/200  (5) |

*Table 2.* The incidence of autopsy-proven central nervous system metastases in patients dying from melanoma

| Reference | $\dfrac{\text{\# of patients with CNS metastases}}{\text{\# of patients with melanoma}}$(%) | | $\dfrac{\text{\# of patients with >1 CNS lesion}}{\text{\# of patients with CNS metastases}}$(%) | |
|---|---|---|---|---|
| Einhorn [2] | 46/85 | (54) | N.S. * | |
| Posner [3] | 50/125 | (40) | 31/50 | (62) |
| Aronson [5] | 13/23 | (57) | N.S. | |
| Chason [6] | 10/11 | (91) | N.S. | |
| Amer [7] | 13/23 | (57) | N.S. | |
| Patel [8] | 118/216 | (55) | N.S. | |
| Beresford [9] | 36/84 | (43) | 32/36 | (89) |
| Das Gupta [10] | 41/105 | (39) | 39/41 | (95) |

* N.S. = Not Stated.

metastatic melanoma harbor CNS metastases and in the majority of these patients there are multiple lesions.

Several authors have noted a higher frequency of CNS metastases from melanoma in males. Fell et al. reported that 74% of 80 patients with metastatic CNS melanoma were males [11]; Amer et al. reported 34 males in a group of 56 patients (61%) [7]; and, in the Duke series of 1341 patients with melanoma, 72 of the 107 who developed clinical evidence of brain metastases were males (67%) in contrast to an equal number of males and females in the overall series [12]. In this same series Bullard et al. reported a higher incidence of nonextremity primary lesions in males, a correlation between the occurrence of CNS metastases and head and neck or oral mucosa primary lesions, and a similar correlation with Clark's level of invasion. It is unlikely that any of these factors are of primary importance with regard to nervous system metastases; rather, male sex, nonextremity primary lesions and more invasive tumors all correlate with an increase in all forms of disseminated disease.

*Table 3.* The incidence of clinically evident metastases outside the nervous system in patients with metastatic CNS melanoma

| Reference | # of patients with extra-CNS metastases / # of patients with CNS metastases | (%) |
|---|---|---|
| Fell [11] | 70/80 | (88) |
| Bullard [12] | 63/107 | (59) |
| Carella [13] | 51/60 | (85) |
| Cooper [14] | 21/30 | (70) |

The great majority of patients presenting with metastatic CNS melanoma have concurrent metastases elsewhere (Table 3). Bullard et al. reported that 63 of 107 patients (59%) had clinically evident involvement of other organs at the time of the diagnosis of CNS disease [12]; in Fell's series, in which the majority of patients were selected as acceptable operative candidates, the incidence of regional or distant metastases was still 88% of 80 patients [11]; Carella et al. [13] and Cooper and Carella [14] reported non-CNS metastatic disease in 70% and 85%, respectively, of patients with melanoma referred for brain radiotherapy. Of course the incidence of additional organ involvement has been even greater in autopsy studies. Amer et al. found that 39 of 40 patients (97%) with CNS metastases had visceral metastases at autopsy [7]. Patel et al. found an incidence of 96% in a similar series of 118 patients [8]. Thus, CNS metastasis from melanoma reflects disseminated systemic disease, and, even if other organ involvement is not evident at the time of neurological presentation, it is soon likely to appear. That this association is not invariable, however, has been shown by isolated case reports of long disease-free survival after excision of a single brain metastasis [15].

Overall, between 5% and 10% of patients with primary dermal melanoma have developed CNS involvement (8% of 1341 patients in the Duke series and 9.6% in the M.D. Anderson series [16]. Because of the unpredictable nature of the disease, the interval from primary diagnosis to the diagnosis of CNS metastasis has varied from immediate to over 15 years. The median interval in Fell's series was 32 months, with 78% of CNS metastases developing within 48 months. These figures are in general agreement with those from other series. This phenomenon of a prolonged interval from primary tumor diagnosis to brain involvement in roughly 20% of cases is in marked contrast to the pattern seen in other forms of CNS metastasis, such as those from lung and testis [17, 18], again reflecting the biology of the neoplasm rather than any peculiarity of nervous system involvement.

*Pathology*

Intraparenchymal brain metastases characteristically occur at the gray–white junction, are well demarcated from surrounding brain and appear in locations in the nervous system which reflect the relative blood supply or mass of the regions. Metastases are often surrounded by considerable brain edema and are often multiple (Figures 1 and 2). Melanoma is often grossly pigmented and is more likely than any other metastatic tumor of the brain, except for choriocarcinoma, to show evidence of hemorrhage. Bremer et al. reported that in seven of 17 craniotomies for parenchymal CNS melanoma "substantial intracerebral hematoma was present" [19]. Hayward reported that ten of 27 patients with CNS melanoma "showed evidence of subarachnoid hemorrhage" [20]. In Fell's series, in 14 of 59 cases examined (24%), there was evidence of hemorrhage in the metastasis [11]. Occasionally, the hemorrhage can be of sufficient severity to obscure the underlying tumor.

*Signs and symptoms*

Most patients with metastatic melanoma of the brain are neurologically symptomatic, and the signs and symptoms reflect the location and extent of their tumors. Altered mental status, headache and focal motor or sensory

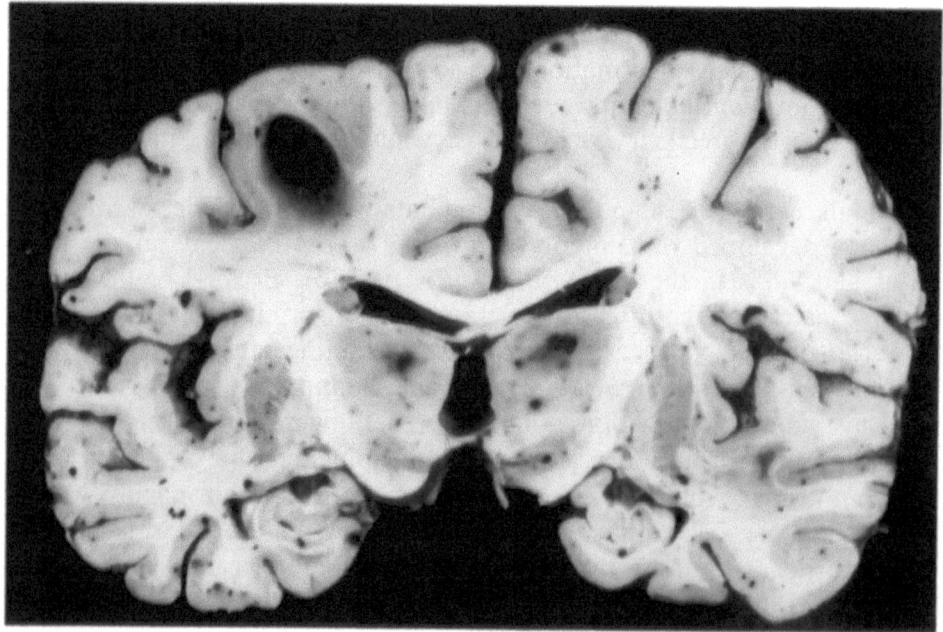

*Figure 1.* Metastatic melanoma of the brain. There are numerous pigmented lesions scattered throughout both cerebral hemispheres.

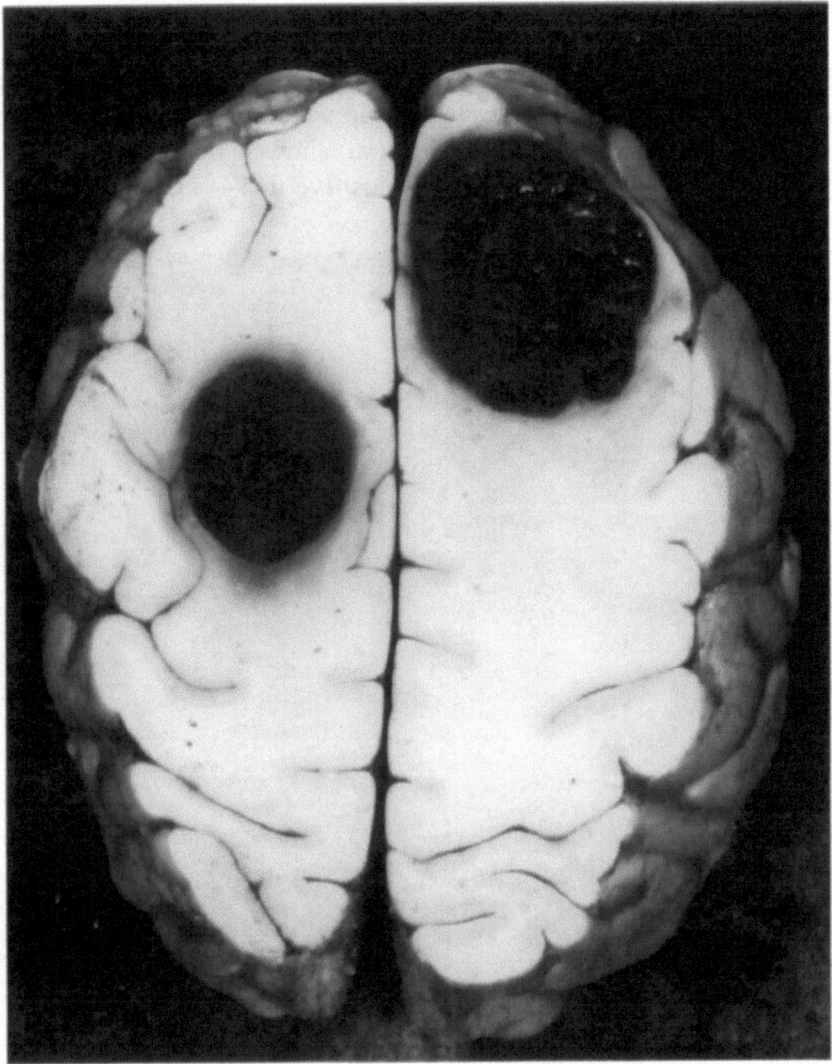

*Figure 2.* Metastatic melanoma of the brain. A large pigmented metastasis is visible in each frontal lobe.

deficits are the most common modes of neurological presentation [7, 13, 19]. Focal seizures have been reported as the initial form of presentation in 11–32% of patients [7, 21]. An abrupt onset of symptoms in patients with CNS melanoma can also be caused by hemorrhage into the tumor.

*Diagnosis*

Metastatic melanoma of the brain is most often diagnosed by the computerized axial tomogram (CAT), a technique which is highly sensitive to the
presence of CNS metastases. Bardfeld et al. showed that the CAT with the
administration of a contrast agent was positive in 94% of 47 patients with

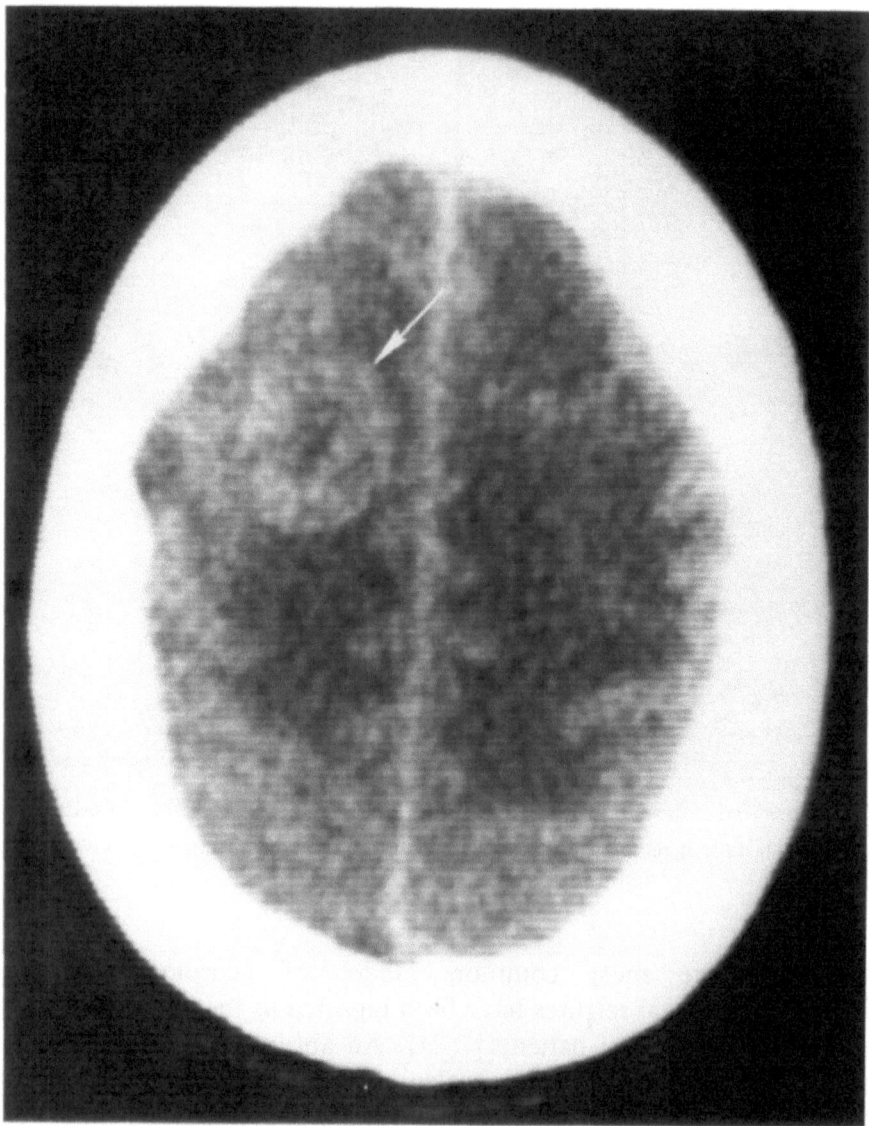

*Figure 3A.* Computerized axial tomogram in metastatic melanoma of the brain (same patient as in
Figure 2). A) Without a contrast agent there is hypodensity of the white matter of both hemispheres as well as an ill-defined hyperdense area in the left frontal lobe (arrow). B) After the
administration of a contrast agent, a metastatic lesion is visible in each frontal lobe. The white
matter hypodensity surrounding the tumors represents cerebral edema.

brain metastases from a variety of primary tumors, including two patients who had negative radioisotope scans [22]. Buell et al. also found that the CAT had greater sensitivity (100 % vs. 81 %) than isotope scans in detecting CNS metastases [23].

Metastatic melanomas in the CNS appear on the CAT as areas of abnormal density which may show enhancement after the administration of a contrast agent (Figures 3A, B) [24]. The lesions are frequently surrounded by a hypodense area which does not change with enhancement and which may

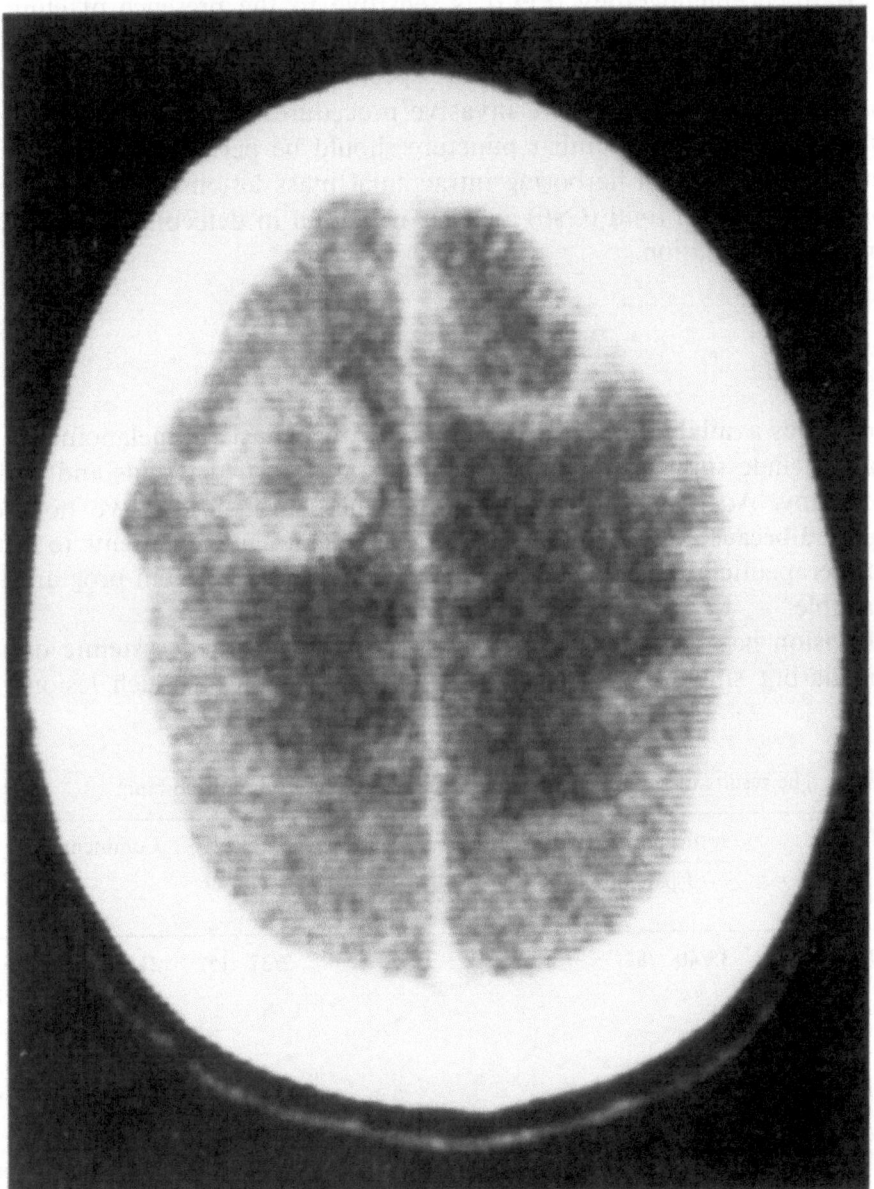

*Figure 3B.*

involve the entire hemisphere; this presumably represents brain edema. If hemorrhage has occurred, the lesions are dense prior to the infusion of the contrast agent, an appearance which may not be distinguishable from primary intracerebral hemorrhage. Radiographic evidence of hemorrhage is often present without a clinical history of abrupt onset of symptoms. All 14 patients in one CAT evaluation of intracerebral metastatic melanoma had lesions which contained a "high absorption area within blood range" [24].

Electroencephalography (EEG) is sensitive to the presence of clinically apparent brain metastases from melanoma [7]. The radionuclide brain scan is somewhat less sensitive but is more specific than EEG. Arteriography and pneumoencephalography are invasive procedures and are usually not required for diagnosis. Lumbar puncture should be performed cautiously in patients suspected of harboring intracranial mass lesions, but when available cerebrospinal fluid (CSF) analysis is helpful in detecting subarachnoid tumor dissemination.

## Treatment

Modalities available for treating patients with metastatic melanoma of the brain include surgery, radiation, chemotherapy, corticosteroids and immunotherapy. Adequate studies comparing these modalities have not been reported because of selection factors in the assignment of patients to different therapeutic groups, but the results of individual treatment programs are available.

Excision has been advocated for patients with limited systemic disease who harbor single, accessible cerebral lesions (Table 4). Such lesions are

Table 4. The results of surgical treatment of metastatic melanoma of the brain

| Reference | # of patients improved / # of patients treated (%) | Median survival (months) | Surgical mortality (%) | Comment |
|---|---|---|---|---|
| Fell [11] | 35/40 (88) | 5 | 2/37 (5) | 21% 1-year survivors, including 1 at 10 years and 1 at 18 years |
| Bremer [19] | 14/19 (74) | 5 | 2/19 (11) | Survival range was 1–15 months |
| Hafstrom [25] | 19/25 (76) | 5 | 3/25 (12) | Longest survivor is alive at 74 months. |

often readily approachable surgically as they are distinct from surrounding uninvolved brain. Hafstrom et al. reported clinical improvement in 19 of 25 patients (76%) with single metastatic melanomas of the brain treated surgically, with a median postoperative survival of five months [25]. Fell et al. reported postoperative clinical improvement in 35 of 40 symptomatic patients (88%) [11]. The median survival of these patients was 20 weeks, a figure which increased to 36 weeks in the 17 patients receiving postoperative whole brain radiotherapy. These investigators also reported a 21% one-year survival, as well as four patients, who "underwent craniotomy for a metastasis that could not be found." Bremer et al. reported clinical improvement in 14 of 19 patients (74%) and a median survival of five months [19]. Surgical mortality in these series was three of 25 (12%), two of 37 (5.4%) and two of 19 (10.5%), respectively. The incidence of negative exploration, reoperation, infection and other complications was not reported in detail in these series, but it has ranged from 19–25% in recently reported series of all forms of metastatic brain tumor [26]. Presumably, these complications will decline with more accurate diagnostic methods and more sophisticated medical support.

A few long-term survivors have been reported among surgically treated patients. McCann et al. described two cases of survival exceeding ten years after excision of metastatic melanoma of the brain [15]. Fell et al. reported two patients alive ten and 18 years after surgery [11]. Despite the occasional long-term survivor, most authorities favor postoperative whole brain radiotherapy because of the high incidence of multiple lesions.

The standard form of treatment of metastatic brain disease is radiation, even for relatively radioresistant tumors such as melanoma (Table 5). Radiation is given to the entire intracranial contents, most commonly in 200–300 rad fractions to a total dose of 3000–4000 rads. Carella et al. reported 60 patients with metastatic CNS melanoma who were treated with whole brain radiotherapy in doses ranging from 1000 rads in one treatment to 4000 rads in four weeks [13]. Forty-three patients received concomitant corticosteroids. Symptomatic improvement was noted in 41 patients (76%) and median survival was between ten and 14 weeks with one patient living at 198 weeks. Nisce et al. reported symptomatic improvement in 22 of 27 patients (81%) with a median response duration of two months [27]. In Gottlieb's series of 41 patients, seven of whom were operated on prior to radiation, symptomatic improvement was observed in 16 (39%) after irradiation, and the median survival was less than three months [21]. Amer et al. reported six responses among 16 patients treated and a mean survival of 7.6 months [7]. Hilaris et al. [28] and Cooper and Carella [14] reported response rates of 67% and 38%, respectively. Thus, patients treated with whole brain radiation for metastatic CNS melanoma have a definite, but short-lived, response rate. Median survival is generally worse than in surgi-

*Table 5.* The results of radiotherapy for metastatic melanoma of the brain

| Reference | # of patients improved / # of patients treated (%) | Median survival (months) | Comment |
|---|---|---|---|
| Einhorn [2] | 8/26 (31) | — | Responders had a 5-month median survival. |
| Amer [7] | 6/16 (38) | 7.6 (mean) | — |
| Carella [13] | 41/54 (76) | ~3 | — |
| Cooper [14] | 11/29 (38) | 3 | 8 of 12 females responded vs. 3 of 17 males. |
| Gottlieb [21] | 16/41 (39) | <3 | Median response duration was 60 days. The longest survivor was 436+ days. |
| Nisce [27] | 22/27 (81) | ~5 | Median response duration was 2 months. 10% survival at 1 year. |
| Hilaris [28] | 18/27 (67) | 4 (mean) | — |

cal series, but the selection of appropriate surgical candidates prohibits comparison of these figures. The morbidity from radiotherapy alone under these circumstances is insignificant.

Chemotherapy alone has essentially not been evaluated as a mode of therapy for CNS melanoma. Because of the relative resistance of this tumor to chemotherapy and the presumed problems of drug delivery to CNS lesions, nearly all patients who are treated for this disease are either operated on or receive radiotherapy. In Fell's series there were 14 patients who received chemotherapy alone (the agents were not specified) with a median survival of four weeks and a 7% six-month survival [11]. In Amer's series, two of 17 patients (11.7%) receiving chemotherapy alone responded, though it was not clear to what extent these represented CNS responses [7]. Fay et al. [29] have recently reported the use of high-dose ($\geq 1200$ mg/m$^2$) BCNU (BCNU = 1,3-bis(2-chloroethyl)-1-nitrosourea) as a single agent in combination with autologous bone marrow transplantation. Four of 12 patients with CNS melanoma responded with response durations of 3, 3.5, 5, and 7.5$^+$ months.

Though not chemotherapy in the usual sense, corticosteroids have a definite place in the management of CNS metastases. Presumably by reducing the peritumoral brain edema, steroids alone produce a significant clinical response. Posner and Shapiro [30] reported a response rate of 60–75%, with symptoms related to increased intracranial pressure, such as headache and altered mental status, most likely to respond. The response is rapid, often within 24 hours, but, unless combined with more direct oncolytic therapy, its benefits are not lasting. Conventionally, 16 mg of dexamethasone in divided doses over 24 hours are administered, but higher doses may be required and equivalent doses of other glucocorticoids may be just as effective. In addition to providing symptomatic relief, the use of steroids has improved operative results by permitting surgical intervention on more stable patients and by reducing postoperative complications. No studies describing the use of steroids in the specific management of CNS metastatic melanoma have been reported, and the extent to which the response in this disease might differ from that in other forms of brain metastasis is not known.

Immunotherapy has received a great deal of attention in melanoma [31]. It is, of course, not employed alone as therapy in metastatic CNS melanoma, but epidemiologic data about the occurrence of CNS metastases in patients treated with immune stimulants for their primary lesions have been reported. In a preliminary report Grooms and Morton [32] found an increased incidence of CNS metastases in patients treated with BCG compared to those receiving no immunotherapy.

The development of brain metastasis from malignant melanoma is a serious complication. Most of these patients have extensive systemic disease at the time of neurological presentation, a significant percentage have multiple CNS lesions, and the median survival is less than six months whatever treatment is employed. Most neurologically symptomatic patients will respond to a combination of corticosteroids and whole brain radiation. Indications for surgical excision include the lack of a primary tissue diagnosis, symptomatic recurrence of a CNS lesion after definitive radiotherapy, and impending herniation due to tumor mass or hemorrhage within the tumor. The management of the unusual patient with relatively stable systemic disease and a single, accessible brain lesion is more controversial. While in this setting there have been a few long-term survivors following surgical excision, the likelihood of rapid CNS or visceral progression is high, and the potential benefit of surgery may be outweighed by its attendant morbidity and the requirement for additional hospitalization. The judgement and experience of the surgeon should influence this decision.

## Leptomeningeal metastases

### Incidence

The cranial and spinal leptomeninges are common sites of metastases from a variety of systemic cancers. The most common neoplasms to involve the meninges are the acute leukemias, the non-Hodgkin's diffuse lymphomas, breast cancer and lung cancer. A number of patients with metastatic melanoma of the meninges have also been described. Five of the 47 patients (10.6%) with leptomeningeal metastases reported by Olson et al. had malignant melanoma [33]. Wasserstrom et al. reported that 11 of 90 adult patients (12.2%) with leptomeningeal metastases from solid tumors had melanoma [34]. In three of 29 (10.3%) and three of 30 (10%) patients with metastatic neoplastic meningitis in two other series, the primary tumor was melanoma [35, 36]. Many patients with metastatic leptomeningeal melanoma have concomitant parenchymal CNS metastases (four of five in the Olson series), and most have disseminated systemic disease.

*Pathology*

Leptomeningeal carcinomatosis consists of sheet-like infiltration of tumor cells over the surface of the brain and spinal cord. The arachnoid of the basal cisterns and the thecal sac are the most common sites of involvement, though any area of the neuraxis can be affected. Occasionally, these masses of tumor cells will coalesce and form discrete nodules; this occurs most often in the cauda equina. The ependymal surfaces of the ventricular system tend to be relatively spared. Hydrocephalus may result from obstruction of the subarachnoid space by tumor. Histologically, tumor cells are arranged in thin layers or small nodules, especially surrounding blood vessels. There is a variable degree of fibroblastic or inflammatory response in the meninges. Involvement of the leptomeninges by melanoma can result in black discoloration of the whole surface of the nervous system (see reference 37 for a particularly striking example).

*Signs and symptoms*

Signs and symptoms of leptomeningeal tumor vary with the site of involvement. If the brain is involved headache, seizures and altered mental status are common findings; if the basal cisterns are the predominant site of tumor, cranial nerve deficits are paramount, with facial palsy, hearing loss and various ophthalmoplegias most common; and low back pain, leg weakness and sphincter disturbances indicate spinal involvement. The presence of concomitant parenchymal metastases produces additional focal disturbances. Evidence of disease disseminated along the neuraxis with a combination of central and peripheral findings is highly suggestive of the diagnosis.

*Diagnosis*

Leptomeningeal metastases are diagnosed by the constellation of appropriate clinical findings and characteristic CSF abnormalities. The CSF is commonly under increased pressure and contains 10–100 white blood cells/mm$^3$, an elevated protein concentration and often a depressed glucose concentration. The diagnosis can be established with certainty, even in the absence of neurological findings, by the presence of malignant cells in the CSF [38]. Any of these variables may be normal in the CSF of a patient with meningeal tumor, though the CSF is abnormal in some way in approximately $\frac{3}{4}$ of patients on the first examination [33]. Anecdotally, a cytologic diagnosis is more difficult in patients with leukemias and lymphomas because of the resemblance of the neoplastic cells to normal blood elements and is often more straightforward in melanoma because of the pigment in the tumor cells. However, the relative sensitivity of CSF cytology in meningeal melanoma has not been specifically addressed.

Other laboratory tests can be of value in the diagnosis of leptomeningeal metastases. The CAT showed pathologic enhancement of the basal cisterns in ten of 45 patients (22%) with documented leptomeningeal metastasis from a variety of tumors [39]. The CATs of both patients with leptomeningeal melanoma in this series were positive. Myelography, with either Pantopaque® or a water-soluble contrast agent, may show nodularity of the spinal nerve roots in a pattern suggestive of arachnoiditis. CSF tumor markers have recently been demonstrated to be of value in the diagnosis of leptomeningeal tumors. Two recent series have documented the presence of increased concentrations of $\beta$-glucuronidase, a lysosomal enzyme, in the CSF of these patients. There were three patients with melanoma in one series [36] and six in the other [40]. Surprisingly, carcinoembryonic antigen was also elevated in the CSF of two patients with leptomeningeal melanoma [40]. This was unexpected as melanoma is not one of the tumors commonly associated with the production of this substance. It suggests that a heavy tumor burden in a relatively small compartment (the ventricular-subarachnoid volume is approximately 125 ml) might allow detection of tumor-related substances not detectable in the blood. Radionuclide uptake [41] and karyotype analysis of CSF cells [42] are two other recently reported diagnostic methods.

*Treatment*

Standard treatment of metastatic leptomeningeal neoplasm consists of radiotherapy and intrathecal chemotherapy, most commonly with methotrexate. Generally, areas of clinical involvement, rather than the whole neuraxis, are radiated, and methotrexate, at a dose of 10–15 mg once or twice weekly, is combined with citrovorum factor, "rescuing" the bone marrow. The ideal route of administration of the drug is intraventricularly via an in-dwelling "Ommaya" reservoir device [43].

Response to this treatment varies with a number of factors, the most important of which are the extent of clinical involvement at the time treatment is initiated and the tumor type. Wasserstrom et al. reported a response rate of 47% (42 of 90 patients stabilized or improved) in patients with a variety of primary tumors. This response was usually brief, though it did correlate with survival. The median survival of all patients in this study was 5.8 months after treatment was initiated; most often, death was due to extensive systemic disease. Eleven patients with melanoma survived from one to 12 months after treatment with clinical improvement reported in two [34]. Engelhardt et al. reported "modest results" with "regression of psychopathological symptoms" in one patient with metastatic leptomeningeal melanoma treated with 25 mg of methotrexate weekly via lumbar puncture [44].

## Spinal cord compression

### Incidence

Spinal cord compression (SCC) from metastatic cancer occurs principally as a result of epidural tumor secondary to vertebral body metastasis. Consequently, the incidence of epidural spinal cord compression reflects the tendency of the primary tumor to involve bone. The most common tumors producing this syndrome are breast cancer, lung cancer, the lymphomas, prostate cancer, various sarcomas and hypernephroma. Melanoma was the tumor of origin in eight of 235 patients (3.4%) in a recent series from MSKCC of patients with epidural spinal cord compression [45]. In a subsequent series from the same institution five of 83 patients (6.0%) had melanoma [46]. Young et al., in a randomized therapeutic study of 29 patients with epidural metastases, reported that in three patients (10.3%) the primary tumor was melanoma [47]. On the other hand, in a surgical series reported by Brice and Mekissock only one of 145 patients had melanoma [48]. Vieth and Odom found that melanoma caused SCC in 5.2% of 78 patients in a series which specifically excluded lymphomas and myeloma [49].

*Pathology*

SCC caused by metastatic tumor is usually secondary to vertebral body metastasis. Since the dura mater acts as an effective barrier to the entrance of tumor from the epidural space, tumor from the vertebrae produces neurological symptoms by compression, rather than invasion, of the spinal cord. If the compression is not relieved, permanent damage results, the pathological consequences of which are necrosis at the site of compression and secondary degeneration of the ascending and descending fiber tracts. Uncommonly, the manifestations of SCC are produced either by localized leptomeningeal tumor or by an intramedullary spinal cord metastasis. In the latter situation a tumor nodule is found within the substance of the cord producing destruction and surrounding edema, analogous to a metastatic nodule in the brain. Any level of the spinal cord or vertebral column can be affected.

*Signs and symptoms*

The most common symptom of patients suffering from SCC from metastatic tumor is pain. In Gilbert's series, 96% of 130 patients had pain at diagnosis [45]; in Greenberg's study 82 of 93 patients (88%) had "significant pain" prior to treatment [46]. The pain is commonly localized to the affected vertebral level, but it may be radicular in character or referred to other areas. It is commonly associated with exquisite tenderness to percussion over the involved vertebra. Other common symptoms in this group of patients are referable to localized spinal cord dysfunction and include weakness, sensory loss and autonomic disturbances, especially incontinence. Once signs and symptoms progress beyond pain and tenderness, rapid progression is the rule. Complete paraplegia can result within hours. When the tumor causing spinal cord dysfunction is intramedullary rather then epidural, pain is less often present and autonomic dysfunction is more prominent, but there is considerable clinical overlap with the more common epidural SCC. No report has focused on melanoma as a cause of SCC; however, it is likely that the clinical syndrome produced by melanoma is similar to that seen with other tumors.

*Diagnosis*

Over 90% of patients with metastatic SCC from solid tumors (excluding lymphomas) have radiographically demonstrable vertebral body metastasis at the appropriate level. Thus, the clinical syndrome of localized spine pain and tenderness, a clinical myelopathy, and vertebral body destruction in a patient with systemic cancer is highly suggestive of the diagnosis of SCC. Definitive diagnosis is made by myelography. If a complete myelographic block is found, it is important to define the upper limit of the block by introducing contrast material through a puncture at the C1–C2 interspace. Cerebrospinal fluid obtained at the time of myelography should be sent for routine studies including cytologic examination, but, if the tumor is restricted to the epidural space, the CSF should be normal except for an elevated protein concentration. A low CSF glucose concentration or malignant cells indicate concomitant leptomeningeal tumor. CSF marker studies have not been helpful in this disease [40]. CAT of the spine may prove to be an accurate, noninvasive method of diagnosis of SCC, but its reliability has not yet approached that of myelography.

*Treatment*

Epidural SCC from metastatic cancer is a neurological emergency. If not treated promptly, neurological dysfunction will rapidly progress, and the success of treatment is directly related to the extent of neurological disability at the time it is instituted. Corticosteroids should be administered immediately once the diagnosis of SCC is established and often before definitive myelography if clinical suspicion is high. This relieves symptoms in the great majority of patients and may reverse or reduce the rate of progression of neurological dysfunction. Once the diagnosis is established, patients are treated either by decompressive laminectomy followed by radiotherapy or by immediate radiotherapy. Whatever treatment is administered, its success is related to the patient's neurological status at its onset and is also correlated with the degree of myelographic block. Indications for surgery include progression after or during adequate radiotherapy, no primary tissue diagnosis and rapid progression without radiotherapeutic facilities immediately available. Many authorities would also recommend laminectomy as the primary form of therapy in patients harboring radioresistant tumors. Gilbert reported that the rate of clinical improvement in the seven melanoma patients in his series was zero of two treated with surgery and radiation and one of five treated with radiation alone [45]; in Greenberg's series, of five patients with melanoma treated with radiation, two improved and three were unchanged [46]. Other studies of SCC do not report the outcome with individual tumor types. However, as in parenchymal brain metastases the immediate radioresistance of melanoma may have been overstated.

## Primary CNS melanoma

### Leptomeningeal pigmentation

The spectrum of primary pigmented lesions of the brain and spinal cord ranges from physiologic hyperpigmentation to frank, rapidly progressive malignant melanoma, distinguishable from the metastatic disease only by the lack of a dermal primary. The pia mater normally contains melanocytes which are concentrated at the base of the brain, especially on the lateral and ventral aspects of the medulla [50]. The degree of physiologic leptomeningeal pigmentation varies widely among individuals paralleling the degree of dermal pigmentation to some extent [51]. It increases during pregnancy, presumably due to increased levels of melanocyte-stimulating hormone [52]. A benign syndrome, which may be familial, of excess leptomeningeal pigmentation is referred to as leptomeningeal melanosis [53].

### Neurocutaneous melanosis (NCM)

NCM is a congenital syndrome in which large or numerous skin nevi are accompanied by excessive numbers of melanocytes in the leptomeninges [53]. It is thus a form of phakomatosis and may occur in association with neurofibromatosis. The skin lesions often follow a dermatomal or "cape" pattern and are histologically benign. Neurological signs and symptoms due to hydrocephalus are common as the thickened leptomeninges interfere with cerebrospinal fluid circulation. Twenty-four percent of cases reviewed by Savitz and Anderson presented neurologically in the first year of life [54]. In most reported cases anaplastic changes are found in the leptomeningeal melanocytes, and the brain parenchyma may be invaded [55]. The malignant neurological condition can be diagnosed in life, but it has been inexorably progressive in most reported cases.

### Primary leptomeningeal melanoma

Most cases of leptomeningeal melanoma are due to metastatic spread from a dermal primary. Primary leptomeningeal melanoma refers to diffuse leptomeningeal invasion by anaplastic melanocytes without evidence of a primary source outside the nervous system. Such a diagnosis cannot be accepted without examination of all possible sources of a primary tumor, including the orbits [56]. So defined, primary leptomeningeal melanoma is a rare disease, with adequately documented cases numbering fewer than 100 according to Savitz and Anderson [54]. Clinical and CSF findings in these patients are identical to those produced by metastatic leptomeningeal melanoma. However, the patients with the primary CNS form of the disease tend to be somewhat younger; Gibson et al. reported that 73% of 59 patients dying from primary CNS melanoma were under 50 and 22% were under 20; in contrast, only 36% of 1395 patients dying from cutaneous melanoma were under 50 [57]. While most patients with primary CNS melanoma do not have associated cutaneous manifestations, there is apparently some overlap with the neurocutaneous syndromes [58]. The patient reported by Savitz et al. [59], for example, had numerous café-au-lait spots, and one of the patients reported by Bojson-Moller had frank neurofibromatosis [60]. Pathologically, this tumor tends to be concentrated at the base of the brain, and there is a spectrum of morphology of the melanocytes, ranging from hyperplasia to typical anaplastic malignant melanoma [57, 61]. The tumor cells often invade the Virchow-Robin spaces and may compress blood vessels. Occasionally, parenchymal nodules in the brain and spinal cord are prominent. The issue of visceral metastases in this disease is controversial, with most authors requiring the disease to be confined to the CNS for the diagnosis of primary CNS melanoma [57]. However, case -7 of Bergdahl et al. [62] in which widespread CNS disease was accompanied by two small hepatic metastases may well represent extra-CNS spread. Primary CNS melanoma is a rapidly progressive disease not unlike metastatic leptomeningeal melanoma. Median survival has been less than six months in most series, though a few cases with survival up to two years have been reported [60]. Treatment has been unsuccessful except when a mass of tumor can be excised. No aggressive chemotherapeutic regimens have been reported.

*Other pigmented CNS tumors*

A number of other primary neoplasms of the CNS may contain melanin. These include meningiomas, medulloblastomas, ependymomas and choroid plexus tumors. Histologic distinction from primary tumors of melanocytic origin is usually not difficult [63].

**Acknowledgments**

Dr. Peter C. Burger kindly supplied the pathological material. Dr. Philip J. DuBois supplied the radiographs.

# References

1. Vieth RG and Odom GL: Intracranial metastases and their neurosurgical treatment. J Neurosurg 23:375-383, 1965.
2. Einborn LH, Burgess MA, Vallejos C, Bodey GP, Sr, Gutterman J, Mavligit G et al: Prognostic correlations and response to treatment in advanced metastatic malignant melanoma. Cancer Res 34:1995-2004, 1974.
3. Posner JB and Chernik NL: Intracranial metastases from systemic cancer. Adv Neurol 19:575-587, 1978.
4. Markesbery WR, Brooks WH, Gupta GD and Young AB: Treatment for patients with cerebral metastases. Arch Neurol 35:754-756, 1978.
5. Aronson SM, Garcia JH and Aronson BE: Metastatic neoplasms of the brain: their frequency in relation to age. Cancer 17:558-563, 1964.
6. Chason JL, Walker FB and Landers JW: Metastatic carcinoma in the central nervous system and dorsal root ganglia: a prospective autopsy study. Cancer 16:781-787, 1963.
7. Amer MH, Al-Sarraf M, Baker LH and Vaitkevicius VK: Malignant melanoma and central nervous system metastases: incidence, diagnosis, treatment and survival. Cancer 42:660-668, 1978.
8. Patel JK, Didolkar MS, Pickren JW and Moore RH: Metastatic pattern of malignant melanoma: a study of 216 autopsy cases. Am J Surg 135:807-810, 1978.
9. Beresford HR: Melanoma of the nervous system: treatment with corticosteroids and radiation. Neurology 19:59-65, 1969.
10. Das Gupta T and Brasfield R: Metastatic melanoma: a clinicopathological study. Cancer 17:1323-1339, 1964.
11. Fell DA, Leavens ME and McBride CM: Surgical versus nonsurgical management of metastatic melanoma of the brain. Neurosurgery 7: 238-242, 1980.
12. Bullard DE, Cox EB and Seigler HF: Central nervous system metastases in malignant melanoma. Neurosurgery 8:26-30, 1981.
13. Carella RJ, Gelber R, Hendrickson F, Berry HC and Cooper JC: Value of radiation therapy in the management of patients with cerebral metastases from malignant melanoma. Cancer 45:679-683, 1980.
14. Cooper JS and Carella R: Radiotherapy of intracerebral metastatic malignant melanoma. Radiology 134:735-738, 1980.
15. McCann WP, Weir BKA and Elvidge AR: Long-term survival after removal of metastatic malignant melanoma of the brain: report of two cases. J Neurosurg 28:483-487, 1968.
16. Harter D, Caderao J and Withers H: The natural history of malignant melanoma metastatic to the brain: the M.D. Anderson experience 1944 through 1973. Proc Am Soc Clin Oncol 22:385, 1981 (abstract).
17. Leavengood JM, Martini N and Posner JB: Brain metastases from non-oat-cell lung carcinoma. Neurology 31, pt 2:68, 1981 (abstract).
18. Schold SC, Vugrin D, Golbey RB and Posner JB: Central nervous system metastases from germ cell carcinoma of the testis. Sem Oncol 6: 102-108, 1979.
19. Bremer AM, West CR and Didolkar MS: An evaluation of the surgical management of melanoma of the brain. J Surg Oncol 10:211-219, 1978.
20. Hayward RD: Secondary malignant melanoma of the brain. Clin Oncol 2:227-232. 1976.
21. Gottlieb JA, Frei E, III and Luce JK: An evaluation of the management of patients with cerebral metastases from malignant melanoma. Cancer 29:701-705, 1972.
22. Bardfeld PA, Passalaqua AM, Braunstein P, Raghavendra BN, Leeds NE and Kricheff II: A comparison of radionuclide scanning and computed tomography in metastatic lesions of the brain. J Comput Assist Tomogr 1:315-318, 1977.

23. Buell U, Niendorf HP, Kazner E, Lanksch W, Wilske J, Steinhoff H et al: Computerized transaxial tomography and cerebral serial scintigraphy in intracranial tumors − rates of detection and tumor type identification. J Nucl Med 19:476–479, 1978.
24. Solis OJ, Davis KR, Adair LB, Roberson GR and Kleinman G: Intracerebral metastatic melanoma: CT evaluation. Comput Tomogr 1:135–143, 1977.
25. Hafstrom L, Jonsson P and Stromblad L: Intracranial metastases of malignant melanoma treated by surgery. Cancer 46:2088–2090, 1980.
26. Black P: Brain metastasis: current status and recommended guidelines for management. Neurosurgery 5:617–631, 1979.
27. Nisce LZ, Hilaris BS and Chu FCH: A review of experience with irradiation of brain metastasis. Am J Roentgenol 111:329–333, 1971.
28. Hilaris B, Raben M, Calabrese A, Phillips R and Henschke UK: Value of radiation therapy for distant metastases from malignant melanoma. Cancer 16:765–773, 1963.
29. Fay JW, Levine MN, Phillips GL, Herzig GP, Herzig RH, Lazarus HM, et al: Treatment of metastatic melanoma with intensive 1,3-bis(2-chloroethyl)-1-nitrosourea (BCNU) and autologous marrow transplantation (AMTX). Proc Am Soc Clin Oncol 22:532, 1981 (abstract).
30. Posner JB and Shapiro WR: The management of intracranial metastases. In: Morley TP (ed) Current Controversies in Neurosurgery, pp 356–366. WB Saunders, Philadelphia, 1976.
31. Gutterman JU, Mavligit GM, Kennedy A, McBride CM, Burgess MA and Hersh EM: Immunotherapy for malignant melanoma. In: Neoplasms of the Skin and Malignant Melanoma, pp 497–531. Year Book Medical Publ, Chicago, 1976.
32. Grooms GA and Morton DL: Failure of adjuvant immunotherapy to prevent brain metastases in malignant melanoma. Proc Am Soc Clin Oncol 16:261, 1975 (abstract).
33. Olson ME, Chernik NL and Posner JB: Infiltration of the leptomeninges by systemic cancer. Arch Neurol 30:122–137, 1974.
34. Wasserstrom WR, Glass JP and Posner JB: Diagnosis and treatment of leptomeningeal metastases from solid tumors: experience with 90 patients. Cancer 49:759–772, 1982.
35. Little JR, Dale AJD and Okazaki H: Meningeal carcinomatosis: clinical manifestations. Arch Neurol 30:138–143, 1974.
36. Shuttleworth E and Allen N: CSF β-glucuronidase assay in the diagnosis of neoplastic meningitis. Arch Neurol 37:684–687, 1980.
37. Shapiro WR, Posner JB, Ushio Y, Chernik NL and Young DF: Treatment of meningeal neoplasms. Cancer Treat Rep 61:733–743, 1977.
38. Glass JP, Melamed M, Chernik NL and Posner JB: Malignant cells in cerebrospinal fluid (CSF): the meaning of a positive CSF cytology. Neurology 29:1369–1375, 1979.
39. Enzmann DR, Krikorian J, Yorke C and Hayward R: Computed tomography in leptomeningeal spread of tumor. J Comput Assist Tomogr 2:448–455, 1978.
40. Schold SC, Wasserstrom WR, Fleisher M, Schwartz MK and Posner JB: Cerebrospinal fluid biochemical markers of central nervous system metastases. Ann Neurol 8:597–604, 1980.
41. Siegal T, Or R, Matzner Y and Samuels LD: Spinal meningeal uptake of technetium-99m methylene diphosphonate in meningeal seeding by malignant lymphoma. Cancer 46:2413–2415, 1980.
42. Kristoffersson U, Dahlquist E and Mitelman F: Cytogenetic diagnosis of meningeal carcinomatosis. N Engl J Med 303:1479, 1980.
43. Ratcheson RA and Ommaya AK: Experience with the subcutaneous cerebrospinal-fluid reservoir. N Engl J Med 279:1025–1031, 1968.
44. Engelhardt P and Lorenz R: Cytostatic treatment of meningeal blastoses. J Neurol 220:279–289, 1979.
45. Gilbert RW, Kim J and Posner JB: Epidural spinal cord compression from metastatic tumor: diagnosis and treatment. Ann Neurol 3:40–51, 1978.

46. Greenberg HS, Kim J and Posner JB: Epidural spinal cord compression from metastatic tumor: results with a new treatment protocol. Ann Neurol 8:361–366, 1980.
47. Young RF, Post EM and King GA: Treatment of spinal epidural metastases: randomized prospective comparison of laminectomy and radiotherapy. J Neurosurg 53:741–748, 1980.
48. Brice J and McKissock W: Surgical treatment of malignant extradural spinal tumours. Br Med J 1:1341–1344, 1965.
49. Vieth RG and Odom GL: Extradural spinal metastases and their neurosurgical management. J Neurosurg 23:501–508, 1965.
50. Russell DS and Rubinstein LJ: Pathology of Tumours of the Nervous System, p 55. Williams & Wilkins, Baltimore, 1977.
51. Das Gupta TK, Brasfield RD and Paglia MA: Primary melanoma in unusual sites. Surg Gynecol Obstet 128:841–848, 1969.
52. Deutsch S and Mescon H: Melanin pigmentation and its endocrine control. N Engl J Med 257:222–226, 1957.
53. Fox H: Neurocutaneous melanosis. In: Vinken PH and Bruyn GW (eds) Handbook of Clinical Neurology, Vol 14, pp 414–428. North-Holland, Amsterdam, 1972.
54. Savitz MH and Anderson PJ: Primary melanoma of the leptomeninges: a review. Mt Sinai J Med N Y 41:774–791, 1974.
55. Lamas E, Lobato RD, Sotelo T, Ricoy JR and Castro S: Neurocutaneous melanosis: report of a case and review of the literature. Acta Neurochir 36:93–105, 1977.
56. Winkelman NW, Gotten N and Silverstein A: Primary melanoblastosis of the meninges. Arch Neurol Psychiatry 35:919–920, 1936.
57. Gibson JB, Burrows D and Weir WP: Primary melanoma of the meninges. J Pathol Bacteriol 74:419–438, 1957.
58. Slaughter JC, Hardman JM, Kempe LG and Earle KM: Neurocutaneous melanosis and leptomeningeal melanomatosis in children. Arch Pathol 88:298–304, 1969.
59. Savitz MH, Gendelman S, Huang YP, Fayemi AO and Anderson PJ: Primary leptomeningeal melanomatosis presenting as carcinomatous meningitis. Mt Sinai J Med 41:812–819, 1974.
60. Bojsen-Moller M: Primary cerebral melanomas: report of six cases and a review of the literature. Acta Pathol Microbiol Scand Sect A 85:447–454, 1977.
61. Bouton J: Primary melanoma of the leptomeninges. J Clin Pathol 11:122–127, 1958.
62. Bergdahl L, Boquist L, Liliequist B, Thulin CA and Toui D: Primary malignant melanoma of the central nervous system: report of 10 cases. Acta Neurochir 26:139–149, 1972.
63. Russell DS and Rubinstein LJ: op cit, p 57.

# 8. Immunobiology of melanoma

GARY M. STUHLMILLER

In discussing the immunobiology of a particular form of human cancer, in this case, melanoma, one makes the tacit assumption that the tumor cells express certain moieties which are not expressed on the normal adult cellular counterpart. Secondly, one also assumes that the host is, to some extent, able to recognize these tumor associated antigens (TAA) as foreign and to respond against them with either a cellular or humoral reaction, or with both. Early studies performed in inbred rodent model systems successfully demonstrated that both virally induced and carcinogen-induced tumors did express such TAA and that, under appropriate conditions, these TAA did provoke a vigorous antitumor immune response [146]. Clinically speaking, the human melanoma TAA of greatest interest are those located on the cell membrane as these would be accessible on the viable tumor cell to the host antitumor immune response. As will be discussed in this chapter, in addition to cell membrane TAA, melanoma cells may also express cytoplasmic and nucleolar TAA. These, however, appear to be of much less importance clinically because of their inaccessibility as targets for immune destruction of the cell.

Melanoma appears to be among the more highly immunogenic of the human cancers, this despite the fact that few human tumors can be as highly invasive and destructive of normal tissues as melanoma. It is of interest that, despite a rapid increase in its rate of incidence, particularly in the Southeastern United States, melanoma still accounts for only 1–3% of all human cancers. This low incidence may, in part, be due to the immunogenic nature of melanoma and to the efficacy of the host immune response to destroy malignantly transformed melanocytes prior to their formation of a clinically evident tumor.

Melanoma has been of great interest since its description in the 19th century, largely because of its bizarre and often unpredictable behavior suggestive of some form of host control of the disease [37]. It is not uncommon for the primary lesion to regress while metastatic lesions persist [31, 64] or for primary and metastatic lesions to regress coincident with the development of new metastases [165, 183]. Despite the fact that it is seldom fully realized, occasional reports of regression of widely disseminated melanoma demonstrate the potential of the immune response to eliminate even large

*Seigler, H. F. (ed.), Clinical Management of Melanoma. ISBN 978-94-009-7495-1*
© 1982, Martinus Nijhoff Publishers, The Hague/Boston/London.

volumes of tumor [164, 174]. A particularly interesting observation is that of delayed onset of metastatic disease in certain ocular melanoma patients, where cases arise in which metastases may appear as many as thirty years after "complete" removal of the primary lesion. Such a delay is strongly suggestive of some form of host control of the disease during this "disease-free" interval.

In this chapter, we will review the evidence which has accumulated to support the existence of human melanoma TAA. Because of the volume of literature on this subject, we can not, in this chapter, possibly evaluate every study which has been conducted. Rather, we will concentrate on those studies which have provided the most informative results, with the hope that due credit will be given to all who have made significant contributions to our understanding of the subject. For further information, the reader is referred to several recent reviews of melanoma immunobiology which treat the subject from different perspectives [171, 45, 111]. In addition to discussing evidence for the existence of the melanoma TAA, we will discuss the potential uses of the TAA in prognosis and diagnosis of melanoma and will also attempt to evaluate potential roles of these TAA in the host–tumor interaction. The use of the TAA as potential targets for immunotherapy will be covered in a separate chapter in this monograph.

Using sera from melanoma patients, it has been possible to demonstrate melanoma TAA in the cytoplasm and nucleolus of melanoma cells as well as on the melanoma cell membrane (Table 1). Lewis provided the first evidence for humoral antimelanoma antibody when he demonstrated a cytotoxic effect of sera from certain melanoma patients upon autologous melanoma cells growing in monolayer culture [96]. Two of his observations are of interest. Each positive serum was reactive only with autologous melanoma cells, a finding which suggested that each melanoma may express individually unique cell membrane TAA. This situation was reminiscent of that of carcinogen-induced murine tumors, where each expressed unique cell membrane TAA. Secondly, Lewis found that only sera from those patients whose disease was localized were antibody-positive. Sera taken from patients with disseminated tumor contained no demonstrable antibody. As will become evident as we progress, these two observations and their significance have been quite controversial. Morton et al. [123], using the same serological procedure, reported quite different results. In his study, sera from 7/7 melanoma patients were positive with autologous cell membrane and cytoplasmic TAA. However, positive results were also obtained in 61% of the homologous serum: cell combinations used and 20% of the normal sera tested were also positive. With regard to cell membrane TAA, Morton's results suggest the possibility of TAA shared by different melanomas. Essentially comparable results were reported by Fossati et al. [48], while several further studies by Lewis and his colleagues have maintained the individu-

Table 1. Serological demonstration of melanoma TAA using human sera

| Investigators | Methods | Results |
|---|---|---|
| Kopf et al., 1966 [89] Lewis, 1967 [96] | Immunofluorescence Complement dependent cytotoxicity | Unable to demonstrate antibody fixed to fresh melanoma cells. Sera from 4/5 patients with localized disease killed autologous melanoma cells. No alloreactivity. |
| Morton et al., 1968 [123] | Immunofluorescence | 7/7 patients sera positive for cell membrane TAA and cytoplasmic TAA of autologous melanoma cells, 61% homologous sera: cell combination positive, 20% normal sera positive |
| Oettgen et al., 1968 [136] | Immunofluorescence | Sera from 61% melanoma patients, 10% patients with nonmelanoma tumors, 11% patients with other nonmalignant diseases were positive melanoma cytoplasmic TAA. |
| Lewis et al., 1969 [97] | Immunofluorescence, complement dependent cytotoxicity, inhibition of RNA synthesis | 1/3 patients positive vs. autologous cells by one or more tests. 80% of patients, with localized disease positive. Both cytoplasmic and membrane TAA were examined. |
| Muna et al., 1969 [125] | Immunofluorescence | Patient sera reactive with cytoplasm of melanoma cells. Very low titers. |
| Romsdahl and Cox 1970 [151] | Immunofluorescence | Antibody demonstrated on melanoma imprints—cytoplasmic and cell membrane TAA demonstrated. |
| Morton et al., 1970 [122] | Complement fixation | Presence of antibody (incidence and titer) correlated with stage of disease. |
| Fossati et al., 1971 [48] | Immunofluorescence | Sera from 13/17 patients positive in autologous combination, 8/10 in allogeneic combinations for cell membrane TAA. |
| Lewis et al., 1971 [100] | Multiple assays | Presence of antibody reactive with antimelanoma antibody as a possible explanation for dissemination and loss of antimelanoma antibody. |
| Hamilton-Fairley et al., 1971 [63] | Complement dependent cytotoxicity, immunofluorescence inhibition of RNA synthesis | Patient sera reactive with autologous cells 5/15 in grade I, 28/44 in grade II, 2/60 in grade III. |
| Lewis and Phillips, 1972a [98] | Immunofluorescence, absorption | Separation of antibody reactive with cell membrane and cytoplasmic TAA — distinct TAA |
| Lewis and Phillips, 1972b [99] | Immunofluorescence | Confirmation of individual specificity of patient sera, need for stringent interpretation of immunofluorescence results. |
| Nairn et al., 1972 [130] | Immunofluorescence, complement dependent cytotoxicity | 2/30 positive in cytotoxicity, 8/34 by immonofluorescence in autologous combinations. Weak cross-reactivity with two allogeneic lines. 14/52 sera positive for cytoplasmic TAA. Cross-reactive. |
| Copeman et al., 1973 [26] | Immunofluorescence | Sera from 1/5 patients with halo nevus reactive with melanoma cytoplasm TAA |
| Hellström et al., 1973c [71] | Antibody dependent cellular cytotoxicity | Sera from four melanoma patients enhanced cell killing. |

*Table 1.* Serological demonstration of melanoma TAA using human sera (continued)

| Investigators | Methods | Results |
|---|---|---|
| Lewis et al., 1973 [95] | Immunofluorescence, complement dependent cytotoxicity | Antimelanoma antibody often detected early in desease, disappears prior to dissemination of tumor. |
| Elliott et al., 1973 [38] | Immunofluorescence, complement dependent cytotoxicity | Sera from patients with nonmelanoma skin lesions did not react with melanoma TAA. |
| Federman et al., 1974 [43] | Immunofluorescence | Four patients with ocular melanoma and two patients with cutaneous melanoma had sera reactive with cytoplasmic TAA, not reactive with normal choroidal melanocytes, normal donor sera nonreactive. |
| Wood and Barth, 1974 [193] | Immunofluorescence | No difference in incidence of antibody reactive with cytoplasmic TAA in sera from melanoma patients, normals and patients with nonmelanoma tumors. Melanoma patients had higher titer—especially late stage patients. |
| Irie et al., 1975 [79] | Mixed hemagglutination | Antibody bound to melanoma cells in vivo. |
| Gupta and Morton, 1975 [59] | Complement fixation | Elution of antibody bound (in vivo) to melanoma cells. |
| Kodera and Bean, 1975 [88] | Antibody dependent cellular cytotoxicity | 4/16 patients sera positive vs. autologous cells; also detected A binding to melanoma cells. |
| Bodurtha et al., 1975 [10] | Complement dependent cytotoxicity | 9/10 autologous positive if disease localized; 1/11 autologous positive if disease disseminated no alloreactivity. |
| DeVries et al., 1975 [34] | Immune adherence | 12/73 sera positive, both autologous and allogeneic combinations, no reactivity on autologous fibroblasts, 0/85 control sera positive. |
| The et al., 1975 [177] | Immunofluorescence | Failed to demonstrate any difference in reactivities between melanoma patient sera and normal sera. |
| Whitehead, 1975 [190] | Immunofluorescence | 32% melanoma patient sera and 17% of control sera positive vs. six melanoma cell lines. Antibody present in 21% stage I, 40% secondary disease, 54% in cured patients. |
| Macher et al., 1975 [105] | Immunofluorescence, immune adherence | Sera from melanoma patients variable, some shared cell membrane TAA. |
| Bowen et al., 1975 [11] | Immunofluorescence | Patient sera reactive with nucleolar TAA—shared by melanoma and some other tumors, TAA is RNA bound. Presence of TAA correlated with latter stage disease, poor prognosis. |
| Cornain et al., 1975 [27] | Immune adherence | 13/73 sera (4/6 autologous) positive 0/50 normal donors positive. No correlation with stage or clinical state. |
| Canevari et al., 1975 [17] | Complement dependent cytotoxicity | 16/52 sera positive—15/40 Stage I and II, 1/12 Stage III, 3/43 controls positive. |
| Kilpatrick and Seigler, 1976 [87] | Complement dependent cytotoxicity | Patients undergoing active immunotherapy have antibody with both auto- and allo-reactivity. |
| Hersey et al., 1976 [74] | Antibody dependent cellular cytotoxicity, absorption | Cross-reactivities for cell membrane TAA variable. |

*Table 1.* Serological demonstration of melanoma TAA using human sera (continued)

| Investigators | Methods | Results |
|---|---|---|
| Minden et al., 1976a [120] | Immunoprecipitation | Melanoma patients have antibody reactive with melanoma and BCG normals also positive. |
| Minden et al., 1976b [119] | Immunoprecipitation | Rabbit antibody vs. melanoma or BCG reacts with both. |
| Carey et al., 1976 [19] | Mixed hemagglutination, absorption | 11/35 patients had antibody vs. melanoma. One serum reactive only with autologous cells (Au). |
| Shiku et al., 1976 [159] | Immune adherence, absorption | 10/18 positive vs. autologous cells. One restricted to autologous (BD). One positive with 5/12 homologous (AH). |
| Irie et al., 1976 [81] | Immune adherence | Sera from melanoma patients detect oncofetal antigen cross-reactive with fetal brain certain other tumor types. |
| Shiku et al., 1977 [160] | Immune adherence, mixed hemagglutination, absorption | Three autologous—positive sera broadly reactive with allogeneic and xenogeneic cells. |
| Siebert et al., 1977 [162] | Immune adherence | Patient antibody reactive primarily with fetal Ag. No common TAA detected. |
| Ferrone and Pelegrino, 1977 [44] | Complement dependent cytotoxicity | 34/90 patient sera positive with allogeneic cells; incidence of antibody in melanoma patients, nonmelanoma or other disease. |
| Leong et al., 1977a [91] | Immunofluorescence, 5 patients Autoimmunized cells and BCG, 5 patients Alloimmunized cells and BCG | 4/5 positive vs. 5/7 melanomas, 5/5 positive vs. 5/7 melanomas, 2/5 positive vs. autologous. |
| Leong et al., 1977b [94] | Immunofluorescence | Sera from treated patients more reactive with methanol-treated cells. TAA embedded in membrane. |
| Liao et al., 1978 [102] | Mixed hemagglutination | Sera from autoimmunized patient reacted with 5/5 melanoma, 2/5 nonmelanomas. KB cells removed nonmelanoma activity. |
| Sidell et al., 1979 [161] | Complement dependent cytotoxicity | Oncofetal Ag on cell membrane—target for immune cytolysis. |
| Irie et al., 1979 [82] | Immune adherence | Oncofetal Ag on cell membrane and immunogenic in patients. |

ality of the cell membrane TAA [95, 97, 98, 63]. Several other groups of investigators have reported either totally negative [89, 177] or highly variable results [105]. The question of whether or not melanomas express certain shared cell membrane TAA is of potentially great therapeutic and diagnostic significance. Indeed, the oncologist is hopeful that one form of therapy might prove highly and equally effective for all patients. This hope is based, in large part, on the assumption of certain identical physiological and biochemical features of the tumor cells. Identity of cell membrane TAA between melanoma cells of different patients makes the task of immunotherapy and immunodiagnosis much less complicated, if not easier.

The weight of evidence now favors at least a partial cross-reactivity between cell membrane TAA of different melanomas (Table 1). With this information in mind, it is useful, at this point, to evaluate possible reasons why different investigators may have arrived at such varied results using the same techniques and comparable materials. A major factor may have been the use of immunofluorescence, a technique which is subject to many variables and has an inherent element of subjectivity. Three criteria have been utilized for evaluation of immunofluorescence, these being intensity of staining, pattern of staining and percentage of cell staining. Lewis has established stringent conditions under which results are interpreted [97]. As such, in his studies, sera from normal donors or patients with tumors of nonmelanoma origin are seldom positive with melanoma cell membrane TAA. It is possible that Morton and others utilized less stringent criteria for interpretation and thus have demonstrated antimelanoma cell membrane TAA alloreactivity and also reactivity in sera from some normal donors. As such, Morton may have obtained some false positive results. However, he may also have detected certain positive results which Lewis, using more stringent conditions, could have failed to detect as positive.

Another possible explanation for divergent findings may be that these early studies were indeed performed with very different sera and cells. Perhaps Lewis' test sera contained only antibody of very restricted specificity while those tested by Morton were more widely reactive. This possibility is supported by the studies of Carey et al. [19] and Shiku et al. [159, 160], as we will discuss in a subsequent paragraph.

Finally, a third possibility, not totally separate from the first two, is the presence, within the test sera, of antibodies against other types of antigens but cross-reactive with melanoma cell membrane TAA. An example is Bacillus Calmette-Guerin (BCG), a mycobacterium used in numerous immunotherapy protocols as a nonspecific immunostimulant. Minden et al. have shown that sera from both normal donors and melanoma patients contain antibody reactive with BCG and with melanoma TAA [120]. Furthermore, rabbit and sera raised against either melanoma cells or BCG, react with antigens from both target cells in immunoprecipitation assays [119]. These studies demonstrate that "natural" anti-BCG antibody in test sera may react with melanoma TAA. A second example is that of natural or immune antiblood group A or B antibodies. Bloom et al. [7] have shown that human tumor cells in tissue culture express a blood group A-like antigen. Kodera and Bean reported that antiblood group A antibody was reactive with melanoma cells [88]. Carcinoembryonic antigen (CEA) has been shown to cross-react with blood group A antigen and Morgan et al. [121] have demonstrated the presence of a CEA-like antigen on melanoma cells. The widespread distribution of anti-blood group A and anti-CEA antibodies in sera from normal donors and the added reactivity of anti-BCG antibodies with melanoma cells make it quite likely that certain of the sera evaluated in these early studies did indeed contain antibodies which were specific for antigens other than melanoma TAA.

Newer serological techniques of greater sensitivity and objectivity have permitted a more detailed evaluation of melanoma cell membrane TAA. In very detailed studies, Carey et al., using mixed hemagglutination and absorption analysis, found sera from 11/35 melanoma patients to contain antibody reactive with melanoma cells [19]. One of these positive sera was examined more extensively and found to react only with autologous tumor cells. Shiku et al. extended these studies using immune adherence and found antibody in 10/18 autologous serum cell combinations [159]. One of these sera described an antigen found solely on autologous melanoma cell membranes while a second serum reacted with 5/12 homologous melanoma cell lines. In one further study, these investigators described three melanoma patient sera which were reactive with autologous tumor, but also with a variety of homologous and heterologous cells [160]. To summarize, these studies have revealed that melanoma cells may express individually unique cell membrane TAA, TAA cross-reactive with or identical to those expressed by homologous melanomas and heterophile antigens as well. In conjunction with results obtained using heteroantisera and monoclonal antibodies and with those from cell mediated immunity studies, these results strongly support the contention that there exists some degree of cross-reactivity between certain of the melanoma cell membrane TAA. Certain melanomas also appear to express individually unique TAA.

From the initial descriptions by Morton et al. [123] and by Oettgen et al. [136] in 1968 and 1969 respectively, there has been general agreement that the melanoma cytoplasmic TAA are shared more or less widely by different melanomas (Table 1). Using absorption analysis, Lewis and Phillips were able to separate antibodies reactive with cell membrane and cytoplasmic TAA, thereby demonstrating that they were indeed two distinct TAA [98]. Most subsequent work involving the cytoplasmic antigen has centered around determining its distribution and specificity for melanoma. Copeman et al. [26] reported that serum from 15 patients with halo nevus reacted to melanoma cytoplasmic TAA, while Elliott et al. [38] found that sera from patients with nonmelanomatous skin lesions did not contain antibody reactive with the cytoplasmic melanoma TAA. Federman et al. [43] found that six melanoma patient sera, all of which were reactive with the cytoplasmic TAA of melanoma cells, failed to react to the cytoplasm of normal choroidal melanocytes. Furthermore, these investigators were unable to demonstrate any anticytoplasmic TAA activity in sera from normal donors. These studies are somewhat in contrast to the original reports of Morton et al. [122] and Oettgen et al. [136] where 20% and 11% of normal sera, respectively, were found to react with melanoma cytoplasm. This author is unaware of any data relating to the use of melanoma patient sera, positive for melanoma cytoplasmic TAA, to study tumors of nonmelanoma origin for their expression of these TAA. In conclusion, although cytoplasmic melanoma TAA have been well described, their specificity for melanoma is still unresolved.

The third serologically described melanoma TAA was identified by Bowen et al. [11]. This TAA is present in the nucleous of melanoma cells but also in cells of certain other tumor types and has been shown to be RNA bound. The investigators who originally defined the antigen have provided the only data to characterize it and no further descriptive data regarding this antigen have been presented.

A discussion of patient antimelanoma cell-mediated immune responsiveness may be easily divided into two sections based upon the nature of the assay used to demonstrate this immunity (Table 2). The first demonstration of cell-mediated antimelanoma immunity was reported by Stewart who used soluble melanoma extract to elicit delayed cutaneous hypersensitivity reactions (DCHR) in melanoma patients [168]. DCHR were found in 1/7 melanoma patients injected with the melanoma extract. As the immunological basis for DCHR is interaction of antigen with specifically sensitized T-lymphocytes followed by secondary release from the T cells of various mediators of inflammation, this study suggested that the responsive patient had been sensitized against melanoma TAA as part of his disease process. Fass et al. [42] and Char et al. [21] quickly followed this report with confirmatory data. Fass et al. demonstrated that melanoma patients having localized disease were responsive to a melanoma extract and Char et al. reported that 18/19 ocular melanoma patients reacted against a melanoma extract while 0/7 controls reacted with the same extract. However, Bluming et al. [8] found that, while 11 patients responded with DCHR to extracts of autologous melanomas, 6/9 of these patients also responded to an extract of autologous skin. This observation suggested that factors other than sensitization to melanoma TAA had a role in DCHR. Hollingshead et al. have utilized partially purified TAA preparations in an attempt to avoid this element of nonspecificity, and have shown that one fraction contained an

Table 2. Demonstration of melanoma TAA by measurements of noncytolytic antimelanoma cell-mediated immune responses

| Investigators | Assays | Results |
|---|---|---|
| Stewart, 1969 [168] | DCHR* | 1/7 melanoma patients showed reaction to melanoma extract. |
| Jehn et al., 1970 [84] | Lymphocyte stimulation | Seven melanoma patients reacted to extract of autologous tumor. TAA shown to be in tumor cyst fluid of one patient. |
| Fass et al., 1970 [42] | DCHR | Eight patients with localized tumor responded to melanoma extract. |
| Char et al., 1970 [21] | DCHR | 18/19 ocular melanoma patients positive with melanoma extract; 0/7 controls positive. |
| Nagel et al., 1971 [129] | Lymphocyte stimulation | Surgical removal of tumor shown to enhance stimulation of PBL by TAA. |
| Bluming et al., 1972 [8] | DCHR | 11 patients reactive with extract of autologous tumor, 6/9 patients reactive with extract of autologous skin. Reactivity did not correlate with stage of disease. |
| Hollingshead et al., 1974 [78] | DCHR | Partially purified melanoma TAA. 17/22 patients with early stage melanoma were positive; 7/19 with late stage melanoma were positive; 1/22 patients with other cancer was positive. A second TAA cross-reactive with breast CA. |
| Hollingshead, 1975 [77] | DCHR | Possible fetal origin of some TAA. |
| Hersh et al., 1975 [76] | Lymphocyte blastogenesis (Stimulation) | 65% positive correlation of blastogenesis to autologous tumor extract with stage of disease. |
| McCoy et al., 1975 [116] | Migration inhibition | 48/79 melanoma patients, 4/27 patients with other disease and 3/50 normal donors were reactive to melanoma extract. |
| Boddie et al., 1975 [9] | Migration inhibition | 19/36 (53%) melanoma patients, 4/23 (17%) patients with nonmelanoma patients and 4/28 (14%) of normals reacted to KCl extract of melanoma. No correlation with stage of disease observed. |
| Cochran et al., 1975 [25] | Migration inhibition | 35/63 melanoma patients showed inhibition and 7/63 enhancement of migration. Patients with localized disease had greater inhibition. 9/59 normal donors and 5/28 breast cancer patients also inhibited. Loss of reactivity in patients preceded recurrences. |
| Halliday et al., 1975 [62] | Leukocyte adherence inhibition | 22/24 melanoma patients, positive; 0/10 normal donors, positive. 50/58 patients sera contained "blocking factor," 3/38 normals' sera also had blocking factor. Presence of blocking factor correlated with stage of disease. |
| Mazuran et al., 1975 [110] | Monocyte spreading inhibition | 24 melanoma patients reactive; six patients with other tumor and 14 normal donors were negative. |
| Weese et al., 1978 [189] | DCHR | Different extracts vary greatly in reactivity. |
| Douwes et al., 1978 [36] | Electrophoretic mobility test | 91% of melanoma patients positive vs. 8.7% controls to KCl extract of melanoma. |
| Vanderbark et al., 1979 [185] | Leukocyte adherence inhibition | Melanoma patients and family members are more highly reactive than control donors. |

* DCHR—delayed cutaneous hypersensitivity reaction.

antigen apparently unique to melanoma cells while a second fraction contained an antigen to which breast cancer patients also responded [77, 78]. This particular assay has fallen into disuse in recent years because of several problems such as variability between antigen preparations [189] and variations in the clinical state and immune responsiveness of the test patients and controls.

Several assays have been utilized to demonstrate antimelanoma cell-mediated immune responsiveness in vitro. Jehn et al. [84] found that a melanoma extract was stimulatory to peripheral blood lymphocyte (PBL) from melanoma patients and that the TAA could be found in tumor cyst fluid of one patient. Nagel et al. [129] demonstrated that in vitro stimulation by soluble TAA could be enhanced by surgical removal of the tumor. McCoy et al. [116], Cochran et al. [23–25], Mackie et al. [106], Mazuran et al. [110] have employed modifications of the migration inhibition assay to show CMI to melanoma TAA in melanoma patients, while Halliday et al. [62], Powell et al. [143], Marti and Thompson [108] and Vanderbark et al. [185] utilized the leukocyte adherence inhibition assay. Each of these assays is dependent upon the liberation of lymphokines by lymphocytes following their interaction with appropriate TAA. Of interest in Vanderbark's study was the fact that family members of melanoma patients exhibited much greater antimelanoma reactivity than did control PBL donors, suggesting that some sort of antimelanoma sensitization had taken place in the family members through close contact with the patients. The sum of results from these studies and numerous others not discussed here provides strong evidence for the existence of both melanoma TAA and the ability of these TAA to sensitize melanoma patients. However, because of the nature of these assays and, specifically, their measurement response to soluble extracts of melanoma tissue, they fail to discriminate between patient responses against cell membrane and those against internal TAA. As has already been discussed, distinct immunogenic TAA may be found in the cytoplasm and on the cell membranes of melanoma cells. It is thus reasonable to assume that melanoma patients would become sensitized to both of these antigens as a result of release of internal TAA from dead tumor cells. Because of this fact, data collected from the assays described here do not provide evidence for a clinically beneficial antimelanoma response. Potential prognostic and diagnostic value of these data will be considered in a subsequent section of this chapter.

The second class of assays we will discuss includes lymphocytotoxicity and its many variations which are designed to measure cell-mediated immune reactivity against cell membrane TAA (Table 3). The initial studies by Hellström et al. [66] created great excitement among tumor immunologists for two reasons. Using colony inhibition, Hellström et al. demonstrated that patients with various forms of cancer had specifically sensitized PBL

Table 3. Demonstration of melanoma TAA using the lymphocytotoxicity assay

| Investigators | Results |
| --- | --- |
| Hellström et al., 1971 [66, 67] | 41/41 melanoma patients positive vs. melanoma targets, blocking factors in serum. |
| Currie et al., 1971 [29] | 5/12 patients had cytotoxic PBL following immunization. |
| Hellström et al., 1971c [68] | Specific antimelanoma killing; abrogated by serum from tumor bearers. |
| Fossati et al., 1971 [48] | 7/12 positive in autologous match; 14/19 in homologous combinations. |
| Nairn et al., 1972 [130] | PBL reactive against melanoma; regional node lymphocytes did not react. |
| Currie and Basham, 1972 [28] | Specific killing blocked by serum factor which acts on PBL. |
| DeVries et al., 1972 [35] | 13/25 patients positive vs. autologous tumor; 31/56 patients positive vs. homologous tumor; 2/50 normals; 1/18 nonmelanoma patients positive, some blocking demonstrated. |
| Hellström et al., 1973a [69] | PBL from healthy blacks killed melanoma targets. |
| Hellström et al., 1973b [70] | Appearance of blocking factor in serum preceded dissemination. |
| Baldwin et al., 1973 [3] | Specific killing. |
| Nind et al., [132] | Regional anergy in five patients. |
| Heppner et al., 1973 [72] | Serum blocking correlated with stage of disease, but results were variable between samples. |
| Takasugi et al., 1973 [175] | PBL from normal donors killed melanoma cells. |
| Takasugi et al., 1974 [176] | PBL from melanoma patients kill a variety of malignant cell types. |
| Parks et al., 1974 [137] | PBL from normal blacks killed allogeneic melanoma and autologous fibroblasts. |
| DeVries et al., 1974 [32] | Long-term cultures were better targets, non-T cells were best effectors. |
| Mukherji et al., 1975 [124] | Specific killing, long-term cultures were better targets. |
| Pavie-Fischer et al., 1975 [140] | PBL from patients and normal donors killed melanoma cells; patients with localized disease were better killers. |
| Embleton and Price, 1975 [39] | Specific killing inhibited by papain-soluble TAA. |
| Roenigk et al., 1975 [150] | No correlation between killing and stage of disease. Patients with regressing halo nevus were better killers. |
| Peter et al., 1975a [141] | PBL from normal donors were more efficient killers. |
| Peter et al., 1975b [142] | K cells were effectors. |
| Heppner et al., 1975 [73] | Variability of results discussed. |
| Canevari et al., 1976 [16] | Short-term cultures were best targets. |
| Golub, 1977 [55] | Sensitized patient PBL vs. melanoma in vitro. Sensitization better if allogeneic cells used. |
| DeVries et al., 1980 [33] | Monocytes required for killing of melanoma targets. |

243

which would kill target tumor cells of the appropriate histologic type. Thus, PBL from 41/41 melanoma patients were shown to kill melanoma target cells, but not tumor cells of nonmelanoma origin. Secondly, Hellström et al. [67] found that sera from melanoma patients with advancing disease could specifically block this cell-mediated tumor cell killing. These studies thus demonstrated that PBL from melanoma patients could indeed kill melanoma cells and that this response could be blocked, in some way, by factors present in sera from patients with growing tumor. Intensive investigation using this assay and its successor, the lymphocytotoxicity assay, were initiated by a host of laboratories. Several subsequent developments and discoveries using this assay will be discussed. Nairn et al. [130] and Nind et al. [132] found that, although PBL from melanoma patients could kill melanoma targets, lymphocytes taken from the regional lymph nodes of patients with tumor failed to kill. Currie and Basham demonstrated that blocking factors acted at the level of the effector cell to prevent killing of targets thereby establishing blocking as an active event, rather than merely as coating of target cell TAA [28]. Hellström et al. demonstrated that blocking factors could be detected prior to clinically evident tumor dissemination thus providing data supporting their contention that blocking factors act to prevent sensitized PBL from killing melanoma cells as a prelude to, rather than a consequence of, metastasis [70]. Hellström et al. also reported that PBL from normal blacks killed melanoma cells, suggesting that blacks have some form of inherent immunity to melanoma [69].

At this point, however, a number of controversial studies were reported, the results of which cast serious doubt upon the significance of the lymphocytotoxicity reaction as a measure of specific cellular immune reactivity. Heppner et al. found wide variability between various samples of sera theoretically containing blocking factors [72]. Takasugi et al. then reported that PBL from normal donors could kill a variety of types of tumor cells and that PBL from cancer patients could also kill a variety of tumor target cells [175, 176]. Parks et al. found that PBL from normal blacks, in addition to killing melanoma cells, also killed autologous fibroblasts [137]. Thus, both the specificity of the lymphocytotoxicity reaction and its significance for cancer patients are questionable. In addition, there exist questions as to whether cells from long-term [32, 124] or from short-term [16] cultures are better target cells, the best procedure for purifying the effector cells [33], the nature of the effector cell [141, 33, 142] etc... These variables and their effects on the interpretation of results from lymphocytotoxicity assay are discussed extensively in an excellent review by Mastrangelo et al. [111] and the interested reader is referred to this source for a more in-depth discussion.

The demonstration of melanoma TAA served as a stimulus for efforts to raise antimelanoma xenoantisera for several reasons. As evident from our discussion of human antimelanoma immune responses, serological analysis has provided much more descriptive information about the TAA than have assays measuring parameters of cellular immunity to TAA. Having described the TAA, interest has turned to isolation and biochemical characterization of the TAA. In this regard, xenoantisera hold an advantage over human sera as they are usually high titered in comparison with sera from patients and, as such, provide more useful reagents to use for isolation procedures. The obvious disadvantage in the use of xenoantisera is that of proving the specificity of the antiserum for TAA. Xenoantisera consequently require extensive absorptions to remove antibodies reactive with human species, tissue and allo-antigens before anti-TAA activity may be determined. In most instances, either rabbits or goats have been utilized to produce antimelanoma xenoantisera (Table 4). Goodwin et al. [56] immunized rabbits with viable melanoma cells and evaluated the resulting antisera by immunofluorescence. The antisera detected an antigen in fixed tissue sections which was shared by different melanomas tested and not related to melanin. The antibody population responsible for this reactivity could be absorbed with whole melanoma cells, suggesting that the TAA are located on the cell membrane. However, this antibody was not cytotoxic for melanoma cells. Ghose et al. [54] immunized a goat with homogenized melanoma tissue. The resulting antibody was shown to react with melanoma cells but not normal tissues of one patient. The IgG of this antiserum was subsequently conjugated with chlorambucil and used for chemoimmunotherapy of this patient. In a series of studies, Viza and colleagues solubilized melanoma TAA with papain and used a partially purified TAA preparation to immunize rabbits [186–188]. The resulting antisera were found to react with extracts of fetal tissue of leukemia and melanoma. Using immunodiffusion and cross-over electrophoresis, it was found that the TAA detected by these antisera could be demonstrated in serum of melanoma patients. However, 8/51 patients free of tumor (16%) were shown to have this serum-borne TAA while only 9/53 (17%) of patients having tumor were positive. The investigators attributed this inability to discriminate between tumor-bearing and tumor-free patients to low sensitivity of the assays used. Carrel and Theilkaes raised rabbit antisera against a urinary melanoma TAA and found that this antiserum reacted with a melanoma extract [20]. In addition, 29/32 urine samples from melanoma patients were shown to contain the TAA while only 3/72 urine samples from normal donors or from patients with other nonmalignant disorders or with malignant disease of nonmelanoma origin were positive.

Our approach to this question has been to utilize nonhuman primates for production of antimelanoma antisera [117, 173]. Nonhuman primates, particularly the chimpanzee, express antigens identical or highly cross-reactive with those of several human species and alloantigen systems [173]. As such,

Table 4. Antimelanoma xenoantisera

| Investigators | Species immunized/Antigen source | Assays | Results |
|---|---|---|---|
| Viza and Phillips, 1971 [186] | Rabbit/Papain-Soluble TAA | Immunodiffusion | Antiserum reactive with extracts of melanomas, leukemias and fetal tissue. |
| Ghose et al., 1972 [54] | Goat/Homogenized fresh tumor | Immunofluorescence | Antiserum absorbed with normal tissues of melanoma patient until nonreactive; used for chemoimmunotherapy of the patient after its conjugation with chlorambucil. |
| Goodwin et al., 1972 [56] | Rabbit/Viable cells | Immunofluorescence | Common TAA detected in tissue sections not related to melanin. Antibody removed by viable melanoma cells, not cytotoxic. |
| Carrel and Theilkaes, 1973 [20] | Rabbit/Urine-borne TAA | Immunodiffusion | Urine of 29/32 melanoma patients, 3/72 control samples positive. |
| Metzgar et al., 1973 [117] | Monkey/Viable cells from melanoma cell lines | Complement dependent cytotoxicity, mixed agglutination | Common TAA demonstrated on four melanoma cell lines. Reactivity with other tumors was removed by absorption. |
| Viza et al., 1973 [188] | Rabbit/Papain-soluble TAA | Crossover electrophoresis | TAA detected in serum of melanoma patients. |
| Viza and Phillips, 1975 [187] | Rabbit/Papain-soluble TAA | Immunodiffusion | TAA found in sera from 8/51 (16%) melanoma patients free of tumor, and 9/53 patients bearing tumor (17%). |
| Stuhlmiller and Seigler, 1975 [173] | Chimpanzee/Fresh tumor | Complement dependent cytotoxicity | TAA found on 14/14 melanomas, 0/8 control tumors, 8/8 fetal fibroblast lines. Melanoma TAA distinct from fetal TAA. |
| Fritze et al., 1976 [50] | Guinea pig/Viable cells | Complement dependent cytotoxicity | Melanoma TAA shared by different lines, cross reactive with antigens on fetal skin. |
| Ghose et al., 1977 [53] | Goat, rabbit/Viable cells | Immunofluorescence | Antibody coupled with chlorambucil; 2/11 patients showed objective response. |
| Brüggen et al., 1978 [12] | Monkeys/Viable cells | Immune adherence | TAA were primarily fetal antigens, little cross-reactivity with different melanomas was once antifetal was removed. |
| Koprowski et al., 1978 [90] | Mouse/Melanoma hybrid | $^{125}$I-anti F(ab)$_2$ binding | Monoclonal antibodies reactive with melanoma. Two distinct cell membrane TAA. |
| Steplewski et al., 1979 [167] | Mouse/Melanoma hybrid | $^{125}$I- anti F(ab)$_2$ binding, mixed hemagglutination | Cells from primary and metastatic lesions express same antigens. |
| Liao et al., 1979 [103] | Monkey/Viable cells | Mixed hemagglutination | Three antisera detected TAA shared by melanomas; fetal antigen unique to melanoma and retinoblastoma. |
| McCabe et al., 1979 [114] | Rabbit/Viable cells | $^{125}$I-Staph protein A binding | Melanoma specific antibody, fetal antigen shared with carcinoma. |
| Mutzner et al., 1980 [127] | Chimpanzee/Viable cells from culture | Immunofluorescence | Common melanoma cell membrane TAA, fetal antigen shared with other tumor types. |
| Gupta et al., 1980 [60] | Rabbit, sheep/Partially purified TAA | Complement fixation | Reactivity with melanoma, sarcoma, carcinoma and fetal extracts, not with extracts of normal skin, liver or muscle. |

immune responses against many human antigens which are normally highly immunogenic in the xeno setting are minimized and antisera may thus be more readily rendered melanoma-specific through absorption. Using antisera-raised chimpanzees, we have demonstrated that human melanoma cells from either continuous cell lines or fresh tumor express common cell membrane TAA [173, 127]. Furthermore, we have demonstrated the presence of fetal antigens which may be unique to melanoma [173] or shared with tumors of other histological origin [127] depending on whether fresh tumor or a cell line was used in the immunization procedure respectively. By absorption analysis, it was shown that there exist at least two TAA which the chimpanzee antisera detect, one being unique to melanoma cells and the other being the fetal antigen. Several other groups of investigators have now turned to the use of nonhuman primates for production of antimelanoma xenoantisera. Leong et al. found that a chimpanzee antiserum raised against whole cells reacted with cell membrane TAA on 4/5 melanomas tested [92]. Laio et al. [103] have reported data to confirm and extend our earlier results. Thus, these investigators have found that monkey antimelanoma antisera detect cell membrane TAA which are shared by melanoma cells and fetal cells as well as by cells from a retinoblastoma. Brüggen et al. have shown that most of the antibody activity in monkey antisera is directed against antigens shared with fetal cells [12].

Fritze et al. have immunized guinea pigs and have demonstrated a melanoma-associated fetal antigen on the cell membrane [50]. McCabe et al., using rabbits, have demonstrated antibody which detects both a melanoma "specific" TAA and a fetal antigen shared by carcinoma [112]. Gupta et al. have immunized rabbits and sheep with partially purified melanoma TAA [60]. The resulting antisera were shown to react with soluble extracts of melanoma, sarcomas and carcinomas, but not with extracts of normal liver, skin or muscle. The recent development of hybridoma technology has also proven useful in the serologic definition of melanoma TAA. Foremost in this area is the work of Koprowski and his colleagues who have produced monoclonal murine antimelanoma antibodies [90]. These monoclonal antibodies detect cell membrane tumor-associated antigens which are shared by melanoma cells. Certain of these TAA appear to be shared with a limited number of tumors of nonmelanoma origin, most notably, astrocytomas.

From this discussion, it is apparent that melanoma cells do express a variety of TAA. Certain of these are antigens also shared with fetal cells. Of greater significance, however, are the combined observations of numerous investigators that melanoma cells do share certain TAA. As such, efforts to isolate these TAA for therapeutic and diagnostic procedures have been undertaken. A discussion of results dealing with purification of melanoma TAA will be made subsequently.

Several possibilities exist regarding the origin of melanoma TAA. Data from several studies have shown that melanoma cells express a variety of cell membrane and cytoplasmic moieties not found on most normal human cell types. For example, the existence of receptors for human estrogen [47, 115] and for human nerve growth factor [41, 158] on melanoma cells has been demonstrated. In addition, melanoma cells may also express Dr (Ia-like) antigens [192]. Wilson et al. [191] have shown these Dr antigens to be immunogenic in rabbits. Most absorption protocols for antimelanoma xenoantisera fail to include cells expressing these potentially immunogenic molecules. As a result, certain of the xenoantisera might contain antibody against these moieties. While it is beyond the scope of this chapter to explore the implications of these findings, it is obvious that their presence on melanoma cells might have profound effects upon the growth parameters of the tumor and in its interaction with the host. Tyrosinase, the enzyme functional in melanin biogenesis, is restricted to melanoma cells and, as such, might also elicit xenoantibody which most absorption protocols would not remove. To this end, Kerney et al. demonstrated that certain melanoma TAA are found in association with melanin granules [86]. A possible viral origin for certain of the melanoma TAA is suggested by studies of Balda et al. [2] and of Parsons et al. [138, 139] which demonstrate the presence of oncornavirus-like particles within melanoma cells. In addition, a RNA-dependent DNA polymerase has been detected [148] and shown to be associated with the virus-like particles and also to be immunogenic in rabbits [6].

As is evident from our discussion of antimelanoma xenoantisera (Table 4), and to a lesser extent from that of sera from melanoma patients (Table 1), a major class of melanoma TAA appear to be oncofetal antigens. For the most part, these appear not to be related to the more prominent oncofetal antigen, carcinoembryonic antigen (CEA) and alphafetoprotein (AFP). Martin et al. have reported elevated CEA levels in serum from only 1/11 melanoma patients [109], but Morgan et al. have been able to detect the presence of CEA on cells from 2/4 melanoma cell lines using a rabbit anti-CEA antiserum [121]. This finding has yet to be confirmed by other investigators. Mihalev et al. were able to detect elevated serum AFP levels in only 2/12 melanoma patients and no studies have been reported regarding the expression of AFP by melanoma cells [118]. Using a rabbit antiserum raised against human carcinoma of the colon, Fritsche and Mach have described a widely distributed oncofetal antigen [49]. This new oncofetal antigen has been termed B-oncofetal antigen due to its B electrophoretic mobility and is distinct from AFP and CEA. It was found on a variety of human carcinomas and in melanomas. Oncofetal antigen I (OFA-I), as described by Irie et al., is a cell membrane antigen found on human melanomas, certain other histologic types of cancer and human fetal brain, but not on fetal spleen, liver or small intestine or in adult tissues [81]. The tissue distribution and demonstrated immunogenicity of OFA-I in the cancer patient distinguish this antigen from CEA and AFP [82]. Of great potential is the observation by Sidell et al. that OFA-I may serve as a target for immune cytolysis of melanoma cells, suggesting that the patient's anti-OFA-I response may have a significant effect on the control of tumor [161]. Bauer et al. have described a pregnancy associated $\alpha_2$-glycoprotein, serum levels of which are elevated in melanoma patients [4]. No function has been determined for this glyco-protein, nor has its origin in the melanoma patient.

Human melanoma oncofetal antigens have proven highly immunogenic in the xeno setting (Table 4). Indeed, in every study designed to assay anti-melanoma xenoantisera for an anti-oncofetal antibody component, such antibody has been demonstrated. In certain studies [173, 103], the oncofetal antigens are detected on a limited number of cell types, most of these having neuroectodermal origin; while in others, the oncofetal antigens are detected on a wide spectrum of tumor types [12, 114, 127, 60]. Oncofetal antigens on melanoma cells have also been identified using rabbit antisera prepared against an extract of human embryo [1].

Results from several studies, however, suggest that caution be exercised in evaluating results describing oncofetal antigens. For example, Irie et al. [80] have found that tumor cells grown in fetal bovine serum (FBS) have a pas-sively adsorbed serum component to which many cancer patients have a natural antibody. This FBS-derived antigen could thus be detected by cer-tain cancer patient sera or xenoantisera and falsely identified as TAA or an oncofetal antigen. Salinas et al. [154] have presented evidence to suggest that cancer patients have an antibody reactive with human fetal liver cells, a finding somewhat at variance with those of Irie et al. [81], who, in the case of OFA-I, could not demonstrate reactivity of cancer patients sera with fetal liver. Thorpe et al. [182] have furthermore demonstrated that maintenance of normal human skin cells in culture results in their acquisition of certain fetal antigens. This latter observation may, in part, explain the above-men-tioned dichotomy of results regarding the distribution of melanoma-asso-ciated oncofetal antigens as detected by xenoantisera. Specifically we have observed that the use of fresh tumor tissue to immunize chimpanzees results in the production of antibody which describes a fetal antigen of very limited distribution [173]. In contrast, antibody elicited by immunization of chim-panzees with melanoma cells maintained in culture reacts with oncofetal antigens present on all tumor cell types we have evaluated [127]. An expla-nation for these observations might be that the oncofetal antigen expression of the melanoma cells was altered by or during in vitro culture (i.e., the melanoma cells acquired an oncofetal antigen not expressed by the parent tumor cells in vivo).

The conclusive demonstration of the existence and immunogenicity of human melanoma TAA and of the ability of certain of these TAA to function as targets for immune destruction of tumor cells leads into discussion regarding why the tumor is able to grow despite the host antitumor reactivity. One possibility is simply that the antimelanoma immune responses, particularly those measured in vitro, may be of no in vivo significance. While this might actually be true for certain assays which measure in vitro parameters of the cell-mediated immune response, it can not account for the antimelanoma antibody responses of patients to their tumor. Numerous reports have demonstrated a correlation between the presence of detectable anti-TAA antibody and the stage of disease in melanoma patients. Lewis first reported the presence of cytotoxic antimelanoma antibody only in sera from patients with localized disease [98]. Lewis and his colleagues have also shown that serum antibody becomes undetectable prior to clinically evident dissemination of tumor [97]. Morton et al. found both the incidence and titer of antimelanoma antibodies to correlate with the extent of disease [122, 123], while Wood and Barth [193] found titer of antibody reactive with the cytoplasmic TAA to be greater in patients in late stages of disease. Bodurtha et al. [10], Whitehead [190], Bowen et al. [11], and Canevari et al. [17] have also reported correlations between detectability of antimelanoma antibodies and extent of disease. In a similar manner, Fass et al. [42], Morton et al. [122], Hollingshead et al. [78], Hersh et al. [76] and Cochran et al. [25] have demonstrated that various parameters of the cell-mediated anti-TAA immune response, particularly DCHR, correlate with disease staging. Such findings suggest that the antitumor immune response and tumor progression may indeed be related. If one makes this assumption, it is then necessary to establish whether tumor dissemination precedes the loss of anti-TAA reactivity and perhaps actually abrogates the reactivity or whether some inherent deficiency, active suppression or circumvention of the anti-TAA response precedes, and thus permits, tumor dissemination. Although, at present, it is not possible to refute either of these explanations, some data have been presented which favor the latter of the two. Lewis et al. have demonstrated a loss of detectable antibody prior to dissemination of tumor and, as a possible explanation, Lewis has proposed a mechanism whereby idiotype regulation of the antitumor antibody response occurs [100]. Specifically, Lewis et al. have shown that an anti-antibody is formed and that this might curtail immune control over tumor. Significant insight into the loss of immune reactivity has been provided by the work of Hellström and colleagues. In the lymphocytotoxicity assay, PBL from melanoma patients with localized tumor and with disseminated disease were found to be equally reactive against target melanoma cells [66]. However, differences were noted in the effects of inclusion, in the assay, of sera from tumor-bearing patients versus nontumor bearers or normal donors. Specifically, when sera from tumor-bearing melanoma patients were used in place of normal sera, the cytotoxicity was abrogated [67]. Furthermore, this "blocking" was specific in that only sera from melanoma patients blocked the cytotoxic activity of PBL from melanoma patients. Sera from patients with other forms of cancer had no effect nor did the sera of melanoma patients have any effect upon the cytotoxic interaction between PBL and appropriate target cells from patients with other forms of cancer. Such blocking factors have also been demonstrated by DeVries et al. [34], Currie and Basham [28], Heppner et al. [72], Halliday et al. [62], and Hersey et al. [77].

Because of the specificity of the effects of blocking factors, they were originally thought to be host-derived antibody which blocked TAA sites on the melanoma cells and prevented their interaction with sensitized PBL. The work of Sjögren et al. led to speculation that blocking factors were actually immune complexes composed of specific anti-TAA antibody and TAA [163]. In addition, free TAA have also been suggested to have blocking activity [28]. Embleton and Price demonstrated that papain-soluble TAA are able to abrogate the cytotoxicity of PBL for target melanoma cells [39]. Although it is impossible at present to state conclusively that "blocking factors" have any in vivo function in regard to tumor growth. One study in a related system suggests that such a mechanism might be functional. Thus, Myburgh and Smit have demonstrated that soluble immune complexes composed of soluble baboon histocompatibility antigens and specific antibody are able to prolong survival of kidney allografts [128].

One prerequisite for a potential in vivo role of blocking factors is the rapid release from the tumor cell of large amounts of TAA. Fine et al. have demonstrated that this shedding may occur with histocompatibility antigens [46]. Long-surviving rat kidney allografts were shown to first bind appropriate alloantibody and then to release it in the form of soluble immune complexes. Studies reported by Theofilopoulos et al. [181], Jerry et al. [85], Gupta et al. [61] and Shepherd [157] have shown that sera from melanoma patients have greatly elevated levels of immune complexes. In vitro studies by Stuhlmiller and Seigler [172], McCabe et al. [114], Leong et al. [91], Jacubovich and Dore [83], Grimm et al. [57] and Gupta et al. [58] have shown rapid release of melanoma TAA into culture fluids. Leong et al. have also demonstrated that cell membrane TAA form caps and are released into the culture fluid following incubation with antimelanoma antisera [94]. Rahman et al. have shown that as much as 50% of incorporated 3H-glucosamine was released from melanoma cells within 96 hours and that 15–30% of the label could be released by trypsinization [147]. Bystryn [14] further demonstrated that melanoma-associated antigens were released more rapidly into the culture medium than were other macromolecules. Further evidence to support the shedding of melanoma TAA comes from studies demonstrating the presence of melanoma TAA in serum [188], urine [20, 84] and cyst fluid [84] of melanoma patients. Thomson et al. have also reported that PBL potentially reactive in LAI assays are coated in vivo by soluble antigen in patients with large tumor burden and are not reactive in vitro until the TAA are removed [180]. Thus, although it is not conclusive, strong evidence exists to suggest a role for soluble TAA either free or in the form of immune complexes in the host–tumor interaction, perhaps by induction of a specific suppressor cell population [130].

In addition to the possible effects of "blocking factors," a number of other factors may exert effects on the host–tumor interaction. As an example, several investigators have evaluated overall immunocompetence of melanoma patients in the hope of uncovering inherent immunological defects in these patients. Results from these studies are inconclusive as some investigators have reported diminished [5, 155], normal [156] or elevated [166] immunocompetence of melanoma patients relative to normal individuals. Snyderman et al. have demonstrated a correlation between abnormal monocyte chemotactic responses and tumor burden [166]. Removal of tumor caused return to normal values for this response. Alteration of monocyte function in conjunction with tumor growth has also been demonstrated by Hedley and Currie [65]. In this study, monocytes from patients with disseminated disease responded poorly to a phagocytic stimulus and had a diminished potential to reduce nitroblue tetrazolium (NBT). Reduction of NBT is an indirect measure of activity in the hexose monophosphate shunt and these data thus suggested a reduced metabolic potential for the monocytes. Because of the complexity of interaction between B cells, T cells and cells of the monocyte series in the generation of immune responses, it is evident that alteration of the capabilities of any of these cell types will have profound effects upon immune responsiveness. Further indication of the pivotal role played by monocytes is provided by Gauci who reported that monocyte content of human tumors showed a close correlation with the extent of dissemination [52].

Local defects may also exist as shown by Nind et al. [132] and Nairn et al. [130]. Despite being able to demonstrate systemic immunocompetence, these investigators found lymphoid cells from within tumor or from regional lymph nodes to be incapable of effecting cytolysis of melanoma targets in vitro. Such anergy might be due to local specific (TAA) or nonspecific immunosuppression. Nimberg et al. [131] have reported that a peptide found in the sera of cancer patients had a nonspecific suppressive effect upon several parameters of immune responsiveness as measured in vitro.

Much interest has recently centered on the isolation and biochemical and physiochemical characterization of melanoma TAA as well as on defining their relationships to other cell membrane constituents. Several reasons exist for this trend. In that the role of the melanoma TAA in the host–tumor interaction is unknown, identification of any relationships with other cell membrane constituents, and in particular, $B_2$-microglobulin, HLA antigens and Dr antigens might provide clues as to possible functions of the TAA. Isolation and characterization of the TAA is a first step in development of sensitive assays for detection of soluble TAA in body fluids. While, at present, it would not be feasible to screen sera for the population at large, such "immunodiagnostic" assays may prove useful for monitoring melanoma patients for recurrent disease. This ability might permit detection of soluble TAA in patient sera prior to clinical presentation of recurrent disease, and thereby permit earler initiation of suitable therapy. In addition, such assays would be of value for evaluating efficacy of various therapeutic regimens for melanoma and for research into possible roles of TAA in the host–tumor interaction. Possible large scale immunizations with purified TAA remains a distant but potential future use for purified TAA, as is specific active immunotherapy.

A variety of procedures have been utilized to obtain soluble TAA for isolation purposes including use of soluble TAA in body fluids of melanoma patients [20, 84, 184], KCl extraction [152] or enzymatic release [170] of TAA from fresh melanoma tissue or melanoma cell lines and use of TAA spontaneously shed into culture medium [112]. Carrel and Theilkaes defined a melanoma TAA in urine which was used to produce a rabbit xenoantiserum [20]. Jehn et al. identified a soluble TAA of B-electrophoretic mobility in melanoma tumor cyst fluid which was antigenically identical to homogeneous urine-borne TAA [84]. Murray et al. examined sera having blocking activity in LDA assays [126]. By gel filtration, two components were identified, these having molecular weights of less than 60 000 daltons and of approximately 300 000 daltons. Both of these TAA were bound by Con A suggesting content of carbohydrate and both were resolved into a single 15 000 mw component by SDS-PAGE analysis. This moiety bound to an antimelanoma antibody resin and was antigenically active in blocking LDA reactions. A similar TAA was purified from melanoma cell membrane extracts and from spent tissue culture fluid. KCl extracts of melanoma TAA have been used as skin test reagents [153] and in leukocyte adherence [62] and migration inhibition assays [9]. Hollingshead et al. found two DCHR-reactive constituents which were separated by gel filtration and SDS-PAGE [77, 78]. One of these also elicited DCHR in breast cancer patients.

Chee et al. [22] adapted a melanoma cell line to growth in serum-free chemically defined medium and used KCl to solubilize TAA active in DCHR. Roth et al. found TAA extracts from this cell line to be resolved into two constituents by gel filtration chromatography, each of which stimulated DCHR in only 1/7 patients with other cancers [152, 153]. Reisfeld et al. demonstrated that KCl-extracted TAA were separable from solubilized HLA antigens by floatation on KBr, thereby showing the distinction between HLA molecules and TAA [149]. McCabe et al. extended these observations by showing that KCl-extracted TAA could be isolated by KBr floatation, ion exchange chromatography and preparative isoelectric focusing [112]. The isolated TAA elicited DCHR in melanoma patients, reacted with antimelanoma antibody and elicited production of xenoantibody. Identical results were obtained using TAA spontaneously shed into culture fluid. Malley et al. found that KCl-extracted melanoma TAA reactive in LAI and in DCHR were bound to an affinity resin bearing antihuman $B_2$-microglobulin [107] suggesting that these TAA contained $B_2$-microglobulin. Embleton et al. have recently shown that KCl-extracted TAA may be substantially purified using affinity chromatographic procedures with specific antimelanoma antibody [40]. TAA spontaneously shed into culture medium have been utilized by Reisfeld et al. [149], Grimm et al. [57], Stuhlmiller and Seigler [172], Leong et al. [91], McCabe et al. [112, 113] and by Gupta et al. [58] for purification purposes. Grimm et al. found that spontaneously shed melanoma TAA reactive in DCHR and complement fixation could be partially purified by gel filtration and ion exchange chromatography [57]. In contrast to the findings of Malley et al. [107], McCabe et al. [113] found no association between melanoma TAA and $B_2u$ by immunoprecipitation analysis. TAA with molecular weights of 94 000 daltons and 240 000 daltons were identified in these immunoprecipitates and these TAA were not precipitated using an anti-$B_2$ microglobulin antiserum. Gupta et al. have successfully separated melanoma TAA from OFA-I in spent culture fluid [58]. In this study, TAA were soluble in chloroform-ethanol while OFA-I was insoluble. Leong et al. [91] demonstrated that spontaneously shed TAA have molecular weights of 70–150 000 daltons as determined by gel filtration chromatography. Viza and Phillips [186], and Embleton and Price [39] demonstrated the antigenicity of papain-solubilized melanoma TAA. Viza and Phillips found these TAA elicited antimelanoma antibody in rabbits while Embleton and Price reported that papain-soluble TAA were able to inhibit cytolysis of melanoma cells by sensitized PBL. Thomson et al. used limited papain digestion to solubilize TAA reactive in the LAI assay [178]. By gel giltration chromatography, these TAA had molecular weights of 70–150 000 daltons. In agreement with the observations of Malley et al. [107], Thomson et al. found that these TAA were bound by an anti-$B_2u$ affinity resin. In subsequent studies, Thomson et al. used SDS-PAGE analysis and chromatography on a 6M-guanidine-HCl column to resolve the TAA into constituents having molecular weights of 40 000 daltons, 25 000 daltons and 12 000 daltons [179]. Carey et al. found that papain-soluble AU melanoma TAA were not precipitated by either anti-$B_2u$ or anti-HLA antisera [18]. Certain of these TAA did bind to a lens culinaiis lectin resin suggesting carbohydrate was present. By gel filtration, these TAA were found to have approximate molecular weights of 20–50 000 daltons. In our studies, we have utilized pronase digestion to release melanoma TAA [170]. These soluble TAA are able to inhibit specifically nonhuman primate antimelanoma antisera in complement-dependent cytotoxicity and in $^{125}$I-SpA binding assays [170]. By gel exclusion chromatography, we have resolved soluble TAA into four distinct molecular weight classes: 48 000 daltons, 25 000 daltons, 17 000 daltons and 13 000 daltons. The three larger molecular weight classes also contain oncofetal antigen-like activity, whereas the 13 000 dalton component containes only melanoma TAA activity. Further purification on DEA-cellulose has permitted separation of TAA from HLA antigens and from $B_2$-microglobulin. The reactive TAA have furthermore been shown not to bind to Con A suggesting that pronase-soluble melanoma TAA lack carbohydrate. The soluble TAA are also stable to prolonged incubation at low pH.

Detergent extracts of melanoma cells have been utilized. Bystryn and Smalley [15] released TAA using NP-40 while Preddie et al. [144] utilized SDS or Triton X-100. Preddie et al. purified the soluble TAA on an affinity resin bearing antimelanoma antibody from patients [145]. Two distinct TAA were obtained, one of which had a molecular weight of 80 000 daltons and was a common melanoma TAA while the second, with a molecular weight of 124 000 daltons, was identified as an "individual" melanoma TAA. Hersey et al. extracted melanoma TAA using urea acetate and isolated the antigens using lectin affinity and gel filtration chromatography and preparative isoelectric focusing [75]. The isolated TAA were acidic glycoproteins (pI 3.5) of 15 000 dalton molecular weight. These TAA were resistant to neuraminidase and heat but susceptible to trypsin. Furthermore, the TAA were shown to be unrelated to CEA, $B_2$-microglobulin or HLA antigens.

As is apparent from the above discussion, a controversy exists over whether or not melanoma TAA contain or are closely associated with $B_2u$. There is now a general agreement that melanoma TAA and HLA antigens are distinct entities. Although no clear-cut answer may be posed to solve this discrepancy, it is possible that certain of the melanoma TAA express $B_2u$ while others do not. The various assays performed may discriminate between different forms of TAA. Thus, melanoma TAA demonstrations using the LAi assay may depend in some way on the presence of $B_2u$ while serological demonstration of the TAA does not. As further proof of the lack of association between melanoma TAA and HLA antigens, Curry et al. have produced hybrids of human melanoma cells and murine fibroblasts and have shown that genes encoding for melanoma TAA segregate independently from those coding for HLA antigens [30].

While development of specific radioimmunoassays for detection of melanoma TAA appears to be a feasible undertaking, alternative means for diagnosis and immunodiagnosis have also been evaluated. In certain cases, melanoma may present as a metastatic lesion in a lymph node and no primary is found. Because melanomas may be nonpigmented, particularly in metastatic lesions, such tumors are often diagnosed as undifferentiated carcinomas. In that different histological forms of cancer are selectively responsive to different forms of therapy, a precise diagnosis is highly desirable. We have utilized chimpanzee antimelanoma antisera in a number of such cases and have demonstrated a correlation between the reactivity of cells from these lesions and their content of tyrosinase and of melanosomes [169]. Such solid tumor diagnosis using operationally specific antisera should prove to be a useful adjunct to conventional pathological evaluation. The levels of tyrosinase in serum may also prove a useful indication for aberrant melanocyte proliferation. Nishioka et al. have found that melanoma patients had elevated tyrosinase levels [134] and that certain tyrosinases may be altered as a result of malignant transformation of the melanocyte [135].

# References

1. Avis P and Lewis MG: Tumor-associated fetal antigens in human tumors. J Natl Cancer Inst 51:1063–1066, 1973.
2. Balda BR, Hehlmann R, Cho JR and Spiegelman S: Oncornavirus-like particles in human skin cancers. Proc Natl Acad Sci 72:3697–3700, 1975.
3. Baldwin RW, Embleton MJ, Jones JSP and Langman MJS: Cell mediated and humoral immune reactions to human tumors. Int J Cancer 12:73–83, 1973.
4. Bauer HW, Deutschmann KEM, Peter HH and Bohn H: Pregnancy associated $\alpha$-2-glycoprotein in malignant melanoma. Eur J Cancer 15:123–126, 1979.
5. Bernengo MG, Capella G, DeMatteis A, Tovo PA and Zina G: The in vitro effects of a calf thymus extract on the peripheral blood lymphocytes of sixty-six melanoma patients. Clin Exp Immunol 36:279–284, 1979.
6. Birkmayer GD, Hammer C, Eberhard HD and Brendel W: A tumor specific antigen associated with reverse transcriptase. Behring Inst Mitt 56:107–115, 1975.
7. Bloom ET, Foley JL, Peterson IA, Geering G, Bernhard M and Trempe G: Anti-tumor activity in human serum: antibodies detecting blood-group.a.like antigen on the surface of tumor cells. Int J Cancer 12:21–31, 1973.
8. Bluming AZ, Vogel CL, Ziegler JL and Kiryabwire JWM: Delayed cutaneous sensitivity reactions to extracts of autologous malignant melanoma: a second look. J Natl Cancer Inst 48:17–24, 1972.
9. Boddie AW, Urist MM, Chee DO, Holmes EC and Morton DL: Inhibition of leukocyte migration in agarose by KCl extracts of a human melanoma cell line grown in serum-free medium. Int J Cancer 16:1035–1041, 1975.
10. Bodurtha AJ, Chee DO, Laucius JF, Mastrangelo MJ and Prehn RT: Clinical and immunological significance of human melanoma cytotoxic antibody. Cancer Res 35:189–193, 1975.
11. Bowen JM, McBride CM, Hersh EM and Miller MF: Nucleolar antigens in tumor cells of patients with malignant melanoma. In: Immunological Aspects of Neoplasia, pp 223–239. Williams & Wilkins, Baltimore, 1975.

12. Brüggen J, Sorg C and Macher E: Membrane associated antigens of malignant melanoma: V. serological typing of cells using antisera from non-human primates. Cancer Immunol Immunother 5:53–62, 1978.

13. Burger DR, Vandenbark AA, Finke P, Malley A, Frikke M, Black J, Acott K, Begley D and Vetto RM: Assessment of reactivity to tumor extracts by leukocyte adherence inhibition and dermal testing. J Natl Cancer Inst 59:317–323, 1977.

14. Bystryn J: Release of cell surface tumor associated antigens by viable melanoma cells from humans. J Natl Cancer Inst 69:325–328, 1977.

15. Bystryn J and Smalley JR: Identification and solubilization of iodinated cell surface human melanoma associated antigens. Int J Cancer 20:165–172, 1977.

16. Canevari S, Fossati G and Della Porta G: Cellular immune reaction to human melanoma and breast carcinoma cells. J Natl Cancer Inst 56:705–709, 1976.

17. Canevari S, Fossati G, DellaPorta G and Balzarini GP: Humoral cytotoxicity in melanoma patients and its correlation to extent of disease. Int J Cancer 16:722–729, 1975.

18. Carey TE, Lloyd KO, Takahashi T, Travassos LR and Old LJ: AU cell surface of human malignant melanoma: solubilization and partial characterization. Proc Nat Acad Sci 76:2898–2902, 1979.

19. Carey TE, Takahashi T, Resnick LA, Oettgen HF and Old LJ: Cell surface antigens of human malignant melanoma: mixed hemadsorption assays for humoral immunity to cultured autologous melanoma cells. Proc Nat Acad Sci 73:3278–3282, 1976.

20. Carrel S and Theilkaes L: Evidence for a tumor-associated antigen in human malignant melanoma. Nature 242:609–610, 1973.

21. Char D, Hollingshead A, Cogan DG, Ballintine EJ, Hogan MJ and Herberman RB: Cutaneous delayed hypersensitivity reactions to soluble melanoma antigen in patients with ocular melanoma. N Engl J Med 291:274–277, 1974.

22. Chee DO, Boddie AW, Roth JA, Holmes EC and Morton DL: Production of melanoma-associated antigens by a defined malignant melanoma cell strain grown in chemically defined medium. Cancer Res 36:1503–1509, 1976.

23. Cochran AJ, Jehn UW and Gothoskar B: Cell mediated immunity in malignant melanoma. Lancet 1:1340–1341, 1972.

24. Cochran AJ, Mackie RM, Thomas CE, Grant RM, Cameron-Mowat DE and Spilg WGS: Cellular immunity to breast carcinoma and malignant melanoma. Br J Cancer Suppl 1:77–81, 1973.

25. Cochran AJ, Ross CE, Mackie RM, Grant RM and Hoyle DE: The immune status of patients with malignant melanoma. Behring Inst Mitt 56:125–130, 1975.

26. Copeman PWM, Lewis MG, Phillips TM and Elliott PG: Immunological associations of the halo nevus with cutaneous malignant melanoma. Br J Dermatol 88:127, 1973.

27. Cornain S, DeVries JE, Collard J, Vennegoor C, van Wingerden I and Rumke P: Antibodies and antigen expression in human melanoma detected by the immune adherence test. Int J Cancer 16:981–997, 1975.

28. Currie GA and Basham C: Serum-mediated inhibition of the immunological reactions of the patient to his own tumor: a possible role for circulating antigen. Br J Cancer 26:427–438, 1972.

29. Currie GA, Lejeune F and Hamilton-Fairley G: Immunization with irradiated tumor cells and specific lymphocyte cytotoxicity in malignant melanoma. Br Med J 2:305–310, 1971.

30. Curry RA, Quaranta V, Pellegrino MA and Ferrone S: Serologically detectable human melanoma associated antigens are not genetically linked to HLA-A and HLA-B antigens. J Immunol 122:2630–2632, 1979.

31. Das Gupta T, Dowden L and Berg TW: Malignant melanoma of unknown primary origin. Surg Gynecol Obstet 117:341–345, 1963.

32. DeVries JE, Cornain S and Rumke PH: Cytotoxicity of non-T versus T-lymphocytes from melanoma patients and healthy donors on short and long-term cultures melanoma cells. Int J Cancer 14:427–434, 1974.

33. DeVries JE, Mendelsohn J and Bont WS: The requirement of monocytes in spontaneous cytotoxicity by lymphocytes from healthy donors and melanoma patients. Int J Cancer 25:73–84, 1980.

34. DeVries JE, Cornain S and Rumke PH: Humoral and cellular immunity in melanoma patients. Behring Inst Mitt 56:148–156, 1975.

35. DeVries JE, Rumke PH and Bernheim JL: Cytotoxic lymphocytes in melanoma patients. Int J Cancer 9:567–576, 1972.

36. Douwes FR, Spellman HJ, Mross K and Wolfrum DI: Immunodiagnostics of malignant disease: VI. electrophoretic mobility test (EMT) in malignant melanoma. Oncology 35:163–167, 1978.

37. Eberman AA: Beitrag zur Casuistik der melanotischen Geschwülste. Dtsch Z Chir 11:498, 1896.

38. Elliott PG, Thurlow B, Needham PRG and Lewis MG: The specificity of the cytoplasmic antigen in human malignant melanoma. Eur J Cancer 9:607–610, 1973.

39. Embleton MJ and Price MR: Inhibition of in vitro lymphocytotoxic reactions against tumor cells by melanoma membrane extract. Behring Inst Mitt 56:157–160, 1975.

40. Embleton MJ, Price MR and Baldwin RW: Demonstration and partial purification of common melanoma associated antigens. Eur J Cancer 16:575–585, 1980.

41. Fabricant RN, DeLarco JE and Todaro GJ: Nerve growth factor receptors on human melanoma cells in culture. Proc Natl Acad Sci 74:565–569, 1977.

42. Fass L, Ziegler JL, Herberman RB and Kiryabwire JWM: Cutaneous hypersensitivity reactions to autologous extracts of malignant melanoma cells. Lancet 1:116–118, 1970.

43. Federman JL, Lewis MG and Clark WH: Tumor-associated antibody to ocular and cutaneous melanomas: negative interaction with normal choroidal melanocytes. J Nat Cancer Inst 52:587–589, 1974.

44. Ferrone S and Pellegrino MA: Cytotoxic antibodies to cultured melanoma cells in the sera of melanoma patients. J Natl Cancer Inst 58:1201–1204, 1978.

45. Ferrone S and Pellegrino MA: Antigens and antibodies in malignant melanoma. In: Waters H (ed) Handbook of Cancer Immunology, Vol 3, pp 291–327. Garland STPM, New York, 1978.

46. Fine RN, Batchelor JR, French ME and Shumak KH: The uptake of $^{125}$I-labeled rat alloantibody and its loss after combination with antigen. Transplantation 16:641–648, 1973.

47. Fisher RI, Neifeld JP and Lippman ME: Estrogen receptors in human malignant melanoma. Lancet 1:337–338, 1976.

48. Fossati G, Colnaghi MI, Della Porta G, Cascinelli N and Veronesi U: Cellular and humoral immunity against human malignant melanoma. Int J Cancer 8:344–350, 1971.

49. Fritsche R and Mach JP: Identification of a new oncofetal antigen associated with several types of human carcinomas. Nature 258:734–737, 1975.

50. Fritze D, Kern DH, Drogemuller CR and Pilch YH: Production of antisera with specificity for malignant melanoma and human fetal skin. Cancer Res 36:458–466, 1976.

51. Fritze D, Kern DH and Pilch YH: Serologic evidence for cross-reacting tumor associated antigens in two chemically induced murine sarcomas and in human malignant melanoma. Behring Inst Mitt 56:90–97, 1975.

52. Gauci CL: The macrophage content of human malignant melanomas. Behring Inst Mitt 56:73–78, 1975.

53. Ghose T, Norvell ST, Guclu A, Bodurtha A, Tai J and MacDonald AS: Immunochemotherapy of malignant melanoma with chlorambucil-bound anti-melanoma globulins: Preliminary results in patients with disseminated disease. J Natl Cancer Inst 58:845–852, 1977.

54. Ghose T, Norvell ST, Guclu A, Cameron D, Bodurtha A and MacDonald AS: Immunotherapy of cancer with chlorambucil-carrying antibody. Br Med J 3:495–499, 1972.

55. Golub SH: In vitro sensitization of human lymphoid cells to antigens on cultured melanoma cells. Cell Immunol 28:379–389, 1977.

56. Goodwin DP, Hornung MO, Leong SPL and Krementz ET: Immune responses induced by human malignant melanoma in the rabbit. Surgery 72:737–743, 1972.

57. Grimm EA, Silver HKB, Roth JH, Chee DO, Gupta RK and Morton DL: Detection of tumor-associated antigen in human melanoma cell line supernatants. Int J Cancer 17:559–564, 1976.

58. Gupta RK, Irie RF, Chee DO, Kern DH and Morton DL: Demonstration of two distinct antigens in spent tissue culture medium of a human malignant cell line. J Natl Cancer Inst 63:347–356, 1979a.

59. Gupta R and Morton DL: Suggestive evidence for in vivo binding of specific antitumor antibodies of human melanoma. Cancer Res 35:58–62, 1975.

60. Gupta RK, Silver HKB and Morton DL: Production and characterization of xenogeneic antisera to tumor-associated antigen. J Surg Oncol 13:75–89, 1980.

61. Gupta RK, Theofilopoulos AN, Dixon FJ and Morton DL: Circulating immune complexes as possible cause for anticomplementary activity in humans with malignant melanoma. Cancer Immunol Immunother 6:211–221, 1979b.

62. Halliday WJ, Maluish AE, Little JH and Davis NC: Leukocyte adherence inhibition and specific immunoreactivity on malignant melanoma. Int J Cancer 16:645–658, 1975.

63. Hamilton-Fairley G, Lewis MG, Ikonopisov RL, Nairn RC and Alexander P: Detection of tumor specific immune reaction in human melanoma. Ann N Y Acad Sci 177:286–289, 1971.

64. Handley WS: The pathology of melanocytic growths. Lancet 1:927, 1907.

65. Hedley DW and Currie GA: Monocytes and macrophages in malignant melanoma: III. reduction of nitroblue tetrazolium by peripheral blood monocytes. Br J Cancer 37:747–752, 1978.

66. Hellström I, Hellström KE, Sjögren HO and Warner GA: Demonstration of cell-mediated immunity to human neoplasms of various histological types. Int J Cancer 7:1–16, 1971a.

67. Hellström I, Sjögren HO, Warner G and Hellström KE: Blocking of cell-mediated tumor immunity by sera from patients with growing neoplasms. Int J Cancer 7:226–237, 1971b.

68. Hellström I, Hellström KE, Sjögren HO and Warner G: Serum factors in tumor-free patients cancelling the blocking of cell-mediated tumor immunity. Int J Cancer 8:185–191, 1971c.

69. Hellström I, Warner GA, Hellström KE and Sjögren HO: Destruction of cultivated melanoma cells by lymphocytes from healthy black (North American Negro donors). Int J Cancer 11:116–122, 1973a.

70. Hellström I, Warner GA, Hellström KE and Sjögren HO: Sequential studies on cell-mediated tumor immunity and blocking serum activity in ten patients with malignant melanoma. Int J Cancer 11:280–292, 1973b.

71. Hellström I, Hellström KE and Warner GA: Increase of lymphocyte-mediated tumor-cell destruction by certain patient sera. Int J Cancer 12:348–353, 1973c.

72. Heppner G, Stolbach HL, Cummings F, McDonough E and Calabresi P: Cell-mediated and serum blocking reactivity to tumor antigens in patients with malignant melanoma. Int J Cancer 11:245–260, 1973.

73. Heppner G, Stolbach H, Cummings F, McDonough E and Calabresi P: Problems in the clinical use of the microcytotoxicity assay for measuring cell-mediated immunity to tumor cells. Cancer Res 35:1931–1937, 1975.

74. Hersey P, Honeyman M, Edwards A, Adams E and McCarthy WH: Antigens on melanoma cells detected by leukocyte dependent antibody assays of human melanoma antisera. Int J Cancer 18:564–573, 1976.

75. Hersey P, Murray E, Werkmeister J and McCarthy WH: Detection of low molecular weight antigen on melanoma cells by human antiserum in leukocyte dependent antibody assays. Br J Cancer 40:615–627, 1979.

76. Hersh EM, Gutterman JV, Mavligit GM, Granatek CH, Reed RC, Ambus V and McBride C: Approaches to the study of tumor antigens and tumor immunity in malignant melanoma. Behring Inst Mitt 56:139–147, 1975.

77. Hollingshead AC: Analysis of soluble melanoma cell membrane antigens in metastatic cells of various organs and further studies of antigens present in primary melanoma. Cancer 36:1282–1288, 1975.

78. Hollingshead AC, Herberman RB, Jaffurs WJ, Alpers LK, Minton JP and Harris JE: Soluble membrane antigens of human malignant melanoma. Cancer 34:1235–1243, 1974.

79. Irie K, Irie RF and Morton DL: Detection of antibody and complement complexed in vivo on membranes of human cancer cells by mixed hemadsorption techniques. Cancer Res 35:1244–1248, 1975.

80. Irie RF, Irie K and Morton DL: Natural antibody in human serum to a neoantigen in human cultured cells grown in fetal bovine serum. J Natl Cancer Inst 52:1051–1058, 1974.

81. Irie RF, Irie K and Morton DL: A membrane antigen common to cancer and fetal brain tissues. Cancer Res 36:3510–3517, 1976.

82. Irie RF, Giuliano AE, Morton DL: Oncofetal antigen: a tumor associated fetal antigen immunogenic in man. J Natl Cancer Inst 63:367–373, 1979.

83. Jacubovich R and Dore JF: Tumor-associated antigens in culture medium of malignant melanoma cell strains. Cancer Immunol Immunother 7:59–64, 1979.

84. Jehn UW, Nathanson L, Schwartz RS and Skinner M: In vitro lymphocyte stimulation by a soluble antigen from malignant melanoma. N Engl J Med 283:329–333, 1970.

85. Jerry LM, Rowden G, Cano PO, Phillips TM, Deutsch GF, Capek A, Hartmann D and Lewis MG: Immune complexes in human melanoma. A consequence of deranged immune regulation. Scand J Immunol 5:845–859, 1976.

86. Kerney SE, Montague PM, Chretien PB, Nicholson JM, Ekel TM and Hearing VJ: Intracellular localization of tumor-associated antigens in murine and human malignant melanoma. Cancer Res 37:1519–1524, 1977.

87. Kilpatrick RJ and Seigler HF: Specific cytotoxic antibody in sera from patients with melanoma. J Surg Res 21:301–305, 1976.

88. Kodera Y and Bean MA: Antibody-dependent cell-mediated cytotoxicity for human monolayer target cells bearing blood group and transplantation antigens and for melanoma cells. Int J Cancer 16:579–592, 1975.

89. Kopf AW, Silberberg I and Cooper NS: Immunohistochemical study of human malignant melanoma for the presence of gamma globulin. J Invest Dermatol 47:83–86, 1966.

90. Koprowski H, Steplewski Z, Herlyn D and Herlyn M: Study of antibodies against human malignant melanoma produced by somatic cell hybrids. Proc Natl Acad Sci 75:3405–3409, 1978.

91. Leong SPL, Cooperbrand SR, Sutherland CM, Krementz ET and Deckers PJ: Detection of human melanoma antigens in cell-free supernatants. J Surg Res 24:245–252, 1978.

92. Leong SPL, Hornung HO and Krementz ET: Immunofluorescent studies on chimpanzee humoral responses to human melanoma cells. Oncology 33:246–249, 1976.

93. Leong SPL, Sutherland CM and Krementz ET: Immunofluorescent detection of common melanoma membrane antigens by sera of melanoma patients immunized against autologous or allogeneic cultured melanoma cells. Cancer Res 37:4035–4042, 1977a.

94. Leong SPL, Sutherland CM and Krementz ET: Changes in distribution of human malignant melanoma membrane antigens in the presence of human antibody by immunofluorescence. Cancer Res 37:293–298, 1977b.

95. Lewis MG, Avis PJG, Phillips TM and Sheikh KMA: Tumor-associated antigens in human malignant melanoma. Yale J Biol Med 46:661–668, 1973.

96. Lewis MG: Possible immunological factors in human malignant melanoma in Uganda. Lancet 2:921–922, 1967.

97. Lewis MG, Ikonopisov RL, Nairn RC, Phillips TM, Hamilton-Fairley G, Bodenham DC and Alexander P: Tumour-specific antibodies in human malignant melanoma and their relationship to the extent of disease. Br Med J 3:547–552, 1969.

98. Lewis MG and Phillips TM: Separation of two distinct tumor-associated antibodies in the serum of melanoma patients. J Natl Cancer Inst 49:915–917, 1972a.

99. Lewis MG and Phillips TM: The specificity of surface membrane immunofluorescence in human malignant melanoma. Int J Cancer 10:105–111, 1972b.

100. Lewis MG, Phillips TM, Cook KB and Blake J: Possible explanations for loss of detectable antibodies in patients with disseminated malignant melanoma. Nature 232:52–54, 1971.

101. Lewis MG and Raymond MJ: Humoral and cellular host reactions to melanoma antigens. Behring Inst Mitt 56:120–125, 1975.

102. Liao S, Leong SPL, Sutherland CM, Dent PB, Kwong PC and Krementz ET: Common human melanoma membrane antigens detected by mixed hemadsorption microassay with serum from a patient undergoing immunotherapy with autologous tumor cells. Cancer Res 38:4395–4400, 1978.

103. Liao S, Kwong PC, Thompson JC and Dent PB: Spectrum of melanoma antigens on cultured human malignant melanoma cells as detected by monkey antibodies. Cancer Res 39:183–192, 1979.

104. Lieberman R, Wybran J and Epstein W: The immunologic and histopathologic changes of BCG-mediated tumor regression in patients with malignant melanoma. Cancer 35:756–777, 1975.

105. Macher E, Muller CHR, Sorg G, Gossen A and Sorg C: Evidence for cross-reacting membrane associated specific melanoma antigens as detected by immunofluorescence and immune adherence. Behring Inst Mitt 56:86–90, 1975.

106. Mackie RM, Spilg WGS, Thomas CE and Cochran AJ: Cell-mediated immunity in patients with malignant melanoma. Br J Dermatol 87:523–528, 1972.

107. Malley A, Burger DR, Vandenbark AA, Frikke P, Begley D, Acott K, Black J and Vetto RM: Association of melanoma tumor antigen with $B_2$-microglobulin. Cancer Res 39:619–623, 1979.

108. Marti JH and Thomson DPM: Anti-tumor immunity in malignant melanoma assayed by tube leukocyte adherence inhibition. Br J Cancer 34:116–133, 1976.

109. Martin EW, Kibbey WE, DeVecchia L, Anderson G, Catalano P and Minton JP: Carcinoembryonic antigen: clinical and historical aspects. Cancer 37:62–81, 1976.

110. Mazuran R, Mujagic H, Malenica B and Silobrcic V: In vitro detection of cellular immunity to melanoma antigens in man by the monocyte spreading inhibition test. Int J Cancer 17:14–20, 1976.

111. Mastrangelo MJ, Bellet RE and Berd D: Immunology and immunotherapy of human cutaneous malignant melanoma. In: Clark WH, Goldman LI and Mastrangelo MJ (eds) Human Malignant Melanoma, pp 355–416. Grune & Stratton, New York, 1979.

112. McCabe RP, Ferrone S, Pellegrino MA, Kern DH, Holmes EC and Reisfeld RA: Purification and immunologic evaluation of human melanoma-associated antigens. J Natl Cancer Inst 60:773–777, 1979.

113. McCabe RP, Indiveri F, Galloway DR, Ferone S and Reisfeld RA: Lack of association of serologically detectable human melanoma-associated antigens with $B_2$-microglobulin: serologic and immunologic evidence. J Natl Cancer Inst 65:707–707, 1980.

114. McCabe RP, Quaranta V, Frugis L, Ferrone S and Reisfeld RA: A radioimmunometric antibody binding assay for evaluation of xenoantisera to melanoma associated antigens. J Natl Cancer Inst, 1979.

115. McCarty KS, Jr, Wortman J, Stowers S, Lubahn DB, McCarty KS, Sr and Seigler HF: Sex steroid receptor analysis in human melanoma. Cancer 46:1463-1470, 1980.

116. McCoy JL, Jerome LF, Dean JH, Perlin E, Oldham RK, Char DH, Cohen MH, Felix EL and Herberman RB: Inhibition of leukocyte migration by tumor associated antigens in soluble extracts of human melanoma. J Natl Cancer Inst 55:19-23, 1975.

117. Metzgar RS, Bergoc PM, Moreno MA and Seigler HF: Melanoma specific antibodies produced in monkeys by immunization with human melanoma cell lines. J Natl Cancer Inst 50:1065-1068, 1973.

118. Mihalev A, Tzingilev D and Sirakov LM: Radioimmunoassay of alphafetoprotein in the serum of patients with leukemia and malignant melanoma. Neoplasma 23:103-107, 1976.

119. Minden P, Jarrett C, McClatchy JK, Gutterman JU and Hersh EM: Antibodies to melanoma cell and BCG antigens in sera from tumor-free individuals and from melanoma patients. Nature 263:774-777, 1976b.

120. Minden P, Sharpton TR and McClatchy JK: Shared antigens between human malignant melanoma cells and mycobacterium bovis (BCG). J Immunol 116:1407-1414, 1976a.

121. Morgan G, McCarthy WH, Hersey P: Detection of carcinoembryonic-like antigen on melanoma cells by leukocyte-dependent antibody assays. Br J Cancer 36:446-452, 1977.

122. Morton DL, Eilber FR, Malmgren RA and Wood WC: Immunological factors which influence response to immunotherapy in malignant melanoma. Surgery 68:158-164, 1970.

123. Morton DL, Malmgren RA, Holmes EC and Ketcham AS: Demonstration of antibodies against human malignant melanoma by immunofluorescence. Surgery 64:233-240, 1968.

124. Mukherji B, Vassos D, Flowers A, Binder SC and Nathanson L: Selective and non-selective lymphocytotoxicity in human melanoma: observation on the effect of long-term culture and fetal bovine serum on target cell sensitivity to lymphocytes. Int J Cancer 16:971-980, 1975.

125. Muna N, Marcus S and Smart C: Detection by immunofluorescence of antibodies specific for human malignant melanoma cells. Cancer 34:1712-1721, 1969.

126. Murray E, Ruygrok S, Milton GW and Hersey P: Analysis of serum blocking factors against leukocyte-dependent antibody in melanoma patients. Int J Cancer 21:578-587, 1978.

127. Mutzner PA, Stuhlmiller GM and Seigler HF: Characterization of melanoma cell membrane tumor associated antigens using xenoserum, alloserum and autoserum: I. immunofluorescence. J Surg Oncol 14:367-377, 1980.

128. Myburgh JA and Smit JA: Prolongation of liver allograft survival by donor-specific soluble transplantation antigens and antigen-antibody complexes. Transplantation 19:64-71, 1975.

129. Nagel GA, Piessens WF, Stilmont MM and Lejeune F: Evidence for tumor-specific immunity in human malignant melanoma. Eur J. Cancer 7:41-47, 1971.

130. Nairm RC, Nind APP, Guli BPG, Davies DJ, Little JH, Davis NC and Whitehead RH: Anti-tumour immunity in patients with malignant melanoma. Med J Aust 1:397-403, 1972.

131. Nimmberg RB, Glasgow AH, Memzoian JO, Constantian MB, Cooperband SR, Mannick JA and Schmid K: Isolation of an immunosuppressive peptide fraction from the serum of cancer patients. Cancer Res 35:1489-1494, 1975.

132. Nind APP, Nairm RC, Rolland JM, Guli EPG and Hughes ESR: Lymphocyte anergy in patients with carcinoma. Br J Cancer 28:108-117, 1973.

133. Ninnemann JB: Melanoma-associated immunosuppression through B-cell activation of suppressor T-cells. J Immunol 120:1573–1579, 1978.

134. Nishioka K, Romsdahl MM, Fritsche HA and McMertrey MH: Tyrosinase activity in the sera of patients with malignant melanoma: method and specificity. Int J Cancer 20:289–293, 1977.

135. Nishioka K, Romsdahl MM and McMertrey MH: Comparative studies of tyrosinases of malignant melanoma and correlation to serum tyrosinase in patients with malignant melanoma. Cancer Biochem Biophys 2:145–150, 1978.

136. Oettgen HF, Aoki T, Old LJ, Boyse EA, DeHarven E and Mills GM: Suspension culture of a pigment-producing cell line derived from a human malignant melanoma. J Natl Cancer Inst 41:827–831, 1969.

137. Parks L, Smith W and Williams G: Distinction of allogeneic immunity from tumor-specific immunity in man. Surgery 76:43–49, 1974.

138. Parsons PG, Goss P and Pope JH: Detection in human melanoma cell lines of particles with some properties in common with RNA tumor viruses. Int J Cancer 13:606–618, 1974.

139. Parsons PG, Klucis E, Goss PD, Pope JH, Little JH and Davis NC: Oncornavirus-like particles in malignant melanoma. Int J Cancer 18:757–763, 1976.

140. Pavie-Fischer J, Kourilsky FM, Banzet P, Puissant A and Levy JP: Investigation of cell-mediated immune reactions in malignant melanoma using the chromium release test. Behring Inst Mitt 56:160–167, 1975.

141. Peter HH, Diehl V, Kalden JR, Seeland P and Eckert G: Humoral and cellular cytotoxicity in vitro against allogeneic human melanoma cells. Behring Inst Mitt 56:167–177, 1975a.

142. Peter HH, Pavie-Fischer J, Fridman WH, Aubert C, Cesarin J, Roubin R and Kourilsky FM: Cell-mediated cytotoxicity in vitro of human lymphocytes against a tissue culture melanoma cell line (IGR3). J Immunol 115:539–548, 1975b.

143. Powell AE, Sloss AM, Smith RN, Makley JT and Hubay CA: Specific responsiveness of leukocytes to soluble extracts of human tumors. Int J Cancer 16:905–913, 1975.

144. Preddie E, Hartmann D and Lewis MG: Human melanoma tumor specific antigens. (1) an allogeneic antigen from patient "PY" melanoma tumor cell plasma membranes. Cancer Biochem Biophys 2:161–167, 1978.

145. Preddie E, Hartmann D, Persad S, Khosravi M, and Lewis M: Isolation of an autologous tumor-specific antigen from tumor cell plasma membranes of a human melanoma patient. Cancer Biochem Biophys 2:199–202, 1978.

146. Prehn RT and Main JM: Immunity to methyl-cholanthrene-induced sarcomas. J Natl Cancer Inst 18:769–778, 1957.

147. Rahman AFR, Liao SK and Dent PB: Characterization of human malignant melanoma cell lines. In Vitro 13:580–583, 1977.

148. Reid T and Albert DM: RNA-dependent DNA polymerase activity in human tumors. Biochem Biophys Res Commun 46:383–390, 1972.

149. Reisfeld RA, David GS, Ferrone S, Pellegrino MA and Holmes EC: Approaches for the isolation of biologically functional tumor-associated antigens. Cancer Res 37:2860–2865, 1977.

150. Roenigk HH, Jr, Deodhar SD and Krebs JA: Microcytotoxicity and serum blocking factors in malignant melanoma and halo nevus. Arch Dermatol III:720–725, 1975.

151. Romsdahl SA and Cox IS: Human malignant melanoma antibodies demonstrated by immunofluorescence. Arch Surg Chicago 100:491–497, 1970.

152. Roth JA, Holmes EC, Reisfeld RA, Slocum HK and Morton DL: Isolation of a soluble tumor associated antigen from human melanoma. Cancer 37:104–110, 1976.

153. Roth JA, Slocum HK, Pellegrino MA, Holmes EC and Reisfeld RA: Purification of soluble human melanoma-associated antigens. Cancer Res 36:2360–2364, 1976.

154. Salinas FA, Sheikh KM and Chandor SB: Serological reactivity in cancer patients to human and mouse fetal liver cells. Cancer Res 38:401–407, 1978.

155. Sample WF, Gertner HR and Chretien PB: Inhibition of phytohemagglutinin-induced in vitro lymphocyte transformation by serum from patients with carcinoma. J Natl Cancer Inst 46:1291–1297, 1971.

156. Seigler HF, Shingleton WW, Metzgar RS, Buckley CE and Bergoc PM: Immunotherapy in patients with melanoma. Ann Surg 178:352–359, 1973.

157. Shepherd PS: A comparison of two $^{125}$I Clq binding tests to detect soluble immune complexes in serum of patients with malignant disease. Clin Exp Immunol 36:250–255, 1979.

158. Sherwin SA, Sliski AH and Todaro GJ: Human melanoma cells have both nerve growth factor and nerve growth factor receptors on their cell surfaces. Proc Natl Acad Sci 76:1288–1292, 1979.

159. Shiku H, Takahashi T, Oettgen HF and Old LJ: Cell surface antigens of human malignant melanoma: II. serologic typing with immune adherence assays and definition of two new surface antigens. J Exp Med 144:873–881, 1976.

160. Shiku H, Takahashi T, Resnick LA, Oettgen HF and Old LJ: Cell surface antigens of human malignant melanoma: III. recognition of autoantibodies with unusual characteristics. J Exp Med 145:784–789, 1977.

161. Sidell N, Irie RF and Morton DL: Oncofetal antigen I: a target for immune cytolysis of human cancer. Br J Cancer 40:950–953, 1979.

162. Siebert E, Sorg C, Happle R and Macher E: Membrane associated antigens of human malignant melanoma: III. specificity of human sera reacting with cultured melanoma cells. Int J Cancer 19:172–178, 1977.

163. Sjögren HO, Hellström I, Bansal SC and Hellström KE: Suggestive evidence that "blocking anibodies" of tumor-bearing individuals may be antigen-antibody complexes. Proc Natl Acad Sci 68:1372–1375, 1971.

164. Smith JL and Stehlin JS: Spontaneous regression of primary malignant melanoma with regional metastases. Cancer 18:1399–1415, 1965.

165. Smithers DW: Spontaneous regression of cancer. Ann R Coll Surg Engl 41:160–162, 1967.

166. Snyderman R, Seigler HF and Meadows L: Abnormalities of monocyte chemotaxis in patients with melanoma: effects of immunotherapy and tumor removal. J Natl Cancer Inst 58:37–41, 1977.

167. Steplewski Z, Herlyn M, Herlyn D, Clark WH and Koprowski H: Reactivity of monoclonal anti-melanoma antibodies with melanoma cells freshly isolated from primary and metastatic melanoma. Eur J Immunol 9:94–96, 1979.

168. Stewart THM: The presence of delayed hypersensitivity reactions in patients toward extracts of their malignant tumors: I. the role of tissue antigen, non-specific reactions of nuclear material and bacterial antigen as a cause for this phenomenon. Cancer 23:1368–1379, 1969.

169. Stuhlmiller GM, Boylston JA, Seigler HF and Fetter BF: Immunodiagnosis of melanoma using chimpanzee antihuman melanoma antiserum. Am J Clin Pathol 67:573–579, 1977.

170. Stuhlmiller GM, Green RW and Seigler HF: Solubilization and partial isolation of human melanoma tumor associated antigens. J Natl Cancer Inst 61:61–67, 1978.

171. Stuhlmiller GM and Seigler HF: Immunology and Immunotherapy of Melanoma. In: Waters H (ed) Handbook of Cancer Immunology, Vol 5, pp 315–343. Garland STPM, New York, 1978.

172. Stuhlmiller GM and Seigler HF: Enzymatic susceptibility and spontaneous release of human melanoma tumor associated antigens. J Natl Cancer Inst 58:215–221, 1977.

173. Stuhlmiller GM and Seigler HF: Characterization of a chimpanzee antihuman melanoma antiserum. Cancer Res 35:2132-2137, 1975.

174. Sumner WC and Foraker AG: Spontaneous regression of human melanoma: clinical and experimental studies. Cancer 13:79-81, 1960.

175. Takasugi M, Mickey M and Terasaki PI: Reactivity of lymphocytes from normal persons on cultured tumor cells. Cancer Res. 33:2898-2901, 1973.

176. Takasugi M, Mickey M and Terasaki PI: Studies on the specificity of cell-mediated immunity to human tumors. J Natl Cancer Inst 53:1527-1538, 1974.

177. The TH, Huiges NA, Schraffordt-Koops H, Lamberts HB and Niewg HO: Surface antigens on cultured malignant melanoma cells as detected by a membrane immunofluorescence method with human sera. Lack of tumor-specific reactions on melanoma lines. Ann N Y Acad Sci 254:528-540, 1975.

178. Thomson DMP, Gold P, Freedman SO and Shuster J: The isolation and characterization of tumor-specific antigens of rodent and human tumors. Cancer Res 36:3518-3525, 1976.

179. Thomson DMP, Rauch JE, Weatherhead JC, Friedlander P, O'Conner R, Grossner N, Shuster J and Gold P: Isolation of tumor-specific antigens associated with $B_2$-microglobulin. Br J Cancer 37:753-775, 1978.

180. Thomson DMP, Tataryn DN, Schwartz R and MacFarlane JK: Abrogation of the phenomenon of leukocyte adherence inhibition by excess circulating tumour antigen. Eur J Cancer 15:1095-1106, 1979.

181. Theofilopoulus AN, Andrews BS, Vrist MM, Morton DL and Dixon FJ: The nature of immune complexes in human cancer sera. J Immunol 119:657-663, 1977.

182. Thorpe WP, Parker GA and Rosenberg SA: Expression of fetal antigen by normal human skin cells grown in tissue culture. J Immunol 119:818-823, 1977.

183. Todd DW, Spencer-Payne W, Farrow GM and Winklemann RK: Spontaneous regression of primary malignant melanoma with regional metastases: report of a case of photographic documentation. Proc Mayo Clin 41:10-17, 1966.

184. Tomecki KJ, Montague PM and Hearing VJ: Serum and urine protein differences in patients with malignant melanoma. J Natl Cancer Inst 64:29-32, 1980.

185. Vanderbark AA, Greene MH, Burger DR, Vetto RM and Reimer RR: Immune response to melanoma extracts in three melanoma-prone families. J Natl Cancer Inst 63:1147-1151, 1979.

186. Viza D and Phillips J: Extraction and solubilization of cell surface antigens from malignant melanomas. Rev Inst Pasteur Lyon 4:339-342, 1971.

187. Viza D and Phillips J: Identification of an antigen associated with malignant melanoma. Int J Cancer 16:312-317, 1975.

188. Viza D, Phillips J and Bourgoin JJ: Detection of specific antigens in the serum of melanoma patients. Rev Inst Pasteur Lyon 6:321-324, 1973.

189. Weese JL, Herberman RB, Hollingshead AC, Cannon GB, Keels M, Kibrite A, Morales A, Char DH and Oldham RK: Specificity of delayed cutaneous hypersensitivity responses to extracts of human tumor cells. J Natl Cancer Inst 60:255-263, 1978.

190. Whitehead RH: Fluorescent antibody studies in malignant melanoma. Br J Cancer 28:525-529, 1973.

191. Wilson BS, Indiveri F, Pellegrino MA and Ferrone S: Dr (Ia-like) antigens on human melanoma cells. J Exp Med 149:658-668, 1979.

192. Winchester RJ, Wang C, Gibofsky A, Kunkel HG, Lloyd KO and Old LJ: Expression of Ia-like antigens on cultured human malignant melanoma cell lines. Proc Natl Acad Sci 75:6235-6239, 1978.

193. Wood GW and Barth RF: Immunofluorescent studies of the serologic reactivity of patients with malignant melanoma against tumor-associated cytoplasmic antigens. J Natl Cancer Inst 53:309-316, 1974.

194. Wood GW and Gollahon KA: Detection and quantitation of macrophage infiltration into primary human tumors with the use of cell surface markers. J Natl Cancer Inst 59:1081–1087, 1977.

# 9. Melanoma of the head and neck

T. BOYCE COLE

Melanoma constitutes 1–3% of all malignancies, with approximately ⅓ of these in the head and neck. Melanoma manifests itself in a variety of ways. It may occur in a preexisting nevus with recent changes. Much more commonly, it develops de novo as a new pigmented lesion or, rarely, as an amelanotic lesion. Metastatic lesions from a known or unknown primary, at times, affect most or almost all structures in the head and neck. Pigmented mucosal lesions or polyps should always be suspect.

Considering the high incidence of benign nevi, certainly all nevi cannot be removed. It has been estimated that 250 000 nevi must be removed to prevent one melanoma [1]. However, prior lesions with a change in character should be removed. These changes include spreading horizontally or vertically, color changes either becoming darker, or gray or tan; itching, bleeding, weeping, or becoming scaly. In addition, lesions exposed to chronic irritation should be removed. Cauterization, curettage or shaving should be discouraged. Giant pigmented nevi, however, have a significant incidence of malignant transformation and many authors in the literature have advocated their removal when possible [2–5].

## Diagnosis

The preferred method is total excisional biopsy. In selected large lesions, incisional biopsy may be adequate and allow better overall management (Figure 1). Each specimen should be properly labeled and examined by a pathologist familiar with the information desired, specifically, tumor thickness and level of invasion.

In 1969, a method of classifying melanoma according to its level of invasion was described and correlated with prognosis [6]. Subsequently, in 1975, a method of measurement of tumor thickness by use of an ocular micrometer was reported [7]. These measurements were related to prognosis and the possibility of developing recurrent disease. Comparing these two methods of classification, it has been found that the thickness of the lesion is quite variable, particularly in Clark's Levels III and IV. Level of invasion has been found to be less predictive of prognosis than tumor thickness [8–

*Seigler, H. F. (ed.), Clinical Management of Melanoma. ISBN 978-94-009-7495-1*
© *1982, Martinus Nijhoff Publishers, The Hague/Boston/London.*

A                                     B

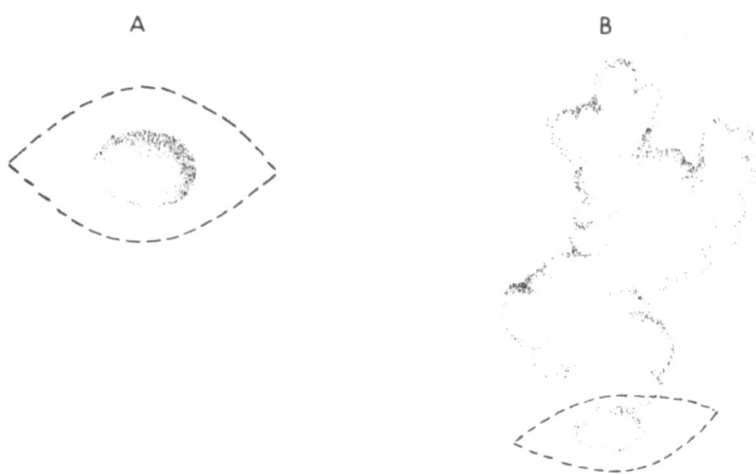

*Figure 1.* (A) Excisional biopsy preferred. (B) Incisional biopsy preferable in selected cases.

11]. Level of invasion and/or tumor thickness are related to risk of nodal metastases, while ulceration of the primary and the presence of nodal metastases correlate inversely with survival [8]. If both classifications are reported, comparison of data is possible and a more dependable method may be used in the future. When patients are seen on a referral basis, desirable information is commonly not available. Often, neither depth of invasion nor tumor thickness can be adequately assessed.

**Treatment**

Lesions less than 0.76 mm in thickness or in Clark's Levels I or II require only local excision. What is an adequate local excision? Wide local excision with skin grafting has not been found to be significantly better than simple local excision with adequate margins [11, 12]. Should the local resection be taken down to and include the underlying fascia, and a skin graft placed? The best approach is to individualize these situations. If a tumor is of the superficial spreading type or develops in a Hutchinson's freckle, a wider skin margin is taken without too much emphasis on excision of the underlying fascia. A deeper excision is performed for nodular types with less emphasis on several centimeters of margin. Recurrent lesions also are treated with more emphasis on wider margins and depth of resection, namely, 4–5 cm of margin and including the deep fascia. Scalp lesions are considered separately and a 5–6 cm margin is taken down to periosteum and skin grafting is recommended. Should removal of the periosteum and/or underlying bone be required, a rotation flap with skin grafting of the donor site is used.

A continuing controversy regarding treatment of melanoma concerns the use of elective neck dissection in Stage I invasive melanoma (Levels III, IV and V). Lesions thicker than 1.5 mm reportedly have a significantly better prognosis with elective neck dissection, but lesions in the 0.76 to 1.5 mm range are not benefited by elective neck dissection [7, 11]. Lesions in this range of thickness may include a very thick Level II through very thin Level IV lesion. Most Level I and II lesions are thinner than 0.76 mm and most Level IV and V lesions are greater than 1.5 mm. Patients with nodal metastases have a very poor prognosis and nodal disease has been the greatest indicator of systemic disease [1, 12–15]. Effective adjuvant therapy in the form of immunotherapy and chemotherapy is being developed. The presence of tumor in nonclinically positive nodes is the earliest indicator of the necessity for instituting these methods of treatment. Local and regional disease control is beneficial in spite of systemic metastasis. Disease in the head and neck area is often both psychologically and physically crippling.

It has been reported that the immediately adjacent nodes are always involved if more distant nodal groups in the neck contain tumor [15]. However, lymph channels bypassing nodes and entire groups of nodes has been described [16]. For patients with lesions in the thickness range of 0.76 to 1.5 mm upon whom a decision cannot be made regarding the desirability of an elective neck dissection based upon ulceration, histologic type, mitotic activity, thickness or depth of invasion, a regional node dissection can be done along with excision or treatment of the primary lesion. Should the nodes be clinically positive, a complete therapeutic dissection can be done at the time or subsequently.

Our treatment plan has included a complete neck dissection for all Stage I, Levels IV, V and most Level III's. The surgical technique is widely used and has been well described [17]. One variation is suggested. The posterior belly of the digastric and stylohyoid muscle should be resected. This allows the internal jugular vein to be transected higher and nodes removed to the base of the skull.

## Lymphatics of the head and neck

Prior to a discussion of specific sites, a brief review of the lymphatics might be helpful. Figure 2 outlines these schematically. The lymphatic drainage of the head and neck has been described in great detail [18].

Superficial occipital nodes drain primarily the occipital portion of the scalp, posterior ear and mastoid area, with the efferents passing to the deep occipital nodes, upper nodes of the superior deep cervical group and spinal accessory nodes.

Postauricular nodes resting upon the mastoid portion of the insertion of

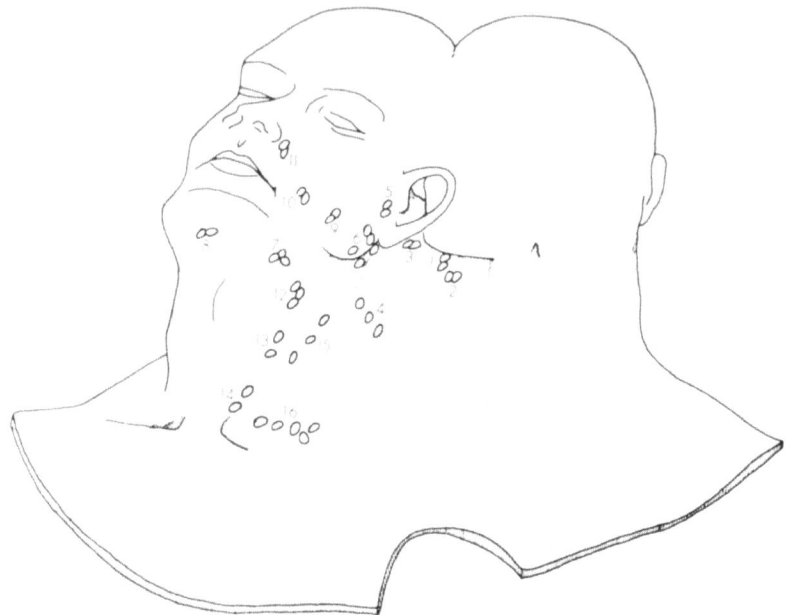

*Figure 2.* Lymphatics of the head and neck: (1) superficial occipital nodes, (2) deep occipital nodes, (3) postauricular nodes, (4) spinal accessory nodes, (5) preauricular nodes, (6) paratid nodes, (7) submandibular nodes, (8) submental nodes, (9) masseter nodes, (10) buccinator nodes, (11) maxillary nodes, (12) upper deep cervical nodes, (13) med deep cervical nodes, (14) lower deep cervical nodes, (15) superficial cervical nodes and (16) transverse cervical nodes.

the sternocleidomastoid muscle received afferents from the posterior temporal and parietal regions of the scalp as well as posterior ear, with efferents to the upper nodes of the superior deep cervical and spinal accessory groups.

Preauricular nodes located in front of the tragus received afferents from the anterior surface of the pinna and the external auditory meatus as well as a portion of the lids, temporal scalp and forehead. Efferents pass to the superior deep cervical and parotid nodes.

Parotid nodes received afferents from the same regions as the preauricular nodes as well as the preauricular nodes themselves. In addition, parotid nodes received afferents from intraoral structures with efferents going to the superior deep cervical nodes.

Submandibular nodes situated along the horizontal ramus of the mandible as well as occasionally within the submandibular gland itself receive afferents from the submental and facial nodes draining the lip, face, nose, cheek, inferior portions of the lids, gums and both jaws, as well as anterior tongue. Efferents go to the superior deep cervical nodes.

Submental nodes are found beneath the chin between the anterior bellies of the two digastric muscles. Afferents come from the integument of the chin, lower lip and floor of the mouth. Efferents pass to the submandibular nodes then to the superior deep cervical nodes.

Facial nodes include nodes along the horizontal portion of the mandible anterior to the masseter, the buccinator group along the surface of the buccinator muscle and maxillary nodes situated in the groove formed by the junction of the nose and cheek. Afferents come from the adjacent facial areas with the efferents passing to the submandibular, parotid and deep cervical nodes.

Retropharyngeal nodes are primarily situated along the junction of the lateral and posterior surface of the pharynx. Afferents come from the upper part of the pharynx as well as mucous membranes of the nose and sinuses. Efferents pass to the upper deep cervical nodes.

Deep cervical lymphatics of the neck are primarily the internal jugular complex divided into superior, middle and inferior groups. Efferents from the deep cervical nodes drain into the thoracic duct.

Superficial cervical nodes are situated along the external jugular vein lateral to the sternocleidomastoid with efferent drainage into the deep cervical nodes. Spinal accessory nodes are situated along the course of the spinal accessory nerve. The transverse cervical nodes are primarily situated along the course of the transverse cervical artery and vein. Efferents from both these groups go to the deep cervical chain.

**Specific sites**

*Scalp*

Melanoma of the scalp is usually of the superficial type, but its diagnosis is often delayed. The scalp is quite vascular and rich in lymphatics with no local lymph barriers to impede spread. The long-term cure rate is quite low, in the range of 10% to 20%. Local lesions are treated with wide resection, usually 5-6 cm margins. The local defect is covered with a skin graft or rotation scalp flap if periosteum and bone are removed. A nodal dissection for scalp lesions varies depending upon the location of the lesion. For temporal and frontal lesions as well as some anterior parietal lesions, a parotidectomy, either superficial or total depending upon whether the nodes are clinically positive, is combined with a routine anterior neck dissection. For patients with grossly positive nodes, a total parotidectomy with facial nerve resection and grafting is preferable.

For posterior parietal, occipital and mastoid scalp lesions, a posterior neck dissection is done with or without an anterior neck dissection. The posterior scalp, posterior ear, mastoid skin and skin of the posterior neck drain through the superficial occipital nodes located in the angle between

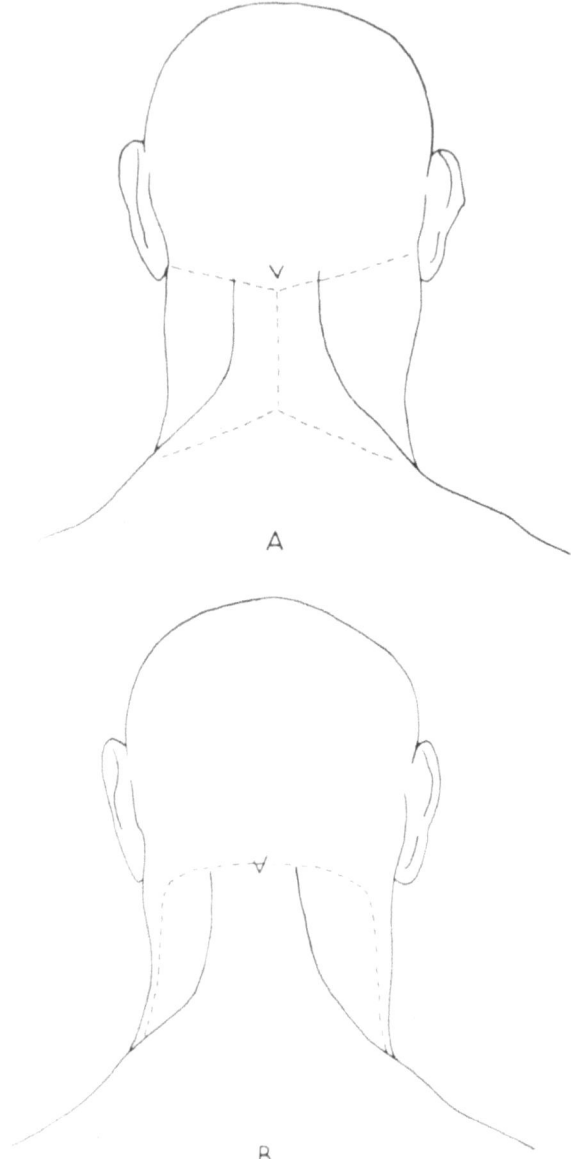

*Figure 3.* Skin incisions for bilateral posterior neck dissection.

the insertion of the trapezius and sternocleidomastoid muscles and superficial to the splenius muscle. The efferent vessels from these superficial nodes drain into the deep occipital and/or spinal accessory nodes. The deep occipital nodes are located beneath the splenius muscle and in the suboccipital triangle. A regional node dissection for lesions in these areas would necessarily include a posterior neck dissection. This should be combined with either the posterior triangle of the anterior neck when the nodes are clini-

cally negative or an anterior neck dissection if the nodes are clinically positive. For midline lesions, a bilateral posterior neck dissection may be done.
Figure 3 illustrates the recommended incisions. The indications for and the
surgical technique of posterior neck dissection have been outlined [19–21].
For lesions near the midline, injection of technetium antimony trisulfide
colloid with subsequent scanning of the suspected nodal drainage areas may
give some direction regarding the type of nodal dissection necessary. This
technique is currently under investigation and should be widely available in
the near future.

The technique of posterior neck dissection is not generally utilized and
will be discussed in more detail. The posterior neck dissection is done in the
prone position if a unilateral or bilateral posterior dissection is performed
alone. The patient is placed on his side for combined posterior and anterior
dissections with the incisions outlined in Figure 4. Flaps are elevated in the
usual manner (Figure 5). The trapezius and splenius capitis muscles are
detached from the superior nuchal line as well as the ligamentum nuchae in
the midline. The trapezius and splenius capitis muscles are retracted laterally allowing dissection of the superficial and deep occipital nodes in the
suboccipital triangle. The suboccipital triangle is bounded by the rectus
capitis major and minor, the superior oblique and inferior oblique muscles,
and the occipit, with the floor formed by the atlanto-occipital membrane
and vertebral artery (Figure 6). The trapezius and splenius capitis muscles
are resected above the scapula proceeding laterally to the clavicle. The

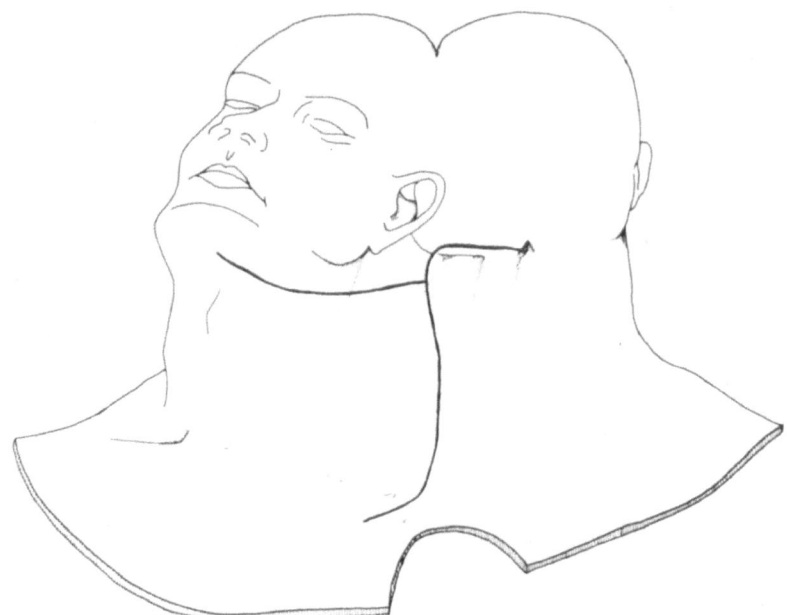

*Figure 4.* Skin incision for combined anterior and posterior neck dissection.

274

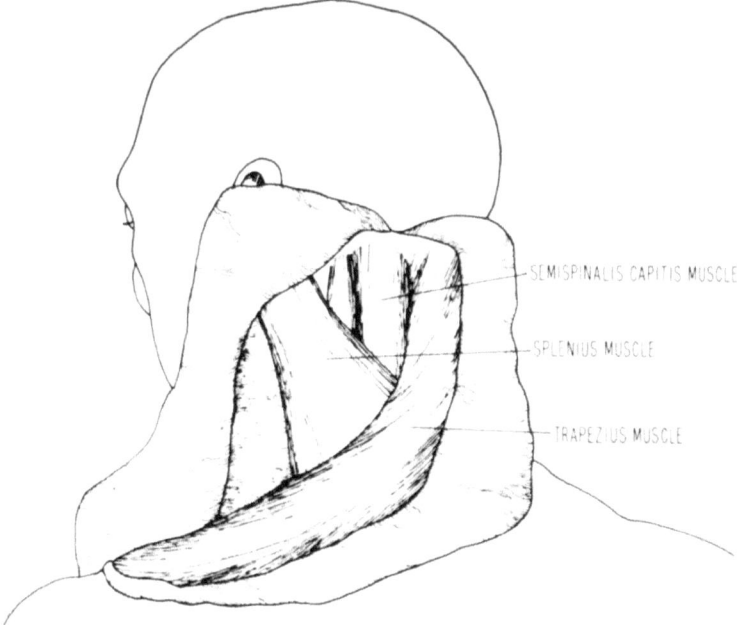

*Figure 5.* Skin flaps elevated for posterior neck dissection.

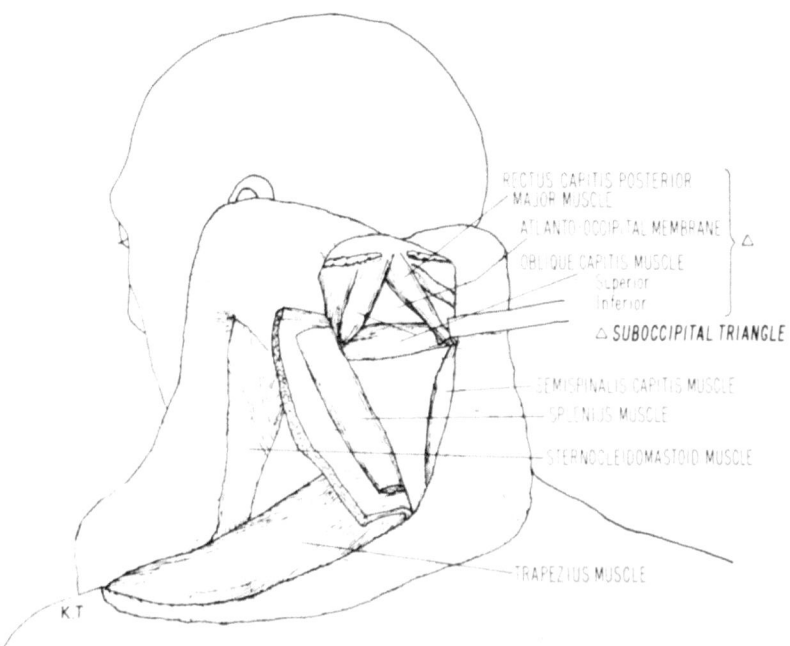

*Figure 6.* Posterior neck dissection.

remainder of the resection depends upon whether the posterior triangle of the anterior neck or standard anterior neck dissection is added to the posterior dissection. In either case, a standard dissection of these areas is performed.

## Face

Local lesions of the forehead are treated in the usual manner and, should a regional node dissection be required, a parotidectomy is combined with the procedure. Lid lesions as well as lateral cheek lesions may also require parotidectomy along with a neck dissection.

Medial cheek lesions, nasal and chin lesions require only inferior parotidectomy unless gross parotid disease is present. Midline lesions of the nose, lip, chin and neck are generally treated locally unless nodes are clinically positive on one side of the neck or the other.

## Ear

Treatment of ear lesions depends on the location of the melanoma with regard to the ear anatomy. Anterior lesions are treated by local resection. If indicated, a regional node dissection requires a parotidectomy as well as an anterior neck dissection. Posterior ear lesions require posterior neck dissections as do lesions on the mastoid aspect of the scalp. Inferior lesions lateral to the ear canal may be treated without total auriculectomy. However, lesions near the canal or deep in the concha require total auriculectomy as do lesions on the upper part of the pinna. Lesions within the canal should be treated much as a squamous cell carcinoma of the ear canal requiring a modified or possibly total temporal bone resection.

## Mucosal

Mucosal melanomas of the head and neck have a very poor prognosis, with reported survival below 20% at five years and below 10% at ten years [22, 23]. Any suspicious pigmented lesion on the mucosa should be biopsied. Mucosal melanomas are usually diagnosed late because of a number of factors. A lesion in the mouth cannot be seen and does not cause symptoms until the melanoma is larger than the usual cutaneous ones. In addition, the symptoms of a nasal or sinus melanoma in the early stages are the same as other common benign conditions related to allergy, upper respiratory infections, etc. Primary symptoms are nasal obstruction, drainage and, later, epistaxis and facial deformity. Differential diagnosis of mucosal pigmented lesions has been well outlined [24, 25]. Dark lesions of the mucosa are usually due to the presence of blood, metallic particles or melanin. Traumatic lesions such as cheek biting or hematoma from whatever etiology are easily distinguished. Hemangiomas, telangiectasia and dilated veins are also easily distinguishable. Metallic particles such as dental amalgam, graphite tattooing secondary to trauma, pigmentation of lead or bismuth are usually easily differentiated. Some of the melanotic lesions such as racial pigmentation, pigmentation with Addison's Disease, post inflammatory pigmentation or drug related pigmentation such as chloroquine are easily distinguished from melanoma. Other lesions such as ephilides (freckles) and lentigines (liver spots) as well as pigmented nevi are not so easily differentiated. A good general rule is to excise solitary brown or black lesions of the mucosa.

Surgically, the approach for oral melanoma is approximately the same as that used for squamous cell carcinoma in these areas. The exception is that a wider margin or surrounding mucosa needs to be obtained along with careful evaluation for local submucosal spread. Primary melanomas have also been reported in the tonsil, pharynx, larynx, esophagus and trachea, and are treated much the same as squamous cell lesions in these areas.

Treatment regimens and survival data obtained from the literature regarding nasal and paranasal sinus melanoma are quite variable. Nasal mucosal melanoma has a potential survival between 27% and 44% with sinus melanoma survival close to zero [23, 26]. Nasal and sinus melanomas usually present with unilateral nasal obstruction, bleeding and/or facial swelling. Pain is an occasional symptom.

Sinus lesions do less well, probably because of later diagnosis. The tumors are larger with more likelihood of metastatic disease. Preoperative evaluation of the extent of the lesion is more difficult than with cutaneous lesions, and a classification of sinus melanoma has been suggested [27]. Radical removal of sinus and nasal mucosa is the preferred method of treatment. Surgical techniques for maxillectomy, septectomy, etc. are published and well known. Regional nodal metastatic disease is not a prominent feature. Regional node dissection is rarely indicated. These tumors develop in an older age group than cutaneous melanoma. Local recurrences are more common than with cutaneous melanoma. Repeated removal with cauterization, cryosurgery or radiation therapy as adjunctive treatment modalities are useful.

# References

1. Seigler HF and Fetter BF: Current management of melanoma. Ann Surg 186:1:1–12, 1977.
2. Pack GT and David J: Nevus giganticus pigmentosus with malignant transformation. Surgery 49:347–354, 1961.
3. Dobson L: Prepubertal malignant melanomas. Am J Surg 89:1128–1135, 1955.
4. Shaw MH: Malignant melanoma arising from a giant hairy naevus. Br J Plast Surg 15:426–431, 1962.
5. Reed WB, Becker SW, Sr, Becker SW, Jr and Nickel WR: Giant pigmented nevi, melanoma, and leptomeningeal melanocytosis. Arch Dermatol 91:100–119, 1965.
6. Clark WH, Jr, From L, Bernardino EA and Mihm MC: The histogenesis and biologic behavior of primary human malignant melanomas of the skin. Cancer Res 29:705–715, 1969.
7. Breslow A: Tumor thickness, level of invasion and node dissection in Stage I cutaneous melanoma. Ann Surg 182:5:572–575, 1975.
8. Balch CM, Soong SJ, Murad TM, Ingalls AL and Maddox WA: A multifactorial analysis of melanoma II, prognostic factors in patients with Stage I (localized) melanoma. Surgery, 86:2:343–351, 1979.
9. Wanebo HJ, Woodruff J and Fortner JG: Malignant melanoma of the extremities: a clinicopathologic study using levels of invasion (microstage). Cancer 35:666–676, 1975.
10. Breslow A, Natale C, Van der Esch EP and Morabito A: Stage I melanoma of the limbs: assessment of prognosis by levels of invasion and maximum thickness. Tumori 64:273–284, 1978. WHO Collaborating Centres for Evaluation of Methods of Diagnosis and Treatment of Melanoma.
11. Hansen MG and McCarten AB: Tumor thickness and lymphocytic infiltration in malignant melanoma of the head and neck. Am J Surg 128:557–561, 1974.
12. Ames FC, Sugarbaker EV and Ballantyne AJ: Analysis of survival and disease control in Stage I melanoma of the head and neck. Am J Surg 132:484–491, 1976.
13. Ballantyne AJ: Malignant melanoma of the skin of the head and neck. Am J Surg 120:4:425–431, 1970.
14. Conrad FG: Treatment of malignant melanoma: wide excision alone vs lymphadenectomy. Arch Surg 104:587–593, 1972.
15. Roses DF, Harris MN, Grunberger I and Gumport S: Selective surgical management of cutaneous melanoma of the head and neck. Ann Surg 192:5:629–632, 1980.
16. Fisch UP and Del Buano MS: Die Lymphographic des Holses. Arch Ohren Nasen Kehlkopf Heilkd 12:311–315, 1963.
17. Martin H, Valle BD, Ehrlick H and Gahan WG: Neck dissection. Cancer 4:441–499, 1951.
18. Rouviere H: Anatomie des Lymphatiques de l'Homme. Masson, 1932.
19. Rochlin DB: Posterolateral neck dissection for malignant melanoma. Surg Gynecol Obstet 115:369–373, 1962.
20. Wander JV and Chaudhuri P: Dissection of the posterior part of the neck. Surg Gynecol Obstet 143:97–100, 1976.
21. Goepfert H, Jesse RH and Ballantyne AJ: Posterolateral neck dissection. Arch Otolaryngol 109:618–620, 1980.
22. Eneroth CM and Lundberg C: Mucosal malignant melanomas of the head and neck. Acta Otolaryngol 80:452–458, 1975.
23. Freedman HM, DeSanto LW, Devine KD and Weiland LH: Malignant melanoma of the nasal cavity and paranasal sinuses. Arch Otolaryngol 97:322–325, 1973.
24. Birt BD, From L and Main JHP: The diagnosis of melanotic and other pigmented lesions of the lip and oral mucosa (dark spots in the mouth). J Otolaryngol 7:3:203–210, 1978.

25. Powell JP and Cummings CW: Melanoma and the differential diagnosis of oral pigmented lesions. Laryngoscope 88:1252–1265, 1978.
26. Harrison DFN: Malignant melanomata arising in the nasal mucous membrane. J Laryngol Otol 90:993–1005, 1976.
27. Sisson GA, Johnson NE, Amiri CS: Cancer of the maxillary sinus: clinical classification and management. Ann Otol Rhinol Laryngol 72:1050–1059, 1963.

# 10. Prognostic factors in malignant melanoma

EDWIN B. COX

## 1. Introduction

Some of the most substantive recent developments regarding malignant melanoma involve the elucidation of prognostic factors in the disease. Formerly, melanoma had the well-justified reputation of being a capricious, unpredictable neoplasm. The advances in prognostic classification are largely due to pathological microstaging guidelines formulated by Clark et al. and Breslow [1, 2]. Their criteria have made it possible to precisely predict which patients have almost certainly been cured by wide local excision alone, which patients are likely to have occult distant metastases with a high risk for recurrence and which patients have occult metastasis confined to regional lymph nodes. Several of the long-standing issues in treating melanoma, such as the efficacy of prophylactic lymph node dissections and the role of various modalities of adjuvant therapy, should be readily resolvable with well-designed studies involving a practical number of subjects now that it is possible to form subgroups of patients with uniform prognostic features.

Parallel with the development of the histologic guidelines of Clark et al. and Breslow, new biostatistical methods have been developed which allow much more efficient extraction of prognostic factor information. These multifactor analysis methods allow simultaneous adjustment for the effects of all known prognostic factors when evaluating treatment efficacy. Use of these methods will minimize differences among treatment trials due to effects of baseline inequalities among treatment groups.

In this chapter we will introduce the concepts of the newer statistical methods, outline the prognostic factors by type and stage of disease, and recommend data collection and reporting standards in studies of melanoma.

*Seigler, H. F. (ed.), Clinical Management of Melanoma. ISBN 978-94-009-7495-1*
*© 1982, Martinus Nijhoff Publishers, The Hague/Boston/London.*

## 2. Methods for prognostic factor analysis

### 2.1 General methods and applications

The methods for prognostic factor evaluation and uses for this type of analysis have undergone a dramatic change in the past decade. An understanding of the spirit of these methods is central to the interpretation of a number of excellent clinical studies which have substantially enhanced our understanding of melanoma. A brief description of these methods follows.

The expression prognostic factor analysis has become associated with a particular set of statistical techniques used to evaluate outcomes in a disease. There are often many outcomes of interest—type of response to treatment, duration of response, duration of survival. Prognostic factor analysis determines the relationship of these outcomes to other characteristics of the host and his environment. Traditionally, "prognostic factors" referred to uncontrollable characteristics of the patient, the underlying or baseline condition of the patient. Formerly, prognostic factors were used simply for stratifying patients prior to treatment allocation or analysis to obtain relatively uniform groups for comparison. A major methodological problem with stratification as the sole means of assuring comparability is the decrease in the size of individual subgroups as the number of subgroups increases. If more than a handful of important prognostic factors are identified, the groups usually contain too few subjects for meaningful comparison. Furthermore, important interactions among variables are easily missed with stratification. Even if individual factors seem equally distributed, the effects of several important variables, each of which is slightly more frequent in one group, may compound to produce a spuriously significant difference in outcome between the groups [3]. Finally, when groups do differ significantly in prognostic factor distribution, conventional methods of comparing the groups cannot be used.

There are new techniques available which circumvent these problems with stratification. The newer methods are referred to as regression techniques. The term *regression* is used in statistics to imply that a change in one variable can be related to a change in another variable. In multiple regression, the possibility that multiple influences contribute to a result simultaneously—some with positive effects, others with negative effects—may be explored by postulating a specific functional relationship ("model") between an outcome and the putative influences. The advantage of regression techniques over simple subgrouping by stratification is the ability to extract more information from the data. Not only does one avoid the loss of statistical power inherent in making multiple comparisons, but interactions among variables which are important to outcome are more readily discerned.

Different outcomes are often of interest in melanoma, such as duration, quality and type of response to treatment. If there is no variation in outcome, there is no need to examine prognostic factors. The uniformity of the outcome implies a direct mechanistic progression of the disease. Certain types and stages of cancer are monotonous in their progression. Unresectable non-small cell bronchogenic carcinomas, pancreatic adenocarcinomas and, indeed, metastatic melanoma behave in a stereotyped fashion, nearly oblivious to host or treatment variations. Prognostic factor analysis is generally unrewarding in these circumstances but advances in treatment are readily detected.

When variations in outcomes are observed, it is worthwhile to ask whether the variation can be explained. Specifically, is a deviation in a disease or patient characteristic away from the norm associated in a systematic way with a difference in the outcome? Certain intellectual traps must be avoided. Prognostic factor analysis reveals associations. Association does not imply causality. If thicker melanomas are found to be associated with a higher recurrence rate and a shorter survival time, it does not follow that thickness per se is responsible for the recurrence. Rather thickness itself may be a rich composite of true determinants of outcome—mitotic rate of the melanoma, its invasiveness, lack of awareness by the patient and probability of tumor cells having been shed to enter lymphatics and blood vessels. Determination of causality is generally not critical except with regard to evaluating effects of treatments. There is a constant danger of attributing to treatment the effects of unrecognized factors which influenced treatment allocation.

As a consequence of the generality of the prognostic factors methods, this chapter will not simply be confined to description of passive underlying factors but will also consider effects of treatments evaluated by these methods. Our best available information on several of the most urgent issues in the treatment of melanoma is derived from such prognostic factor studies, as will be described.

## 2.2. Multifactor survival regression analysis

The effect of prognostic factors on remission duration, or survival time, is evaluated with survival regression methods. In general, the factors are thought of as influencing the force of mortality (death rate) rather than predicting individual survival times. In one popular method, the proportional hazard model, the force of mortality for the individual, $\lambda_i$, is related to that of the overall group, $\lambda_o$, by an equation linear in the regression coefficients. Thus if $x_1$ and $x_2$ are two factors, say, age and thickness of the primary lesion, $\beta_1$ and $\beta_2$ are the coefficients (weights) for the influence of those factors to be estimated from the data. The combined effect of the two factors is given by $\beta_1 x_1 + \beta_2 x_2$. A final statement of the force of mortality ("hazard") function is then

$$\log_e (\lambda_i) = \log_e (\lambda_o) + \beta_o + \beta_1 x_1 + \beta_2 x_2,$$

where $\beta_o$ is the intercept coefficient.

It is easily seen that if $\beta_o$, $\beta_1 x_1$ and $\beta_2 x_2$ sum to 0, the individual patient has a projected death rate of the overall group; he is the typical group member. A sum greater than 0 signifies a higher expected death rate for that individual relative to the overall group, while a sum less than 0 indicates a lower projected death rate. Tests of significance on the coefficients evaluate their relative prognostic importance. This particular formulation, developed by Cox [4], is very general and widely used, although a number of other models have been developed with the assumption of specific hazard functions. Several excellent references are available regarding the details and uses of these methods [5-7].

## 2.3. Endpoints in melanoma reporting

The traditional endpoint for evaluation of cancer treatments is the five-year survival rate, and this has been most commonly used in melanoma studies. Some authors have reported five-year recurrence-free survival as the endpoint, and still others have also reported ten-year survival or disease-free status. Some studies give only direct survival estimates while others use actuarial estimates based on life tables. The many different reporting policies compound the problem of comparing various studies.

Actuarial methods give survival estimates which make the most efficient use of available information, particularly if some patients have had relatively short follow-up. The only limitation on their use is the requirement that follow-up be very aggressive and complete. If there is any important lag in ascertaining recurrence or death of patients and more than a very few patients are recorded as alive or disease-free when in fact they have died or recurred, the initial survival estimates will be unduly optimistic and will gradually decrease as the failures finally get reported. Nevertheless, whenever feasible we favor actuarial methods because of their more efficient use of the data, i.e., smaller confidence intervals about survival estimates.

With regard to the use of disease-free interval and survival, it is highly recommended that both be reported in studies of primary melanoma. We have found that the survival curves in melanoma closely parallel the time to recurrence curves with a lag of 12-16 months at all Clark's levels and thicknesses. This finding implies that the average survival following relapse is about 14 months, with no important variation across prognostic groups. This being the case, time to recurrence gives the desired information regarding the efficacy of initial treatment and adjuvant therapy and shortens the time to study endpoint by about 14 months. Clinical trials can be shortened by this much if time to recurrence is used as the end point rather than survival. Time to recurrence should generally be to systemic recurrence. Patients who have had adequate lymph node dissections are at very low risk for nodal recurrence, the most common site of first relapse in patients who do not have elective lymph node dissections. Comparisons of time to first recurrence without regard to site of recurrence would therefore be very misleading.

It is well known that five years is an inadequate length of time to follow melanoma patients, since an important number of recurrences still occur after this point, and clear divergence of survival curves using different treatments is sometimes seen only after 5–7 years or more. Survival rates given at a single time point (e.g., five years or ten years) fail to convey the pattern of failure over time, which itself is often informative. We favor reporting results in the form of survival or time to recurrence curves, either by the Kaplan-Meier method [8] or the Berkson-Gage method [9]. Whenever possible, 95 % confidence intervals should be included to indicate the variability associated with the data.

## 3. Overview of prognostic factors in melanoma

Melanoma has the reputation of being a capricious neoplasm. Certain obvious and well-known signs—large ulcerated lesions, multiple lesions, mucocutaneous primary sites, lymph node or distant metastases—have long been recognized for their ominous nature. Relatively few patients have these features. Of the large remaining group with a single cutaneous lesion, many are cured by local excision. Others are disease-free for only a brief time and suffer rapid progression and death. An intermediate group goes for years free of disease, only to experience delayed recurrence and death . Until relatively recently, no means existed for predicting which patients in this clinically homogenous group were at high risk for recurrence or likely to be cured. It is understandable that melanoma has been considered so frustrating.

A classic paper by Allen and Spitz in 1953 described the diagnostic criteria and prognostic factors for melanoma that they gleaned from the literature and from their landmark review of 934 cases [10]. Their discussion focused upon the differentiation of malignant melanoma from benign pigmented lesions and the histologic distinction between primary and metastatic lesions. Virtually every prognostic factor which has proven useful in prognostication was presaged in their discussion.

Prognostic factors in melanoma fall into five general categories (Table 1).

*Table 1.* Prognostic factors of primary melanoma

CLINICAL

| | |
|---|---|
| Clinical stage | Race |
| Primary site | Metastatic site |
| Sex | Delay from appearance to treatment |
| Age | |

HISTOPATHOLOGIC

| | |
|---|---|
| Pathological stage | Ulceration |
| Number of involved regional nodes | Partial regression |
| Histogenetic type | Lymphocytic infiltration |
| Level of invasion | Pigmentation |
| Thickness | Mitotic activity |

IMMUNOLOGIC

| | |
|---|---|
| Antimelanoma antibody | Nonspecific immunologic reactivity |
| Melanoma antigens | |

TREATMENT

| | |
|---|---|
| Elective lymph node dissection | Adjuvant therapy |

MISCELLANEOUS

| | |
|---|---|
| Temporal trends | Psychologic factors |

The clinical factors are obvious and have been well characterized for a long time. Among the more intriguing issues is why women have such a substantial advantage over men in this disease [11]. Although they have been quantitatively studied only in the past decade, the histopathologic factors have come to play a central role in the evaluation of prognosis in melanoma. In particular, the work of Clark and Breslow in particular defining the prognostic importance of depth of invasion and thickness have stimulated a number of excellent studies sorting out various therapeutic and prognostic issues among Stage I patients. The prognostic implications of immune competence or lack thereof are still quite uncertain, possibly because the tests employed are so nonspecific and means of measuring specific antimelanoma immunity are incompletely developed. Treatment is not a prognostic factor in the usual sense. However, the statistical methods described allow a comparison of the relative importance of alternative types of treatment in relationship to other factors influencing outcome. Finally, several miscellaneous factors have been associated with prognosis in melanoma, including time trends and psychological factors, which are not immediately explained in terms of other known prognostic factors.

# 4. Clinical factors

## 4.1. Staging in melanoma

The staging of a malignancy is an attempt to determine the anatomical extent of tumor spread. If it is possible to ascertain that all tumor is confined to tissue which may be surgically removed without undue morbidity, treatment may safely be limited to surgery. The extent of surgery—how large a margin of surrounding normal tissue should be removed with the primary, whether to remove regional areas of potential spread such as lymph nodes—is based upon the best determination of the probable extent of disease. Distant spread of tumor calls for the use of adjunctive systemic treatment in addition to the removal of known bulk disease.

Unfortunately, there is presently no practical way to detect micrometastasis, although such means as scintiscanning after the administration of labeled antibodies to melanoma specific antigens holds promise for the future. The most satisfactory way to approximate true stage is to make retrospective associations between patterns of recurrence and initial descriptors of disease. This is the essence of prognostic factor analysis, to use indirect indicators to infer, on a statistical basis, the likely extent of disease.

Melanoma follows the classical pattern of spread and dissemination of malignant tumors from primary to regional nodes to distant metastatic sites. The neoplasm is thought to arise from a single cell and grow as a single, locally confined mass until a critical size is reached. At this point, cells shed from the periphery of the mass are carried along the lymphatics to regional lymph nodes. The metastatic foci proliferate in the nodes, apparently confined to them, until a threshold size is reached at which cells break away and are carried into the venous circulation. Recent evidence suggests that metastatic cells lodge in the pulmonary circulation, grow until a threshold size is attained, and finally gain access to the systemic circulation whereby they seed virtually every organ. About 10–15% of patients behave as though they have hematogenous dissemination from the primary. These are the patients with thin to intermediate lesions who should have disease confined to regional nodes but relapse with distant disease despite lymph node dissection.

The evidence for this cascade concept of tumor spread is as follows. Many patients are cured by local excision alone. This finding implies that no viable tumor cells have escaped the vicinity of the primary by the time of surgery, or if they have, are destroyed by the immune system. For other patients, who have a wide local excision only, disease recurs first in the regional nodes. Some of these patients have long survivals following node resection and are presumably cured by removal of all remaining viable tumor confined to the nodes. This observation indicates that microscopic tumor was present in the lymph nodes at initial diagnosis and continued to grow without giving rise to further dissemination of viable cells during the latent period of growth. The disagreement among surgeons over efficacy of elective lymph node dissections (ELND) pivots on whether this group of patients is relatively large, in which case a substantial percentage of patients may be helped, or relatively small, in which case a large number of ELND must be performed to salvage just a few patients.

Apparently the lungs are a second way station in the spread of melanoma. Gromet et al. carefully followed a large series of melanoma patients for evidence of progression using serial lung tomography [12]. Twelve of 13 patients found to have disseminated disease in the interval showed first evidence of metastases in the lungs, thus implicating the lungs as an obligatory intermediate in the spread of melanoma. The practical implication of this findings is that follow-up of primarily treated patients should focus carefully on the lungs, possibly including the removal of isolated lesions in the absence of extra-pulmonary recurrence. Gromet et al. provided preliminary data supporting the value of this treatment strategy.

## 4.2. The practice of staging in melanoma

Practical staging in melanoma is an attempt to determine the true stage of disease as described above. The staging system in common use is shown in

RIGHT CERVICAL AREA

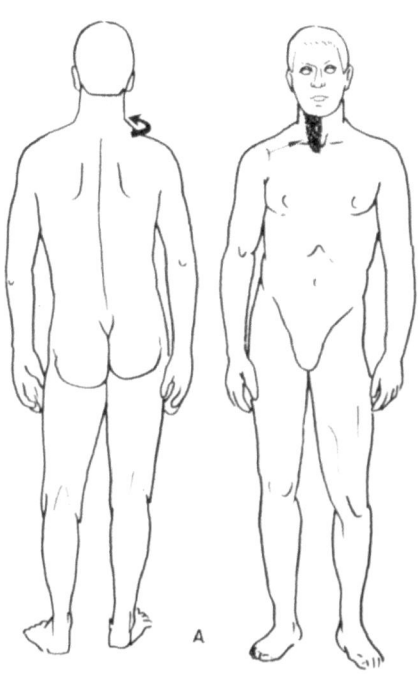

A

## RIGHT AXILLA

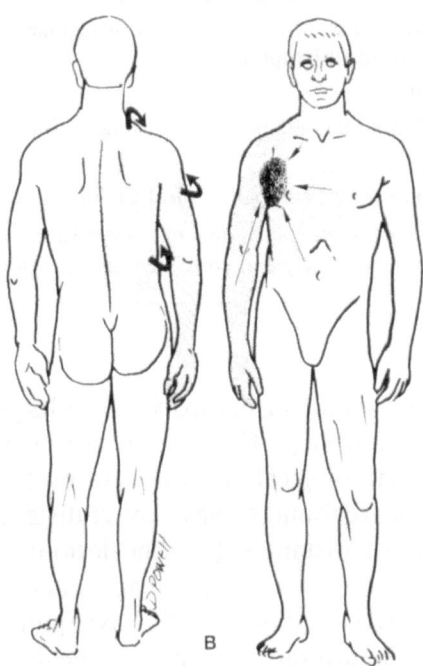

## RIGHT GROIN

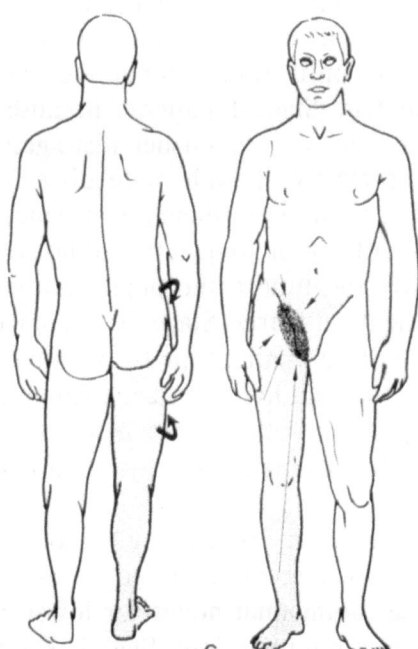

*Figure 1.* Distribution of primary lesions known to have metastasized to right cervical nodes (A), right axillary nodes (B) and right groin nodes (C).

*Table 2.* Common staging of malignant melanoma

---

  I. Localized melanoma without metastases to distant or regional lymph nodes
 II. Metastases confined to regional lymph nodes
III. Disseminated melanoma

Clinical stage: Based on information obtained prior to surgery, including physical examination, scans, X-rays, lab studies

Pathological stage: Based on surgical and pathological findings subsequent to surgery

True stage: The actual extent of disease, including micrometastases, although not observable in practice. May be inferred retrospectively and correlated with prognostic factors

---

Table 2. One must be careful in comparing results from various studies, since the terms Stage I and Stage II are often used without qualification as to whether clinical or pathological criteria were used.

About 4% of patients are found to have overt distant metastases at initial diagnosis on the basis of distant soft tissue lesions, positive chest x-ray, bone scan or x-ray, liver scan or brain scan. Their staging is direct and simple (clinical Stage III). Another 18% have palpably enlarged lymph nodes, of which 80–95% turn out to be pathologically positive and are thus clinical Stage II. Few long-term survivors are seen in this group even after resection of the involved nodes. This indicates a strong likelihood that microscopic distant metastases have occurred by the time macroscopic lymph node involvement has been recognized (true Stage III). Those who are truly Stage II (disease confined to regional nodes) generally are clinically indistinguishable from true Stage I patients because their nodes are not palpably enlarged. The only way to further distinguish true Stage II from true Stage I patients is elective lymph node dissection with pathological exam of the nodes. Even this is problematical, since microscopic disease consisting of small foci of tumor frequently cannot be detected on routine histological sections. By the time a thorough removal of lymph nodes is accomplished, the patient with true Stage II has virtually the same treatment outcome as a true Stage I patient treated with wide local excision only. Consequently, we have the paradox that stage distinctions are of less importance in a treatment program which includes elective lymph node dissections, although this method of management gives a better approximation to the true staging.

The final aspect to staging is determining the possible escape routes for tumor cells if lymph node resections are to be attempted. The common routes are generally the ilioinguinal nodes for lower extremity lesions and axillary nodes for upper extremity lesions. Sugarbaker and McBride [13] and McNeer and Das Gupta [14] have provided guidelines to expected sites of metastasis from trunk primaries based upon sites of nodal recurrence observed in large series of Stage I patients (Figure 1). A number of centers are now evaluating the lymph node areas at risk in trunk melanoma by following the pattern of spread of radioactive colloidal gold or other tracers injected about the lesion with scintigrams [15].

## 4.3. Stage of disease

The lowest common denominator among studies of melanoma is clinical stage of disease. About 4% of patients present with clinical Stage III (distant metastasis), about 18% with clinical Stage II (palpably involved regional lymph nodes) and the remaining 78% are in clinical Stage I. Survival curves for clinical Stages I and II, pathologically positive and negative (Figure 2), demonstrate a highly significant difference among them. The difference between Stage II and Stage III (not shown) largely reflects the time required

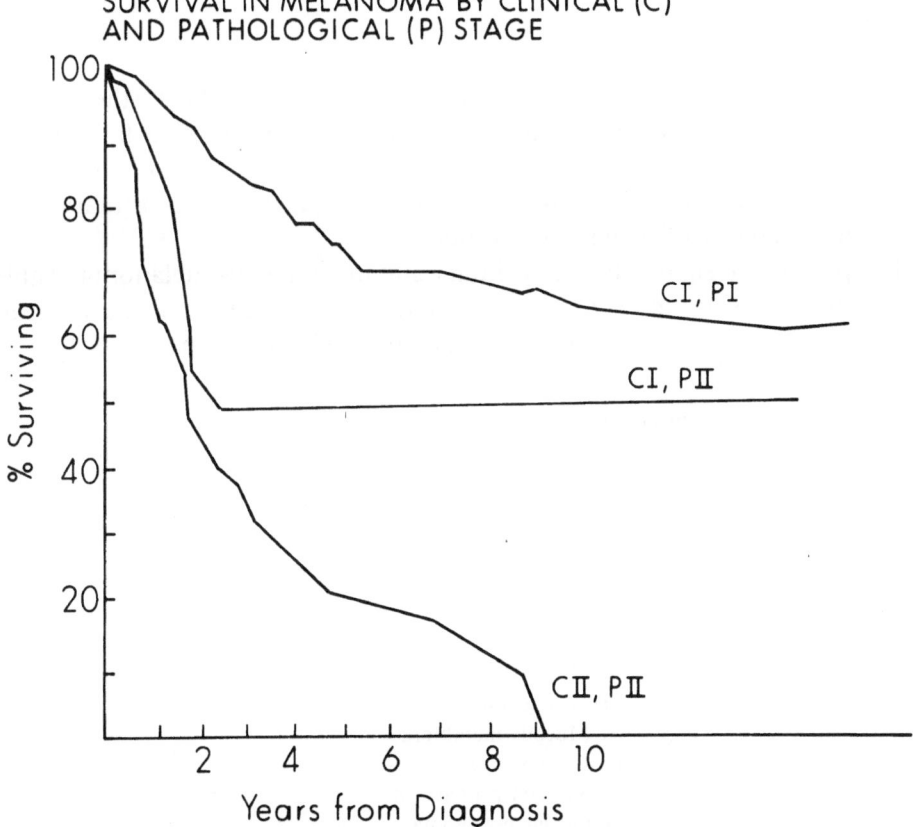

*Figure 2.* Comparison of survival from diagnosis by clinical and pathological stage.

for the systemic micrometastases almost universally present in clinical Stage II patients to become clinically apparent.

A practice which causes some confusion in reading the literature of melanoma is that of restaging. If a patient who was initially clinical Stage I has a recurrence in the regional nodes with no sign of distant metastasis, the patient is "restaged" to clinical Stage II at that point. Many treatment trials for adjuvant therapy of clinical Stage II include such patients once they have had therapeutic lymph node dissections and refer to them as clinical Stage II alongside patients who made their initial presentation in clinical Stage II. Whether this practice introduces more variability or improves the study through the availability of more subjects is hard to determine from available information. The study of Stage II patients by Balch and associates suggests that they are a rather uniform group, even including pathologically defined Stage II patients, if one takes the date of diagnosis of regional node involvement as the index date and takes into account the prognostic factors they described including number of nodes involved and presence of ulceration in the primary lesion [16].

### 4.4. Primary site

Melanomas fall into two general categories, which may be further subdivided with respect to primary site (Table 3). The largest number fall into the category of cutaneous melanomas, while extracutaneous primary sites make up the remainder. Cures are uncommon for extracutaneous primary sites with the exception of ocular melanoma.

The prognostic significance of primary site in cutaneous melanoma (Table 4)—whether arising upon upper extremity, lower extremity, trunk or head and neck area—is difficult to determine from published reports because of

Table 3. Primary site of melanoma

I. Cutaneous
  A. Extremities
     (other than volar/subungual)
  B. Trunk
  C. Head and neck
  D. Volar
  E. Subungual

II. Extracutaneous
  A. Mucous membrane
  B. Unknown primary site
  C. Visceral primary site
  D. Ocular melanoma

*Table 4.* Five-year survival of cutaneous melanoma by primary site

| Head/Neck | Upper extremity | Lower extremity | Extremities combined | Trunk | Reference |
|-----------|-----------------|-----------------|----------------------|-------|-----------|
| 31 %      | 12 %            | 26 %            | —                    | 20 %  | 10        |
| 68        | —               | —               | 81 %                 | 71    | 17        |
| 41        | 43              | 13              | —                    | 19    | 18        |
| 50        | 37              | 38              | —                    | 38    | 19        |
| 69        | —               | 50              | —                    | 40    | 20        |
| 43        | 52              | 56              | —                    | 39    | 21        |
| 33        | 37              | 51              | —                    | 17    | 22        |
| 53        | 71              | 53              | —                    | 57    | 23        |
| 79        | 89              | 86              | —                    | 73    | 24        |
| —         | —               | —               | 75                   | 45    | 25        |
| 81        | 82              | 74              | —                    | 68    | 26        |
|           |                 | "No differences" |                     |       | 27        |
| —         | 50              | 72              | —                    | —     | 28        |
| 65        | 88              | 70              | —                    | 60    | 29        |
| —         | —               | —               | —                    | 66    | 13        |

variations in etiology and treatment which are not clearly accounted for in most reports [10, 13, 17–29]. However, primary site probably has little independent influence on prognosis. Correlations between primary site and other factors may have made the primary site seem significant in some studies. For example, surgeons are more often willing to do regional node dissections in patients with extremity lesions, where lymphatic drainage is predictable, than in trunk lesions, where the lymph node drainage is frequently ambiguous. If lymph node dissections are truly beneficial, this selection factor would make trunk primaries appear worse when in fact the difference is due to the treatment.

Head and neck primary melanoma is difficult to compare with other sites. Many melanomas arising on the face are lentigo maligna melanomas arising in an Hutchinson's mole. These are generally thin melanomas and even the thicker lesions have a good prognosis. Most series reported do not divide the head and neck group by histogenetic type, thus making it impossible to determine the moderating influence of lentigo maligna class on overall head and neck survival.

Women account for a distinct majority of extremity primary lesions, particularly lower extremity, whereas men predominate among trunk primaries. This difference has been attributed to differences in dressing habits. Women traditionally have worn skirts, thus exposing their legs, but wear several layers of clothing on the torso. Men, on the other hand, wear pants but wear fewer layers of garments on the torso. The marked preponderance of chest and upper back lesions are a sharp contrast to the scarcity of abdomen and lower back lesions in both sexes, areas traditionally doubly covered. This observation suggests that differential exposure to solar radiation explains much of the variation in distribution of melanoma primaries. The ease and frequency of looking at different areas of the body may result in more advanced lesions at diagnosis in the areas which are not often seen, such as the back.

Volar (palm and sole) and subungual melanomas are a special subgroup of extremity melanomas, distinguished by the predominance of a particular histogenetic pattern, acral lentiginous melanoma. These lesions tend to be more deeply invasive at diagnosis than other extremity lesions and have a correspondingly poorer prognosis. Whether this difference represents a different biologic behavior of ALM or is due to delayed recognition and treatment of these sites is not clear. Volar and subungual melanomas are discussed further under histogenetic types.

## 4.5. Sex

One of the most intriguing prognostic relationships in melanoma is the better survival of women compared to men (Table 5). This finding is consistent across published studies [10, 11, 17–19, 21–24, 27–33]. Explanations which have been offered include hormonal influences upon the growth of melanoma, predominance of extremity (particularly lower extremity) primary lesions among women and earlier recognition of lesions due to increased

*Table 5.* Five-year survival of cutaneous melanoma by sex

| Male | Female | Reference |
|------|--------|-----------|
| 13% | 26% | 10 |
| 21 | 31 | 18 |
| Female survival twice that of men | | 19 |
| 44 | 57 | 21 |
| 28 | 58 | 30 |
| 43 | 63 | 23 |
| 46 | 67 | 31 |
| 30 | 63 | 32 |
| 20 | 41 | 22 |
| 32 | 48 | 27 |
| 58 | 84 | 17 |
| 67 | 83 | 11 |
| 65 | 82 | 24 |
| 61 | 73 | 28 |
| 65 | 75 | 29 |
| 29 | 38 | 33 |

*Table 6.* Multifactorial survival regression (Cox model) analysis of time to recurrence and time to death in melanoma

| | Trunk and extremity primary site, minimum 3-year follow-up N = 259 | | |
| --- | --- | --- | --- |
| | Time to recurrence | | Time to death |
| Variable | Univariate [1] | Adjusted [2] | Adjusted [2] |
| | p | p | p |
| Clark's level | 0.0002 | 0.0002 | 0.008 |
| Stage (I vs. II) | 0.04 | 0.01 | 0.08 |
| Sex | 0.34 | 0.19 | 0.05 |
| Primary site | | | |
| (Trunk vs. extremities) | 0.60 | 0.49 | 0.41 |
| Age | 0.75 | 0.59 | 0.75 |

[1] p value for this variable with no other variable accounted for.
[2] p value for this variable once other 4 variables are accounted for.

awareness of skin blemishes resulting in thinner lesions at diagnosis. Data regarding hormonal influences are critically evaluated in Chapter 12. Adjustment for thickness and primary site removes most, but not all, of the female advantage.

In the Duke series, no difference was found by sex in the rate of recurrence. However, among those in whom there was recurrence, the duration of remaining survival was significantly better for women (Table 6). This finding is consistent with the report of Shaw et al. that the residual difference found between men and women once thickness and primary site were adjusted for was confined to the patients with the thickest lesions (>3 mm) or Stage II disease [11].

These studies suggest some sex-related factor which delays the progression of established disseminated disease. Otherwise any remaining sex differences are probably explained by differential etiologic factors (i.e., dressing practices) and increased awareness of skin lesions in women.

## 4.6. Race

Melanoma is considerably less common among blacks than whites. U.S. mortality statistics from 1950 to 1969 show a death rate of 1.31 per 100 000 for whites versus 0.34 for nonwhites [34]. Because of their smaller representation in the population, however, nonwhites accounted for only 1056 deaths (2.4% of the total) from melanoma over this 20-year period. Melanoma in blacks is largely restricted to volar, subungual and mucosal surfaces. These are the sites for which acral lentiginous melanoma (ALM) is the

*Table 7.* Age distribution of melanoma patients by sex: Duke Melanoma Clinic series

| Age at diagnosis | Male | | Female | |
|---|---|---|---|---|
| | # | % | # | % |
| <10 | 1 | 0.1 | 3 | 0.3 |
| 10-19 | 19 | 1.9 | 23 | 2.4 |
| 20-29 | 132 | 13.2 | 143 | 15.1 |
| 30-39 | 182 | 18.2 | 186 | 19.7 |
| 40-49 | 210 | 21.0 | 183 | 19.3 |
| 50-59 | 239 | 23.9 | 179 | 18.9 |
| 60-69 | 149 | 14.9 | 149 | 15.8 |
| 70-79 | 64 | 6.4 | 67 | 7.1 |
| 80-89 | 6 | 0.6 | 11 | 1.2 |
| 90-99 | 0 | 0 | 2 | 0.2 |
| Total | 1002 | | 946 | |

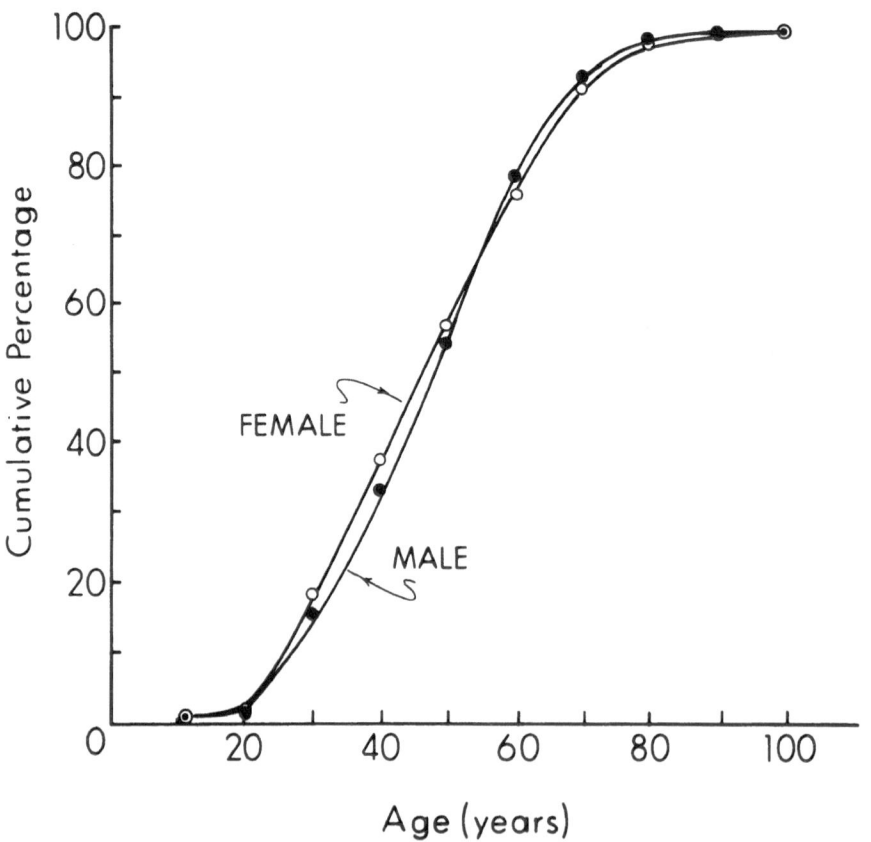

*Figure 3.* Cumulative percentage of melanoma patients by age (Duke series). (● Male, N = 1002; o Female, n = 946).

predominant histogenetic type. Twenty-three of 33 patients with volar melanomas, including 18 of the 27 classified as ALM, reported by Arrington et al. were blacks [35].

## 4.7. Age

The distribution of age at diagnosis for melanoma patients (Table 7, Figure 3) includes 90% of patients within the range of 20 to 70 years, with a median age of 47 years. No difference is seen in the age distribution between men and women (Figure 3), despite the other substantial differences, such as primary site and survival between the sexes.

*Table 8.* Relationship between age and survival of malignant melanoma

| | 20-29 | 30-39 | 40-49 | 50-59 | 60-69 | 70-79 | 80-89 | Reference |
|---|---|---|---|---|---|---|---|---|
| | 66% | 67% | 61% | 60% | 40% | 12% | | 21 |
| | 50 | 60 | 52 | 50 | 47 | 40 | 20 | 36 |
| ♂ | 16 | 11 | 16 | 13 | 17 | 5 | | 10 |
| ♀ | 13 | 30 | 16 | 40 | 30 | 22 | | |
| ♂ | 78 | 69 | | | 53 | 31 | | 37 |
| ♀ | 86 | 83 | | | 75 | 48 | | |
| | 93 | | 83 | | | 60 | | 38 |

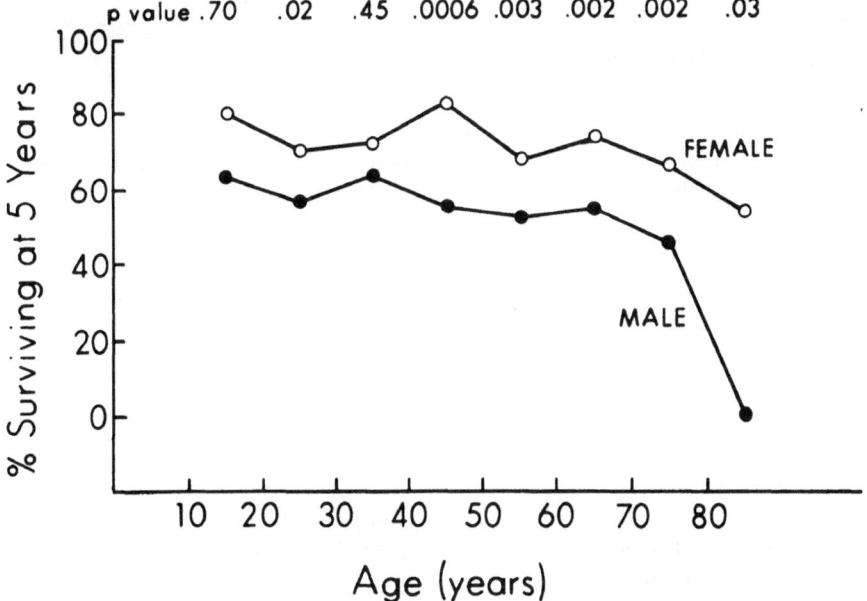

*Figure 4.* Five-year survival in melanoma by age in men and women (Duke series).

Numerous reports underscore the poorer survival of patients older than 70 years at diagnosis (Figure 4, Table 8), although it is not clear that the mortality is solely due to melanoma in these elderly patients [10, 21, 36–38]. Balch et al. observed increasing thickness of primary lesions with age [39]. Patients in the third decade had a median thickness of 1.1 mm, compared to 1.5 mm in the fifth decade and 2.8 mm in the seventh decade. This finding suggests that pigmented lesions are more likely to be ignored in an elderly population, that there is a lapse of host-defense mechanisms allowing early vertical-phase growth or that a differing hormonal milieu may be responsible for the finding of thick lesions in elderly patients.

## 5. Histopathologic factors

### 5.1. Histogenetic types of melanoma

Twelve distinct histogenetic types of malignant melanoma (Table 9) have been recognized, although some types may simply be variants of others [40]. Only seven types are sufficiently common that substantial numbers of patients have been available to ascertain reliable prognostic data.

By far the most common histogenetic type is superficial-spreading melanoma (SSM), not to be confused with the "superficial" melanomas referred

*Table 9.* Histogenetic types of malignant melanoma

| Histogenetic type | Comment |
| --- | --- |
| GENERAL CUTANEOUS | |
| Superficial-spreading melanoma (SSM) | |
| Nodular melanoma (NM) | |
| Unclassifiable radial growth phase | Borderline SSM-NM, inadequate specimen |
| Prepubertal noncongenital | Probably same biology as adult type |
| SPECIALIZED CUTANEOUS | |
| Lentigo maligna melanoma (LMM) | Exposed areas (face), actinic damage |
| Acral lentiginous melanoma (ALM) | Volar (palm, sole), subungual |
| Arising from congenital nevus | Primarily giant hairy nevus, infancy |
| Arising from blue nevus | |
| NONCUTANEOUS | |
| Unknown primary melanoma | Probably most have spontaneous regression of primary lesion |
| Mucous membrane melanoma | Related to ALM |
| Arising from visceral melanocytic rests | |
| Ocular melanoma | |

to by earlier authors [10]. SSM is characterized by a prolonged phase of radial growth, that is, growth outwardly from the primary lesion in a plane parallel to the surface of the skin, mostly within the epidermis but with some areas of intrusion into the papillary dermis. Inflammatory cells are often seen at the deep border of this lesion, leading dermatopathologists to postulate that the melanoma attempts to grow in all directions, including vertically, but is repelled by the immune system, with the net result of growth restricted to a plane parallel to the surface.

If left intact long enough, a transition occurs in the behavior of the SSM or the host defense fails, allowing predominant vertical growth of the lesion, that is, growth perpendicular to the surface of the skin. This is a focal process, so that the pathologist may recognize a surrounding annulus confined to epidermis and papillary dermis indicating the previously dominant radial growth phase.

Nodular melanoma (NM), the next most common general histogenetic type, differs from superficial-spreading melanoma in its total lack of radial growth. Because of the absence of evidence of a period of indolent superficial growth, NM is sometimes referred to as a "de novo" lesion. Inflammatory reaction is usually minimal or absent. Possibly these lesions arose in the same manner as SSM but achieved vertical growth too early for substantial radial growth to have occurred. NM is usually invasive into the deeper levels of the dermis or subcutaneous tissues at diagnosis. Occasional lesions may not be clearly distinguished between SSM and NM, usually due to inadequate material for review, and are referred to as having "unclassified radial growth phase."

A third common and distinctive histogenetic type is the lentigo maligna melanoma. This lesion is similar to SSM in that there is a long period of radial growth during which its potential for distant spread is nil. It is entirely confined to epidermis and is considered a benign process at this stage, referred to as *lentigo maligna*. The radial component is distinct from that of SSM in its pleomorphic melanocytic composition, which contrasts with the uniform population of large epitheloid melanoma cells in SSM. With transition to vertical growth, the lesion is then called *lentigo maligna melanoma* (LMM) and its metastatic potential increases, although this potential is apparently less at any given level of invasion than that of SSM. LMM invariably is found in exposed areas, typically the face, of elderly patients whose skin shows actinic damage.

The final common cutaneous melanoma is variously referred to as acral lentiginous melanoma (ALM) or plantar lentiginous melanoma. ALM, only recognized as a distinct type about five years ago by Reed [41] and Arrington et al. [35], is the histogenetic type most closely associated with volar (palm and sole) primary lesions, subungual melanoma, and melanomas arising from mucous membrane of the oral cavity, vagina and anorectal area. This type has a radial growth phase which mimics that of LMM. However, the lesion has almost invariably transformed into a vertical growth phase by the time of diagnosis. The biologic behavior, especially its propensity to metastasis, is much more like that of SSM than LMM. Hence the emphasis in dealing with this type is on avoiding the false sense of security that goes with an appearance similar to LMM and choosing more aggressive treatment appropriate to SSM or NM.

Most nevi do not become apparent before puberty, and melanoma is uncommon in childhood. The congenital nevi are exceptions and are important in that the incidence of melanoma arising in these nevi is considerable, of the order of 2–13%, making up 40% of the melanomas seen in childhood [40]. The large, complex hairy nevus ("bathing trunk nevus") is particularly prone to malignant transformation. Excision of small nevi and careful follow-up of the larger lesions are indicated. The prognosis for melanomas arising from congenital nevi is generally poor. Melanomas in childhood not associated with congenital nevi have been singled out as a special class, although Clark feels that the instances he has seen are clinically and biologically indistinguishable from melanoma in adults of the same histogenetic type, usually superficial spreading [40].

A substantial number of patients present with melanoma metastatic to lymph nodes or subcutaneous tissues for whom no primary lesion is found after an exhaustive search. A careful interview sometimes uncovers the history of previous pigmented lesions in the drainage area of the involved node, which disappeared spontaneously or following trauma. Smith and Stehlin [42] found evidence of spontaneous regression of these primary lesions in a number of patients, giving credence to the notion that most unknown primary lesions arise from primary lesions which themselves undergo spontaneous regression subsequent to spawning metastases.

## 5.2. Level of invasion and thickness

The seminal work of Allen and Spitz [10] summarized the information available on prognosis in melanoma in 1954. They clearly demonstrated that, while definitely malignant and capable of metastasis, superficial melanomas have a very low propensity to metastasis compared to invasive melanoma. However, these workers failed to provide an operational definition of the terms "superficial" and "invasive."

Over the next 15 years, there was a gradual realization that lesions could be subdivided by depth of penetration (Table 10). Lund and Ihnen divided the invasive lesions into intradermal and subcutaneous with very distinct five-year survival rates [18]. Menhert and Heard demonstrated that, among those with intradermal presentation, half of the melanomas penetrated no

*Table 10.* Evolution of level of invasion in the histopathologic staging of melanoma

| Allen<br>Spitz<br>1953 (10) | Lund<br>Ihnen<br>1955 (18) | Mehnert<br>Heard<br>1965 (21) | Clark<br>From<br>Bernardino<br>Mihm<br>1969 (1) |
|---|---|---|---|
| Pre invasive<br>(100%) | Pre invasive<br>(100%) | Ø In situ<br>11 (100%) | I In situ<br>(100%) |
| Superficial<br>dermis<br>27 (74%)* | Superficial<br>dermis<br>4 (75%) | 1 Superficial<br>dermis<br>58 (78%) | Within papillary<br>II dermis<br>36 (72%) |
| Invasive<br>337 (29%) | Dermal<br>42 (29%) | 2 Intradermal<br>57 (39%) | To papillary-reticular<br>III dermis junction<br>71 (47%)<br><br>Invading<br>IV reticular dermis<br>76 (32%) |
| | Subcutaneous<br>18 (11%) | 3 Subcutaneous<br>25 (8%) | V Subcutaneous<br>25 (12%) |

\* Number of patients (% surviving at 5 years).

further than the deepest extent of the rete pegs [21]. Five-year survival was 78% when so confined, compared to 39% among patients with lesions penetrating more deeply within the dermis. Patients with subcutaneous penetration in their series had only an 8% survival at five years.

Clark et al. further subdivided Mehnert and Heard's classification [1]. Level I corresponded to the previous description of preinvasive or in situ melanoma, whereas remaining Levels II–V were the invasive melanomas (Table 10). Clark's analysis of 208 cases demonstrated these levels to be of prognostic importance in his hands, and Clark's level of invasion soon came into widespread use. Many studies have now been reported in which survival is stratified by Clark's level (Figure 5), clearly demonstrating the prognostic importance of level of invasion.

In 1970, Breslow [2] suggested adding to Clark's level an ocular micrometer reading of the maximal tumor thickness as a guide to prognosis. This procedure was justified by his demonstration in 98 patients that, within a given Clark's level, there was often a marked variation in thickness (Figure 6) and a gradient of survival by thickness within levels (Table 11). Breslow's

300

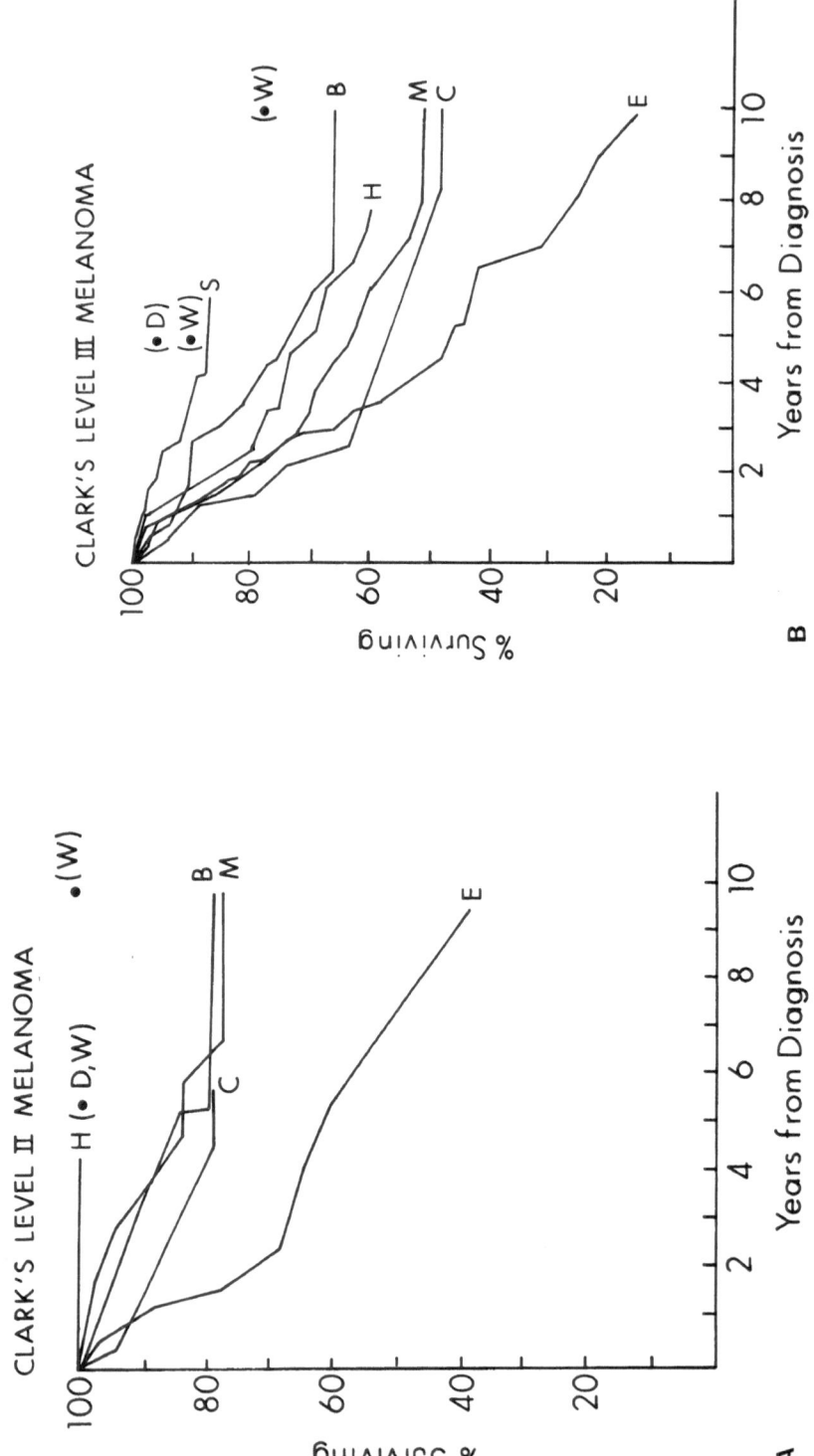

*Figure 5.* Survival from first treatment in melanoma by Clark's level. (A) Level II; (B) Level III; (C) Level IV; (D) Level V; (E) composite of published studies at each level. (Reference: H = 17, D = 26, W = 43, B = 29, M = 72, C = 25, E = 27, S = Duke specific active immunotherapy series)

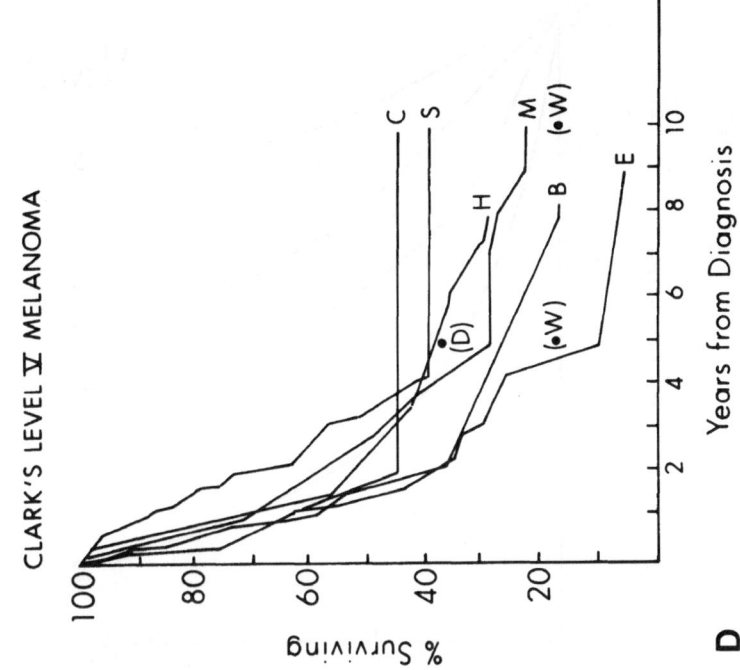

CLARK'S LEVEL V MELANOMA

% Surviving

Years from Diagnosis

D

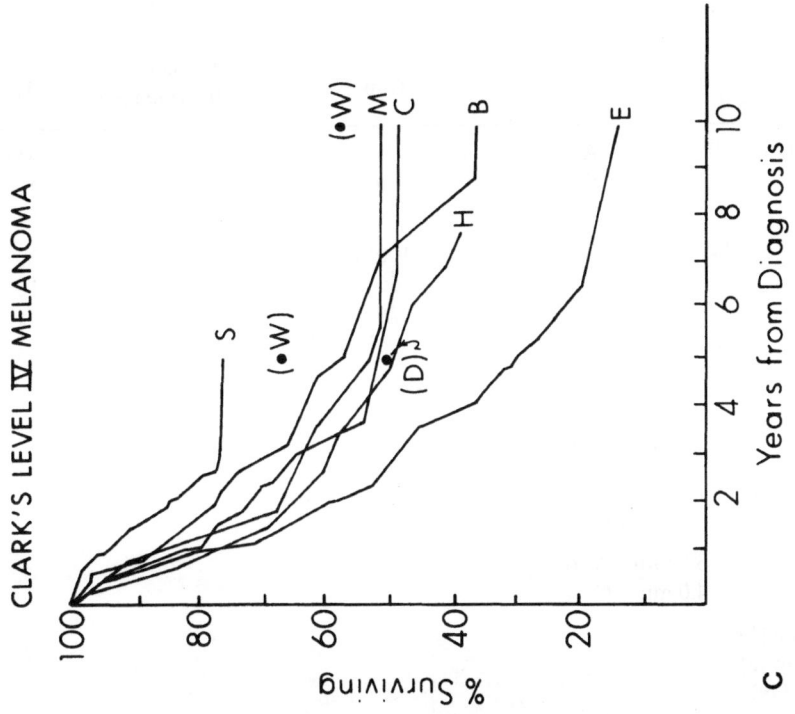

CLARK'S LEVEL IV MELANOMA

% Surviving

Years from Diagnosis

C

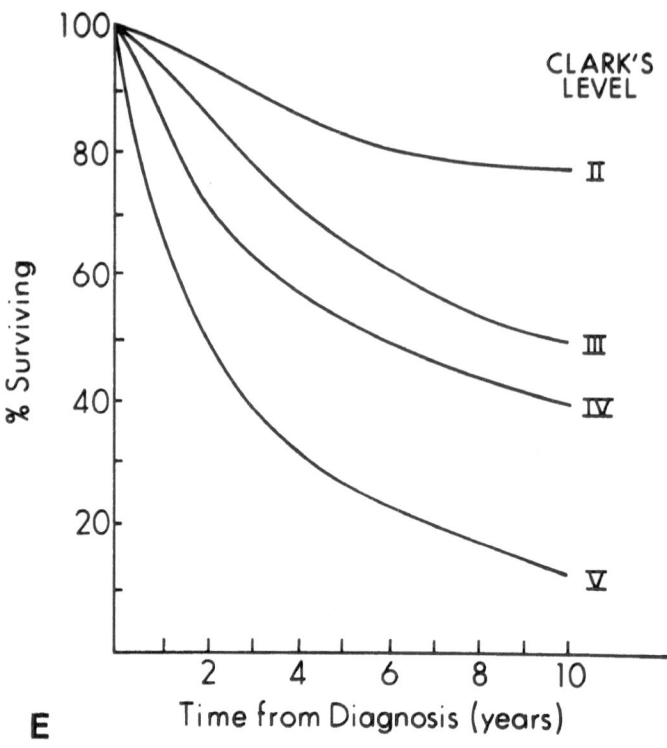

E

*Table 11.* Variation in survival of melanoma by thickness within Clark's level

|  |  |  | Thin | Thickness Intermediate | Thick |
|---|---|---|---|---|---|
| Clark's Level III |  | A | 75% | 75% | 45% |
|  |  | B | 80 | 75 | 50 |
|  |  | C | 71 | 65 | — |
|  | IV | A | 100% | 75% | 30% |
|  |  | B | 66 | 57 | 18 |
|  |  | C | 76 | 67 | 25 |
|  | V | B | — | 100% | 20% |
|  |  | C | — | 52 | 0 |

| | | |
|---|---|---|
| Thin | <1.5 mm A, B | 0.77–1.5 mm C |
| Intermediate | 1.5–3.0 mm A, B | |
| | 1.5–4.0 mm C | |
| Thick | >3.0 mm A, B | |
| | >4.0 mm C | |

A  Hanson [17]
B  Breslow [2]
C  Balch [29]

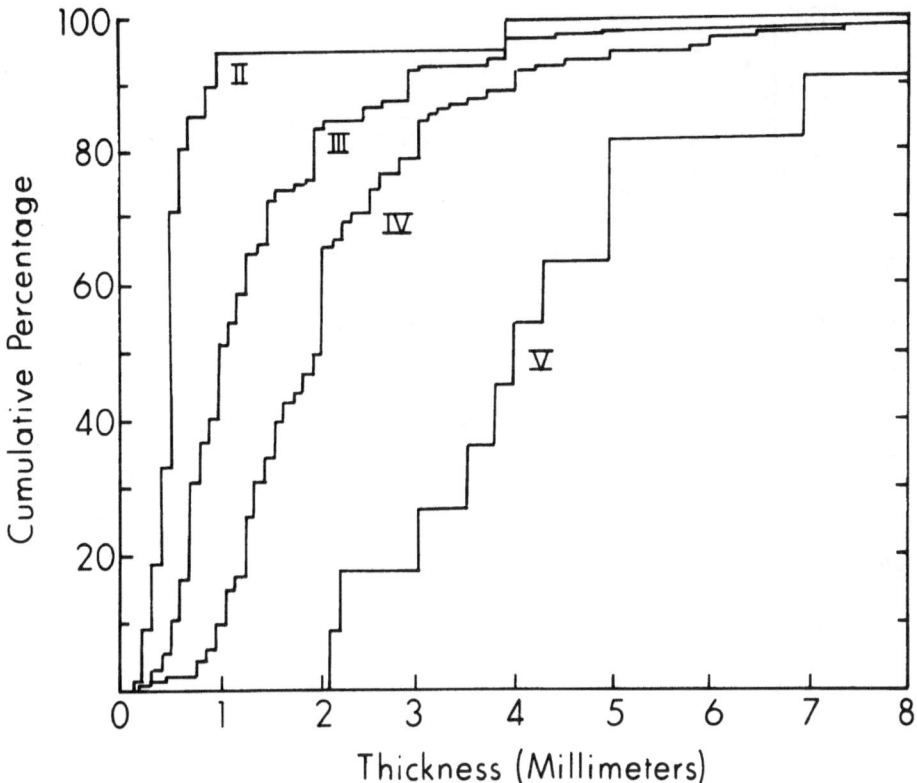

*Figure 6.* Distribution of thickness within Clark's levels (Duke series).

work was met with some skepticism and many authors continued to report their results solely by Clark's levels because their biological intuition convinced them that thick lesions in thick skin should be no more likely to metastasize than thin lesions in thin skin, as long as the anatomic level of penetration was held constant. In 1974, Hansen and McCarten [17] reported 154 patients with cutaneous melanoma who were jointly staged by level of invasion and measured thickness. Their results confirmed Breslow's finding of a gradation of prognosis by thickness within each Clark's level. Wanebo and co-workers [43] further corroborated the added prognostic usefulness of the thickness measurement. Unfortunately, the number of patients in these series was relatively small so as to limit the statistical validity of their findings.

Subsequent results have provided convincing evidence that thickness is a powerful prognostic indicator which, as a single factor, is substantially more informative than Clark's level (Figure 7). Balch and co-workers have provided the most comprehensive and statistically satisfactory analysis of the comparative prognostic power of anatomic level of invasion and the measured thickness [29, 39]. When Stage I and II patients were grouped by

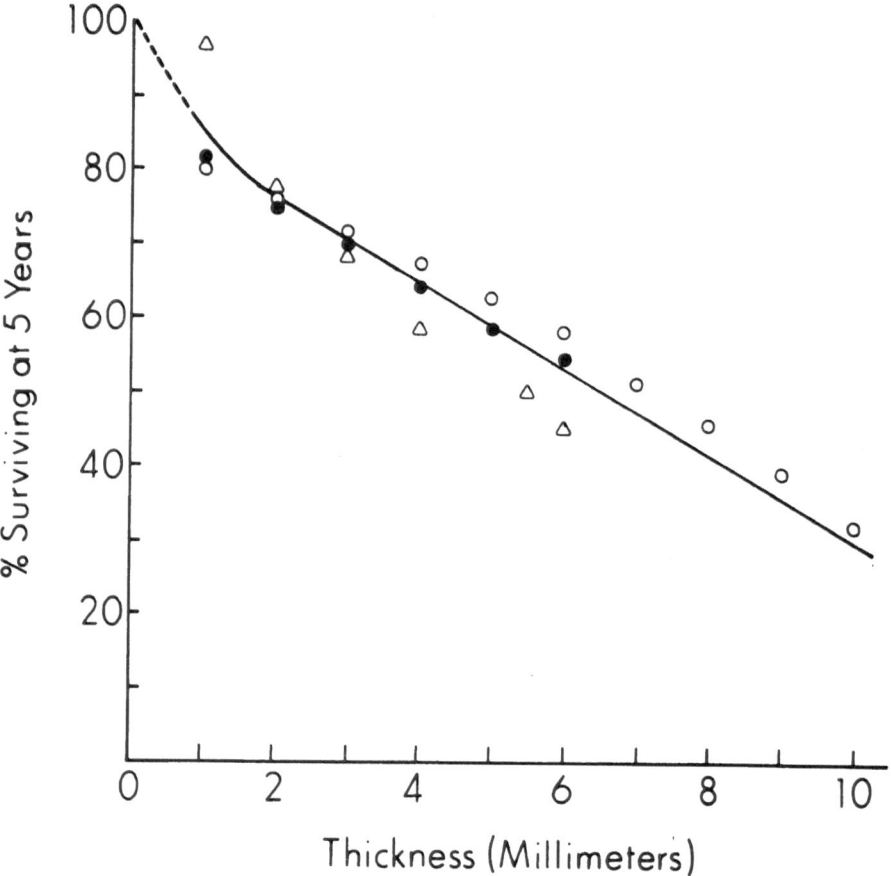

*Figure 7.* Five-year survival by primary melanoma thickness (o = Breslow (72), • = McGovern (46), △ = Wanebo (43)).

Clark's levels, there was an orderly progression to significantly poorer prognosis with deeper levels. However, there was a statistically significant spectrum of survival within each Clark's level when further subdivided by thickness. For example, five-year survival ranged from 45% to 92% in Level II, from 65% to 100% in Level III, from 25% to 76% in Level IV and from 0% to 52% in Level V, according to whether the lesions were less than 0.76 mm, 0.77–1.50 mm, 1.50–3.99 mm or greater than 4.00 mm in thickness. When stratified first by thickness, however, there were no significant differences by Clark's level in any thickness group. Multiple regression analysis of five-year survival revealed thickness as the single most powerful factor. Much of the importance of thickness was in predicting pathologically involved nodes. Once pathological stage and other factors were accounted for, thickness diminished considerably in significance ($p = 0.032$). The moderate significance of Clark's level when considered by itself ($p = 0.003$) was entirely abolished by prior information about thickness.

In an analysis of time to recurrence in 187 patients with trunk and extremity cutaneous primary melanomas for whom both Clark's level and thickness were recorded, we have confirmed the preeminence of thickness as a prognostic factor. In single factor analysis, thickness and Clark's level were both significant ($p = 0.001$ and 0.03, respectively). After accounting for Clark's level, thickness diminished minimally in significance. Prior accounting for thickness, however, left no information to be conveyed by Clark's level. In an analysis confined to clinical Stage I patients, thickness accounted for virtually all of the variation in survival in Balch's series [39]. Once thickness was accounted for, Clark's level was again not significant. When analyzed within the group treated with an ELND, thickness was reduced in significance ($p = 0.04$). The authors imply that much of the information in thickness relates to the likelihood of microscopic lymph node metastases. If the nodes are removed, the chance of disease recurrence is diminished and the prognostic importance of thickness is thereby lessened. The authors suggest that the residual significance of thickness in ELND patients is conferred by its prediction of micrometastases at distant sites, especially in patients whose melanomas are more than 4.00 mm thick.

It is perhaps surprising that a simple measurement of tumor thickness should be such a powerful prognostic indicator, especially in view of the considerable variation in thickness of the epidermis in different areas of the body. A priori biological reasoning might suggest that the anatomical layer of the dermis to which tumor has penetrated would be the dominant controlling factor in whether tumor cells have escaped the primary site. The papillary dermis is quite vascular, so any melanoma reaching this layer would pose a threat of dissemination. It is possible that, as long as the melanoma remains thin, sufficient nutrients and oxygen can be supplied to the tumor from existing vessels. A tumor exceeding the maximal distance for diffusion would stimulate the formation of new blood vessels and lymphatics, increasing the risk of metastasis [44].

Another contrast between thickness and Clark's level has to do with the reproducibility of the observation. Thickness is a strictly objective measurement whose reliability is affected by relatively few technical factors, such as making certain that the histological section through the thickest part of the tumor is examined, that the section is oriented exactly perpendicular to the surface of the skin and that thickness is properly interpreted in the presence of ulceration and regressing lesions. Clark's level, on the other hand, is a subjective measure requiring the identification of a cleavage between papillary and reticular dermis, which is indistinct in some areas of the skin. Moreover, precisely how many cells may be found in the reticular dermis while still classifying the lesion as Level III is a matter of interpretation. Substantial disagreement in classification is observed between pathologists, or even the same pathologist upon reexamination, unless special pains are taken to further standardize specific presentations. Biological differences aside for the moment, thickness would appear to have definite technical advantages in reliability and reproducibility of measurement. How much of the difference between the prognostic significance of thickness and Clark's level can be explained by these purely technical considerations is up to now unknown.

One should not conclude that Clark's level may be disregarded. It may be found in future studies that Clark's level adds further information. At some primary sites (e.g., head and neck) and with more attention to reproducibility of readings, it may add some independent information. In fact, some centers are reporting that Clark's level has become a more significant prognostic factor over the past five years, suggesting an improvement in standardization of its interpretation [45]. Finally, there is a considerable body of information on treatment results based mainly or solely on level of invasion with which future studies may need to be compared.

Thickness is a composite of biological characteristics of the tumor and the host rather than a primary biological factor itself. Such factors as histogenetic type, mitotic rate, lymphocytic infiltration, evidence of partial regression, sex, age, primary site and pigmentation have all been recognized as prognostic factors in melanoma when evaluated individually. Virtually every one of the factors mentioned is eliminated from prognostic significance by prior adjustment for thickness. That thickness is not eliminated by the composite of these factors indicates its incorporation of other, unaccounted factors, such as the latency between evolution and treatment of the lesion. The fact that thickness can provide the information contained in the other prognostic factors is a tremendous simplifying influence. However, it should not restrain the clinician from recording these other factors and testing them for special subgroups, as we have recommended for Clark's level. Only if one of these studies is expensive, time consuming or otherwise difficult to obtain, should it be omitted from a data collection protocol.

Finally, it should be remembered that the prognostic information in thickness is probably most strongly tied to its prediction of nodal metastasis. When the nodes are uniformly removed as part of the treatment plan, the relative importance of thickness and other prognostic factors may be considerably altered.

## 5.3. Ulceration

Ulceration of the epidermis overlying a primary melanoma was defined as an adverse prognostic factor by Allan and Spitz [10]. Some ulceration is undoubtedly a reflection of trauma to a thick, protuberant nodular tumor.

307

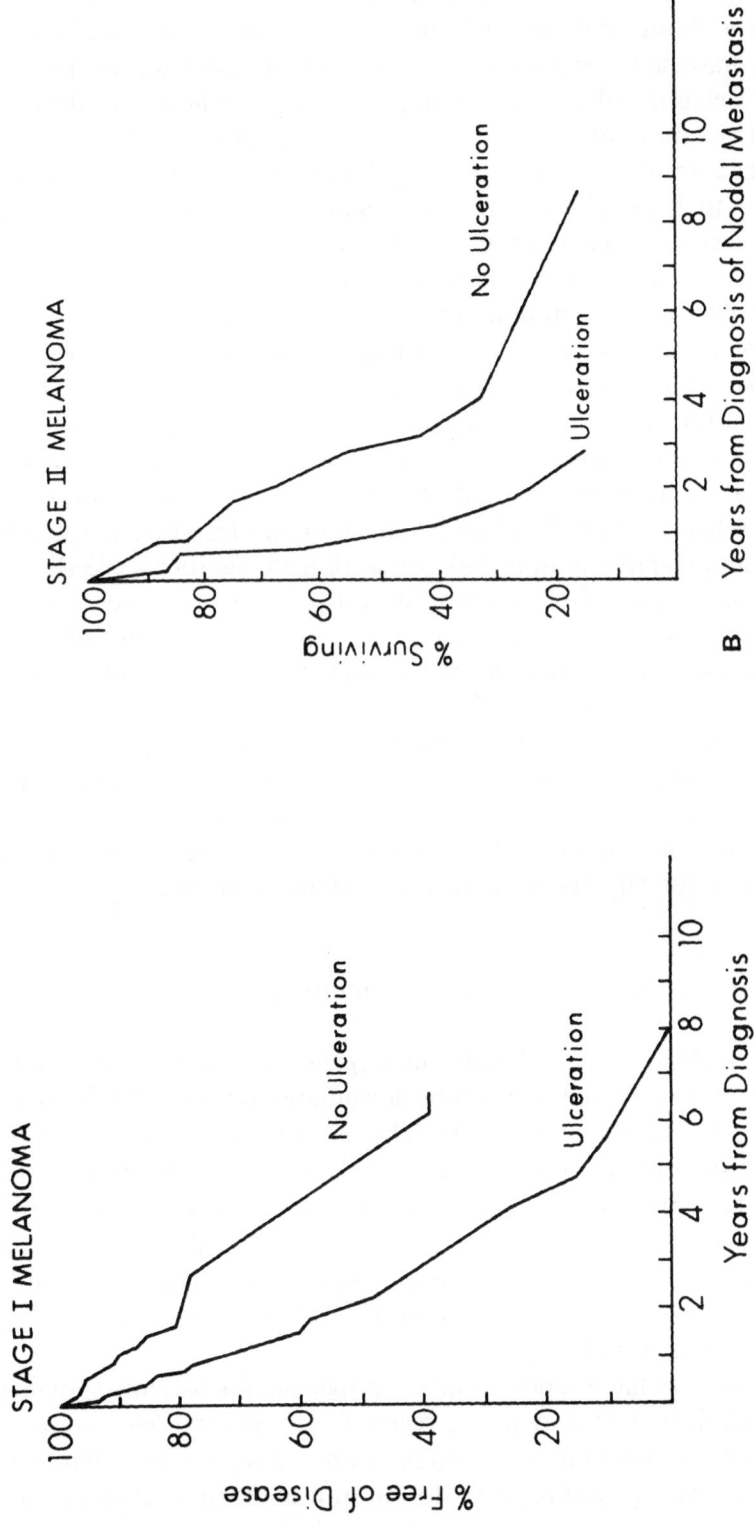

*Figure 8.* Survival from diagnosis by ulceration (A) Clinical Stage I, Duke series; (B) Stage II, Balch et al. [16].

Since many thinner, flat lesions also demonstrate microscopically defined ulceration without evidence of trauma, these authors postulated that such ulceration may be a consequence of acantholysis associated with a "spreading factor" elaborated by the tumor. This spreading factor would be analogous to the hyaluronidases and other enzymes promoting the spread of certain virulent strains of bacteria by dissolving connective tissue. Tumor cells preceded in their path by an enzymatic vanguard should have an easier time gaining access to vascular channels, they reasoned.

Whatever the underlying mechanism it represents, ulceration is a very important prognostic factor in cutaneous melanoma (Figure 8). Balch and co-workers found ulceration to be among the five highly significant factors when considering Stage I and II melanoma together [29]. Of great interest is the fact that ulceration hardly diminished in significance once other factors were accounted for and was the second most significant factor, just behind pathological stage, in the amount of independent prognostic information it supplied. When evaluated in Stage I melanoma, ulceration fell just behind thickness and elective lymph node dissection in significance [39].

In the Duke series of 216 clinical Stage I patients with thickness between 0.77 mm and 3.90 mm, ulceration was the single most significant individual factor. Moreover, after adjustment for other factors, its significance diminished but little.

The striking significance of ulceration and its independence from other prognostic factors are highly suggestive of an inherent biological property of melanomas which is expressed in 40% of primary lesions. This property is apparently responsible for higher likelihood of metastasis and more aggressive behavior for any given anatomical extent of disease.

## 5.4. Partial regression and lymphocytic infiltration

Malignant melanoma occasionally undergoes some degree of lymphocytic infiltration and/or partial regression, presumably reflecting an immunologic response to the tumor by the host. The end result of this process is areas adjacent to the tumor, rich in blood vessels but devoid of tumor cells. The presence of melanin-laden macrophages implies the prior presence of melanoma cells. Partial regression has been reported in 20–35% of patients in different large series which were otherwise quite comparable [29, 46]. This degree of variation is probably a reflection of the subjective nature of the interpretation of partial regression.

Several authors have reported better prognosis for patients showing lymphocytic infiltration or evidence of regression. In general, melanomas showing lymphocytic infiltration or regression are thin lesions. That they owe their thinness and good prognosis to the immunologic response is conceivable, but no additional prognostic information is gained by taking these factors into account once thickness is known [29].

One possible exception to the foregoing statement concerns the very thin lesion (<0.77 mm). Gromet reported an unusually high rate of metastasis (22%) among 23 thin melanomas showing obvious regression, whereas only two of 98 patients lacking regression developed metastases [47]. Regression presumably results in reversion of the tumor to a thinner lesion than its maximum thickness during its evolution, while its potential for metastasis appears to relate more closely to its thickness prior to regression. Thin melanomas should be carefully examined for regression and those in which it is found should be thought of as having thicker lesions for prognosis and treatment purposes.

## 5.5. Mitotic activity

The mitotic activity of a melanoma is a reflection of its proliferative rate and should therefore be of prognostic value. Allen and Spitz found this to be the case [10]. Mitoses were found in 46% of their patients who succumbed to melanoma, whereas only 28% of patients surviving has more than a rare mitotic figure. McGovern et al. has recently reviewed the significance of several histologic features of melanoma while simultaneously accounting for thickness [46]. There was a decrease in five-year survival rate with increasing mitotic activity (Table 12). However, Grade I patients were almost totally confined to thin lesions of 2 mm or less, whereas patients in Grade III almost always had thicker lesions. After accounting for thickness, no difference in survival remained among the groups.

One possible exception to the foregoing occurs in acral lentiginous melanoma. Feibleman and co-workers found that most of their volar and subun-

Table 12. Five-year survival of cutaneous melanoma by mitotic activity

| | Number of patients (%) | 5-year survival |
|---|---|---|
| Grade I (no mitoses found) | 241 (35) | 84% |
| Grade II (<1 mitosis/h.p.f.) | 295 (42) | 77% |
| Grade III (>1 mitosis/h.p.f.) | 158 (23) | 61% |
| | 694 (100) | |

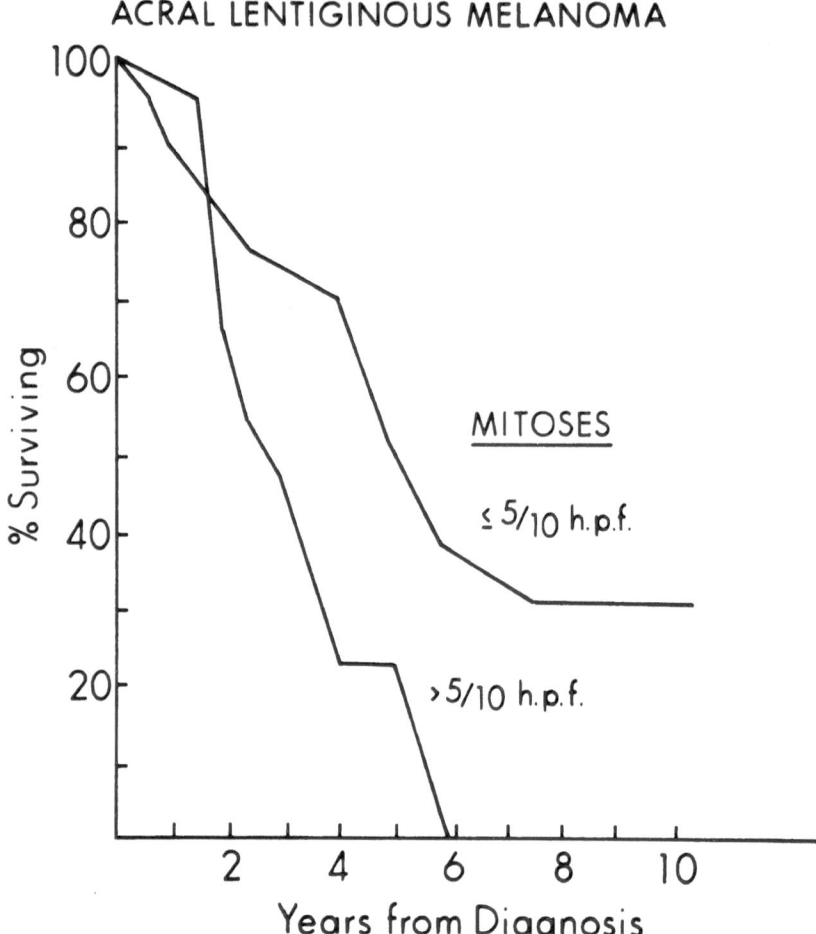

Figure 9. Survival in acral lentiginous melanoma by mitotic rate.

gual melanomas were thick lesions, with 21/31 (68%) greater than 3 mm and all but one at Levels IV and V [48]. Thickness and level of invasion are somewhat difficult to measure and subjective in many of these patients. No variation in survival was seen by thickness or level of invasion. However, the number of mitoses separated patients into two groups, greater than and less than five mitoses per 10 h.p.f., which had 2.75 year and 5.0 year median survival (Figure 9). Other than stage of disease, mitotic rate was the only significant prognostic factor identified in their study.

## 5.6. Pigmentation

About 10–20% of melanomas lack normal pigmentation. This is a difficult distinction to make histologically, since virtually no melanomas are entirely amelanotic at the ultrastructural level. No satisfactory criteria have been established to allow reproducibility of this finding. Lack of pigmentation is an adverse prognostic sign when considered by itself [29]. However, depigmentation is highly associated with thicker lesions. Once thickness is accounted for, pigmentation yields no additional prognostic information. In patients with Stage II disease, depigmentation is similarly of no additional prognostic significance. Lack of pigmentation may be indicative of a less differentiated and biologically more aggressive neoplasm. For practical purposes, this information is reflected in stage of disease and thickness of the primary lesion so that no additional independent information is gained from it.

## 6.   Treatment and miscellaneous factors

### 6.1. Elective lymph node dissection

The thorniest issue in the surgical management of clinical Stage I melanoma is the question of what to do with the regional lymph nodes draining the area of the primary. It is well established that most patients who have no initial node dissection and subsequently relapse have the first site of recurrence in the regional nodes. Thus, the most frequent pattern of spread is via regional nodes and only then to the systemic circulation. The source of lymph node relapse is viable tumor cells not removed by the wide excision of the primary—either in transit between the primary and the nodes or microscopically involving the nodes at the time of original disease. Proponents of lymph node dissection contend that systematic removal of at-risk node groups (when possible, with an in-continuity en bloc dissection including tissues between the primary and the nodes in the specimen) can provide additional cures in patients whose disease has not become established beyond the nodes.

Objections to this notion have been raised by surgeons who feel that lymph nodes act as a natural barrier to dissemination in many patients and that lymph stasis subsequent to lymph node dissection promotes the entrenchment of in transit metastases to form satellite lesions. That the discussion over the desirability of ELND is not a new one is indicated from the Hunterian Lecture delivered by Mr. W. Sampson Handley in 1907 [49]. Based on the finding of frequent regional node involvement with melanoma, he had exhorted his colleagues to routinely remove the nodes. Yet a review of the practice in his own Middlesex Hospital revealed "in nearly every case that the primary growth was removed and the lymphatic glands were left!" He expressed hope that "we are not in all cases restricted to the helpless recognition of accomplished facts, and even in dealing with malignant melanoma an intelligent anticipation of the trend of events may sometimes avail to stay the finger of Fate. There can be little doubt that the failure of surgery to deal successfully with melanoma is partly due to causes within the surgeon's control, in other words, to defective methods of operation."

The controversy has not abated with time. Many workers report improved survival with ELND [26, 33, 50–54]. Most of these studies involved retrospective review of inadequately controlled surgical experience before the availability of the precise prognostication by microstaging. Small case numbers and inadequate statistical methods have combined to generate skepticism in the results. Critics of ELND claim that, with careful follow-up, therapeutic dissections can produce as good end results as elective dissections and limit surgical morbidity to patients actually needing surgery. They point out that in transit metastases are undoubtedly left behind after ELND, that resection of nodes removes a potentially important immunologic defense mechanism and that mechanical alteration of lymphatic dynamics may promote entrapment of in transit cells, producing satellite lesions. They point out the relatively low rate (20%) of pathologically identified metastases in lymph node resection specimens and imply that this sets an upper bound on the therapeutic effect of ELND.

Very recently, five separate studies have provided fresh data on this issue, including two prospective randomized trials and three retrospective studies using multiple regression techniques. Since results of the two methods produced different conclusions and are based on prognostic factor analysis methods, it is appropriate to devote attention to them at this point.

A group of 17 cancer institutions in 12 countries mounted a cooperative clinical trial in 1967 under the aegis of the World Health Organization to address the issue of elective vs. therapeutic regional dissections in patients with distal extremity melanoma [28]. The study was limited to Stage I patients with lesions of the distal two-thirds of the leg or distal one-half of the arm. Patients were randomized between immediate (elective) lymph node dissection (Group I) and monthly follow-up with therapeutic excision of clinically recognized nodal metastases (Group II). The initial report on these 553 cases showed no difference between the survival curves of these two groups. Twenty-four percent of patients with five year follow-up in Group II had nodal recurrence, while no patient in Group I had nodal recurrence (20% had pathologically positive nodes at ELND). While no survival differences were seen for patients with thin (1.5 mm) or thick (4.6 mm) lesions, there was a small, but not significantly different, five-year survival benefit for ELND patients (78.5% vs. 69.7%) in the intermediate thickness group (1.6–4.5 mm).

In 1972, Sim and colleagues at the Mayo Clinic began a prospective study randomizing Stage I melanoma patients among their treatment groups [55].

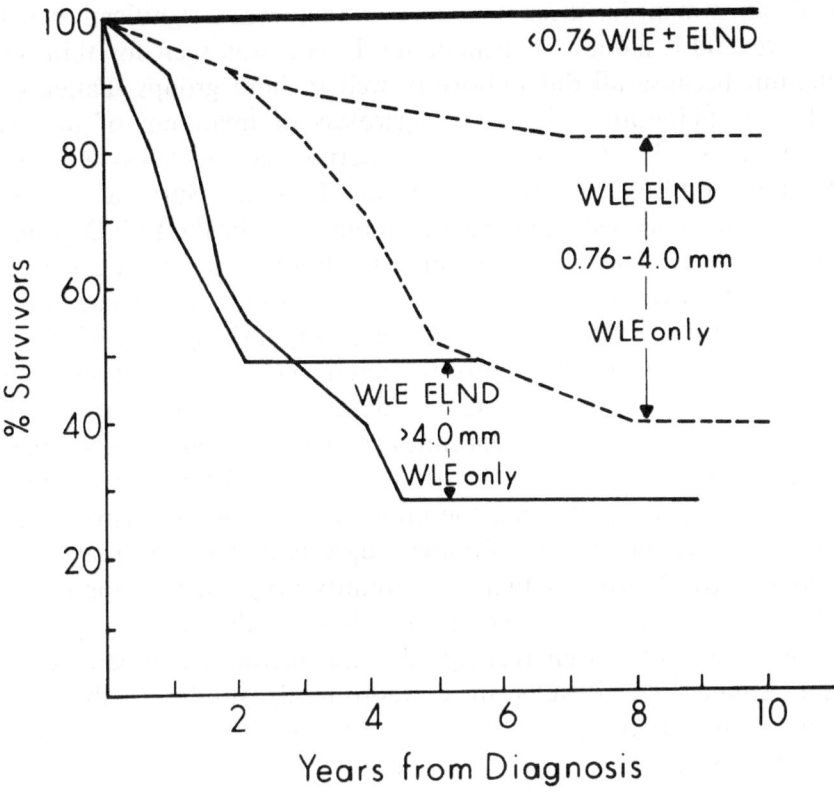

*Figure 10.* Survival for clinical Stage I melanoma within thickness groups by treatment (WLE = wide local excision, ELND = elective lymph node dissection).

Group I (63 patients) had node dissections only if clinical signs of nodal metastasis developed. Group II (56 patients) received an ELND delayed an interval of two to four months following excision of the primary lesion, and Group III (54 patients) had an immediate ELND. With follow-up out to a maximum of five years, no significant differences had emerged among their groups. The number of patients with distant metastasis was quite small (20/173) and only five of these were in patients with thin or intermediate thickness lesions (<3.0 mm).

Balch and co-workers retrospectively reviewed their 20-year experience in 394 Stage I patients at the University of Alabama in 1979 [39]. Enthusiasm for ELND waxed and waned over the 20-year period, with the net result that about half of the patients underwent ELND (164) and the other half had only wide local excision (WLE). Thickness, ulceration and primary site were the only independent prognostic factors identified using multiple regression survival analysis. Together they accounted for most of the observed variation in survival. When ELND was evaluated by regression analysis with adjustment for these three factors, there was a significant benefit to ELND over WLE alone. No benefit for ELND was seen for thin lesions (<0.76 mm) because all did uniformly well in both groups. Patients with thick lesions (4.0 mm) did poorly regardless of treatment of the lymph nodes. It was solely the patients with intermediate thickness lesions who benefited from ELND, but the effect was dramatic. Survival curves appeared to plateau beyond eight years at about 80% for the ELND group and 40% for the WLE only group (Figure 10). Both WLE and ELND curves looked equally favorable out to $3\frac{1}{2}$ years, and a clear divergence of these curves was not discernible before five years, emphasizing the need for long-term follow-up in the evaluation of treatment results in melanoma. For all patients with lesions thicker than 0.75 mm, the relative death rate of patients in the WLE group was 3.4 times greater than that of ELND patients having comparable prognostic factors ($p = 0.004$). ELND was somewhat less significant ($p = 0.05$) when the group with extremity primary lesions was evaluated separately. This findings suggests that ELND may be more efficacious in trunk primary than in extremity primary, just opposite from the usual supposition. The experience of Milton with over 1000 patients in Australia has recently been reanalyzed using methods comparable to the Alabama studies [56]. Results are extraordinarily similar to those of the Alabama group with regard both to the prognostic factors for Stage I and the benefit of ELND.

The final retrospective multifactor analysis comes from the Duke series. Among 216 patients in clinical Stage I trunk or extremity melanoma with primary lesions of intermediate thickness ($0.76 <$ thickness $< 4.00$ mm), 44 had ELND while 172 had only WLE. All patients were given inoculations of irradiated, neuraminidase treated autochthonous tumor cells and BCG in an effort to induce specific immunity. Follow-up is relatively short but 45 patients have had recurrence or recognition of metastatic disease after initial WLE. Five of these were among the ELND group (11%), all identified as having microscopic nodal metastases at the time of ELND. Only one of these patients has had distant metastasis and is the single death from disease in the ELND group. Forty patients in the WLE-only group have developed recurrence or metastases (23%) and 12 died from their disease. There was a suggestive advantage in time to recurrence among the ELND group ($p = 0.16$). Patients in the ELND group were found to be at somewhat higher underlying risk of recurrence due to thicker lesions than the WLE-only group. The mean thickness was 1.93 mm in the ELND group and only 1.68 mm in the WLE-only group. Similarly, 64% of patients had Clark's levels IV and V lesions in the ELND group while only 54% had levels IV and V in the WLE-only group. Once thickness and ulceration were adjusted for in multiple regression analysis, ELND patients fared significantly better than WLE-only patients ($p = 0.03$) and had a relative death rate of 0.39

compared to WLE-only patients with otherwise comparable prognostic factors.

The difficulty in establishing the effectiveness of ELND in a clinical trial involving all Stage I patients is easily demonstrated by an example. Assume that ELND adds nothing to the treatment of patients with lesions <0.75 mm because all are cured by WLE. Further assume that patients with lesions

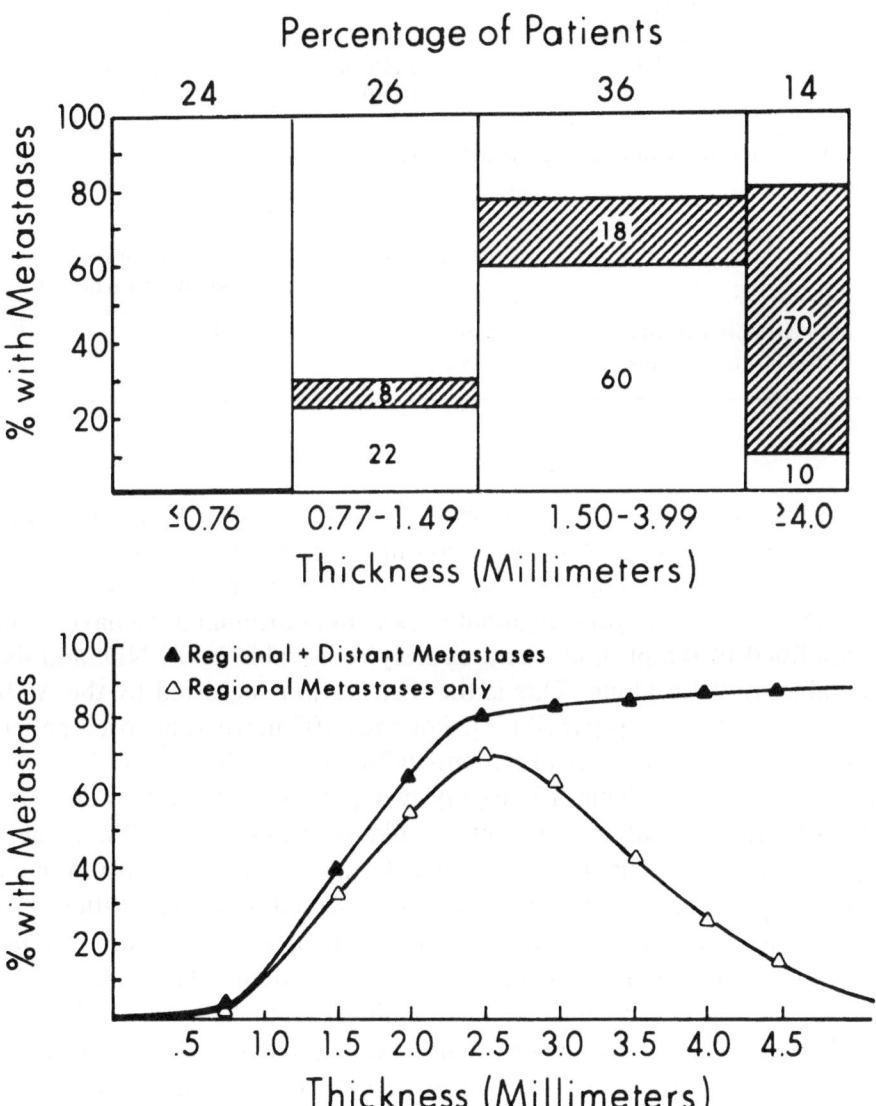

*Figure 11.* Incidence of regional (open area) and distant metastases (shaded area) at diagnosis of clinical Stage I melanoma by thickness. (Top panel) within thickness groups, estimated from ultimate percentage of regional and distant metastases with and without elective node dissection [57]. (Bottom panel) Interpretation of (top panel) plotted as percent metastatic vs. thickness.

*Table 13.* Numbers of patients required in controlled trials of prophylactic lymph node dissection in Stage I melanoma involving all thicknesses or intermediate thickness lesion only

| Thickness | Patients entered | 5 years free of distant metastasis | |
| --- | --- | --- | --- |
| | | WLE | WLE+ELND |
| <0.75 | 24 | 24 | 24 |
| 0.75–4.0 | 62 | 31 | 54 |
| >0.4 | 14 | 3 | 4 |
| Study all | 100 | 58 (58%) | 82 (82%) |
| Study 0.75–4.00 | 62 | 31 (49%) | 54 (87%) |

A controlled trial capable of detecting the differences seen above at $\alpha = 0.05$, $\beta = 0.1$, 1 tailed test are:

| | Patients required | Total melanoma population required |
| --- | --- | --- |
| Study all melanoma patients — | 116 | 116 |
| Study 0.75–4.00 mm patients — | 48 | 77 |

>4.0 mm have nothing to gain from ELND because all are metastatic beyond regional nodes at diagnosis and only 20% will be disease-free at five years. Finally assume that 13% of patients in the intermediate thickness group are metastatic beyond regional nodes, an additional 38% have metastasis confined to lymph nodes and entirely removable by ELND, and 49% are curable by WLE alone. This is the distribution suggested by the Alabama study (Figure 11, top panel) [57]. For each 100 newly diagnosed patients with melanoma, the number of patients falling into each category is approximately as given in Table 13. Eighty-two patients would be cured with WLE+ELND, but only 58 patients would be cured with WLE alone. A study of all patients must be able to detect a 25% improvement in the cure rate from 58% to 82%. A randomized trial designed to detect a difference of 25% with a probability of false positive (alpha) error of 0.05 and false negative (beta) error of 0.1 would require 116 patients. This assumes that the study would not be analyzed until all patients had been followed a minimum of seven to ten years so that most all recurrences will have occurred. A smaller treatment effect, shorter period of follow-up, or other compromise would require correspondingly more patients. On the other hand, if the study were restricted to the intermediate thickness group, a 40% improvement is anticipated, which requires only 24 patients in each treatment arm to detect. Since 62% of new patients fall into the intermediate thickness group, 77 new melanoma patients would yield 48 intermediate

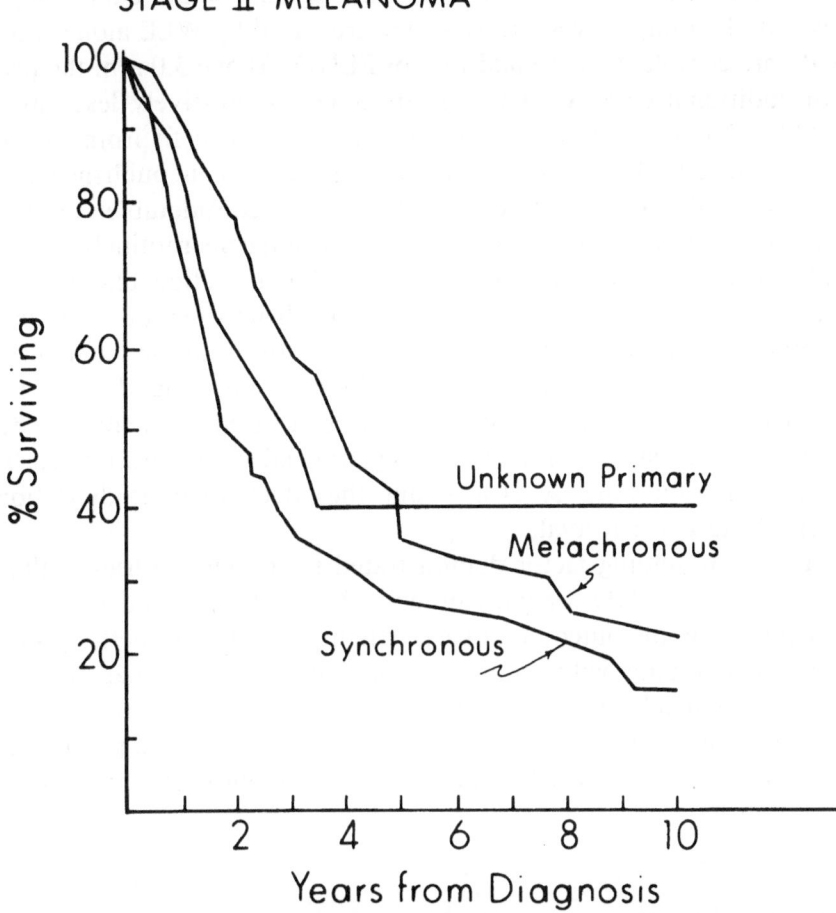

*Figure 12.* Survival from diagnosis in Stage II melanoma by time of discovery (synchronous vs. metachronous vs. unknown primary).

thickness patients for the study, resulting in a 33% decrease in number of new melanoma patients needed for such a study. This example makes the point that all clinical trials need to be as narrowly focused as biological reasoning and other evidence allows so as not to subject patients to ineffective treatments but moreover to avoid diluting treatment effects with irrelevant data.

An interpretation of the findings from the retrospective studies is given in Figure 11 (bottom panel). Virtually no patient with a primary lesion less than 0.76 mm develops metastases. Above 0.76 mm, a steadily increasing percentage of patients have regional node metastases, but up to perhaps 2.5 mm the percentage of those with spread beyond lymph nodes is small—possibly 10% or less. This group has the most to gain from ELND according to this interpretation. In the most striking regions of this curve (approximately 2.0–3.0 mm) only some 10–20% are cured by WLE alone, whereas 80–90% are curable with the addition of ELND. Above 3.0 mm the percentage of additional cures with ELND becomes progressively less until less than 20% of patients above 4.5 mm get additional benefit from ELND.

Several aspects of ELND need better clarification in published reports than has been the practice. For example, there is considerable variation in the type of lymph node dissection done. Some surgeons routinely perform a radical dissection, others perform a superficial dissection and perform a radical dissection only if nodes are positive on frozen section examination, while others guide their procedure on the basis of examining a small sampling of nodes. Each of these procedures—biopsy, superficial dissection, and radical dissection—may get included in series of ELND patients in variable proportions, whereas only those patients getting adequate dissections should be included for the purpose of assessing the effects of node dissection on recurrence rate and survival.

Another confounding factor demonstrated in the Duke series is the tendency to reserve ELND for patients with thicker lesions and poorer prognosis. Comparing the outcome of such patients with that of better prognosis patients treated only with local excision has a built-in bias which will obscure a beneficial effect of lymph node dissection. The role of elective lymph node surgery is far from settled, but it should now be possible to do proper, focused trials with numbers of patients sufficient to resolve the issues involved.

## 6.2. Temporal trends

Myers and Hankey compared the relative five-year survival for patients diagnosed with melanoma in 1970–73 with that for patients diagnosed in 1960–63 based upon data from participants in the End Results Group [58]. A significant increase in survival was found for both men (62% vs. 51%) and women (75% vs. 68%). It is not clear whether this difference reflects earlier diagnosis, better treatment and supportive care, or some effects relating to differential etiology and histogenetic type over time. Based on experience in other types of cancer, it is not safe to assume that the difference is necessarily due to improved treatment [59].

## 6.3. Psychological factors

Folk wisdom has long maintained that will to live and other psychological factors are important to survival of patients with cancer as well as other conditions. Hard data to support this point are in short supply. Qualities such as indomitability are difficult to study objectively.

Rogentine and co-workers at the NCI have reported an interesting association between one particular measure, something they call the melanoma adjustment score (MAS), and the probability of remaining disease free for one year after local excision and lymph node dissection with curative intent, in Stage II or poor prognosis Stage I melanoma patients [60]. These patients were enrolled in an immunochemotherapy adjuvant study. Patients were asked to rate on a scale of 1 to 100 the amount of personal adjustment needed to handle or cope with their disease. A high score indicated a lot of adjustment required, a low score, little adjustment required. All patients were immediately postoperative and disease free when the psychological testing was done. The group of patients who remained in remission had a mean of 80 in their MAS compared with a mean of 53 among patients who did relapse ($p<0.001$). This result was repeated on a second independent set of patients, again showing a significantly higher mean MAS of 79 in 22 patients remaining disease free at one year compared to a mean of 56 in 11 relapsers ($p = 0.05$). By the use of a model based on results in the first group, the outcome of patients in the second group was prospectively predicted and was correct in 76% of the patients ($p = 0.03$). This result could not be explained by correlation with any of the known biological prognostic factors. However, if a patient had seven or more positive nodes, patients had a high relapse rate regardless of MAS. It was solely in the group with fewer than seven nodes that MAS had its predictive value. Relapse-free survival of the 43 patients with MAS > 65 was distinctively better than that for the 24 with scores < 65 ($p = 0.001$).

The interpretation given to these data by the authors was that patients with low MAS use denial or repression of disease impact as a mechanism of coping, whereas those with high MAS had a more realistic appraisal of the profound implications of their disease. The low MAS group perhaps could be considered more resigned or passive, while the high MAS patients were more active. Additional psychological scales relating to other factors such as depression did not correlate with relapse rate. The authors speculated that psychophysiologic mechanisms, such as the relationship of stress to the endocrine system and its modulation of the immune system, were responsible for the finding. This interesting study should be considered very tentative, but points to an interesting direction for further study.

## 7.  Prognostic factors by stage of disease

### 7.1. Stage I

Patients who present without clinical evidence of regional node or distant metastasis make up by far the largest subgroup of melanoma patients. This group also shows an extraordinary range of outcomes. Many patients are cured by surgery, while others who are clinically indistinguishable relapse and die of melanoma in short order. Prognostic factor analysis has made its most important contribution to melanoma in identifying and quantifying the effect of factors associated with the wide variation in prognosis in Stage I disease.

Clearly the most profound adverse finding is the presence of tumor in regional nodes removed electively. Pathologically identified nodal metastases are indicative of a high likelihood of systemic metastases. At least half of such patients will die of melanoma at a rate similar to that of Clinical Stage II patients (Figure 2). Much of the prognostic information contained in the other prognostic factors is due to their prediction of nodal metastases and, consequently, systemic metastases.

A major shortcoming in the practical use of nodal metastasis as a prognostic factor is the necessity for routinely performing elective lymph node dissection in order to determine it. Attempts to compare results in Stage I patients from surgeons routinely performing ELND with those of surgeons who are not are complicated by the fact that site of first recurrence is most often the regional nodes in patients with intact nodes but is of necessity distant in lymphadenectomized patients. The second major difficulty with the use of pathologically defined node involvement is the high false negative rate due to technical factors. Histologic assessment of the nodes is tedious and time-consuming, and small foci of melanoma can escape a meticulous examination. Typically 20% of clinical Stage I patients are found to have histologically positive lymph nodes, whereas 60% of Stage I patients actually have nodal involvement as estimated from the difference in recurrence rate with and without lymph node dissection [57]. The pathologist's estimate of the probability of finding metastases by routine techniques is about one-third of involved nodes, corroborating the impression that two-thirds of tumor-containing nodes are read as negative [61].

The most useful current strategy is to retrospectively correlate nodal recurrence patterns in patients with intact nodes with other more accessible factors which can then be used to predict nodal status. The factors most highly correlated with nodal status, and thus with recurrence rate, are depth of invasion as measured by Breslow's thickness or by Clark's level. Of these, thickness has been shown to contain the most independent prognostic information. Lesions 0.75 mm and less in thickness rarely metastasize even with just local excision, whereas lesions thicker than 4.0 mm almost invariably have spawned systemic metastases by the time of diagnosis. The possibility of benefit from ELND is thus almost entirely confined to the intermediate thickness group, 0.75–4.00 mm. Thickness appears to predict primarily for the probability of metastases, for when pathological stage is adjusted for in multiple regression analysis, thickness loses much of its significance.

Ulceration is the next most important factor in Stage I prognosis. Unlike thickness, it retains its full significance even after all other factors are accounted for, suggesting that ulceration is a marker for a distinct biological property of the tumor or host response. Other factors, such as primary site, histogenetic pattern, sex, age, regression, lymphocytic infiltration, pigmentation and mitotic rate, have all been reported to be of prognostic significance in Stage I melanoma. Each is correlated with thickness, however. Once the effect of thickness is adjusted for, none continues to be independently informative [29, 46]. Finally, treatment has been described as a significant prognostic factor in survival regression analysis. Elective regional lymph node dissection (ELND) is associated with a favorable outcome in patients with tumor thickness greater than 0.75 mm. Elaboration upon these individual factors is presented in preceding sections.

## 7.2. Stage II

Stage II is defined by the presence of metastases in regional lymph nodes. Several distinct situations are encompassed by this stage, which should be carefully distinguished, because of possibly differing prognoses. Patients with pathologically positive nodes (P+) at initial diagnosis are said to have synchronous metastases and make up substage IIA. Patients with palpable regional lymph nodes at the initial diagnosis, considered by the surgeon most likely to be involved with tumor (C+), are clinical Stage II. Most patients in this situation undergo a therapeutic lymph node dissection whereupon histologic confirmation of melanoma is obtained in up to 90% of patients considered clinically positive. The small number who are found to be histologically negative are restaged to pathological Stage I and presumably are at no greater risk for recurrence than patients found pathologically negative at routine lymphadenectomy, although Karakousis et al. have reported a worse prognosis in the clinically positive patients with pathologically negative nodes compared to path positive nodes [62]. Patients with clinically negative nodes (C−) in whom the nodes are found to be P+ at elective node dissection are included in pathological Stage IIA. Patients who have clinically normal regional nodes at diagnosis, do not have an elective node dissection, and subsequently develop palpable nodes, are referred to as having delayed metastases (substage IIB). Finally, patients with nodal metastases from an unknown primary site are classified as substage IIC.

Long-term survival is poor for Stage II disease [16]. Only 30% survive more than five years after the diagnosis of nodal metastases and less than 20% survive beyond ten years. If survival is calculated from the date of initial diagnosis, Stage IIB patients survive longer than IIA patients (Figure 12). However, if survival is calculated from the date of recognition of nodal metastasis, the survival curves are similar. This finding suggests that the only difference between groups IIA and IIB is that patients are at different stages of the evolution of the disease with different body tumor burden when the initial diagnosis is made. Substage IIC is rare, but based on a small number of patients the survival is probably at least as good and possibly better than in IIA patients. Among Stage IIA patients, there is a trend toward better survival among clinical Stage I patients compared to clinical

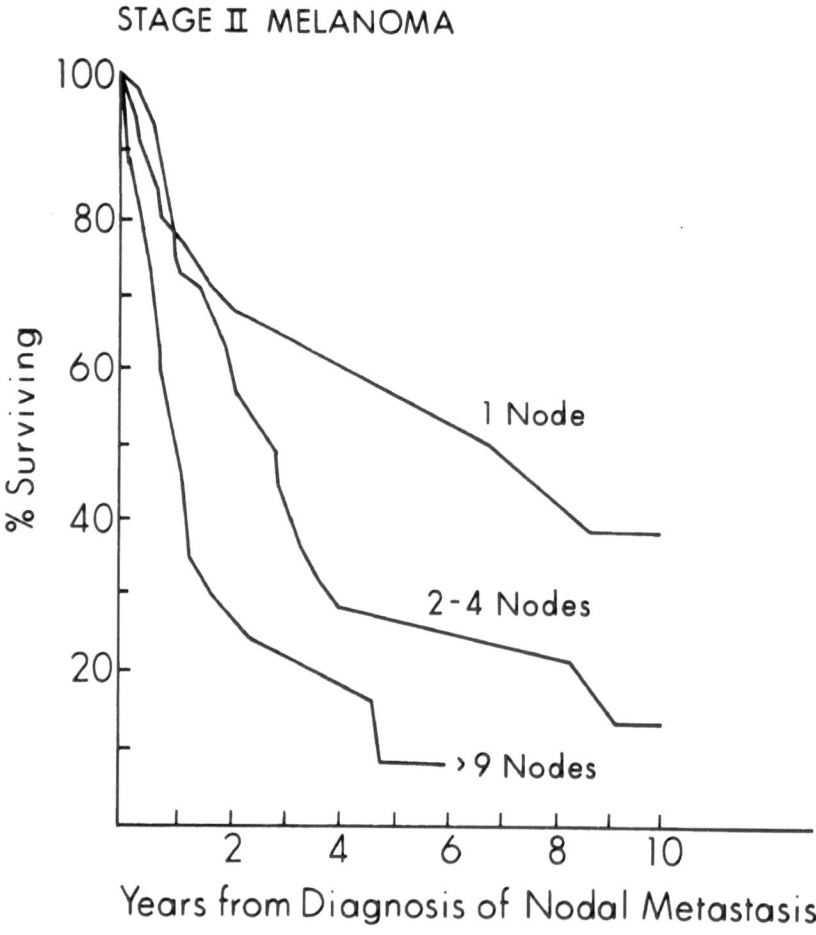

*Figure 13.* Survival from nodal metastasis in Stage II melanoma by number of nodes involved.

Stage II patients. Age, sex, primary site, thickness and disease-free interval among Stage IIB patients yield no significant prognostic information.

The two prognostic factors which Balch et al. found to be most useful were number of nodes involved and the presence of ulceration in the primary lesion [16]. A larger number of positive nodes probably indicates a higher body tumor burden by the time of node resection and is associated with shorter survival [16, 25]. Five-year survival was less than 10% for those with five or more positive nodes, while ten-year survival was 40% for those with only one positive node and an intermediate curve was seen for those with 2-4 nodes involved (Figure 13). Ulceration is the only other factor significantly correlated with survival [16, 63]. Ulceration retains virtually all its prognostic information in Stage I patients after accounting for thickness. It is the only prognostic factor common to Stages I and II (Figure 8). These facts suggest that ulceration is not merely a reflection of a thick, protruding or traumatized lesion but is a marker linked to a distinct biological property of the tumor related to more aggressive behavior.

The Melanoma Clinical Cooperative Group studied 325 clinical Stage I patients undergoing elective lymphadenectomy, of whom 46 proved to be histologically positive [64]. In contrast to the studies of Balch, which involved mostly clinical Stage II patients, primary tumor characteristics remained informative in the pathologically positive, clinically negative node group. Thickness and Clark's level, lymphocytic response, vascular invasion, regression and mitotic rate were individually significant, whereas ulceration, sex, age, histogenetic type, location and number of positive nodes did not influence prognosis. Using multiple regression analysis for time to disease recurrence, thickness ($p = 0.0001$), percentage of nodes positive ($p = 0.0013$) and lymphocytic infiltration ($p = 0.02$) were the three independent factors forming the optimal predictive model.

## 7.3. Advanced disease

Disseminated melanoma is among the most relentlessly progressive neoplasms. Its course is monotonous, with a minimum of variation. As would be expected from this finding, few prognostic factors have been identified and their significance is relatively low.

Einhorn and associates at M.D. Anderson Hospital reported on prognostic factors in 426 patients with disseminated melanoma, all of whom received chemotherapy [65]. Median survival for all patients from the beginning of chemotherapy was 4.7 months, and the overall response rate was 18% (75/426). Ninety patients with only skin, nodal or other soft tissue metastases had a response rate of 28% and a median survival of eight months. Patients with unknown primary site had median survival of 18 months if all known disease could be resected, but only seven months if the disease was unresectable. CNS metastases foretold exceptionally poor prognosis—less than three months median survival—in the 11% showing clinical evidence of CNS lesions when dissemination was diagnosed. Women showed a higher response rate to chemotherapy, a slightly better survival from beginning of chemotherapy (five vs. four months) and survived nearly twice as long from original diagnosis. No further data were presented to help explain whether this long survival was due to longer disease-free interval or better survival once dissemination occurred. In the Duke series, the latter was observed to be the case.

Among 324 patients followed by Gromet and co-workers over a 24 month period, 12 of the 13 experiencing dissemination had their first identified distant metastasis in the lung [12]. An aggressive surgical approach was taken to patients with resectable lesions (5/12) and all were alive and well from five to 27 months after wedge resection or lobectomy. Einhorn also recorded a better survival for 39 patients having pulmonary involvement as the only manifestation, with a median survival of ten months [65]. These studies suggest that the lungs might be the second major way-station for melanoma dissemination, the first being regional lymph nodes. After a sojourn in the lungs, the second wave of dissemination then spreads by the hematogenous route to virtually every organ in the body. The one exception to this pattern is ocular melanoma, which almost always (74%) spreads first to the liver, according to Einhorn.

Liver function tests were surveyed by Einhorn for correlation with liver scans. Thirty-two percent of patients had abnormal scans. SGOT and alkaline phosphatase were falsely negative in 17 and 10% of these patients, but LDH was normal in only 2% of patients found to have liver metastases. However, LDH was additionally positive in 46% of patients with normal liver scans, indicating its general usefulness as a marker for metastatic disease, but inadequacy as a specific indication of hepatic involvement. No patient without hepatic metastasis had an elevation of total bilirubin, although 30% of those with liver involvement had normal bilirubin levels.

The patterns of metastasis found at autopsy indicate widespread dissemination in virtually every patient. Less than one percent of patients in Patel's series had involvement confined to a single organ at death [66]. Besides skin, lymph nodes and subcutaneous tissue involvement, the highly vascular organs—lungs, liver, kidneys, heart, adrenals and brain—were each involved in a majority of cases in the Einhorn series. A predilection exists for small bowel and peritoneum, not uncommonly presenting with intestinal obstruction during life. On the other hand, there is a curious tendency for melanoma to avoid the bone marrow, a common site of metastasis for other solid tumors which commonly spread via the hematogenous route. Most patients with disseminated melanoma die of organ decompensation due to infiltration with tumor [67, 68]. Failure of lungs (39%), CNS (20%), heart (10%) or liver (7%) account for three-quarters of the deaths.

## 8. Conduct and reporting of clinical trials in melanoma

### 8.1. Dataset for melanoma

The items listed in Table 1 constitutes a basic dataset for categorizing the malanoma patient with regard to all known important prognostic variables. These data can be used to derive the American Joint Committee TNM coding for melanoma [69]. The dataset is not designed for epidemiologic purposes, although a limited number of epidemiologic variables have been included, which may be available from routine clinical histories.

### 8.2. Reporting

Many reports of melanoma series in the literature could be more informative if more data detailing patient characteristics were included. Both clinical and pathological staging should be included when available. Because lymphadenectomy is not routinely done, pathological stage may not be relied upon for controlling interstudy comparisons. The most practical approach is to separate patients by clinical stage and further specify reporting within each stage.

In Stage I melanoma, the most important factor, thickness, is quantitative and the risk of metastasis rises continuously with increasing thickness. However, various authors have used different grouping intervals for presenting their results, thereby compromising comparability among studies. The most consistent grouping reported is 0–0.75 mm, 0.76–1.50 mm, 1.51–3.00 mm and all greater than 3.00 mm, following Breslow's original description. Balch reported that patients with thickness between 3 and 4 mm have survivals more compatible with the group 1.5–3.0 mm thick than with those greater than 4.0 mm, suggesting that they be combined with the former into a group 1.5–4.0 mm rather than be grouped as all greater than 3.0 mm, as has been the usual case. Ulceration is the other independently significant underlying factor. Our current recommendation is to report time to recurrence and survival times in groups less than 0.76, 0.76–1.50, 1.51–3.00 and greater than 3.0, as well as in these intervals separated into ulcerated and nonulcerated categories. Treatment policies, such as elective lymph node dissection, should be commented upon in detail.

The usual method of grouping for comparisons does not fully use the information contained in a dataset [70]. Furthermore the small number of patients in individual cells leads to wide chance variation in survival estimates. A more fruitful approach is to form regression models which use the composite information from a study. If a standard regression model were available, say from a multi-institutional study, a risk score could be developed for each individual from a composite of prognostic factors. Patients could be grouped by risk scores into any convenient number of categories, say five, within each of which survival is reasonably uniform. Estimated survival curves for each risk group based on the regression model could be compared with actual survival curves on the new treatment. More rigorously, data from the new treatment group could be merged with the reference population data, with the addition of a variable signifying the group to which the patient belongs. A regression analysis on the combined dataset can test the difference of experimental versus reference treatment while controlling for all known factors. Unfortunately, no such reference dataset currently exists, but a project is underway among the U.S. Comprehensive Cancer Centers to compile a data base of this type for melanoma.

In clinical Stage I melanoma, various studies have found sex, primary site, age, regression, histogenetic type, lymphocytic infiltration, vascular invasion, pigmentation and mitotic rate to be of prognostic value. Most investigators now agree that the information in these variables is available from thickness alone. Nevertheless, these variables should be obtained if readily accessible and included in study reports in case future studies show interactions between them and new types of treatment or other identified factors. In clinical Stage II melanoma, the most important factors appear to be the presence of ulceration and number of nodes. Primary site and duration of remission prior to occurrence of positive nodes for those who were clinical Stage I at initial diagnosis were other weak factors. Patients with advanced disease should be categorized by site of metastasis and sex.

## 8.3. Stratification

Stratification prior to treatment allocation in clinical trials has the effect of more nearly balancing prognostic factors between treatment groups than simple randomization would achieve. If the number of factors upon which to stratify is more than a two or three, subgroups often get so small that more imbalance may be created than prevented [3]. Furthermore, if stratification imposes an operational stumbling block such as inhibiting patient accrual, it can actually be a detriment to the study [71]. In most situations, it is preferable not to stratify prior to allocation, but to make use of regression analysis in evaluating the study to adjust for imbalance between groups which may have occurred by chance.

# References

1. Clark WH, From L, Bernardino E and Mihm M: The histogenesis and biologic behavior of primary human malignant melanomas of the skin. Cancer Res 29:705–726, 1969.
2. Breslow A: Thickness, cross-sectional areas and depth of invasion in the prognosis of cutaneous melanoma. Ann Surg 172:902–908, 1970.
3. Lee KL, McNeer JF, Starmer CF, Harris PJ and Rosati RA: Clinical judgement and statistics. Lessons from a simulated randomized trial in coronary artery disease. Circulation 61:508–515, 1980.
4. Cox DR: Regression models and life tables. J R Stat Soc B 34:187–220, 1972.
5. Breslow N: Covariance analysis of censored survival data. Biometrics 30:89–100, 1974.
6. Kalbfleisch JD and Prentice RL: The Statistical Analysis of Failure Time Data. John Wiley, New York, 1980.
7. Armitage P and Gehan EA: Statistical methods for the identification and use of prognostic factors. Int J Cancer 13:16–36, 1974.
8. Kaplan EL and Meier P: Non-parametric estimation from incomplete observations. J Am Stat Assoc 53:457–481, 1958.
9. Berkson J and Gage R: Calculation of survival rates for cancer. Proc Mayo Clin 25:270–286, 1950.
10. Allen AC and Spitz S: Malignant melanoma. A clinicopathological analysis of the criteria for diagnosis and prognosis. Cancer 6:1–45, 1953.
11. Shaw HM, McGovern VJ, Milton GW, Farago GA and McCarthy WH: Malignant melanoma: influence of site of lesion and age of patient in the female superiority in survival. Cancer 46:2731–2735, 1980.
12. Gromet MA, Ominsky SH, Epstein WL and Blois MS: The thorax as the initial site for systemic relapse in malignant melanoma. A prospective study of 324 patients. Cancer 44:776–784, 1979.
13. Sugarbaker EV and McBride CM: Melanoma of the trunk: the results of surgical excision and anatomic guidelines for predicting nodal metastasis. Surgery 80:22–30, 1976.
14. McNeer G and Das Gupta T: Routes of lympatic spread of malignant melanoma. Cancer 15:158–174, 1965.
15. Holmes E, Carmack MH, Morton DL, Clark W, Robinson D and Urist MM: A rational approach to the surgical management of melanoma. Ann Surg 186:481–490, 1977.
16. Balch CM, Soong S-J, Murad TM, Ingalls AL and Maddox WA: A multifactorial analysis of melanoma III. Prognostic factors in melanoma patients with lymph node metastases (Stage II). Ann Surg 193:377–388, 1981.
17. Hansen MG and McCarten AB: Tumor thickness and lymphocytic infiltration in malignant melanoma of the head and neck. Am J Surg 128:557–561, 1974.
18. Lund RH and Ihnen M: Malignant melanoma. Clinical and pathological analysis of 93 cases. Is prophylactic lymph node dissection indicated? Surgery 38:652–659, 1955.
19. Lane N, Lattes R and Malm J: Clinicopathological correlations in a series of 117 malignant melanomas of the skin of adults. Cancer 11:1025–1043, 1958.
20. Petersen NC, Bodenham DC and Lloyd OC: Malignant melanoma of the skin. A study of the origin, development, aetiology, spread, treatment, and prognosis. Part I. Br J Plast Surg 15:49–94, 1962.
21. Mehnert JH and Heard JL: Staging of malignant melanomas by depth of invasion. A proposed index to prognosis. Am J Surg 110:168–176, 1965.
22. Knutson CO, Hori JM and Spratt JS, Jr: Melanoma: Current Problems in Surgery (a series of monthly clinical monographs). Year Book Medical Publ, Chicago, 1971.
23. Perzik SL and Baum RK: Individualization in the management of melanoma: a review of 164 consecutive cases. Am Surg 35:177–180, 1969.

24. Davis NC, McLeod GR, Beardmore GL, Little JH, Quinn RL and Holt J: Primary cutaneous melanoma: a report from the Queensland Melanoma Project. CA Cancer J Clin 26:80–107, 1976.

25. Cohen MH, Ketcham AS, Felix EL, Li S-H, Tomaszewski M-M, Costa J, Rabson AS, Simon RM and Rosenberg SA: Prognostic factors in patients undergoing lymphadenectomy for malignant melanoma. Ann Surg 186:635–642, 1977.

26. Das Gupta TK: Results of treatment of 269 patients with primary cutaneous melanoma: a five-year prospective study. Ann Surg 186:201–209, 1977.

27. Elias EG, Didolkar MS, Goel IP, Formeister JF, Valenzuela LA, Pickren JL and Moore RH: A clinicopathologic study of prognostic factors in cutaneous malignant melanoma. Surg Gynecol Obstet 144:327–334, 1977.

28. Veronesi U et al: Inefficacy of immediate node dissection in Stage I melanoma of the limbs. N Engl J Med 297:627–665, 1977.

29. Balch CM, Murad TM, Soong S-J, Ingalls AL, Halpern NB and Maddox WA: A multifactorial analysis of melanoma: prognostic histopathological features comparing Clark's and Breslow's staging methods. Ann Surg 188:732–742, 1978.

30. Olsen G: The malignant melanoma of the skin. Acta Chir Scand Suppl 365:1–222, 1966.

31. Bodenham DC: A study of 650 observed malignant melanomas in the southwest region. Ann R Coll Surg Engl 43:218–240, 1968.

32. Cochran AJ: Malignant melanoma: a review of 10 years' experience in Glasgow, Scotland. Cancer 23:1190–1199, 1969.

33. Fortner JG, Booher RJ and Pack GT: Results of groin dissection for malignant melanoma in 220 patients. Surgery 55:485–494, 1964.

34. U.S. Department of Health, Education and Welfare, National Institutes of Health: US Cancer Mortality by County: 1950–1969. Government Printing Office, Washington, 1974.

35. Arrington JH, III, Reed RJ, Ichinose H and Krementz ET: Plantar lentiginous melanoma: a distinctive variant of human cutaneous malignant melanoma. Am J Surg Path 1:131–143, 1977.

36. Shah JP and Goldsmith HS: Prognosis of malignant melanoma in relation to clinical presentation. Am J Surg 123:286–288, 1972.

37. Magnus K: Prognosis in malignant melanoma of the skin. Significance of stage of disease, anatomical site, sex, age and period of diagnosis. Cancer 40:389–397, 1977.

38. Eldh J, Boeryd B and Peterson L-E: Prognostic factors in cutaneous malignant melanoma in Stage I. A clinical, morphological and multivariate analysis. Scand J Plast Reconstr Surg 12:243–255, 1978.

39. Balch CM, Soong S-J, Murad TM, Ingalls AL and Maddox WA: A multifactorial analysis of melanoma. II: prognostic factors in patients with Stage I (localized) melanoma. Surgery 86:343–351, 1979.

40. Clark WH, Jr, Ainsworth AM, Bernardino EA, Yang C-H, Mihm MC, Jr and Reed RJ: The developmental biology of primary human malignant melanomas. Semin Oncol 2:83–103, 1975.

41. Reed RJ: New Concepts in Surgical Pathology of the Skin, pp 89–90. John Wiley, New York, 1976.

42. Smith JL and Stehlin JS: Spontaneous regression of primary malignant melanomas with regional metastases. Cancer 18:1399–1415, 1965.

43. Wanebo HJ, Fortner JG, Woodruff J, MacLean B and Binkowski E: Selection of the optimum surgical treatment of Stage I melanoma by depth of microinvasion: use of the combined microstage technique (Clark-Breslow). Ann Surg 182:302–315, 1975.

44. Breslow A: Histologic grading of melanoma by thickness. In: Kumar S (ed) Advances in Medical Oncology, Research, and Education, Vol X, pp 87–92. Proceedings of the 12th International Cancer Congress, Buenos Aires, 1978. Pergamon, New York, 1979.

45. Soong S-J: personal communication.

46. McGovern VJ, Shaw HM, Milton GW and Farago GA: Prognostic significance of the histological features of malignant melanoma. Histopathology 3:385–393, 1979.

47. Gromet MA, Epstein WL and Blois MS: The regressing thin malignant melanoma. A distinctive lesion with metastatic potential. Cancer 42:2282–2292, 1978.

48. Feibleman CE, Stoll H and Maize JC: Melanomas of the palm, sole, and nailbed: a clinicopathologic study. Cancer 46:2492–2504, 1980.

49. Handley WS: The pathology of melanotic growths in relation to their operative treatment. Lancet 13:996–1003, 1907.

50. Southwick HW, Slaughter DP, Hinkamp JF and Johnson FE: The role of regional node dissection in the treatment of malignant melanoma. Arch Surg 85:63–69, 1962.

51. Fortner JG, Woodruff J, Schottenfeld D and MacLean B: Biostatistical basis of elective node dissection for malignant melanoma. Ann Surg 186:101–103, 1977.

52. Gumport SL and Harris MN: Results of regional lymph node dissection of melanoma. Ann Surg 179:105–108, 1974.

53. McCarthy JA, Haagensen CD and Herter FP: The role of groin dissection in the management of melanoma of the lower extremity. Ann Surg 179:156–159, 1974.

54. McNeer G and Das Gupta TK: Prognosis in malignant melanoma. Surgery 56:512–518, 1964.

55. Sim FH, Taylor WF, Ivins JC, Pritchard DJ and Soule EH: A prospective randomized study of the efficacy of routine elective lymphadenectomy in management of malignant melanoma. Preliminary results. Cancer 41:948–956, 1978.

56. Soong S-J: personal communication.

57. Balch CM, Murad TM, Soong S-J, Ingalls AL, Richards PC and Maddox WA: Tumor thickness as a guide to surgical management of clinical Stage I melanoma patients. Cancer 43:883–888, 1979.

58. Myers MH and Hankey BF: Cancer patient survival experience: trends in survival 1960–63 to 1970–73. U.S. Department of Health and Human Services, NIH Publication No 80–2148, 1980.

59. Taylor WF, Ivins JC, Dahlin DC and Pritchard DJ: Osteogenic sarcoma experience at the Mayo Clinic, 1963–1974. In: Terry WD and Windhorst D (eds) Immunotherapy of Cancer: Present Status of Trials in Man, pp 257–269. Raven, New York, 1978.

60. Rogentine GN, Jr, Van Kammen DP, Fox BH, Docherty JP, Rosenblatt JE, Boyd SC and Bunney WE, Jr: Psychological factors in the prognosis of malignant melanoma: a prospective study. Psychosom Med 41:647–655, 1979.

61. McCarty KS, Jr: personal communication.

62. Karakousis CP, Stahl L, Moore R and Holyoke ED: Lymph node dissection in malignant melanoma. J Surg Oncol 13:245–252, 1980.

63. Balch CM, Wilkerson JA, Murad TM, Soong S-J, Ingalls AL and Maddox WA: The prognostic significance of ulceration of cutaneous melanoma. Cancer 45:3012–3017, 1980.

64. Day CL, Jr, Sober AJ, Lew RA, Mihm MC, Jr et al: Malignant melanoma patients with positive nodes and relatively good prognoses: microstaging retains prognostic significance in clinical Stage I melanoma patients with metastases to regional nodes. Cancer 47:955–962, 1981.

65. Einhorn LH et al: Prognostic correlations and response to treatment in advanced metastatic malignant melanoma. Cancer Res 34:1995–2004, 1974.

66. Patel JK, Didolkar, MS, Pickren JW and Moore RH: Metastatic pattern of malignant melanoma. A study of 216 autopsy cases. Am J Surg 135:807–810, 1978.

67. Das Gupta T and Brasfield R: Metastatic melanoma. A clinicopathological study. Cancer 17:1323–1339, 1964.

68. Lee Y-T N (M): Malignant melanoma: pattern of metastasis. CA Cancer J Clin 30:137–142, 1980.

330

69. American Joint Committee: Manual for Staging of Cancer. American Joint Committee for Cancer Staging and End-Results Reporting, Chicago, 1978.
70. Cox EB, Laszlo J and Freiman A: Classification of cancer patients: beyond TNM. J Am Med Assoc 242:2691–2695, 1979.
71. Peto R, Pike MC, Armitage P, Breslow NE et al: Design and analysis of randomized clinical trials requiring prolonged observation of each patient. II: analysis and examples. Br J Cancer 35:1–39, 1977.
72. McGovern VJ: Malignant Melanoma: Clinical and Histological Diagnosis, p 125. John Wiley, New York, 1976.

# 11. Radionuclide studies in malignant melanoma

DANIEL C. SULLIVAN

Since melanoma disseminates widely, a variety of scintigraphic procedures have been used to detect lesions in various sites. These include scans of specific organs, such as liver, brain and bone, as well as generalized tumor imaging, such as gallium-67-citrate studies. In addition, procedures such as lymphoscintigraphy and the P-32 uptake test have played a role in the evaluation of the patient with malignant melanoma.

## Liver and spleen scintigraphy

Despite recent advances in several areas of imaging technology, such as ultrasound and computed tomography, detection of hepatic metastases remains a difficult problem. This is especially true in the early stages of disease when the lesions are small and few. However, for several reasons including cost and availability, radionuclide imaging remains the primary imaging test for metastatic liver disease. The absorbed irradiation from technetium-99m-sulfur colloid scintigraphy is approximately 1 rad to the liver and 0.1 rads to the whole body [1].

Several investigators have reported their results with liver scintigraphy in patients with malignant melanoma. Roth et al. found no positive liver scans in 68 patients with Stage I or II disease and four positive in 22 Stage III patients [2]. In 99 patients with all stages of melanoma, Felix et al. found 11 positive scans; nine patients had metastatic disease and two had benign focal lesions [3]. Seigler and Fetter reported positive liver scans in 2% of patients without evidence of systemic disease and in 25% of patients with evidence of widespread disease [4]. Aranha et al. found no positive liver scans in 50 patients with Stage I or II disease, but three scans were false negatives [5]. Thomas et al. reviewed 128 liver scans and found that six of six abnormal scans in Stage I and II patients were false positive, whereas ten of 11 abnormal scans in Stage III patients were true positive [6]. Evans et al. found no true positive scans in patients with Stage I disease, but nine in 137 patients with Stage III disease [7]. Muss et al. reported that 14 of 78 patients with advanced melanoma had positive liver scans and 11 more subsequently developed abnormal scans [8].

*Seigler, H. F. (ed.), Clinical Management of Melanoma. ISBN 978-94-009-7495-1*
*© 1982, Martinus Nijhoff Publishers, The Hague/Boston/London.*

332

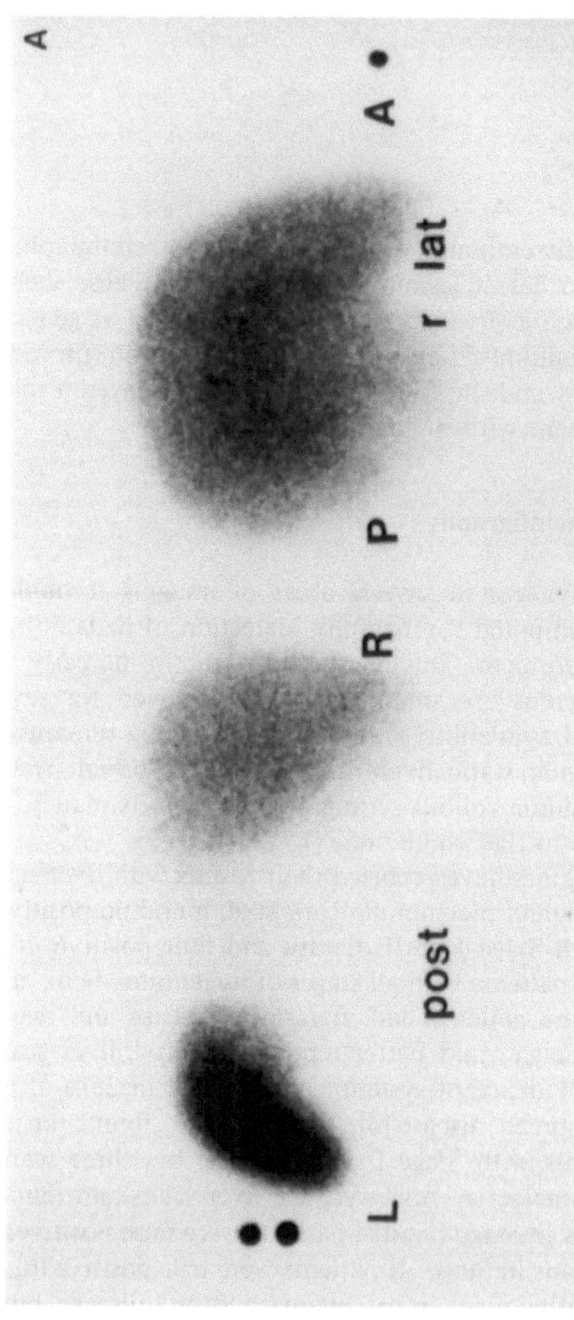

*Figure 1A.* Posterior and right lateral scintigraphs of the liver which show typical findings in a patient presenting with a Clark's Level III melanoma. No focal lesions are present, but there is increased uptake of colloid in the spleen.

333

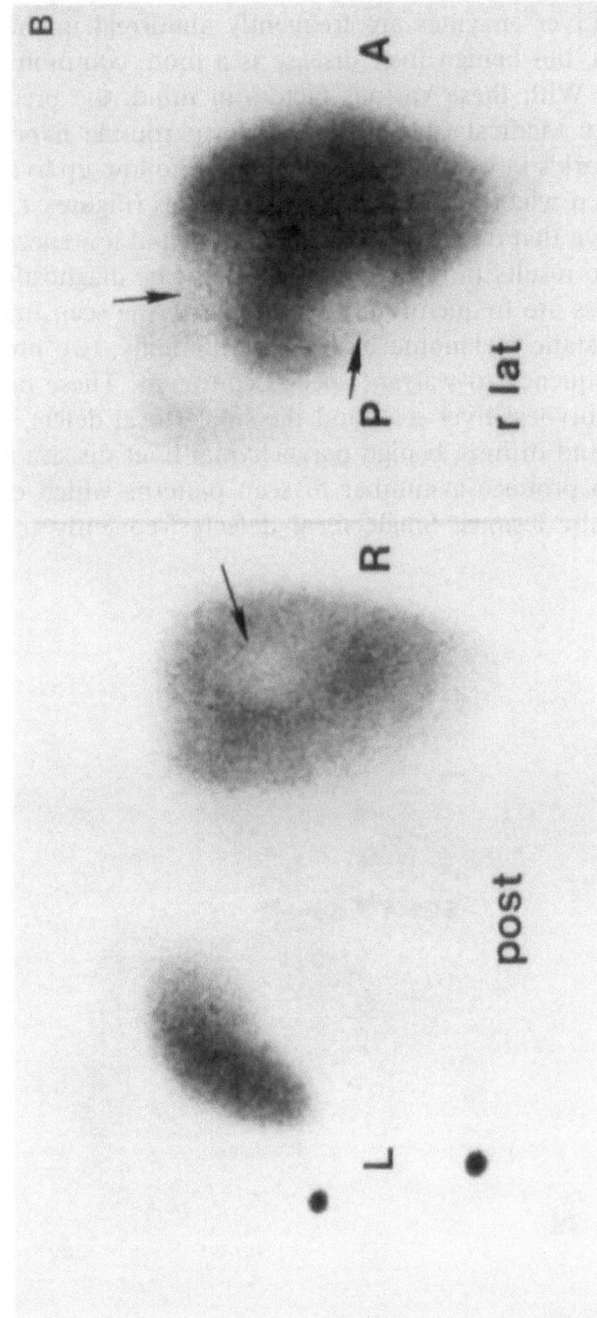

*Figure 1B.* One year later, a repeat study shows at least two metastatic lesions posteriorly in the liver.

334

The findings of the above investigators indicate that occult liver metastases are uncommon in patients with early disease. However, unlike bone or brain lesions, liver metastases rarely produce clinical symptoms until they are advanced. Liver enzymes are frequently abnormal in the presence of liver metastases, but benign liver disease is a more common cause of elevated enzymes. With these various factors in mind, the present policy at Duke University Medical Center is to perform routine liver scans on all patients with Clark's Level III lesions or greater. Follow-up liver scintigrams are then obtained when the clinical status changes (Figures 1, 2).

It is well known that due to the high sensitivity and low specificity of liver scintigraphy, the results in a given case may not be diagnostic. Additional diagnostic studies are frequently needed to clarify the scan findings. In the search for metastatic melanoma by liver scintigraphy, two problems occur with enough frequency to warrant special comment. These problem situations are the equivocal liver scan and the single focal defect. Normal anatomic variants and diffuse, benign parenchymal liver disease are common, and combine to produce a number of scan patterns which can mimic or obscure metastatic lesions. Single focal defects frequently turn out to be

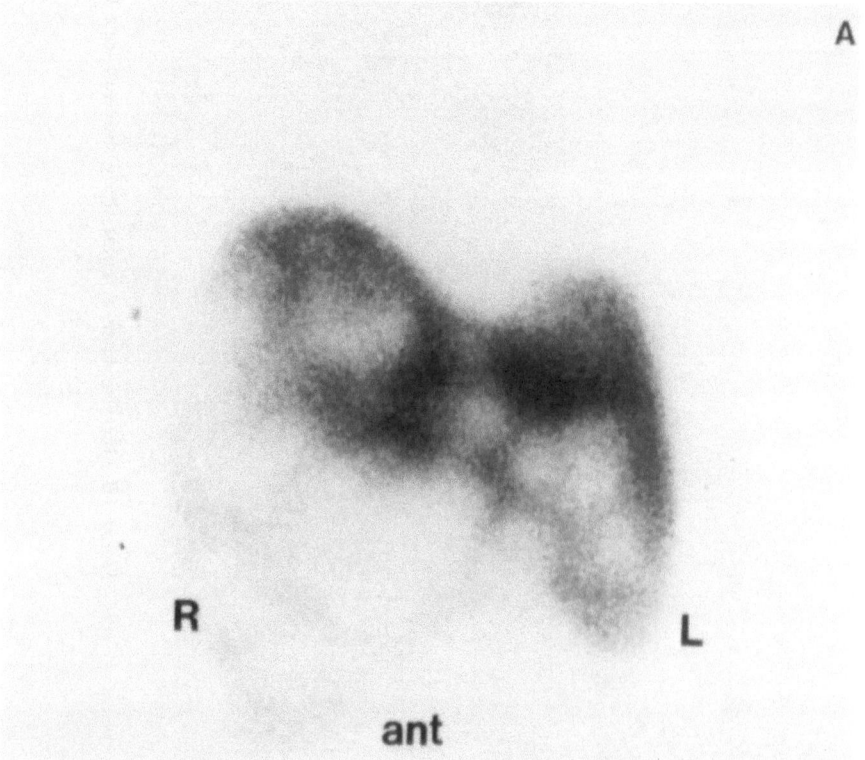

*Figure 2.* Anterior scintigraph illustrating how extensive liver involvement can be in a patient with advanced melanoma. The liver is almost entirely replaced with metastases.

benign lesions such as cysts, hemangiomas or hamartomas (Figures 3, 4). In most of these situations either ultrasound or computed tomography can indicate whether a lesion is present and whether the lesion is cystic or solid [9, 10]. If it is solid, a directed needle biopsy of the lesion is useful to establish the diagnosis.

Melanoma also metastasizes to the spleen and such lesions produce focal defects on scan (Figure 5). Berjian et al. found six of 66 patients had splenic metastases [11]. The size of the spleen and the degree of colloid uptake did not correlate with the presence or absence of metastases. Increased splenic uptake of colloid is a common finding in patients with melanoma and is probably related to some immunologic stimulation.

## Bone scintigraphy

Bone scanning performed with $^{99m}$Tc-phosphate compounds is widely accepted as being more sensitive than radiography for detecting early bone lesions. Several investigators have reported their experience with bone scintigraphy in patients with malignant melanoma.

Roth et al. reviewed bone scans on 100 patients with melanoma and found no positive studies in 16 patients with Stage I disease, one positive study in 35 with Stage II disease and two positive in 13 patients with Stage III disease [2]. Felix et al. reported on bone scan results in 61 patients with all clinical stages of melanoma, who had no symptoms relative to the skeleton [12]. They found no true positive scans, but five false positive studies. Seigler and Fetter found in their experience that bone scans done routinely were positive in 12% of asymptomatic patients as opposed to 57% of symptomatic cases [4].

Aranha et al. reviewed 30 patients with Stage I and 20 patients with Stage II disease and found no positive scans [5]. Thomas et al. found 20 abnormal bone scans in 105 patients with malignant melanoma [6]. Six of the abnormal scans were in patients with Stage I or II disease and these all proved to be false positive studies. Four of the 14 abnormal scans in Stage III patients were false positive. The ten patients with true positive studies had clinical evidence compatible with the scanning results. Muss et al. reviewed bone scans in 49 patients with advanced melanoma (recurrent or metastatic disease) [8]. Twenty-eight patients had bone pain and 15 of these had positive scans. Of the 21 patients without bone pain, only one had a positive scan. The authors concluded that some patients with advanced melanoma may have symptoms resembling bone pain but the symptoms are due to other problems. The bone scan is useful to distinguish these two groups of symptomatic patients.

It is the unanimous conclusion of the above investigators that routine bone scans are not indicated in patients with melanoma who have no symptoms referable to the skeletal system. In particular, the bone scan is not useful in the staging of asymptomatic patients at the time of presentation. When a patient develops clinical signs or symptoms suggesting bone involvement, then the bone scan will be very helpful. A normal scan will suggest that the symptoms are secondary to a nonbone problem, while a positive scan will indicate the sites and extent of bone disease (Figure 6).

The findings on bone scintigraphy are nonspecific in terms of benign vs. malignant disease. However, the distribution of lesions is sometimes char-

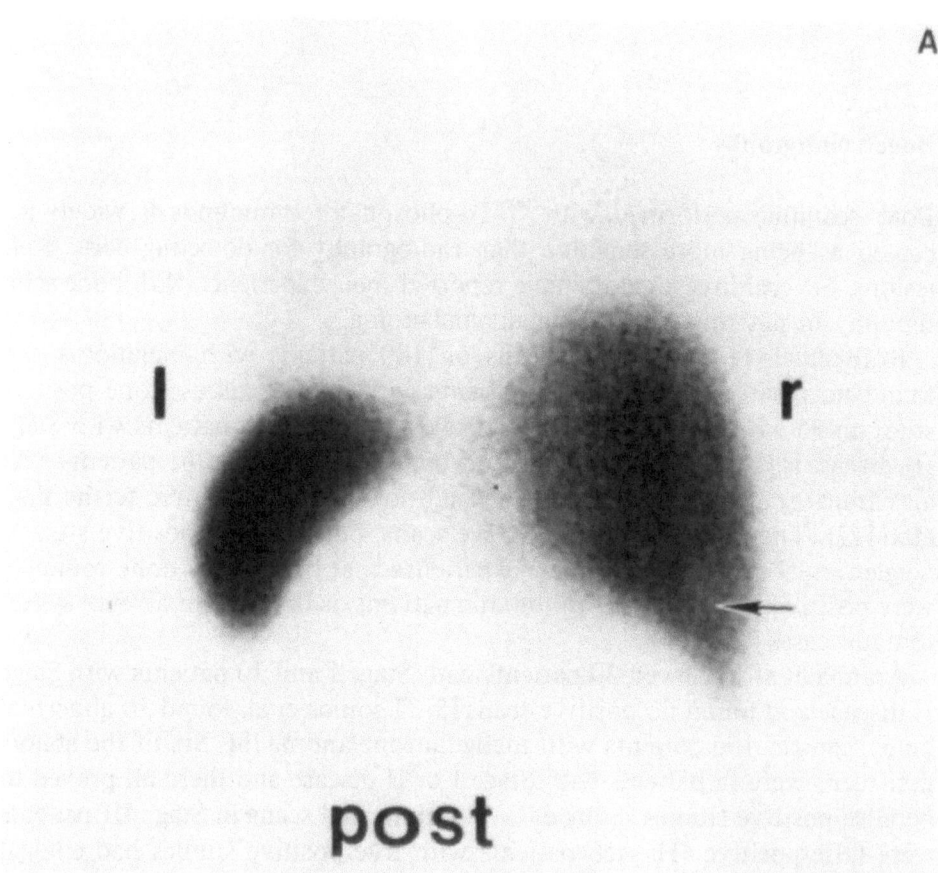

*Figure 3A.* Equivocal findings on liver scintigraphy can often be clarified by ultrasound or computed tomography. (Figure 3A) Posterior scintigraph from a patient with malignant melanoma shows a questionable area of decreased activity in the inferior portion of the right lobe (arrow). All other views appeared normal. (Figure 3B, next page) Ultrasound section shows two small cysts (arrows) adjacent to the diaphragm (D) in the posterior-inferior portion of the right lobe of the liver (L). (Figure 3C, next page) Computed tomographic section gives the same information. One cyst and a portion of the second (arrows) are seen laterally and posteriorly in the liver. In this case, either ultrasound or computed tomography would have been sufficient to confirm the presence of the lesions and indicate their benign nature.

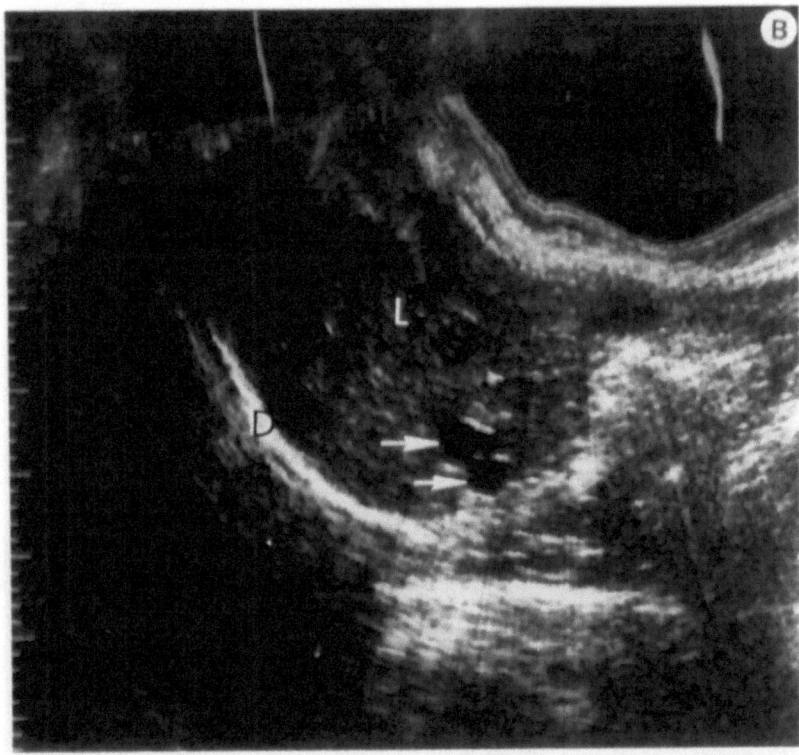

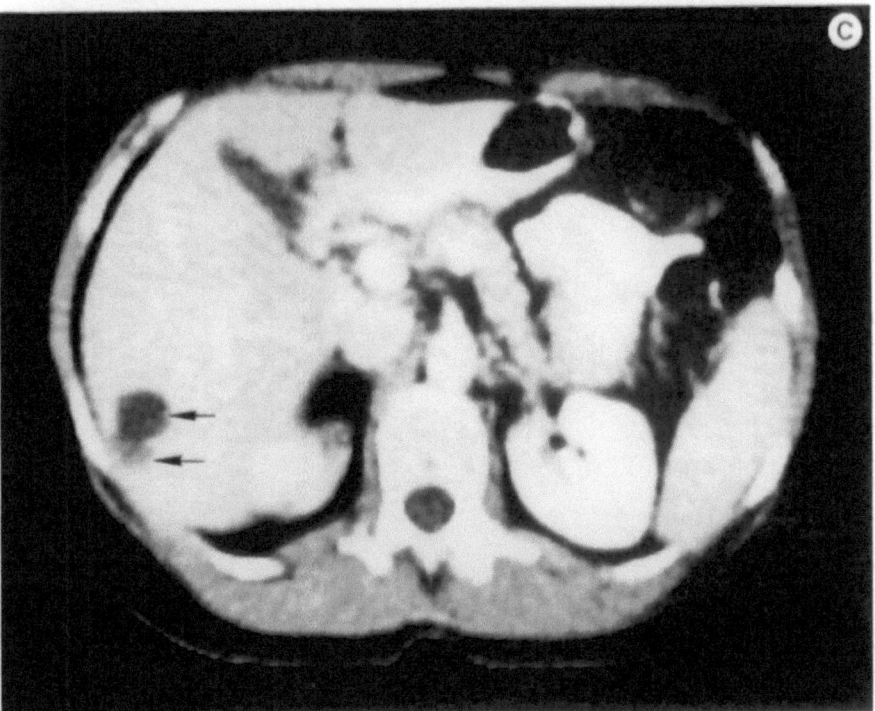

*Figures 3B, C.*

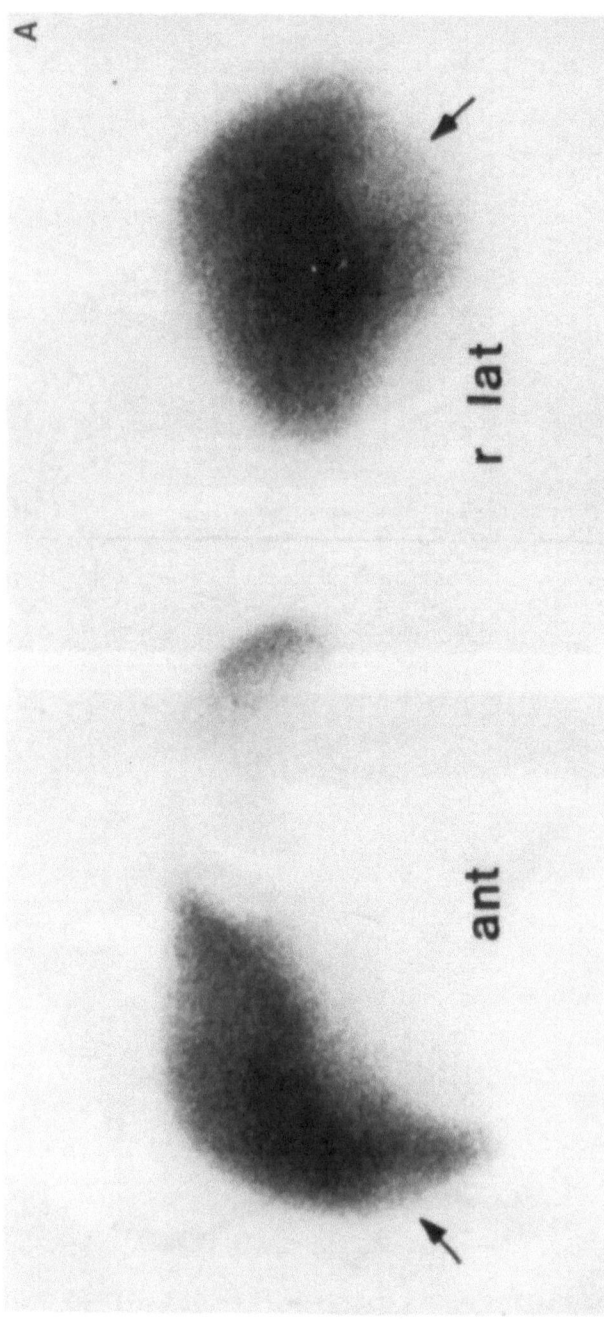

*Figure 4A.* Single focal lesion in the liver may be benign rather than malignant. (Figure 4A) Anterior and right lateral scintigraphs from a patient with malignant melanoma show a single focal lesion in the anterolateral portion of the right lobe (arrows). (Figure 4B, next page) Ultrasound examination demonstrates the lesion to be solid (arrows) (L = liver; D = diaphragm). Laparoscopic biopsy was performed and a benign hamartoma was found.

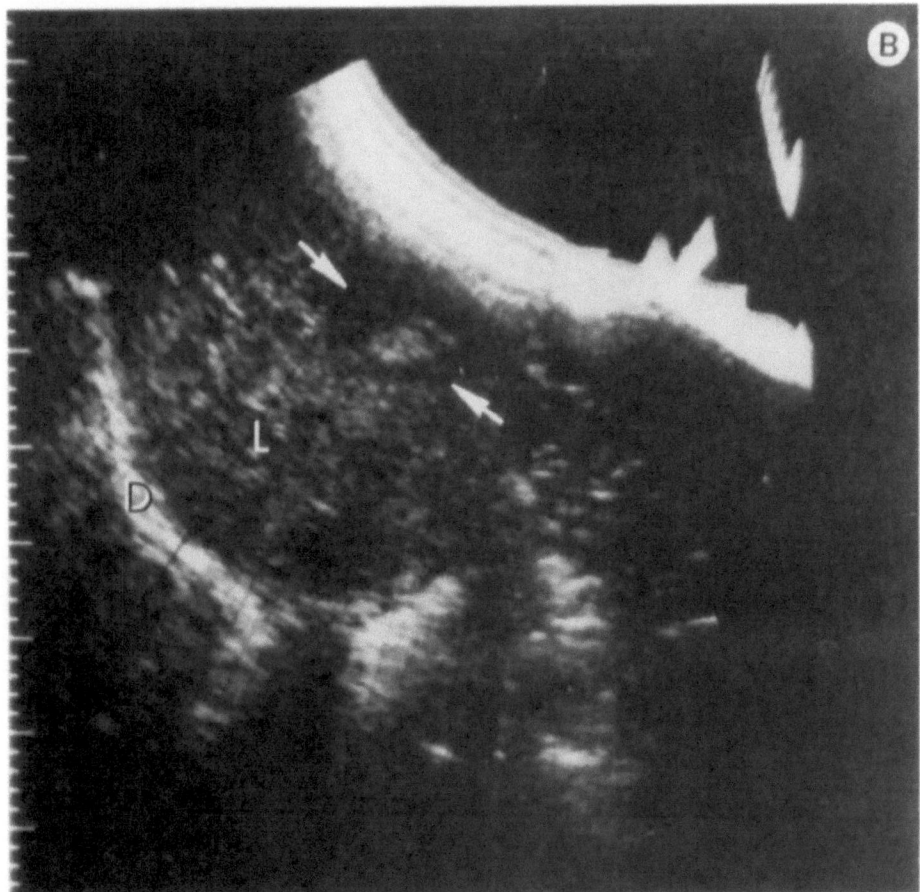

*Figure 4B.*

acteristic for either benign or malignant disease and no further studies are necessary. In other cases, appropriate radiographs will add specificity. In still others, the radiographs will be normal and the cause of an abnormal scan may remain in doubt. In such cases, the lesions may be biopsied, or serial scans or radiographs may be performed to establish the diagnosis by the presence or absence of progression.

The absorbed irradiation from contemporary bone scintigraphy is approximately 0.24 rads to the whole body and 1 rad to bones [13].

## Brain scintigraphy

Brain scanning has been widely used for many years to detect brain metastases. In those institutions where computed tomography (CT) is available, it has largely supplanted brain scintigraphy in recent years for imaging central

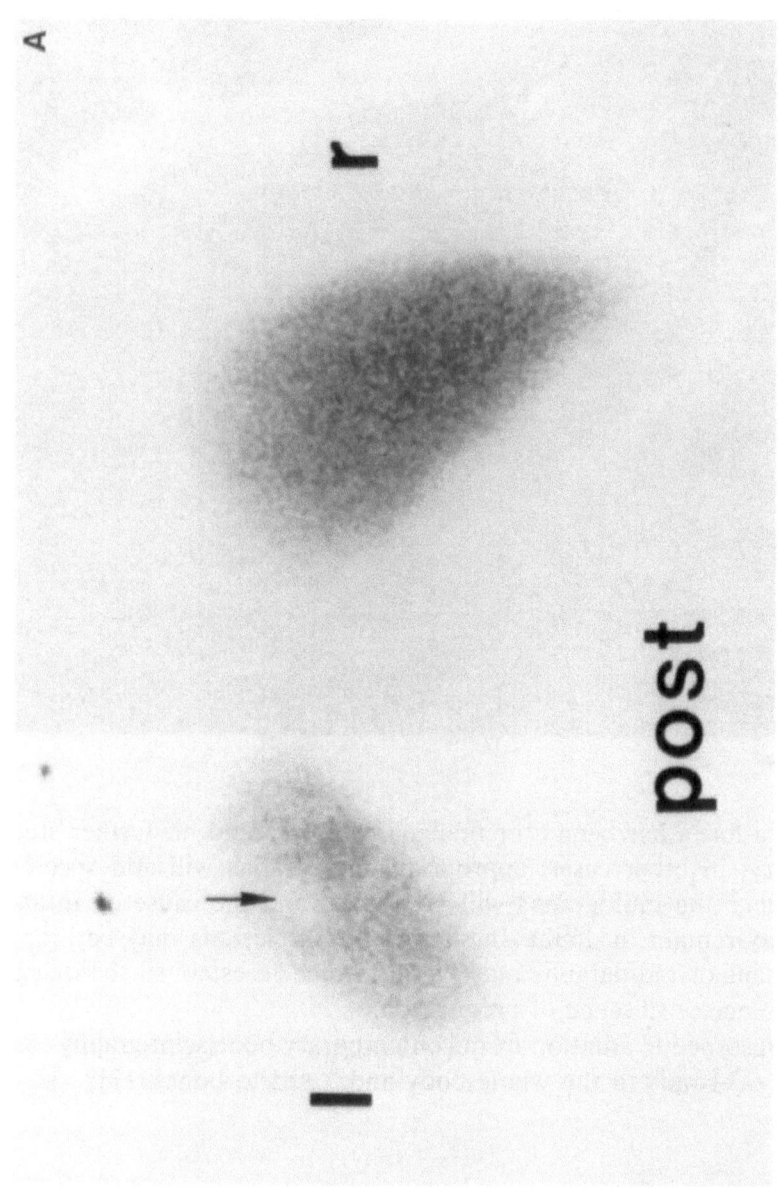

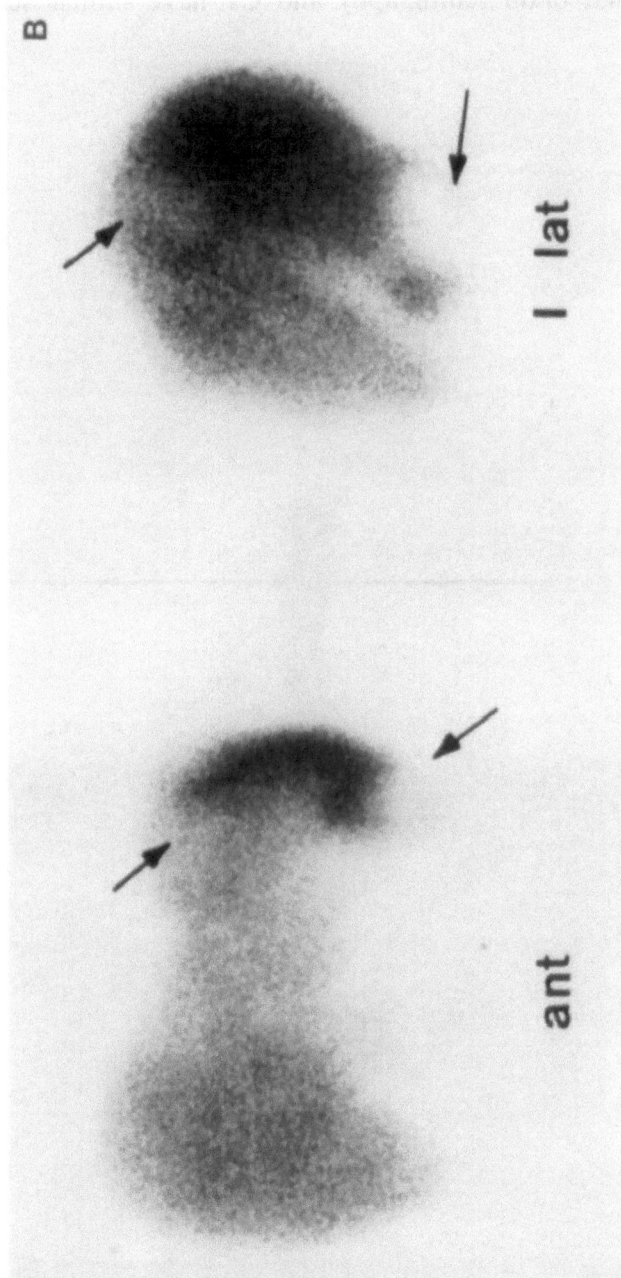

*Figure 5.* Examples of splenic metastases (arrows) in two different patients with malignant melanoma.

nervous system (CNS) disease. Several investigators have published their results with brain scintigraphy in malignant melanoma, but there is not yet a large reported experience with CT in this disease. However, several studies have shown that brain scintigraphy and CT have similar sensitivity for

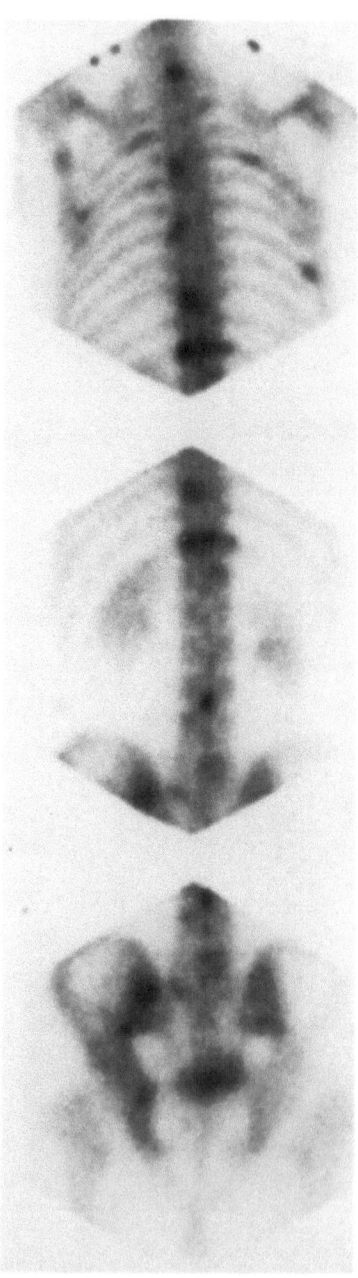

*Figure 6.* Posterior views from bone scintigraphy illustrating typical findings in metastatic melanoma. There are lesions (areas of increased blackness) involving the ribs, scapula, spine and pelvis.

detecting focal CNS lesions. It remains to be seen what the clinical role of CT will be in patients with melanoma, but present experience suggests that it will not be significantly different from the role of brain scintigraphy.

Roth et al. found no positive brain scans in 55 patients with Stage I or II disease and three positive in 19 patients with Stage III disease [2]. Felix et al. reviewed brain scans in 60 patients and reported 59 as true negative and one, in a patient with Stage II disease, as false negative [12]. Aranha et al. found similar results in 50 patients with Stage I or II disease: 49 brain scans were true negative and one was false negative [5]. Seigler and Fetter ordered brain scans only in patients with neurologic signs or symptoms and found them positive in 24% of such cases [4]. Thomas et al. reviewed brain scans in 116 patients and found four false positive and three true positive results [6]. The true positive scans were all in Stage III patients with neurologic signs or symptoms. Muss et al. reviewed scans in 65 patients and found negative studies in 44 of 45 patients without symptoms and nine true positive scans in 21 patients with symptoms [8]. Evans et al. found 156 of 158 Stage I patients had true negative scans [7]. In 137 Stage III patients they found four true positive scans and in 121 Stage IV patients there were 27 positive brain scans.

The above investigators concur that routine brain scintigraphy is not indicated as a staging procedure in patients without neurologic signs or symptoms. The yield for detecting occult metastases is very low.

Brain scanning, like other nuclear medicine procedures, is nonspecific. Multiple lesions in a patient with a known primary are generally presumed to be metastases (Figure 7). Single lesions in the same setting usually represent metastatic disease, but the possibility of a second primary or other CNS lesion must also be kept in mind. The absorbed irradiation from brain scintigraphy is approximately 0.4 rads to the whole body [1].

**Tumor imaging**

Several radiopharmaceuticals have been investigated as agents which will specifically label tumor at any site in the body. Two that have shown some clinical utility in patients with melanoma are indium-111-bleomycin and gallium-67-citrate. Both are tracers which have a greater affinity for tumor cells than for normal tissue. Neither agent is specific for melanoma or for tumor in general; both will localize in inflammatory as well as neoplastic lesions. Therefore, false negative and false positive results limit their clinical usefulness.

Lilien et al., utilizing $^{111}$In-bleomycin, reported an 87% true negative rate in 22 patients with malignant melanoma [14]. Jones and Salmon suggested that such scans might be useful to determine the extent of disease in patients who have regional node involvement, invasive primary lesions or their first recurrence [15].

Gallium-67 scintigraphy is more widely used clinically for tumor scanning, and several groups have reported their experience with melanoma. Langhammer et al. found eight positive studies in 11 patients with melanoma [16]. Midler et al. correlated scan findings with sites of disease in 44 patients and found a 54% detection rate with a 2% incidence of false positive results [17]. They noted that tumor size was important and that lesions smaller than 2 cm in diameter were seldom detected. Jackson et al. studied 36 patients and found a true positive rate of 69% and a false positive rate of 5.7% [18]. Based on these results and on his own experience, Hoffer concluded that the specificity of gallium scintigraphy in malignant melanoma is high (greater than 90%) and that the sensitivity is low (less than 90%) [19].

Romolo and Fisher compared gallium scans with physical examination to determine the presence or absence of tumor in regional lymph nodes [20].

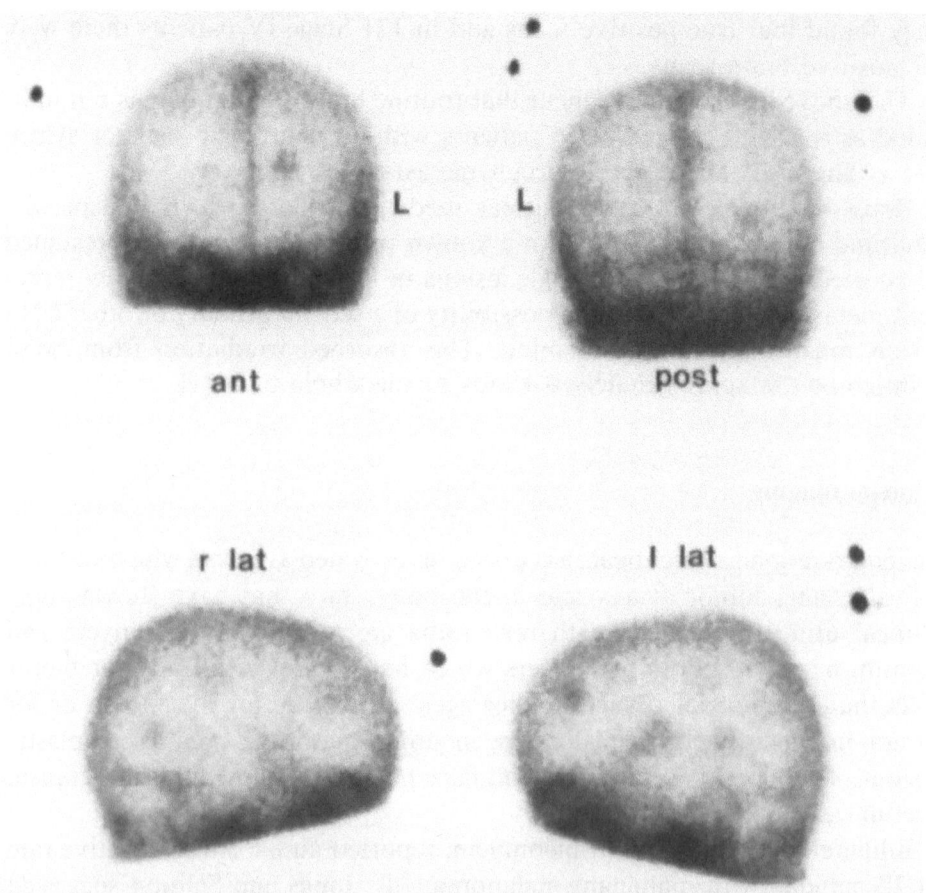

*Figure 7.* Two patients with brain metastases from malignant melanoma.

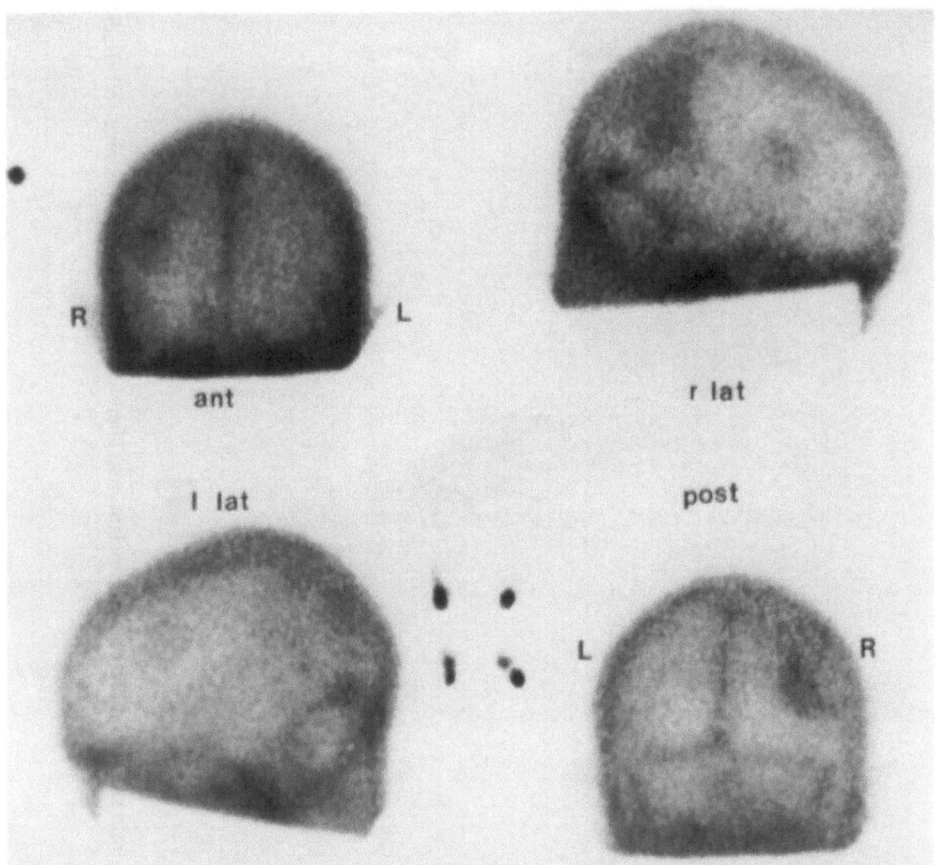

Figure 7A shows a patient with multiple small lesions in both hemispheres, and Figure 7B shows a patient with two large lesions in the right hemisphere.

They evaluated 60 patients with Stage II malignant melanoma or with Clark's Level IV or V primary lesions. Physical examination and gallium scintigraphy showed equal specificity (92% and 96%, respectively) but palpation was significantly more sensitive than scanning for detecting positive nodes (70% vs. 39%). The authors concluded that gallium scintigraphy is not useful as a routine preoperative test in staging malignant melanoma.

Wilson and Boyd compared gallium-67 scintigraphy with P-32 uptake and fluorescein angiography in five patients with choroidal melanomas [21]. The gallium images were negative in every case, whereas the P-32 test was positive in each case. Thus the gallium study is not useful in evaluating suspicious choroidal lesions.

Because gallium scans may fail to detect all sites of melanoma, most clinicians feel they are not indicated as routine studies. On occasion, however, the scan provides dramatic demonstration of clinically unsuspected metastases. Hoffer adds a word of caution that fresh skin grafts and sites of

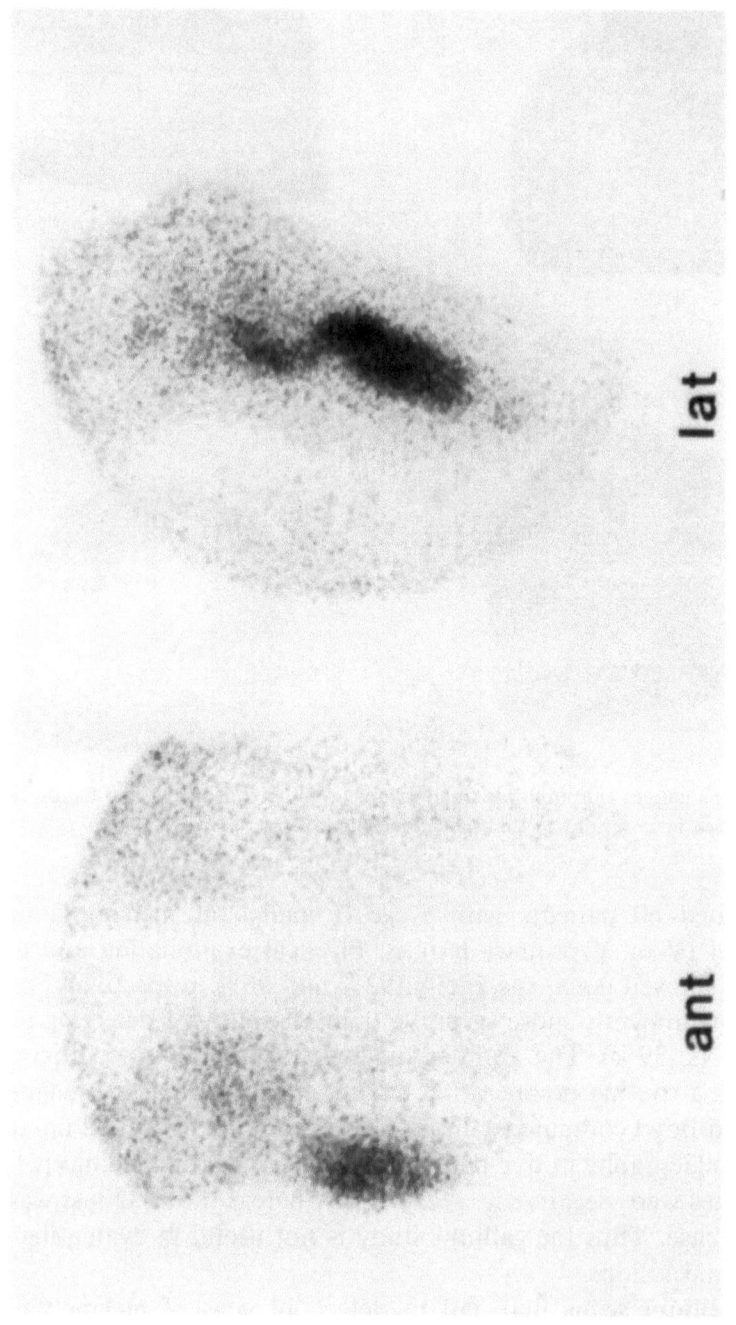

*Figure 8.* Anterior and lateral views of the legs from a gallium-67-citrate study in a patient with melanoma. There is intense uptake in a large soft tissue site of melanoma in the lateral aspect of the right calf.

BCG administration will be positive on gallium scans and should not be mistaken for recurrent or metastatic disease [19].

When gallium scintigraphy is performed, best results are obtained by using high doses (6 to 10 mCi) of gallium-67-citrate and high resolution imaging devices (gamma cameras or tomoscanners with multiple pulse-height analyzers) (Figure 8). Absorbed radiation is approximately 1.5 to 2.5 rad to the whole body and 6 to 10 rad to the spleen, colon and bone marrow [22].

Radiopharmaceuticals which would localize specifically in one type of malignancy have long been sought. Some have shown promise, but none has yet proved to be clinically useful. Beierwaltes et al. reported some early results with an I-125-labeled analog of chloroquine [23]. This quinoline derivative has a strong affinity for melanin and accumulates in pigmented melanomas. Melanoma deposits in several patients were successfully imaged.

Several groups are working to isolate and characterize melanoma-specific antigens and antibodies. Preliminary work in animals suggests that radiolabeled antimelanoma antibodies have potential value as tumor-scanning agents [24]. However, further elucidation of several aspects of tumor immunology is necessary before the diagnostic potential of this technique can be fully realized.

## Lymphoscintigraphy

The lymphatics draining a site of cutaneous melanoma provide an important pathway for dissemination of malignant cells. Prophylactic resection of regional lymph node groups is recommended in patients with advanced Clark's-level lesions. However, the wide variability in lymph system anatomy frequently makes it impossible to know which node groups are at risk. For example, truncal lesions near the midline may drain to ipsilateral or bilateral nodal groups. Scalp lesions near the vertex may drain to either or both sides, and anterior as well as posterior to the ear. Extremity lesions occasionally drain to epitrochlear or popliteal nodes as well as axillary or inguinal nodes.

These anatomic pathways of lymph drainage can be determined scintigraphically by injecting radio-labeled colloid material into the tissue of interest. Radioactive particles of appropriate size (2 to 20 m$\mu$) will enter the lymphatics and be carried to the regional nodes where may will be trapped. Robinson et al. reported the results of lymphoscintigraphy in 77 patients with primary melanoma of the trunk or proximal extremity [25]. They injected gold-198 colloid intradermally around the primary site and scanned the patients 24 hours later. Many patients with lesions near the midline, or near

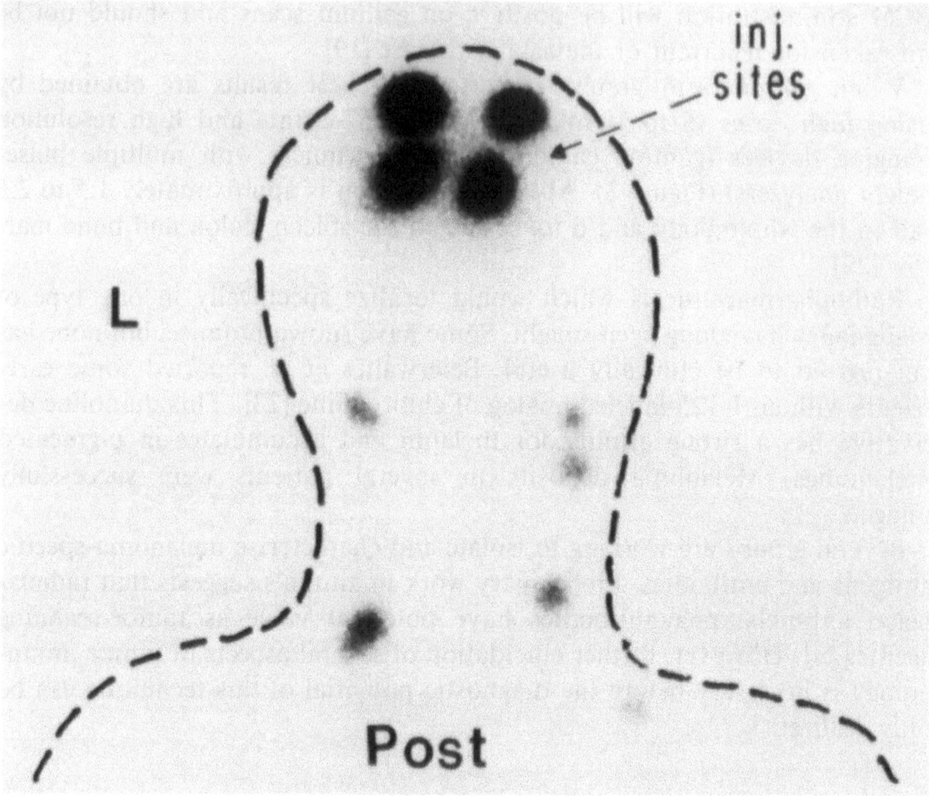

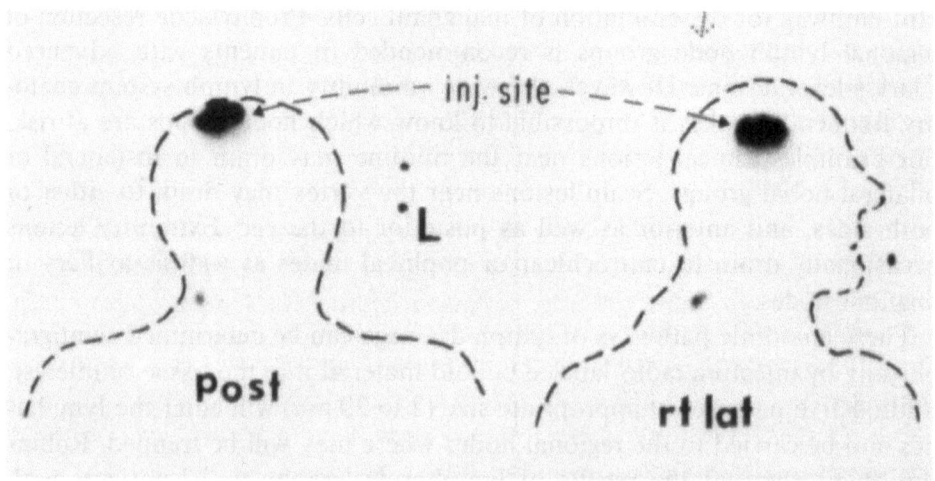

*Figure 9.* Lymphoscintigrams from two patients with scalp melanoma.

(Figure 9A) Posterior view from a patient with a lesion near the midline shows activity in posterior cervical node groups bilaterally. (Figure 9B) Posterior and right lateral views from a patient with a right occipital melanoma. Lymph drainage is demonstrated only to the posterior lymph nodes on the right side. There is no activity anterior to the ear.

"Sappey's line," exhibited variation that did not conform to established patterns [26]. These investigators concluded that lymphoscintigraphy would be useful to the surgeon in planning lymphadenectomies when the primary was in a region of variable lymph drainage. Fee et al. subsequently reported that in 32 patients followed for up to 55 weeks, none developed metastatic disease in node groups other than those which showed colloidal gold uptake on lymphoscintigraphy [27]. This provided evidence that the procedure accurately identifies the nodal groups at risk.

Recently, colloidal preparations of technetium-99m ($^{99m}$Tc), a radionuclide with more favorable imaging and dosimetry properties than gold-198, have been evaluated. Meyer et al. reported using $^{99m}$Tc-sulfur colloid for lymphoscintigraphy in 11 patients with malignant melanoma [28]. We and others are now utilizing $^{99m}$Tc-antimony sulfur colloid. This agent has a more uniformly small particle size (3 to 12 m$\mu$) than other $^{99m}$Tc-colloid preparations, and evidence to date suggests it is the agent of choice for lymphoscintigraphy [29, 30].

The total dose of 1 m$\mu$ of $^{99m}$Tc-antimony sulfur colloid is subdivided into two to four intradermal injections around the edge of the primary lesion, or biopsy site. The total volume injected is less than 1.0 cm$^3$. We use a large-field gamma camera and obtain approximately 100 000 counts per image. An image of the injection site taken within the first few minutes after injection will show linear strands of activity radiating from the lesion toward regional node groups. This picture reflects the transport of colloid via intradermal lymphatics. The clearance of interstitial colloid is rapid and imaging of the systemic reticuloendothelial system can be accomplished by two to four hours after injection. At the time of imaging, a large amount of activity will still be present at the injection site, but much of this is fixed in tissue macrophages and is no longer available for transport [31]. Evidence from rabbit and patient studies indicate that images delayed longer than four to six hours after injection contribute no additional diagnostic information [28, 32].

We obtain images of all regional node groups at three to four hours after injection. Other areas of interest are also imaged, such as palpable, subcutaneous, "in-transit" masses. Lateral views are frequently useful in localizing the nodal groups involved. In some cases it is helpful to the referring physicians to mark the skin over the nodes which show activity. We have found the procedure useful not only in patients with truncal lesions, as described by previous authors, but also in patients with scalp lesions. In these latter patients the results of lymphoscintigraphy frequently lead to a more conservative operation than would be performed without such information.

The procedure will not be accurate in the presence of lymphatic obstruction or lymphedema. If a wide excision has been carried out, the lymphatics within the margins of the resected area will, of course, be abnormal. Injection of the colloid material can be made outside the area of surgery, but the pattern of lymph drainage thus identified may be different than that from the primary site. Therefore, we must be cautious about the significance of results obtained in patients with extensive prior surgery.

There is not yet enough experience with this technique in patients with malignant melanoma to be certain about its clinical value. The technique does not identify abnormal nodes or metastatic disease, but only indicates the normal anatomic pathways of lymph drainage from a given site. Therefore, it promises to be useful in the planning of surgical lymphadenectomies.

### P-32 uptake test

Because of its higher metabolic rate, neoplastic tissue will incorporate more of an administered dose of inorganic phosphate than will normal tissue. This differential uptake can be exploited in the evaluation of certain ocular lesions.

Radioactive phosphorus P-32 emits beta particles which have a short average range in tissue (2 to 3 mm). Therefore, with appropriate Geiger-Müller or solid-state detectors it is possible to determine the activity in a relatively small lesion and in correspondingly small control areas of normal tissue (Figure 10). When originally developed, the P-32 uptake test was generally performed without surgically-provided access to the lesion, and posterior lesions were viewed through the intact globe. This technique is poor for evaluating posterior lesions (because of the short range of the beta particles) and so the procedure fell into disfavor. In recent years, the use of routine surgical access to posterior lesions has improved the diagnostic value of the P-32 uptake test.

The test is performed with 700 microcuries of P-32 sodium phosphate administered intravenously. The absorbed irradiation is approximately 7 rads to the whole body and 25 rads to the bone marrow[33]. Forty-eight hours after administration, counts are made over the lesion and control sites. For anterior lesions, counts are made transconjunctivally, and control areas are often selected in the contralateral eye. For posterior lesions, the conjunctiva is incised so that the detector can be inserted posterior to the globe and positioned directly over the lesion. Ultrasound is sometimes used to aid in positioning, especially in eyes with opaque media. Control sites are selected in the involved eye, but at some distance from any lesion. We try to obtain five 60-second counts over each area, alternating the probe from the lesion to the control site.

Various investigators have used different threshold levels to define a positive test. We consider a ratio of 2:1 (lesion:control) or greater to represent a positive test for malignancy. Lesions which give a ratio of 1.3:1 or less are benign lesions. Results which fall in the range of 1.3:1 to 2:1 are equivocal.

Shields, in a review of 500 cases, found an accuracy rate of 96% to 99%, depending on the anatomic location of the lesion [34]. The test was particularly useful in confirming malignancy in lesions of the ciliary body and choroid. False negative results were more common in lesions of the iris and Shields suggests the test not be performed on such lesions. False positive results have been reported in isolated cases of a wide variety of benign lesions, but no single benign condition commonly causes false positive results. Many of the reported false positive cases have yielded ratios in the range of 1.5:1 to 2:1. If ratio of 2:1 or greater is required to define a positive test, the incidence of false positive results will be very low. Management decisions concerning lesions in the equivocal range should rest on other available information; often they are lesions which can be followed and observed closely for change. It must also be remembered that the test cannot differentiate between malignant melanoma and metastatic tumor.

Acknowledging the limitations of the test, many ophthalmologists still find the procedure useful in confirming the malignant nature of suspicious lesions of the ciliary body or choroid.

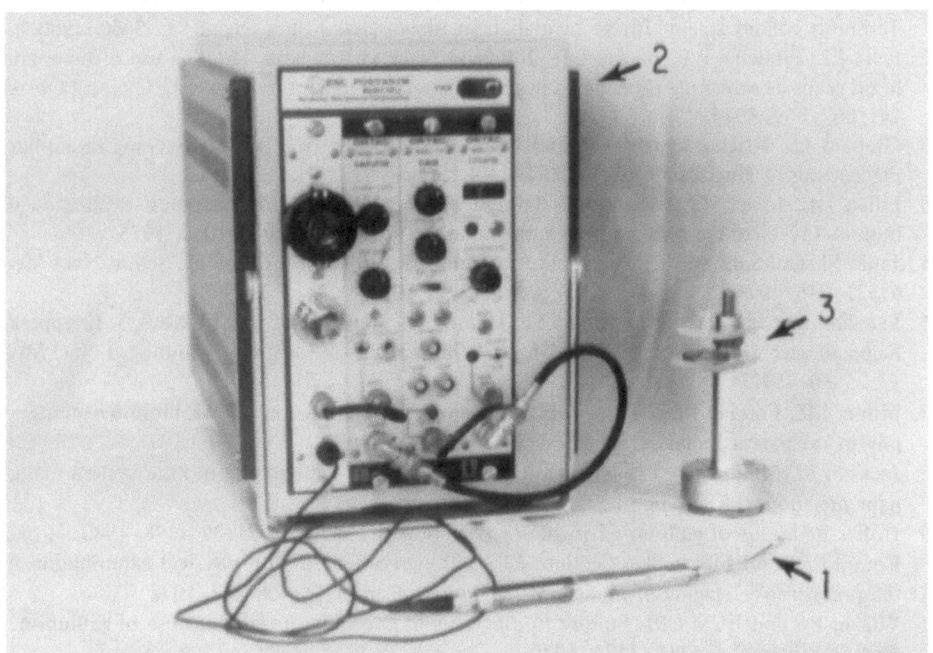

*Figure 10.* Apparatus for detecting P-32 (beta) activity from ocular lesions. Number 1 indicates a solid-state probe which can be placed behind the globe, directly over a lesion; 2 indicates the amplifier and scaler (counter); and 3 indicates a reference source for checking and calibrating the equipment.

# References

1. Gottschalk A and Potchen EJ (ed): Diagnostic Nuclear Medicine, Williams & Wilkins, Baltimore, 1976.
2. Roth JA, Eilber FR, Bennett LR and Morton DL: Radionuclide photoscanning: usefulness in preoperative evaluation of melanoma patients. Arch Surg 110:1211-1212, 1975.
3. Felix.EL, Bagley DH, Sindelar WF, Johnston GS and Ketcham AS: The value of the liver scan in preoperative screening of patients with malignancies. Cancer 38:1137-1141, 1976.
4. Seigler HF and Fetter BF: Current management of melanoma. Ann Surg 186:1-12, 1977.
5. Aranha GV, Simmons RL, Gunnarsson A, Grage TB and McKhann CF: The value of preoperative screening procedures in Stage I and II malignant melanoma. J Surg Oncol 11:1-6, 1979.
6. Thomas JH, Panoussopoulous D, Liesmann GE, Jewell WR and Preston DF: Scintiscans in the evaluation of patients with malignant melanomas. Surg Gynecol Obstet 149:574-576, 1979.
7. Evans RA, Bland KI, McMurtrey MJ and Ballantyne AJ: Radionuclide scans not indicated for clinical Stage I melanoma. Surg Gynecol Obstet 150:532-534, 1980.
8. Muss HB, Richards F, Barnes PL, Willard VV and Cowan RJ: Radionuclide scanning in patients with advanced malignant melanoma. Clin Nucl Med 4:516-518, 1979.
9. Sullivan DC, Taylor KJW and Gottschalk A: The use of ultrasound to enhance the diagnostic utility of the equivocal liver scintigraph. Radiology 128:727-732, 1978.
10. Snow JH, Goldstein HM and Wallace S: Comparison of scintigraphy, sonography, and computed tomography in the evaluation of hepatic neoplasms. Am J Roentgenol 132:915-918, 1979.
11. Berjian RA, Parthasarathy KL, Didolkar MS, Bakshi SP and Moore RH: Significance of $^{99m}$Tc-Sulfur colloid splenic image in malignant melanoma. J Surg Oncol 13:53-60, 1980.
12. Felix EL, Sindelar WF, Bagley DH, Johnston GS and Ketcham AS: The use of bone and brain scans as screening procedures in patients with malignant lesions. Surg Gynecol Obstet 141:867-869, 1975.
13. Graham LS, Krishnamurthy GT and Blahd BH: Dosimetry of skeletal-seeking radiopharmaceuticals. J Nucl Med 15:496, 1974.
14. Lilien DL, Jones SE, O'Mara RE, Salmon SE and Durie BGM: A clinical evaluation of indium-111 bleomycin as a tumor-imaging agent. Cancer 35:1036-1049, 1975.
15. Jones SE and Salmon SE: The role of radionuclides in clinical oncology. Semin Nucl Med 6:331-346, 1976.
16. Langhammer H, Glaubitt G, Grebe SF, Hampe JF, Haubold U, Hor G, Kaul A, Koeppe P, Koppenhagen J, Roedler HD and Van der Schoot JB: $^{67}$Ga for tumor scanning. J Nucl Med 13:25-30, 1972.
17. Milder MS, Frankel RS, Bulkley GB, Ketcham AS and Johnston GS: Gallium-67 scintigraphy in malignant melanoma. Cancer 32:1350-1356, 1973.
18. Jackson FI, McPherson TA and Lentle BC: Gallium-67 scintigraphy in multisystem malignant melanoma. Radiology 122:163-167, 1977.
19. Hoffer P: Status of gallium-67 in tumor detection. J Nucl Med 21:394-498, 1980.
20. Romolo JL and Fisher SG: Gallium-67 scanning compared with physical examination in the preoperative staging of malignant melanoma. Cancer 44:468-472, 1978.
21. Wilson RS and Boyd CM: Studies in diagnosis of choroidal melanoma: use of gallium-67. Ann Ophthalmol 8:1119-1124, 1976.
22. MIRD/Dose estimate report no 2. J Nucl Med 14:755-756, 1973.
23. Beierwaltes WH, Lieberman LM, Varma VM and Counsell RE: Visualizing human malignant melanoma and metastases: use of chloroquine analog tagged with iodine-125. J Am Med Assoc 206:97-102, 1968.

24. Stuhmiller GM, Sullivan DC, Vervaert CE, Croker BP, Harris CC, Stumpf WE, Sar M and Seigler HF: In vivo tumor localization utilizing tumor specific xenoantibody, alloantibody, and monoclonal antibody. Ann Surg 194:592–601, 1981.
25. Robinson DS, Sample WF, Fee HJ, Holmes EC and Morton DL: Regional lymphatic drainage in primary malignant melanoma of the trunk determined by colloidal gold scanning. Surg Forum 28:147–148, 1977.
26. Sugarbaker EV and McBride CM: Melanoma of the trunk: the results of surgical excision and anatomic guidelines for predicting nodal metastasis. Surgery 80:22–30, 1976.
27. Fee HJ, Robinson DS, Sample WF, Graham LS, Holmes EC and Morton DL: The determination of lymph shed by colloidal gold scanning in patients with malignant melanoma: a preliminary study. Surgery 84:626–632, 1978.
28. Meyer CM, Lecklitner ML, Logic JR, Balch CE, Bessey PQ and Tauxe WN: Technetium-99m sulfur-colloid cutaneous lymphoscintigraphy in the management of truncal melanoma. Radiology 131:205–209, 1979.
29. Ege GM and Warbick A: Lymphoscintigraphy: a comparison of $^{99m}$Tc-antimony sulphide colloid and $^{99m}$Tc-stannous phytate. Br J Radiol 52:124–129, 1979.
30. Kaplan WD, Davis MA and Rose CM: A comparison of two technetium-99m-labeled radiopharmaceuticals for lymphoscintigraphy: concise communication. J Nucl Med 20:933–937, 1979.
31. Prassavinichai S, Honda T, Nedwich A, Lam S and Brady LW: Observations on the transport mechanism of colloidal gold. Radiol Clin Biol 42:460–467, 1973.
32. Ege GN: Radiocolloid lymphoscintigraphy in neoplastic disease. Cancer Res 40:3065–3071, 1980.
33. Packer S, Lambrecht RM, Christman DR, Ansari AN, Wolf AP and Atkins HL: Metal isotopes used as radioactive indicators of ocular melanoma. Am J Ophthalmol 83:80–94, 1977.
34. Shields JA: Accuracy and limitation of the $^{32}$P test in the diagnosis of ocular tumors: an analysis of 500 cases. Ophthalmology 85:950–966, 1978.

# 12. Hormonal aspects of melanoma

KENNETH SCOTT McCARTY, Jr.,*+ DOUGLAS EDWARD
PAULL*+ and KENNETH SCOTT McCARTY, Sr.**

## I. Introduction

Several lines of evidence suggest a relationship between the biologic behavior of melanoma and hormone action. Epidemiologic observations have included sex-associated differences in survival and incidence, rarity of melanoma in prepubescent individuals and studies of the effects of pregnancy on melanoma growth. Attempts to define the specificity of hormonal influence on melanoma have included various regimens of endocrine manipulation as well as investigations to evaluate the presence of hormone receptors in melanoma tissues. Laboratory, clinical and epidemiologic evidence has implicated sex steroids, melanocyte stimulating hormone (MSH), adrenocorticotropin (ACTH) and other peptide hormones in the growth and development of melanoma. This chapter will consider the historical evidence for hormonal influence on melanoma and review evidence for specific steroid and peptide hormone interaction with melanoma.

## II. Historical aspects

### A. *Epidemiology*

Epidemiologic evidence suggesting an influence of hormones on melanoma include: (1) the better prognosis of the female patient as compared to male patients [1–4]; (2) the rarity of melanoma in prepubertal children [5–10]; (3) the increased survival for premenopausal women compared to postmenopausal women [3, 4, 11]; and (4) the better prognosis for multiparous females [12].

White observed an overall five-year survival rate for females with melanoma of 43.5% compared to a 28.2% rate for males [1] in a study of patients with cutaneous melanoma recorded in the California Tumor Registry from 1942 to 1961. A comparison between male and female survival for

From the Endocrine Oncology Laboratory, Departments of Medicine*, Pathology+ and Biochemistry** Duke University Medical Center, Duke University, Durham, N.C. 27710

*Seigler, H. F. (ed.), Clinical Management of Melanoma. ISBN 978-94-009-7495-1*

periods greater than five years showed an improved survival among females as compared to males. Moreover, female survival in any age group was as good or better than male survival. In a compilation of reported cases of melanoma through 1959, one thousand nine hundred one patients were identified (985 males, 916 females). Female five-year survival rate was 34.5% while male survival ratio was 23.4% [1]. Data reported from Stanford utilizing 73 patients with cutaneous melanoma and 58 patients with ocular melanoma confirmed White's observation that females have a more favorable prognosis [1]. On the basis of these studies, White reiterated the suggestion that melanoma might be hormonally responsive and/or dependent.

The survival differences between males and females appear to be independent of the stage of disease. A study comparing survival, sex and stage of disease, consisting of 140 male and 205 female patients seen at the M.D. Anderson Hospital, noted that patients with primary melanoma demonstrated a five-year survival rate of 79.0% for females compared to 62.9% for males and ten-year survival rates of 60.6% and 49.4% for females and males respectively [2]. In a series of 256 males and 213 females with metastases on admission, female and male five-year survival rates were 15.8% and 9.8%, respectively, and ten-year survival rates were 14.2% and 7.0% for females and males, respectively [2]. Additional studies on large series of patients support the conclusion that females with melanoma have an improved survival as compared to age-matched males with melanoma [3, 4].

Melanoma is rare in prepubescent children. Out of 1014 patients with melanoma (Norway Cancer Registry, 1953–1962) only four patients were less than 14 years of age [5]. In Pack's experience with 900 pigmented tumors observed in infants and young children, there were no cases in which metastases to regional lymph nodes were observed [6]. This served to emphasize the distinction between melanoma in adults and the pigmented tumors, termed juvenile melanomas, observed in children. Several other authors have confirmed the fact that "melanoma" with malignant behavior is rare in prepubertal children [7–10]. Survival rates for children with true malignant melanoma are comparable to those for adults with the disease [7].

Postmenopausal women have decreased survival compared to premenopausal women. While age influences survival, the pre- vs. post-menopausal difference in survival is not due to aging alone, as the difference is noted even when Kaplan-Meier survival curves are utilized including only patients who die of melanoma. Wright et al. reviewed the records of 132 patients with melanoma (85 females, 47 males) treated in the training hospitals of Glasgow from 1939 to 1949. The five-year survival rate for females aged less than 50 years was 77% compared to 23% for females over 50 years of age. However it must be noted that this age differential also applied to male patients. Males below 50 had a five-year survival rate of 45 % while males over 50 had a rate of 27 % [11]. Nathanson et al. studied 164 patients with melanoma. The mean survival of premenopausal females exceeded that of males in the fourth decade of life (55 compared to 26 months, respectively). This difference was no longer apparent in the fifth and sixth decade of life [3]. It was also noted that four of 21 women within 12 months of the menopause in the study had an exacerbation of disseminated melanoma [3], a finding which has been reported by other investigators.

Evidence contradicting the importance of menopausal status in prognosis was provided by Shaw et al. They reported a series of 1861 patients with melanoma. The difference in survival rates between male and female patients below 50 years of age was similar to the difference between male and female survival in patients over 50 years of age [4]. A difference in five-year survival rates of men and women of 11.8 % was observed in patients less than 50 years old, which was similar to the difference of 11.1 % in survival rates between men and women over 50 years of age [4]. Thus, the data, while all suggesting differences between male and female survival, are conflicting with regard to changes in the biologic behavior of melanoma, as reflected in survival rates of patients with melanoma, who are identified into cohorts based on the pituitary-ovarian changes associated with the menopause.

Additional support for a relationship of hormones to melanoma growth is the observation that multiparous women with melanoma have higher survival rates than nulliparous women with melanoma [12]. Women who had had a previous pregnancy had a five-year survival rate of 77 % compared to 68 % for nulliparous women with melanoma ($p<0.10$). Multiparous women with Stage I disease (localized) had a five-year survival rate of 84 % versus a five-year survival rate of 75 % in nulliparous women with Stage I disease. For Stage II disease (nodal involvement) the five-year survival rates were 38 % and 29 % for multiparous and nulliparous women respectively (difference not statistically significant). On the basis of these data, as well as observations of fetal antigens on melanoma cels, Hersey et al. proposed that previous exposure to fetal antigens in multiparous females might represent an immunologic explanation of the observed differences in survival [12].

The epidemiologic evidence for hormonal influence on melanoma thus includes: (1) the better prognosis for female patients with melanoma; (2) the rarity of melanoma in childhood; (3) the suggested improved prognosis for premenopausal females with melanoma; and (4) the suggested improved prognosis for multiparous females. The effect of intercurrent pregnancy upon melanoma behavior will be considered separately.

358

## B. *Pregnancy*

Relatively few studies have addressed the question of what effects, if any, pregnancy has on human melanoma. In 1950, Pack and Scharnagel described 32 patients, out of their total series of 1050 patients with melanoma, in whom pregnancy was associated with the growth or development of a melanoma [13]. These 32 women were categorized into three groups: (1) pregnant women with coexistent active melanoma, (2) postpartum patients with melanoma who had observed changes in nevi during pregnancy and (3) patients treated for melanoma who subsequently became pregnant. At the time of that report, five of ten pregnant patients with coexistent melanoma had died within $2\frac{1}{2}$ years of surgical treatment for their disease, two of the ten were too recently treated for evaluation, and the remaining three patients showed no evidence of disease at 5, 9, and 16 months following surgical treatment respectively. Of the 32 patients in the series, 14 died of melanoma within three years of diagnosis, two patients survived eight and 13 years, and the remaining 16 had insufficient duration of follow-up from the time of surgical treatment for melanoma. Despite this suggestive evidence for changes in melanoma behavior during pregnancy, Pack reported that clinical attempts to alter the disease by gonadectomy, testesterone administration, pituitary ablation or adrenalectomy were not effective. Therapeutic abortion in pregnant women with coexistent active melanoma showed no evidence of altering the course of the disease.

The rarity of melanoma occurring during pregnancy has been emphasized by several anecdotal reports on the subject. Hadley reviewed several case reports of this phenomenon reported before 1949 [14]. He described the account fo a 27-year-old female who died from unsuspected metastatic melanoma during the third trimester of a pregnancy, some five years after a pigmented mole was removed from her arm. He expressed the belief that the tumor growth was accelerated by pregnancy. Byrd and McGanity in 1954 reported the case of a 25-year-old pregnant woman whose condition deteriorated and who ultimately died from disseminated melanoma during her fifth pregnancy after having a melanoma removed from her thigh three years earlier during her fourth pregnancy [15].

Controlled clinical studies show little to no difference in prognosis between pregnant and nonpregnant women with melanoma. George et al. in 1959 reported on a study group of 115 pregnant female patients with melanoma who were compared to a control group of 330 nonpregnant females with melanoma, both groups of women having been seen at the Memorial Center for Cancer in New York during the period from 1917 to 1957 [16]. Of 115 pregnant patients, 77 had primary melanoma clinically apparent during the 9 months of pregnancy, and 38 patients became pregnant after definitive treatment of primary melanoma. The study group and control group were further subdivided according to stage of disease at the time of surgical intervention. There was no difference in the overall five- or ten-year survival rates among pregnant patients as compared to nonpregnant patients. However, the pregnancy-associated melanoma patients had a statistically significant higher percentage of regional lymph node involvement at the time of treatment than did the nonpregnant control group. Despite this difference in nodal status at surgery, there was no evidence of any increase in the incidence of generalized metastases among the study group as compared to controls.

Shiu et al. in 1976 performed a retrospective analysis of 251 women of child-bearing age with melanoma in an attempt to resolve the conflict concerning pregnancy and survival in melanoma patients [17]. These patients with melanoma were divided into groups according to the following conditions documented at the time of admission: multiparous women (group A); parous women with no activation of lesion during previous pregnancy (group B); parous women with apparent activation of a lesion during a previous pregnancy (group C); and women with melanoma admitted and treated during a pregnancy (group D). "Activation" referred to symptoms and signs such as elevation, itching or increase in size of a lesion. The groups were subdivided into stages of disease. Considering only those patients with Stage II disease and considering groups A and B together, the five-year survival rate was 52% as compared to a five-year survival rate of only 25% for groups C and D ($p<0.05$).

Such differences in survival were used to argue for a less favorable prognosis for patients with pregnancy-associated activation of melanoma when the disease was Stage II (node involvement) at the time of diagnosis as compared to Stage II patients in which no change during pregnancy was noted. No difference in survival was observed for patients with Stage I disease in whom lesions had not shown pregnancy associated changes (A and B) and those in whom some change in the lesion was associated with pregnancy(C and D). One question which remains to be resolved is whether the definition of the subgroups used for dichotomization in these studies influenced the outcome. Shiu et al. proposed several theories to explain the poorer prognosis of males vs. females, pregnant women vs. nonpregnant women and postmenopausal vs. premenopausal females. They theorized that the hormonal environment of the premenopausal and nonparous period might have an inhibitory influence on melanoma which would be altered at the menopause or as a result of pregnancy. Alternatively, they suggested androgenic hormones might promote melanoma growth. To support such a theory, they cited studies on melanoma cell cultures which had increased activity when testosterone was added to the medium. However, the several reports currently in the literature do not concur on the influence of pregnancy on survival of females with melanoma.

Observations cited as suggesting an effect of pregnancy on melanoma include: (1) pigmentary changes observed in lesions during pregnancy; (2) reports of decreased survival among pregnant patients with melanoma; and (3) the increase in serum concentrations of MSH and similar hormones during pregnancy [18].

## C. *Endocrine manipulation*

Several reports regarding apparent effects or lack of effect of hormonal manipulation on melanoma have been published. Hawes, in 1943, reported that bilateral orchiectomy did not lead to improvement in the condition of a 47-year-old male with metastatic melanoma, and cautioned surgeons of the hazards of such surgery as an approach to the male patient with meatstatic melanoma [19, 20]. In 1952, Levi and Lewison described the clinical course of a patient with ovarian agenesis (Turner's syndrome) and metastatic melanoma. The patient survived 52 months from the time of grossly evident metastases until death [21]. During the course of her illness, the patient had the spontaneous regression of metastatic lesions of the buttock, thoracic wall and axilla. These authors suggested that the prolonged survival and spontaneous regression of the tumors in this patient with melanoma and ovarian agenesis reflected her prepubertal hormonal status.

Pack and Scharnagel reported no effect of castration in males and females on the natural history of melanoma. Similarly, testosterone treatment in females, pituitary irradiation or bilateral adrenalectomy did not favorably affect melanoma [13]. Pack and Scharnagel as well as Levi and Lewison believed that the possible hormonal factors which induce melanoma formation may not be the same factors which promote its further growth and neoplastic dissemination [13, 21]. Meyer and Gumpert, in a 1953 review of the treatment of melanoma, reiterated the lack of effect of various forms of hormone therapy [22].

Reasoning that MSH from the pituitary gland might stimulate abnormal growth of melanocytes, Wigley and Metz decided to employ radiation to the pituitary in patients with melanoma [23]. An initial case report described the reduction in size and number of subcutaneous melanoma metastases and the clinical improvement in a patient following delivery of 1560 rads to the pituitary over a one-month period. However, in a study of four additional patients with advanced melanoma, similar radiation therapy did not produce significant clinical response.

Several reports have explored the relationship between exogenous hormones and melanoma behavior. Johnson et al. reported objective remissions in five of 44 (11%) patients with metastatic melanoma treated with a 200–600 mg daily dose of 6-$\alpha$-methyl preg-4-ene-3,11,20-trione (an antiestrogenic compound) for an 8-week period [24]. In 1968, Ellerbroek reported the case of a 25-year-old woman who noted the growth and darkening of a pigmented lesion on her arm two months after she had started taking ethynodiol diacetate with mestranol (ovulen-21) and protriptylene hydrochloride, 5 mg daily [25]. Excisional biopsy revealed melanoma. Sadoff et al. (1973) published a report of five patients in whom melanoma arose or became worse following administration of exogenous estrogens [26]. Two patients were males with adenocarcinoma of the prostate gland who developed melanoma after having received diethylstilbestrol postoperatively.

The relationship of melanoma to oral contraceptive use was evaluated by Beral et al. who accumulated data on 17 942 women aged 17–59 who were members of the Kaiser Foundation Health Plan between 1968 and 1972. Twenty-two new cases of melanoma were diagnosed among these women during this period. The age adjusted incidence rate of melanoma per 100 000 women years was 29.5 for patients who used oral contraceptives for four years or more as compared to an incidence of 17.6 for nonusers. This observed difference in melanoma incidence was not statistically significant. Patients who used oral contraceptives for four or more years had a greater age adjusted rate of a past history of skin cancer (14.6 per 1000) as compared to nonusers who had a rate of 7.8 per 1000 ($p<0.05$). In a case-control study of 37 female melanoma patients and randomly selected age matched control female patients without melanoma 60% of the patients with melanoma had used oral contraceptives; while only 45% of patients without melanoma had used oral contraceptives, although this difference did not achieve statistical significance. The relative risk of a user of oral contraceptives having melanoma compared to patients who had never used oral contraceptives was 1.8:1 [27]. Shaw et al., in 1978, reported on the five-year survival rate among 113 melanoma patients who had taken oral contraceptives for a period $\geq 24$ months and within 12 months of diagnosis (users), compared to the five-year survival rates among 237 melanoma patients who had either never used oral contraceptives or used oral contraceptives for <24 months or not within 12 months of diagnosis (nonusers) [4]. The average age and the number of previous pregnancies were similar among users and nonusers. The five-year survival of melanoma patients who were oral contraceptive users and those who did not use oral contraceptives was not significantly different.

Bodenham and Hale described the use of the Geiger probe technique in determining if a given melanoma was sensitive to estrogen [28]. A Geiger probe is placed within the tumor, radioactive phosphorus is given orally to the patient, and radioactive uptake measured. The patient is given stilbestrol, 15 mg orally three times per day, and radioactive uptake again measured. An increase in radioactive uptake presumably indicates an estrogen sensitive melanoma. This study described several examples of temporary remissions following hypophysectomy in patients whose tumors were suggested to be estrogen sensitive by the Geiger probe method [28].

## III. Sex steroid effects on melanoma

The observation of high affinity sex steroid binding proteins in animal melanoma tissue cultures added considerably to evidence suggesting the possibility of endocrine responsiveness of melanoma. For this binding to be considered a biologically significant steroid hormone receptor, the following basic criteria must be met: (1) saturable binding, (2) specific binding, (3) distinct molecular weight species and (4) correlation with some biologic response to the hormone [29].

### A. *In vitro and in vivo animal experiemnts*

Based on the observations that (1) transplanted melanomas appeared to grow faster in female Syrian hamsters than in male Syrian hamsters and that (2) pregnancy and lactation could partly inhibit the melanoma growth in female hamsters, Lipkin (1970) investigated the direct effects of steroid hormones on the growth of cultured hamster melanoma cells [30]. He attempted to correlate the in vivo sex differences of melanoma in hamsters with in vitro melanoma cell culture growth responses to steroid hormones. Matched groups of four-week-old male and female hamsters were inoculated with aliquots of melanoma cells, and the cumulative mortality among males as compared to female hamsters was recorded. At each melanoma inoculum concentration, females had a *higher* cumulative mortality than males. Other experiments addressing this issue included cultures of hamster amelanotic melanoma carried out under three conditions: (1) melanoma cells cultured in testosterone containing medium, (2) melanoma cells cultured in an estrogen containing medium and (3) melanoma cell cultures serving as controls. Cell counts were made daily. Cells exposed to testosterone containing media had the slowest rate of proliferation, whereas control cell cultures grew most rapidly. Cell cultures grown in estradiol grew at intermediate rates. Lipkin noted that the direct inhibitory effect of testosterone an melanoma cell cultures in vitro could be a partial explanation for the faster growth of the melanoma in female hamsters in vivo.

Walker et al. investigated the effects of steroid hormones on the growth of in vitro golden hamster melanoma cell cultures. Testosterone and estradiol in physiologic concentrations in the medium resulted in inhibition of cell culture growth. Growth of hamster melanoma cells was 68 % of control in a medium containing $10^{-12}$M testosterone, while growth of the melanoma cells was 67 % of controls if they were placed in a $10^{-12}$M estradiol medium ($p<0.01$) [31]. Corticosterone and progesterone had no effects on in vitro melanoma growth over a concentration range of $10^{-6}$M to $10^{-12}$M. The authors suggested that hamster melanoma was hormonally responsive and that gonadal steroids exerted a direct effect on melanoma growth.

Results of several studies on mice, unlike hamster studies, but similar to effects observed in humans, show that melanoma grows faster in male mice than in female mice [32]. Proctor et al. inoculated six- to eight-week-old male and female mice with equal numbers of B16 melanoma tumor cells at weekly intervals. At 35 days following the final inoculation the animals were sacrificed, primary tumors weighed and metastases to the lungs counted. Prior to tumor inoculation, various groups of female mice underwent oophorectomy, adrenalectomy or laparotomy, alone or in combination. Groups of male mice were previously subjected to orchidectomy, adrenalectomy or laparotomy, alone or in combination. Groups of male and female mice, which served as controls, were also inoculated with similar aliquots of melanoma cells. The average weight of the primary tumors for female controls was 1.83 g, whereas for oophorectomized females it was 5.19 g ($p<0.005$). Furthermore, tumors grew more slowly in control, laparotomized or adrenalectomized female mice than in any group of male mice. These results were interpreted as showing that female sex hormone significantly suppressed the growth of B16 melanoma in mice. Oophorectomized female mice also had a higher incidence of lung metastases as compared to females undergoing laparotomy or adrenalectomy. Orchidectomy had no effect upon melanoma growth or incidence of lung metastases in male mice. Finally, after groups of male and female animals were operated upon, serum was taken from these animals. In vitro colonies of melanoma cells (100 cells per plate) were grown in a medium containing 25 % serum from either control, oophorectomized, orchidectomized or adrenalectomized mice. Colony formation was counted at 72 hours. Colony formation was similar between cells grown in sera from any group, male or female, regardless of the operative procedure the mouse had undergone. This latter finding was interpreted as suggesting that the hormonal factors may not be acting directly on melanoma cells in the mouse [32]. It should also be noted that other studies have shown that exogenous estrogen may actually stimulate B16 melanoma growth in mice.

Lopez et al. (1978) investigated the effect of estrogen on the in vivo growth of B16 melanoma in mice [33]. Female and male mice were inoculated with $1 \times 10^5$ B16 melanoma cells subcutaneously. The study groups of male and female mice received 1 μg estradiol-17β (E2) subcutaneously daily for three weeks while the controls were injected with saline. After a three-week period of estrogen or saline injection, tumor weights were measured among the experimental groups of mice. The average tumor size for female controls was 2.97 g compared to the 5.25 g average tumor weight for E2 treated female mice ($p<0.01$). For male mice, average tumor weights were 3.24 g and 5.74 g for control and E2 treated mice, respectively ($p<0.01$). Moreover, the stimulation of melanoma growth by estradiol in the mice was dose related. The incidence of lung metastases was significantly higher for both sexes among E2 treated mice as compared to controls injected with saline. Female mice inoculated with $1 \times 10^5$ melanoma cells were treated with 10 $\mu$g E2 daily for three weeks while a control group of female mice inoculated with melanoma received saline. The incidence of lung metastases was 0/12 in controls vs. 8/12 in the E2 treated group ($p<0.002$). Finally, Lopez et al. reported that the antiestrogen nafoxidine impaired melanoma growth in female mice. The data suggested that in mice with B16 melanoma, (1) exogenous estrogen enhances tumor growth and incidence of pulmonary metastases, (2) this stimulation of melanoma growth by estrogen was dose related and (3) antiestrogenic compounds decrease the growth rate of melanoma [33]. These results do not agree with the Proctor et al. study of estrogen influence on B16 mouse melanoma previously cited.

## B. *Steroid receptors in animal melanoma*

With the various lines of evidence suggesting an influence of sex steroid on the behavior of melanoma in animal systems, investigations were initiated to establish the presence of steroid hormone receptors in animal melanoma.

1. *Steroid receptors in B16 mouse melanoma.* Markland and Horn have analyzed the binding characteristics of the estrogen receptor in B16 melanoma using both the dextran coated charcoal assay (DCCA) and sucrose density gradient centrifugation (SDGA) procedures [34, 35]. Their data showed that the B16 melanoma contained an estrogen binding protein that was saturable at 1-2 nM $^3$H estradiol. The Scatchard analysis of titration data suggested a single class of estradiol binding sites with high affinity ($K_d = 5.5 \times 10^{-10}$M). The average total binding was 10.1 fmol/mg protein of B16 melanoma cytosol. The binding was estrogen specific and sedimented as an 8S species.

B16 mouse melanoma appears to contain estrogen binding which is (1) saturable, (2) highly specific and (3) of a unique molecular weight. This data in combination with the biologic response of B16 melanoma in vivo and in vitro, which has already been cited [32, 33], confirms the presence of estrogen receptor in mouse B16 melanoma cytosol. The characteristics of the B16 melanoma estrogen receptor were consistent with the characteristics of estrogen receptor from uterine and other tissues [34, 36, 37].

B16 mouse melanoma cytosols studied by Markland and Horn also showed suppressible dexamethasone binding in the 8S and 4S region [34]. B16 melanoma cytosols showed no suppressible binding indicative of progesterone or androgen receptors. Bhakoo et al. had reported the presence of a specific high affinity glucocorticoid receptor in B16 melanoma. To study the biologic response of B16 melanoma to dexamethasone in vivo, Bhakoo et al. treated mice which had received tumor transplants with a three-week course of either dexamethasone or saline after which the mice were sacrificed and tumor weights and number of lung metastases recorded. Dexamethasone appeared to suppress B16 melanoma growth but did not effect the incidence of lung metastases [38]. Thus, B16 mouse melanoma appears to contain estrogen and glucocorticoid cytoplasmic steroid receptors.

2. *Steroid receptors in syrian hamster.* Markland and Horn analyzed Syrian hamster melanoma cytosols by DCCA and SDGA methods for evidence of steroid receptors [34]. The data detected only glucocorticoid receptors in Syrian hamster melanomas. The observed dexamethasone binding was saturable at 10–16 nM $^3$H dexamethasone. High affinity binding was shown by Scatchard analysis to yield a linear plot, with a slope of $K_d = 2.9 \times 10^{-9}$M, and total binding of 533 fmol/mg melanoma cytosol protein. Specificity of binding of $^3$H dexamethasone was shown by failure of androgens, estrogens, or progestins to inhibit the binding equivalent to that of radioinert glucocorticoids. The saturable binding included 7–8S molecular weight species.

The molecular characteristics of the hamster melanoma glucocorticoid receptor were similar to those of glucocorticoid receptors in other animal systems including rat mammary tissue [39]. Having obtained data on the saturability, high affinity binding and unique molecular weight of the glucocorticoid binding component of hamster melanoma, Markland and Horn investigated the biologic response of Syrian hamster melanoma cells in vitro to dexamethasone [34, 40]. Hamster melanoma cells grown in the absence of dexamethasone had a doubling time of 18 hours, whereas hamster melanoma cells grown in a medium containing $10^{-8}$M dexamethasone had a doubling time of 25 hours. Thus both the biochemical and biological evidence from hamster melanomas in vitro, argue in favor of the presence of a glucocorticoid receptor in Syrian hamster melanoma.

Additional studies have also suggested the possibility of an estrogen receptor in hamster melanoma. Snyder and Das Gupta analyzed hamster melanoma extracts by the dextran coated charcoal assay [41]. The estrogen binding they found in these extracts was saturable, of a high affinity ($K_D = 5.5 \times 10^{-9}$M), with about 35 fmol/mg tumor protein of binding present. Sucrose density gradient analysis was not performed. To test for a biologic response of hamster melanoma, estradiol benzoate, 100 mg per day

366

for three weeks, was administered to female hamsters previously inoculated with melanoma. Estradiol treated hamsters had a 50% increase in melanoma weight as compared to oil injected controls ($p<0.05$) [41]. Other studies previously cited suggested a biologic response of Syrian hamster melanoma to estrogen in vivo and in vitro [30, 31].

In summary, although there is evidence of a true glucocorticoid receptor in Syrian hamster melanoma by dextran coated charcoal and sucrose density gradient assays, there are conflicting reports on the presence of a biologic response of Syrian hamster melanoma cells to glucocorticoid in in vivo and in vitro studies [31, 34]. In addition to the discrepancies regarding the pattern of the biologic response among Syrian hamster melanoma to estrogen in vivo and in vitro, there are conflicting results from biochemical studies on the possible presence of an estrogen receptor [30, 31, 34, 41].

## C. Steroid receptors in human melanoma

Studies reporting the apparent presence of estrogen receptors in human melanoma preceded many of the studies of estrogen receptor in B16 mouse melanoma [34, 35, 42]. In 1976, Fischer, Neifeld and Lippman reported that 16 of 35 patients (46%) with melanoma had apparent estrogen receptor activity in biopsy specimens [42]. They used a dextran-coated charcoal assay to analyze cytosol prepared from histopathologically confirmed melanoma biopsies. The presence of estrogen receptor protein was considered positive when there was $\geqq 5$ fmol of estrogen binding protein per mg of cytosol protein. Their Scatchard analyses of the DCCA data apparently yielded straight lines suggestive of a single class of saturable estrogen binding sites. From the Scatchard analysis of the binding data the $K_D$ was $4.9 \times 10^{-9}$M. The 46% of patients whose biopsied melanomas contained >5 fmol of estrogen binding were nearly equally distributed among the sexes and positive assays were found among primary lesions, lymph node metastases, skin metastases and visceral metastases. Sucrose density gradient analysis was not performed on these melanoma cytosols.

Further studies by Neifeld, Lippman and Fischer suggested the presence of androgen, progesterone, and glucocorticoid receptors in human melanomas [43]. Again, using a DCCA procedure on melanoma cytosols six of 27 patients had progesterone receptor, and melanoma from five of 26 patients were glucocorticoid receptor positive. A protamine sulfate assay revealed androgen binding activity in five of 30 patients with melanoma. A number of patients had more than one steroid-binding activity present in their melanoma cytosols. The authors reiterated the potential usefulness of a steroid receptor assay which could identify a subset of melanoma patients who might be responsive to endocrine therapy in a manner analogous to the procedure used for breast cancer patients.

Fischer and Lippman expanded their series of melanoma patients whose melanomas were analyzed for specific steroid binding activity using the DCCA procedure [44]. Twenty-six of 77 patients (34%) had estrogen-specific, saturable binding with most patient tumors with detectable estrogen binding containing between five and 35 fmol/mg melanoma cytosol protein. Progesterone binding was detected in 19 of 58 patients (33%) and androgen binding in 15 of 57 patients (26%). Fisher and Lippman noted that the binding components had not been analyzed by the SDGA and remarked "for these reasons it is probably not completely justified to refer to these binding components as 'receptors'" [44].

Chaudhuri et al. (1979) investigated steroid receptor in cloned human melanoma cell lines in vitro, testing for correlations between the presence of a particular steroid receptor and the biologic response to that steroid [45]. A dextran coated charcoal technique was used to analyze the cytosols. Positive hormone binding was considered $\geq 3$ fmol/mg protein. Three out of the six cloned cell lines contained saturable, high affinity, specific estrogen and progesterone binding, while a 4th cell line was positive for estrogen binding alone. Calculated $K_D$ from the Scatchard plot for the steroid binding was in physiologic range of $10^{-10}$–$10^{-9}$M. Two out of the six cell lines did not contain specific estrogen or progesterone binding. No cell lines showed androgen binding. Several of the cell lines were then analyzed for their response to steroid hormones in the culture medium. A melanoma cell line which lacked any estrogen and progesterone binding activity did not respond to estradiol, progesterone or testesterone in the culture medium. Based on cell counts, two cell lines which were positive for specific estrogen and progesterone binding showed an apparent increased growth response to $10^{-9}$–$10^{-12}$M estradiol and a decrease growth response to $10^{-6}$–$10^{-12}$M progesterone. However, one cell line which was positive for specific estrogen and progesterone binding showed an increased growth response to the same concentrations of progesterone. Chaudhuri et al. interpreted the data as suggesting the presence of saturable, high affinity, specific estrogen and progesterone receptors in cell lines of human melanoma, but realized that the mere presence of such receptors in a melanoma does not necessarily predict the biologic response (in this case increased or decreased growth) of the melanoma to the specific steroid hormone [45].

When cytosols from human melanomas were evaluated for the presence of estrogen and progesterone binding using both the dextran coated charcoal technique (DCCA) and the sucrose density gradient procedure, seven out of 20 melanoma tumors examined had >3 fmol/mg cytosol protein of specifically inhibitable estrogen binding by DCCA [29]. For these seven tumors with >3 fmol/mg cytosol protein of estrogen binding the $K_D$ was calculated to be between $3.3 \times 10^{-9}$M and $1.5 \times 10^{-10}$M. None of these 20 tumors showed evidence of saturable, high affinity binding specific for progesterone in the DCCA. Furthermore sucrose density gradient analyses of the melanoma cytosols showed poor patterns without distinct 8S estrogen binding. A partially inhibitable (~2.2S) peak was consistently observed in those cytosols in which measurable estrogen binding of more than 4 fmol/mg was present as assessed by the DCCA.

Because of this finding purified tryosinase was subjected to the dextran coated charcoal and sucrose density gradient analyses to evaluate its ability to bind estrogens. Scatchard analyses of the DCCA data showed an apparent estrogen binding of 297 fmol/0.01 mg purified tryosinase. The tryosinase-estradiol binding gave the appearance of high affinity ($K_D = 10^{-9}M$), and specifically inhibition by diethylstilbestrol. Sucrose density gradient analysis of estradiol binding to purified tryosinase revealed a partially inhibitable 2.2S peak which resembled the SDGA pattern of estradiol binding in human melanoma cytosol. Furthermore, the addition of L-DOPA to the estradiol/purified tryosinase DCCA incubation led to a concentration dependent inhibition of the observed binding of estradiol to tyosinase. In contrast L-DOPA did not inhibit binding of estradiol to partially purified uterine estrogen receptor.

The concept that the apparent binding of estrogen in melanoma might be due to a protein other than a steroid receptor was supported by the findings that (1) estrogen binding analysis of purified tyrosinase revealed an inhibitable, high affinity, estrogen specific binding closely resembling that seen in human melanoma, (2) none of the five amelanotic melanoma cytosols studied had estradiol binding, (3) L-DOPA inhibited the estradiol binding to melanoma cytosol but did not inhibit estradiol binding to uterine estrogen receptor and (4) the SDGA of estradiol-tyrosinase binding closely resembled the SDGA pattern for estradiol melanoma cytosol binding. It was suggested that the resemblance of the A ring of estradiol to tyrosine might allow for recognition of estradiol by tyrosinase [29].

The study of steroid receptors in human melanoma is in its early phases. Preliminary studies suggest the presence of estrogen binding in 34–46% of human melanoma [42–44]. The reports on the presence of progesterone receptors in melanoma are conflicting [29, 44]. Recent studies using SDGA suggest the possibility that the apparent estrogen binding in human melanoma may represent an interfering substance mimicking receptor, but do not exclude the possibility of estrogen receptor protein in melanoma. The possibility of a catechol-estrogen effect on these tumors has also been raised [29].

## D. *Clinical studies with hormone therapy*

Fisher, Young and Lippman studied the therapeutic effectiveness of diethylstilbestrol in the treatment of surgically nonresectable melanoma [44, 46].

Twenty-four patients with nonresectable melanoma and clinically measurable disease were entered in the study. Only males and postmenopausal females were selected for the study (21 males, three females). Melanoma biopsies from each patient were obtained and analyzed for steroid receptor. Estrogen binding was present in five of 24 (21%) patients while progesterone binding was present in eight of 22 (36%) of the patients. The patients were treated with DES 5 mg P.O./t.i.d. for a minimum of six weeks or until the disease progressed. Two out of the 24 patients showed objective responses to this treatment. Melanoma biopsies from these two responders had *not* demonstrated estrogen or progesterone binding activity. According to the authors, the lack of estrogen receptor activity among responders suggested that the DES may have an indirect mode of action upon the regression of melanoma [44, 46].

Nesbit et al. (1979) treated 26 patients with tamoxifen. The five women and 21 men received 20–40 mg/day of tamoxifen [47]. Four of 26 patients (14%) had a complete or partial response to tamoxifen treatment. One 83-year-old woman had complete regression of five subcutaneous nodules while being treated with 20 mg tamoxifen b.i.d. The tamoxifen was discontinued after 12 weeks due to alopecia but the patient remained disease free at one year follow-up. These tumors, however, had not been analyzed for estrogen receptor.

Karakbusis et al. studied the correlation of estrogen receptor status of patients with stage IV melanoma with clinical response to tamoxifen [48]. Seventeen patients (six males, 11 females) whose melanomas had been assayed for estrogen receptor were treated with 20 mg tamoxifen P.O./t.i.d. Of the 17 patients studied, seven had positive estrogen receptor activity ($\geq 5$ fmol/mg protein). Three out of the 17 patients had objective remission. All three responders were females. One responder had estrogen binding of 19 fmol/mg protein, a second had a level of 4.3 fmol/mg protein. The third responder did not have detectable estrogen receptor activity.

Until the sex steroid binding observed in human melanoma is more fully characterized, clinical studies correlating the response to endocrine therapy to estrogen receptor status should be interpreted cautiously.

## IV. Peptide hormones and melanoma

The regulation of melanogenesis and melanocyte cell growth by MSH has been elucidated on a molecular level in Cloudman S91 mouse melanoma cells in vitro [49]. MSH effects appear to be cAMP mediated. MSH binding is associated with (1) increased intracellular cAMP; (2) increased tyrosinase activity; (3) inhibition of cell growth; and (4) morphologic changes in wild type mouse melanoma cells capable of responding to MSH [49]. ACTH and corticosterone are also implicated in control of melanoma cell function [50]. Several experiments exploiting the peptide hormone-induced responses among mouse melanoma cells in vitro have been conducted on both in vivo and in vitro animal systems, and studies have been proposed for human melanoma [49].

## A. *MSH—in vitro and in vivo effects*

Cultured mammalian melanoma cells have been used extensively in the study of gene regulation in eukaryotic cells. The advantages of such systems include: (1) quantifiable tyrosinase activity; (2) the availability of amelanotic mutants and (3) large numbers of melanoma cells which can be generated [49]. Mouse melanoma cells demonstrate increased intracellular cAMP within minutes of exposure to MSH and, after a lag phase of 6–9 hours, show an increased tyrosinase activity followed by increased melanin content [49, 51]. MSH activates adenylate cyclase in membrane preparations from mouse melanoma [52]. Activation of adenyl cyclase by MSH is lowered by calcium chelators and restored by calcium, a finding common to peptide hormone activation of cyclase in other tissues [52]. It appears that MSH causes an increase in tyrosinase activity and melaninization by elevated intracellular cAMP. Further support for this relationship of cAMP to melanin production comes from the observation of tyrosinase activity and melaninization in mouse melanoma following exposure to cAMP elevating chemical agents. These include: (1) cAMP; (2) cAMP analogues; (3) methyl xanthine; (4) prostaglandin E1; and (5) cholera toxin [49, 51–54].

An important issue is whether or not RNA transcription and/or translation is necessary for the increased tyrosinase activity caused by MSH via cAMP. Nonsynchronized Cloudman mouse melanoma cells were exposed to MSH for 24 hours followed by removal of MSH from the culture medium. Tyrosinase activity was assayed from 0–48 hours. Cycloheximide inhibited the response to MSH regardless as to whether the cells were exposed to cycloheximide between 0–24 hours *or* 24–48 hours. Actinomycin D inhibited the response to MSH only if the cells were exposed to it within the 0–24 hour period. Pawelek et al. concluded that protein synthesis was continually necessary for the increase in the tyrosinase activity in nonsynchronized melanoma cells following MSH exposure and furthermore, that genetic expression was required [51]. However, further studies on synchronized Cloudman melanoma cell cultures have yielded conflicting results [55].

When Cloudman melanoma cells were synchronized using colchicine, neither cycloheximide nor actinomycin D inhibited the increased tyrosinase activity following MSH stimulation. There was no difference in the intracellular concentration of tyrosinase between control cells and cells exposed to MSH. Crude extracts of melanoma cells not exposed to MSH lowered tyrosinase activity when added to extracts of MSH treated cells. On the basis of these and other observations, Wong and Pawelek suggested that MSH might act to increase tyrosinase activity via cAMP by inactivation of an enzyme inhibitor at the post-translational level. Such regulation would not require transcription or protein synthesis [55].

Fuller and Viskochil found that both cycloheximide and actinomycin D inhibited the increase in tyrosinase activity in melanoma cells following stimulation by (1) MSH, (2) dibutyl cAMP and (3) theophylline [54]. To further study the cellular site of action of MSH via cAMP in increasing tyrosinase activity, double labelling experiments were performed. Melanoma cells were cultured for four days in $^3$H leucine followed by a 30 hour incubation with $^{14}$C leucine with or without MSH. Purified tyrosinase from cells treated with MSH had a $^{14}$C leucine to $^3$H leucine ratio which was greater than in cells not treated with MSH. This suggested that MSH promoted de novo synthesis of tyrosinase, a conclusion inconsistent with the post-translational regulatory model proposed by Wong and Pawelek [54, 55]. Additional studies will be required to illuminate the role of transcriptional and translational control in the MSH stimulated increase in tyrosinase activity in the mouse melanoma model.

In order to assess cell cycle specificity of the response of melanoma cells to MSH, Wong et al. studied the effects of MSH on tyrosinase activity and cAMP levels in colchicine synchronized mouse melanoma cells. Following incubation with MSH, maximal tyrosinase activity and maximal cAMP levels were found to correspond only to the G2 phase of the cell cycle [56].

Varga et al. studied the plasma membrane receptor for MSH among mouse melanoma cells [57]. The MSH receptor was localized to the cell surface. MSH linked covalently to Sepharose beads stimulated tyrosinase activity in the same manner as free MSH. $^{125}$I labeled MSH binding experiments performed using sucrose density gradient analysis revealed that the major part of radiolabeled MSH binding occurred in the plasma membrane fraction of melanoma cells. The receptor was saturable, with $10^4$ sites per cell, had a $K_A = 3 \times 10^8$ l/m and was sensitive to proteolysis. Significantly, colchicine synchronized mouse melanoma cells displayed the majority of radiolabeled MSH binding in G2 [57]. When considered in light of the earlier studies showing maximal MSH sensitive tyrosinase activity occurring also in G2, it appeared as though the mouse melanoma cells were regulating melaninization and sensitivity to MSH by increasing available MSH receptors in the G2 phase of the cell cycle [56, 57]. Varga et al. provided further support for this theory by showing that colchicine synchronized mouse melanoma cells respond to exogenous cAMP continually throughout the entire cell cycle suggesting therefore that the availability of the MSH receptor was the regulating factor [57].

In studies using synchronization techniques other than colchicine the findings are in conflict with the data of Varga et al. and Wong et al. Fuller and Brooks studied synchronized mouse melanoma cells by the percent labeled mitoses (PLM) technique which obviates the need for colchicine treatment of cells [58]. Their results showed that melanoma cells synchronized in this manner were continuously sensitive to MSH throughout the cell cycle as monitored by increased tyrosinase activity. Moreover, cycloheximide inhibited the response to MSH in the PLM synchronized cells, whereas it did not inhibit the MSH response in colchicine synchronized cells [55, 58]. Fuller and Brooks suggested that colchicine may alter the normal metabolism of the mouse melanoma cells leading to differences in MSH sensitivity among colchicine synchronized vs. PLM synchronized melanoma cells.

Not only does MSH exert an effect on tyrosinase activity and melanization, but it appears also to influence melanoma cell growth and morphology. Wong and Pawelek reported that Cloudman S91 melanoma cells exposed to MSH for three days became flattened and dendritic, and there is no further increase in DNA content or cell number in MSH exposed vs. control melanoma cells [59]. Exposure to cAMP could mimic the MSH induced growth and morphological changes.

Further experiments using various melanoma mutants investigated the relationship between the MSH induced changes in tyrosinase activity, growth and morphology [60]. Two mutant melanoma cell types which grew despite the presence of MSH were selected out, amel-1 and mel-1. These two mutants differed in that one was melanotic, one amelanotic. Three Cloudman S91 mouse melanoma cell types were utilized for study: (1) *wild type* melanoma which had MSH inducible tyrosinase activity, as well as MSH inducible inhibition of cell growth; (2) a *mel-1* melanoma mutant variant which was amelanotic in the absence of MSH but became melanotic in the presence of MSH; (3) a *amel-1* melanoma mutant which was amelanotic even in the presence of MSH. MSH inhibited cell growth in wild type cells but had no effect on continual cell growth among the mel-1 and amel-1 mutants as expected. Wild type cells had high values for basal tyrosine activity which could be even further increased by exposure to MSH or cAMP. Mutant amel-1 had very low basal tyrosinase levels which did not increase upon MSH or cAMP stimulation. Mutant mel-1 had low basal tyrosinase levels which increased strikingly upon stimulation by MSH or cAMP. This loss of basal tyrosinase activity in the mel-1 mutant was unexpected, because the mel-1 mutant was originally selected only for its resistance to MSH inhibition of growth. This finding implied that the control of basal tyrosinase activity and the MSH control of growth were somehow related.

MSH and cAMP caused the wild type melanoma cells to flatten and become dendritic in morphology. Although MSH and cAMP caused increased tyrosinase activity and melanization in the mel-1 mutant, there were no changes in morphology. It appeared that the MSH effects on growth, morphology and basal tyrosinase levels were regulated by a mechanism separate from the induction of tyrosinase activity by MSH [60]. In summary, MSH increases levels of intracellular cAMP, promoting increased tyrosinase activity, melanization, inhibition of growth and characteristic morphological changes. However, mutant studies have shown that the underlying regulatory processes governing MSH inducible tyrosinase activity are different from the processes regulating growth and morphologic responses to MSH. Growth and morphological responses to MSH, while not related to MSH inducible tyrosinase activity, are related to basal tyrosinase activity. Pawelek suggested that these vairous mutants may lack certain cAMP dependent protein kinases. For example, one protein kinase might be involved in regulating growth, morphology and basal tyrosinase activity, while a distinct protein kinase might control MSH inducible tyrosinase activity. In fact, there is some evidence for different patterns of protein phosphorylation between wild type and mutant melanoma cells [49].

Although MSH inhibits the growth of melanoma cells in vitro, it has not shown significant pharmacologic inhibition of mouse melanoma growth in vivo [49, 61]. Melanomas from MSH treated mice showed a large increase in tyrosinase activity compared to control mice, whereas tumor weights of MSH treated and untreated mice were similar [61].

The metastatic potential of various melanoma cell lines in vivo have been studied with respect to MSH control of melaninization and growth. Inducible tyrosinase activity and cell growth inhibition was measured in three types of B16 mouse melanoma cell cultures which differed in their propensity to form pulmonary metastases in mice [62]. The three melanoma cell lines included (1) $B16\text{-}F_1$ low metastatic potential, (2) $B16\text{-}F_5$ intermediate metastatic potential, and (3) $B16\text{-}F_{10}$ high metastatic potential. The three cell types were exposed to MSH for 48 hours and tyrosinase activity and cell growth measured. Compared to controls, MSH caused an 11.8-fold increase in tyrosinase activity ($p<0.005$) and a 35% inhibition of cell growth ($p<0.05$) in $F_1$ cells of low metastatic potential. On the other hand, MSH caused only a 1.5-fold increase in tyrosinase activity ($p<0.05$) and an insignificant 3% inhibition of cell growth among $F_{10}$ cells of high metastatic potential. $F_5$ cells responded to MSH with intermediate levels of tyrosinase activity and cell growth inhibition. Apparently, the loss of regulatory control of melaninization and growth by MSH correlated with the increased invasive and metastatic potential of the various B16 mouse melanoma cell lines [62]. Further studies on these metastatic variants showed that as melanoma cells became more metastatic they showed progressive decreases in the peak endogenous cAMP level generated by exposure to MSH [63].

Although all three metastatic variants responded to MSH by elevating cAMP levels, there were significant quantitative differences. For example, $F_1$ low metastatic potential cells had a 3.6-fold higher cyclic AMP level than $F_{10}$ high metastatic potential cells after both types of cells were exposed to 0.2 $\mu$g MSH/ml. Similar quantitative differences in cAMP levels were found between the metastatic variants following ACTH exposure [63]. As is the case with other tumors and biochemical markers, it appears that as melanoma cells become more aggressive in terms of invasiveness and metastatic potential they tend to lose metabolic control mechanisms [62, 63].

Before leaving the topic of MSH and melaninization in melanoma it is important from a chemotherapeutic approach to review the cytotoxicity of melanin precursors to melanoma cells. Hochstein and Cohen proposed a cytotoxic mechanism of action for the phenolic and quinoid intermediates in the conversion of tyrosine to melanin upon the melanoma cell [64]. These phenolic agents were postulated to auto-oxidize, forming hydrogen peroxide which subsequently inactivates sulfhydryl dependent enzymes such as glyceraldehyde 3-phosphate dehydrogenase resulting in inhibition of glycolysis. The melanocyte protects itself from self destruction by a glucose linked glutathione peroxidase pathway whereby hydrogen peroxide is eliminated by oxidation of reduced glutathione. The protective levels of reduced glutathione are dependent on the presence of glucose. Studies showed that tyrosine exerted a cytotoxic effect (decreased rate of anaerobic glycolysis) upon melanoma cells in vitro when the cells were deprived of glucose. The tyrosine cytotoxic effect was abolished by the addition of excess glucose. Hochstein and Cohen suggested that this theory might be applied as a rational basis for chemotherapy in melanoma [64].

Lerner reiterated the cytotoxic effects of phenolic compounds upon melanocytes [65]. He emphasized the concept that the greater the pigment producing activity of a melanocyte, the less likely its chances for survival and cited clinical conditions such as vitiligo and Addison's disease to support his theory of self destruction. Vitiligo often occurs in those areas of the skin that were at one time hyperpigmented. In Addison's disease the increased levels of ACTH lead to skin darkening, and these same patients are more susceptible to vitiligo (hypopigmentation). He postulated that tyrosine or other phenolic intermediates became cytotoxic when normal protective mechanisms are disrupted. Interestingly, Lerner suggested that MSH and cAMP, by darkening melanocytes, should make cells more sensitive to phenol cytotoxicity [65].

Pawelek et al. studied the effects of tyrosine on the growth of melanoma cells in vivo and in vitro [51]. Tyrosine had selective toxicity for melanotic mouse melanoma cells in vitro, having little effect on amelanotic mouse melanoma cells. Mice, injected with melanotic melanoma cells and placed on a four-week diet of chow containing 33% tyrosine, had a 2–5-fold reduction in tumor size as compared to melanoma injected mice on a control diet ($p = 0.05$). Moreover, daily injection of MSH resulted in an even greater tumor size reduction among mice on the high tyrosine diet [51].


## B. *ACTH and melanoma*

The first 13 N-terminal amino acid residues of ACTH are identical to $\alpha$ MSH. ACTH appears to influence melanoma metabolism in a fashion similar to MSH. Although cAMP is involved, the modulation of tyrosinase by ACTH in vivo appears to require glucocorticoids [50, 66]. Other peptide hormones including prolactin, GH, LH and TSH have not been shown to influence tyrosinase activity in melanoma [67].

Abramowitz and Chavin studied the role of ACTH and corticosterone in melanogenesis in Cloudman S91 melanoma in vitro. They utilized cell suspensions in synthetic media to reduce experimental errors associated with contaminant naturally occurring hormones in the serum used for standard in vitro studies [66]. Tyrosinase activity was determined as melanoma cells were exposed to hormones for fairly brief periods. ACTH and corticosterone together, tyrosinase activity increased to a peak at 15 min (4.4X control, $p<0.01$), declined somewhat between 15–30 min and increased steadily thereafter. Cyclic AMP levels peaked at 15 in (19.6X control, $p<0.01$) and returned to control levels by 30 min. This study elucidated several points and raised several questions: (1) the possibility that serum included in the culture media for mouse melanoma experiments in the past may have contained significant concentrations of endogenous ACTH and corticosterone; (2) although ACTH alone led to increased levels of cAMP it did not lead to an increase in tyrosinase activity; (3) the cAMP peak generated by ACTH and corticosterone was quantitatively nearly four times as large as the cAMP peak following ACTH treatment alone; and (4) melanoma in vivo is exposed to both ACTH and corticosterone, since the former promotes the adrenal output of the latter. Abramowitz and Chavin suggested that corticosterone may have a permissive effect upon melanoma cell growth and development [66].

ACTH, corticosterone, cAMP *and* cFMP all influenced tyrosinase activity in Harding-Passey mouse melanoma in vitro [50]. Although ACTH and corticosterone combined hormone treatment results in an increase in tyrosinase activity correlated with increased melanin content in B16, Cloudman S91 and Harding-Passey murine melanomas in vitro, the same hormonal treatment does not lead to an increase in peroxidase activity. Tyrosinase rather than peroxidase appears to be the enzyme of physiologic importance in melanogenesis [68].

## C. *Peptide hormones and human melanoma*

Several studies suggest that human melanoma cell lines in vitro can respond to MSH, cAMP, theophylline and prostaglandin $E_1$ as demonstrated by increased tyrosinase activity [69, 70]. Few studies have measured serum levels of these peptide hormones in patients with melanoma. One such study measured serum levels of the $\alpha$-subunit of the glycoprotein hormones (FSH, LH, TSH and HCG) in patients with metastatic melanoma. Alpha subunit levels were measured before, during and after chemoimmunotherapy in 55 patients with metastatic melanoma. Ten of 20 premenopausal female patients had elevated pretreatment serum $\alpha$-subunit levels (>2.3 ng/ml) whereas the other ten premenopausal females had normal pretreatment $\alpha$-subunit levels. There was a statistically significant reduction in survival among premenopausal melanoma patients with elevated pretreatment $\alpha$-subunit levels as compared to premenopausal melanoma patients with normal pretreatment $\alpha$-subunit levels, with median survivals of 19 weeks and 83 weeks, respectively ($p = 0.015$). The apparent association between elevated $\alpha$-subunit levels and survival in patients with metastatic melanoma could not be explained by transient ovulatory increases in $\alpha$-subunit levels [71].

Pregnancy associated $\alpha_2$ glycoprotein ($\alpha_2$ PAG) is a high molecular weight glycoprotein with an unknown biologic function. Serum levels of $\alpha_2$ PAG have been correlated with the stage of disease in breast and bronchial carcinoma. In a case control study of 97 melanoma patients and 97 healthy controls, it was found that serum $\alpha_2$ PAG levels increased with advancing clinical stage of disease. This increase in $\alpha_2$ PAG levels as disease progressed was most striking in female patients. Female patients with stage III melanoma had a mean $\alpha_2$ PAG level of 6.42 mg% compared to 3.07 mg% for patients with Stage I disease ($p<0.001$). Bauer et al. suggested the possible role of $\alpha_2$ PAG as a screening test to monitor melanoma [72].

Local or systemic factors may be implicated in the activation of nevi in patients with melanoma [73]. Tucker et al. (1980) examined 48 nevi from patients with melanoma and compared them histopathologically with 100 nevi from patients without melanoma. Nevi were scored for activation based on the presence of activated junctional nests of melanocytes, lack of margination of junctional nests, inflammatory infiltration, increased pigmentation, mitotic activity and cytologic atypia. Nevi from melanoma patients had higher activation scores than nevi from controls. Furthermore, considering only nevi from melanoma patients, nevi taken from areas within the lymph drainage area of the primary melanoma had higher activation scores than nevi located outside the area. The data suggested the operation of exogenous or endogenous systemic factors which activated nevi in melanoma patients or the release of local factors from the melanoma which might activate nevi in adjacent regions.

## V. Summary

The epidemiologic, laboratory and clinical evidence for steroid and peptide hormone influence on melanoma have been reviewed. The epidemiologic studies of melanoma suggest that males, postmenopausal females and nulliparous women have poorer survival as compared to females, premenopausal females and multiparous women respectively. Studies on the effects of pregnancy and oral contraceptives either show a worse prognosis or the same prognosis in populations of pregnant patients or those who used oral contraceptives as compared to nonpregnant or non-pill users with melanoma. Several animal model melanomas appear to contain cytoplasmic steroid receptors as well as showing responsivity to steroids. The presence of estrogen receptors in human melanoma has not been conclusively established and various forms of endocrine surgery and chemotherapy have not favorably altered the clinical course of melanoma. The interaction of MSH and ACTH with melanoma is being established on a molecular level. Further research into the endocrine aspects of melanoma may eventually lead to the design of improved treatment modalities for subpopulations of melanoma patients (e.g. those with positive steroid receptors, although this remains to be shown.

## References

1. White LP: Studies on melanoma. II: sex and survival in human melanoma. N Engl J Med 260:789-797, 1959.
2. MacDonald E: Epidemiology of melanoma. Ann N Y Acad Sci 100:4-15, 1963.
3. Nathanson L, Hall TC and Fiarber S: Biological aspects of human malignant melanoma. Cancer 20:650-655, 1967.
4. Shaw HM, Milton GW, Farago G and McCarthy WH: Endocrine influences on survival from malignant melanoma. Cancer 42:669-677, 1978.
5. Myhre E. Malignant melanoma in children. Acta Pathol Microbiol Scand 59:184-188, 1963.
6. Pack GT: Prepubertal melanoma of the skin. Surg 86:374-375, 1948.
7. Skov-Jensen T, Hastrup J and Lambrethsen E: Malignant melanoma in children. Cancer 19:620-626, 1966.
8. Coffey RJ and Berkeley WT: Prepubertal malignant melanoma. J Am Med Assoc 147:846-849, 1951.
9. Dobson L: Pububertal malignant melanoma. Am J Surg 89:1128-1135, 1955.
10. Haagland PW and Hughes CW: Melanocarcinoma of childhood. Arch Surg 81:957-960, 1960.
11. Wright RB, Clark DH and Milne JA: Malignant cutaneous melanoma: a review. Br J Surg 40:360-368, 1953.
12. Hersey P, Stone DE, Milton GW, Morgan G and McCarthy WH: Previous pregnancy as a protective factor against death from melanoma. Lancet 1:451-452, 1977.
13. Pack GT and Scharnagel IM: The prognosis for malignant melanoma in the pregnant woman. Cancer 4:324-334, 1951.

14. Hedley JA: A case of malignant melanoma in pregnancy. J Obstet Gynaecol Br Commonw 59:217–219, 1952.

15. Byrd BT and McGanity WJ: The effect of pregnancy on the clinical course of malignant melanoma. South Med J 47:196–200, 1954.

16. George PA, Fortner JG and Pack GT: Melanoma with pregnancy. Cancer 4:854–859, 1960.

17. Shiu MH, Schottenfield D, Maclean B and Fortner JG: Adverse effect of pregnancy on melanoma. Cancer 37:181–187, 1976.

18. Ances IG and Pomerantz SH: Serum concentrations of B melanocyte stimulating hormone in human pregnancy. Am J Obstet Gynecol 119:1062–1068, 1974.

19. Hawes WE: Removal of testes in treatment of melanoma. J Am Med Assoc 123:304, 1943.

20. Hawes WE: Castration for advanced malignant growth. Radiology 43:272–274, 1944.

21. Levi JE and Lewison EF: Malignant melanoma in a patient with ovarian agenesis. Case report of prolonged survival. J Clin Endocrinol 12:901–907, 1952.

22. Meyer HW and Gumpert SL: Malignant melanoma. Ann Surg 138:643–658, 1953.

23. Wigley PE and Metz MH: Striking regression of generalized subcutaneous and visceral metastases of malignant melanoma following intensive high voltage roentgen irradiation of the pituitary gland. Am J Roentgenol 41:415–419, 1939.

24. Johnson RO, Bisel H, Andrews N, Wilson W, Nochlin D, Segalaff A, Krementz E, Aust J and Ansfield F: Phase I clinical study of 6-$\alpha$-methylpreg-4-ene-3,11,20-trione. Cancer Chemother Rep 50:671–673, 1966.

25. Ellerbroek WC: Oral contraceptives and melanoma. J Am Med Assoc 206:649–650, 1968.

26. Sadoff L, Winkley J and Tyson S: Is malignant melanoma an endocrine-dependent tumor? Oncology 27:244–257, 1973.

27. Beral V, Ramcharon S and Faris R: Malignant melanoma and oral contraceptive use among women in California. Br J Cancer 36:804–809, 1977.

28. Bodenham DC and Hale B: Malignant melanoma. In: Stoll BA (ed) Endocrine Therapy in Malignant Disease, pp 377–383. WB Saunders, London, 1972.

29. McCarty KS, Jr, Wortman J, Stowers S, Lubahn DB, McCarty KS, Sr and Seigler HT: Sex steroid receptor analysis in melanoma. Cancer 46:157–164, 1980.

30. Lipkin G: Sex factors in growth of malignant melanoma in hamsters in vivo and in vitro correlation. Cancer Res 30:1928–1930, 1970.

31. Walker MJ, Chaudhuri PK, Beattie CW, Tito WA and Das Gupta TK: Neuroendocrine and endocrine correlates to hamster melanoma growth in vitro. Surg Forum 29:151–152, 1978.

32. Proctor T, Auclair BG and Stokowski L: Endocrine factors and the growth and spread of B16 melanoma. J Nat Cancer Inst 57:1197–1198, 1976.

33. Lopez RE, Bhakoo H, Palolini NS, Rosen F, Halyoke ED and Goldrosen MH: Effect of estrogen on the growth of B16 melanoma. Surg Forum 29:153–154, 1978.

34. Markland FS, Jr and Horn D: Steroid hormone receptors in melanoma (in press).

35. Markland FS and Horn D: Malignant melanoma: steroid hormone receptor studies. J Cell Biol 77:194a, 1977.

36. Taft D, Shyamala G and Gorski J: A receptor molecule for estrogen: studies using a cell free system. Proc Natl Acad Sci 57:1740–1743, 1967.

37. Jensen EV and DeSombre ER: Mechanisms of action of the female sex hormones. Ann Rev Biochem 41:203–230, 1972.

38. Bhakoo HS, DiCioccio RA and Rosen F: B16 melanoma: glucocorticoid receptors and the effects of glucocorticoids on tumor growth. Proc Am Assoc Cancer Res 20:201, 1979.

39. Goral JE and Wittliff JL: Comparison of glucocorticoid binding proteins in normal and neoplastic mammary tissues of the rat. Biochemistry 14:2944–2952, 1975.

40. Horn D and Schmidhauser TJ: Inhibition of growth by dexamethasone in Syrian hamster melanoma cell: modulation by BRDU. J Cell Biol 79:193a, 1978.

41. Snyder J and Das Gupta TK: Estrogen receptors in hamster melanoma. Fed Proc Fed Am Soc Exp Biol 36:349, 1977.

42. Tischer RI, Neifeld JP and Lippman ME: Estrogen receptors in human malignant melanoma. Lancet 2:337–338, 1976.

43. Neifeld JP, Lippman ME and Fisher RI: Receptors for steroid hormones in human melanoma. Surg Forum 27:108–109, 1976.

44. Fisher RI and Lippman ME: Stroid receptors in malignant melanoma. In: Thompson EB and Lippman ME (eds) Steroid Receptors and the Managment of Cancer. CRC Press, St. Louis, 1979.

45. Chaudhuri PK, Walker MJ, Beattie CW and Das Gupta TK: Endocrine correlates of human malignant melanoma. J Surg Res 26:214–219, 1979.

46. Fisher RI, Young RC and Lippman ME: Diethylstilbestrol therapy of surgically nonresectable malignant melanoma. Proc Am Soc Clin Oncol 58:339, 1978 (abstract).

47. Nesbit RA, Woods RL, Tattersall MHN and Fox RM: Tamoxifen in malignant melanoma. 301:1241–1242, 1979.

48. Karakousis CP, Lopez R, Bhakoo HS, Rosen F and Moore R: Steroid hormone receptor and tamoxifen treatment in malignant melanoma. Proc Am Soc Clin Oncol 60:345, 1980 (abstract).

49. Pawelek JM: Factors regulating growth and pigmentation of melanoma cells. J Invest Dermatol 66:201–209, 1976.

50. Abramowitz J and Chavin W: Interaction of ACTH, corticosterone, and cyclic nucleotides in Harding-Passey melanoma melanogenesis. Arch Dermatol Res 261:303–309, 1978.

51. Pawelek J, Wong G, Sansone M and Morowitz J: Molecular controls in mammalian pigmentation. Yale J Biol Med 46:430–443, 1973.

52. Kreiner PW, Gold CJ, Keirns JJ, Brooks WA and Betinsky MW: MSH-sensitive adenyl cyclase in the Cloudman melanoma. Yale J Biol Med 46:583–591, 1973.

53. O'Keyle E and Cratrecasas P: Cholera toxin mimics melanocyte stimulating hormone in inducing differentiation in melanoma cells. Proc Natl Acad Sci 71:2500–2504, 1974.

54. Fuller BB and Viskochil DH: The role of RNA and protein synthesis in mediating the action of MSH on mouse melanoma cells. Life Sci 24:2405–2416, 1979.

55. Wong G and Pawelek J: Melanocyte stimulating hormone promotes activation of preexisting tyrosinase molecules in Cloudman S91 melanoma cells. Nature 255:644–646, 1975.

56. Wong G, Pawelek J, Sansone M and Morowitz J: Response of mouse melanoma cells to melanocyte stimulating hormone. Nature 248:351–354, 1974.

57. Varga JM, Depasquale A, Pawelek J, McGuire JS and Lerner AB: Regulation of melanocyte stimulating hormone action at the receptor level: discontinuous binding of hormone to synchronized mouse melanoma cells during the cell cycle. Proc Natl Acad Sci 71:1590–1593, 1974.

58. Fuller BB and Brooks BA: Application of percent labeled mitoses (PLM) analysis to the investigation of melanoma cell responsiveness to MSH stimulation throughout the cell cycle. Exp Cell Res 126:183–190, 1980.

59. Wong G and Pawelek J: Control of cultured melanoma cells by melanocyte stimulating hormone. J Cell Biol 55:288a, 1972.

60. Pawelek J, Sansone M, Koch N, Christie G, Halaban R, Hendee J, Lerner AB and Varga JM: Melanoma cells resistant to inhibition of growth by melanocyte stimulating hormone. Proc Nat Acad Sci 72:951–955, 1975.

61. Lee FH, Lee MS and Lu MY: Effects of a $\alpha$ MSH on melanogenesis and tyrosinase of B-16 melanoma. Endocrinology 91:1180–1188, 1972.

62. Niles RM and Makarski JS: Control of melanogenesis in mouse melanoma cells of varying metastatic potential. J Natl Cancer Inst 61:523–526, 1978.

380

63. Niles RM and Makarski JS: Hormonal activation of adenylate cyclase in mouse melanoma metastatic variants. J Cell Physiol 96:355–360, 1978.

64. Hochstein P and Cohen G: The cytotoxicity of melanin precursors. Ann N Y Acad Sci 100:876–886, 1963.

65. Lerner AB: On the etiology of vitiligo and gray hair. Am J Med 51:141–147, 1971.

66. Abramowitz J and Chavin W: Glucocorticoid modulation of adrenocorticotropin-induced melanogenesis in the Cloudman S91 melanoma in vitro. Exp Cell Biol 46:268–276, 1978.

67. Pomerantz SH and Chuang L: Effects of $\beta$MSH, cortisol, and ACTH on tyrosinase in the skin of newborn hamsters and mice. Endocrinology 87:302–310, 1970.

68. Abramowitz J and Chavin W: In vitro effects of hormonal stimuli upon tyrosinase and peroxidase activates in murine melanomas. Biochem Biophys Res Commun 85:1067–1073, 1978.

69. Fuller BB and Meyskens FL: Endocrine responsiveness of normal and malignant human melanocytes in culture. Proc Am Assoc Cancer Res 20:93, 1979.

70. Warrick HM and Kuckerlapati RS: The regulation of tyrosinase activity in human melanoma cell lines. Yale J Biol Med 50, 1977 (abstract # 145).

71. MacFarlane IA, Thatcher N, Swindell R, Beardwell CG, Hayward E and Crawther D: Serum glycoprotein hormone alpha subunit values and survival in metastatic melanoma patients. Eur J Cancer 15:1497–1501, 1979.

72. Bauer HW, Deutschmann KEM, Peter HH, Bohn H: Pregnancy associated $\alpha_2$ glycoprotein in malignant melanoma. Eur J Cancer 15:123–126, 1979.

73. Tucker SB, Harstmann JP, Hertel B, Aranha G and Rosai J: Activation of nevi in patients with malignant melanoma. Cancer 46:822–827, 1980.

# 13. Chemotherapy of melanoma *

VIRGIL S. LUCAS, Jr. and ANDREW T. HUANG

Melanoma is traditionally managed by surgery. High potential for distant recurrence in disease with invasion of deeper levels of skin have forced the oncologist to look for other effective means of controlling the disease at presentation or at recurrence. Various new treatment modalities have been and are still being tested for their efficacy in melanoma. Chemotherapy for melanoma became active approximately twenty years ago at the time when immunotherapy had begun to be widely employed. The efficacy of chemotherapy, however, has not gained a firm hold in the clinical therapy of melanoma, partly attributable to the lack of effective chemotherapeutic agents or combinations thereof, and partly because of the absence of a comprehensive understanding of pathophysiology of the disease. Presently, chemotherapy is reserved for the patients with progressive, metastatic disease and for those who are symptomatic from their metastatic melanomas. Adjuvant chemotherapy has not been demonstrated to be justified on the basis of reported studies. Chemotherapy interphased with efforts to modulate or modify the immune system of the patient is an attractive approach for metastatic melanoma for the future [5].

In this chapter we will review trials of older single agents, new agents and combination regimens. Also we will discuss adjuvant chemotherapy, chemoimmunotherapy and perfusion chemotherapy trials. Finally new chemotherapeutic approaches will be reviewed.

In reviewing the literature on treatment of melanoma many studies were found to be inadequate in lacking (1) sufficient patient numbers (less than ten evaluable patients); (2) a clear definition of response; (3) information on dosage and (4) definition of patient selection. Studies demonstrating any of these flaws were not included in this review. Also studies using doses of agents significantly less than those accepted currently were not included.

## Single agents

Table 1 outlines the response data of single agents which have been tried in metastatic melanoma. Other drugs, tried in small numbers of patients and

* Supported by NIH grants CA 11265 and CA 14236.

Seigler, H. F. (ed.), Clinical Management of Melanoma. ISBN 978-94-009-7495-1
© 1982, Martinus Nijhoff Publishers, The Hague/Boston/London.

382

*Table 1.* Single agents

| References | Agent | Evaluable patients | Responders | Observed response rate |
|---|---|---|---|---|
| 6,7 | DTIC | 1,188 | 278 | 23.4 |
| 8–14 | Methyl-CCNU | 158 | 24 | 15.2 |
| 15,16 | Pregnentrone (Pregnone) | 155 | 11 | 7.1 |
| 17–23 | Lomustine | 153 | 17 | 11.1 |
| 24–26 | Carmustine | 140 | 24 | 17.1 |
| 27–29 | Piperazinedione | 118 | 6 | 5.0 |
| 30,31 | TMCA | 90 | 13 | 14.4 |
| 101,111,112 | Chlorozotocin | 88 | 11 | 12.5 |
| 32–39 | Hydroxyurea | 86 | 7 | 8.1 |
| 40–42 | Methotrexate (High Dose) | 73 | 10 | 13.7 |
| 43–45 | Dianhydrogalactitol | 68 | 1 | 1.5 |
| 46,47 | Mitomycin–C | 65 | 9 | 13.8 |
| 48–54 | Vinblastine | 58 | 7 | 12.1 |
| 107–110 | Cisplatin | 57 | 9 | 15.8 |
| 87,105,106 | Melphalan | 49 | 8 | 20.0 |
| 55,56 | Vindesine | 47 | 7 | 14.9 |
| 86,104 | Mechlorethamine | 45 | 3 | 7.0 |
| 57–59 | Dibromodulcitol | 43 | 8 | 18.6 |
| 60 | Hexamethylmelamine | 42 | 2 | 4.8 |
| 61,62 | Bleomycin | 40 | 1 | 2.5 |
| 96,110 | ICRF-159 | 37 | 0 | 0 |
| 63,64 | Doxorubicin | 32 | 0 | 0 |
| 75–71 | Cyclophosphamide | 32 | 4 | 12.5 |
| 72,73 | Dectinomycin | 30 | 0 | 0 |
| 113 | AMSA | 30 | 2 | 6.5 |
| 74–76 | 6-Mercaptopurine | 29 | 2 | 6.9 |
| 77 | Cyclocytidine | 29 | 1 | 3.4 |
| 78,79 | Cytosine Arabinoside | 27 | 3 | 11.1 |
| 80 | Estramustine P04 | 26 | 1 | 3.8 |
| 81-85 | Vincristine | 26 | 3 | 11.0 |
| 86,88,104 | Thio-TEPA | 24 | 5 | 20.8 |
| 92 | Chlorambucil | 22 | 2 | 9.1 |
| 93 | Pyrazofuran | 21 | 0 | 0 |
| 94 | VM-26 | 21 | 0 | 0 |
| 95 | 5-Fluorouracil | 20 | 1 | 5.0 |
| 43 | VP16-213 | 19 | 0 | 0 |
| 97,98 | Streptozotocin | 19 | 2 | 10.5 |
| 87,89-91 | TEPA | 16 | 3 | 18.8 |
| 99,100 | 5-Azacytidine | 16 | 3 | 18.8 |
| 102,103 | Methotrexate (Low Dose) | 13 | 2 | 15.4 |

too insufficient to give meaningful response data, were not included in this table.

Bellet et al. in an excellent review of melanoma chemotherapy published in 1978 ranked many of these agents into four categories based on their true response rates (TRR) [1]. Dacarbazine (DTIC) was the only agent of which the TRR was greater than 20% and was classified as effective. Carmustine (BCNU), seumustine (methyl CCNU) and thiophosphoramide (Thio-Tepa) were classified as clinically useful (>95% probability of TRR >10%). Trimethylcolchicinic acid (TMCA), triethylenemelamine (TEPA), melphlan, dibromodulcitol (DBD), mitomycin-C (mito-c) and methotrexate (MTX) were listed as potentially useful (80–94.9% probability of TRR>10%). Agents determined as probably not useful (50–79.9% probability of TRR>10%) were cyclophosphamide (CTX), vinblastine (VLB), vincristine (VCR), TIC-mustard, lomustine (CCNU), cytarabine (ARA-C), streptozotocin and chlorambucil. Inactive agents (less than 50% probability of TRR >10%) include mercaptopurine (6-MP), fluorouracil (5-FU), hydroxyurea, hexamethylemelamine (HMM), ICRF-159, pregnane, bleomycin, mechlorethamine (HN2), dactinomycin and doxorubicin.

*Table 2.* Classification of single agents

| Status | Agent | Evaluable patients | Objective responders | Observed response rate | Probability of TRR >10% |
|---|---|---|---|---|---|
| 1 | DBD | 43 | 8 | 18.6 | 98.0 |
| | Cisplatin | 57 | 9 | 15.8 | 95.0 |
| | Melphalan | 49 | 8 | 20.0 | 95.0 |
| | 5-Azacytidine | 16 | 3 | 18.8 | 93.0 |
| 2 | Vindesine | 47 | 7 | 14.9 | 91.0 |
| | Methotrexate (High Dose) | 73 | 10 | 13.7 | 89.0 |
| 3 | Chlorozotocin | 88 | 11 | 12.5 | 83.0 |
| | AMSA | 30 | 2 | 6.5 | 41.0 |
| | Mechlorethamine | 45 | 3 | 7.0 | 32.9 |
| | Cyclocytidine | 29 | 1 | 3.4 | 19.9 |
| | VP16-213 | 19 | 0 | 0 | 10.0 |
| 4 | Pyrazofuran | 21 | 0 | 0 | 10.0 |
| | VM-26 | 21 | 0 | 0 | 10.0 |
| | Piperazinedione | 118 | 6 | 5.0 | 4.3 |
| | Dianhydrogalactitol | 68 | 1 | 1.5 | 6.06 |

TRR = True Response Rate
Status: 1 = Clinically useful (>95% probability of TRR >10%)
2 = Potentially useful (80–94% probability of TRR >10%)
3 = Probably not useful 50–79.9% probability of TRR >10%)
4 = Inactive (<50% probability of TRR >10%)

384

Several agents listed in Table 1 were not evaluated by Bellet and his co-workers because at that time insufficient number of patients had been treated or the drugs were not available. Table 2 lists these agents and some other drugs listed by Bellet with updated patient numbers. Following some new trials DBD, melphalan and cisplatin have currently been relisted as clinically useful. In the authors' hands DBD has not shown any clinical activity in 12 patients studied. More data are needed to determine if cis-platin and melplan in usual doses are truly useful in melanoma. The use-fulness of agents such as chlorozotocin, high-dose MTX, vindesine, 5-aza-cytidine and other new drugs requires further study.

## Combination chemotherapy

On reviewing combination chemotherapy for melanoma, one finds a myriad of regimens which are similar. It is useful to divide them into eight catego-ries. The first category is made up of regimens containing DTIC and a nitrosourea (Table 3). The second category contains regimens with DTIC, and a nitrosourea (many of these regimens chose BCNU) and vincristine (Table 4). The doses of drugs and stage of disease are similar in studies in category 2 except for data from Beretta et al. [120, 124] in which somewhat lower doses of DTIC were used. Differences in patient selection are also noted. Patients reported by Cohen et al. [118] have mostly subcutaneous disease. Although some studies in these two categories show responses high-er than 30%, the overall observed rate is not significantly higher than that from DTIC alone.

Table 5 shows the third category of combination regimens containing DTIC, a nitrosourea and miscellaneous other agents. It is difficult to com-

*Table 3.* DTIC and nitrosourea

| References | Regimen | Eval pts. | # Res-ponders | ORR % | Prob. of TRR >20% | Comments |
|---|---|---|---|---|---|---|
| 114 | DTIC-BCNU | 61 | 12 | 20 | 0.55 | |
| 115 | DTIC-CCNU | 29 | 7 | 24 | 0.79 | |
| 116 | DTIC-Me-CCNU | 122 | 18 | 14 | 0.88 | |
| 117 | DTIC-Me-CCNU | 21 | 6 | 28.6 | 0.89 | |
| | | 233 | 43 | 18.5 | 0.31 | Totals |

ORR = observed response rate

*Table 4.* DTIC, combinations of nitrosourea and vincristine

| Refer-ences | Regimen | Eval. pts | # Res-ponders | ORR % | Prob. of TRR >20% | Comments |
|---|---|---|---|---|---|---|
| 118 | DTIC-BCNU-VCR | 16 | 10 | 63 | 0.99 | Mostly sub-a disease |
| 119 | DTIC-BCNU-VCR | 40 | 17 | 42.5 | 0.99 | |
| 120 | DTIC-BCNU-VCR | 59 | 16 | 27 | 0.93 | |
| 121 | DTIC-BCNU-VCR | 65 | 15 | 23.1 | 0.78 | |
| 122 | DTIC-BCNU-VCR | 22 | 5 | 22.7 | 0.74 | |
| 123 | DTIC-BCNU-VCR | 20 | 7 | 35 | 0.96 | |
| 124 | DTIC-BCNU-VCR | 129 | 27 | 20.9 | 0.65 | |
| 125 | DTIC-BCNU-VCR | 135 | 31 | 23 | 0.83 | |
| 121 | DTIC-CCNU-VCR | 67 | 11 | 16.4 | 0.29 | |
| 126 | DTIC-Me-CCNU-VCR | 30 | 9 | 30 | 0.94 | |
| | | 599 | 157 | 26 | 0.99 | Totals |

*Table 5.* DTIC combination regimes with nitrosourea and miscellaneous other agents

| Refer-ences | Regimen | Eval pts | # Res-ponders | ORR % | Prob of TRR >20% | Comments |
|---|---|---|---|---|---|---|
| 127 | DTIC-BCNU-HU | 89 | 24 | 27 | 0.96 | |
| 128 | DTIC-BCNU-VCR-Chloropromazine | 127 | 27 | 22 | 0.78 | +Chloropromazine |
| 129 | DTIC-BCNU-VCR-Procarbazine | 25 | 6 | 24 | 0.78 | |
| 124 | DTIC-BCNU-Act-D | 61 | 19 | 31 | 0.98 | |
| 121 | DTIC-BCNU-HU | 63 | 8 | 12.5 | 0.094 | |
| 127 | DTIC-BCNU-HU-VCR | 89 | 27 | 30 | 0.99 | |
| 130 | DTIC-CCNU-Bleo-VCR | 72 | 29 | 40 | 0.99 | |
| | | 520 | 140 | 26.9 | 0.58 | Totals |

ORR = observed response rate

pare among these regimens due to their differences in doses chosen. The overall observed response rates are again not significantly better than those combinations listed in Tables 2–4 or DTIC alone.

DTIC is the most active and the most studied single agent. Many other drugs than those mentioned in categories 1–3 have also been combined with it to attempt to increase the response rate of the tumor. Table 6 shows these combinations (category 4). The overall observed response rate is not different from the combinations which include DTIC and a nitrosourea, or DTIC alone.

As a single agent, cisplatin has shown a response rate of 15.8%. Table 7 shows results of different studies with the combination of DTIC and cisplatin at variable doses (category 5). Studies reported by Karakousis et al. and by Friedman et al. [140, 141] show responses that are greater than DTIC as a single agent. Response rates of the other combination studies, on the contrary, are worse. A careful study of cisplatin-DTIC combination against DTIC alone is mandatory. If this new combination is not found to be more effective than those containing no cisplatin, it should be avoided as the emetogenic side effect in this combination is compounded to the gravest extent.

Table 8 lists miscellaneous combination regimens of category 6. Most of these regimens have too few patients studied. Stages of disease in these patients are also variable. De Wasch et al. [147] report a high response rate of 48.5% in their patients with stage III disease. Contanzi et al. [144] and

*Table 6.* DTIC and miscellaneous other agents

| References | Regimen | Eval pts | # Responders | ORR % | Prob of TRR >20% | Comments |
|---|---|---|---|---|---|---|
| 131 | DTIC (Bom D) Bleo-VCR-MTX | 14 | 5 | 35 | 0.95 | |
| 115 | DTIC-Adria- | 27 | 5 | 18.5 | 0.53 | |
| | DTIC-HU | 28 | 5 | 17.8 | 0.50 | |
| 124 | DTIC-HU-VCR | 84 | 17 | 0.20 | 0.59 | |
| 132 | DTIC-Act-D | 22 | 5 | 22.7 | 0.73 | |
| 133 | DTIC-VCR | 18 | 4 | 22.2 | 0.71 | |
| 134 | DTIC-Act-D | 69 | 14 | 20 | 0.59 | |
| 135 | DTIC-CTX | 17 | 3 | 17.6 | 0.55 | |
| 136 | DTIC-CTX | 51 | 7 | 14 | 0.17 | |
| | DTIC-CTX-Dip | 46 | 9 | 20 | 0.56 | |
| 137 | DTIC-HMM | 16 | 2 | 12.5 | 0.35 | |
| 138 | DTIC-VCR | 16 | 6 | 37.5 | 0.97 | |
| 9 | DTIC-VLB | 34 | 6 | 18 | 0.47 | |
| | DTIC-Procarb | 29 | 7 | 24 | 0.79 | |
| | DTIC-CTX | 32 | 4 | 13 | 0.20 | |
| 10 | DTIC-VCR | 18 | 2 | 11.1 | | |
| | | 503 | 99 | 19.6 | 0.45 | Totals |

*Table 7.* DTIC and cisplatin

| References | Regimen (DDP Dosage) | Eval pts | # Responders | ORR % | Prob of TRR >20% | Comments |
|---|---|---|---|---|---|---|
| 139 | DTIC-DDP (40 mg/m$^2$) | 20 | 2 | 10 | 0.21 | |
| 140 | DTIC-DDP (40 mg/m$^2$) | 16 | 6 | 42.5 | 0.97 | |
| | DTIC-DDP-Procarbazine (40 mg/m$^2$) | 13 | 2 | 15.4 | 0.50 | |
| 141 | DTIC-DDP (75 mg/m$^2$) | 18 | 6 | 33 | 0.95 | |
| 107 | DTIC-DDP (15 mg/m$^2$ × 5 days) | 11 | 1 | 9 | 0.32 | |
| | | 78 | 17 | 21.7 | 0.71 | Totals |

*Table 8.* Combination miscellaneous agents

| References | Regimen | Eval pts | # Responders | ORR % | Prob TRR >20% | Comments |
|---|---|---|---|---|---|---|
| 142 | BCNU-VCR | 51 | 8 | 24 | 0.28 | |
| 143 | VIB-Act-D-Procarb. | 13 | 5 | 38 | 0.47 | |
| 144 | CTX-VCR-5FU-MTX | 10 | 5 | 50 | 0.99 | |
| 145 | BCNU-VCR | 20 | 12 | 60 | 0.99 | |
| 146 | Me-CCNU Procarb. | 17 | 1 | 5.8 | 0.12 | (DTIC failures) |
| 147 | CCNU-VCR-Bleo | 35 | 17 | 48.5 | 0.99 | (stage III patients) |
| 148 | CCNU-VCR-Bleo | 13 | 5 | 38 | 0.97 | (DTIC failures) |
| R | Me-CCNU-CTX | 18 | 1 | 5.5 | 0.99 | |

Moon [145] report an unusually high response rate in small numbers of patients (ten and 20 patients respectively). Patient selection in these studies is also of concern as the patients have predominantly skin or nodal metastasis. The 38% response rate reported by Everall et al. [148] is of special interest as all of their 13 patients had failed DTIC prior to the trial of lomustine-vincristine-bleomycin combination.

Only six combination regimens reviewed above report response rates equal to or greater than 40% [119, 130, 140, 144, 145, 147]. One report by De Wasch et al. [147] was on Stage III patients, and the remaining five regimens dealt with metastatic melanoma. Of these five, only two regimens have 40 or more evaluable patients [119, 130] and only one [145] of the remaining three has a significant number of evaluable patients (20 patients). For reports of studies on small numbers of evaluable patients, it is perhaps wise to interpret the data cautiously.

Two combination regimens in the above category having observed response rates greater than 40% in 40 or more evaluable patients deserve some discussion. Cohen et al. reported results of a triple combination regimen of DTIC, carmustine and vincristine [119] on 40 evaluable patients in stage IV melanoma. Three complete and 14 partial responses seen mainly in nodal, skin and pulmonary lesions were noted. One of four patients with cerebral involvement also responded. Nine patients with liver involvement did not respond. The median response duration was four months and median survival of responders was 9.5 months compared to two months for nonresponders. Toxicity was mild to moderate with no drug related deaths. Nausea and vomiting were well controlled with standard antiemetics in most cases.

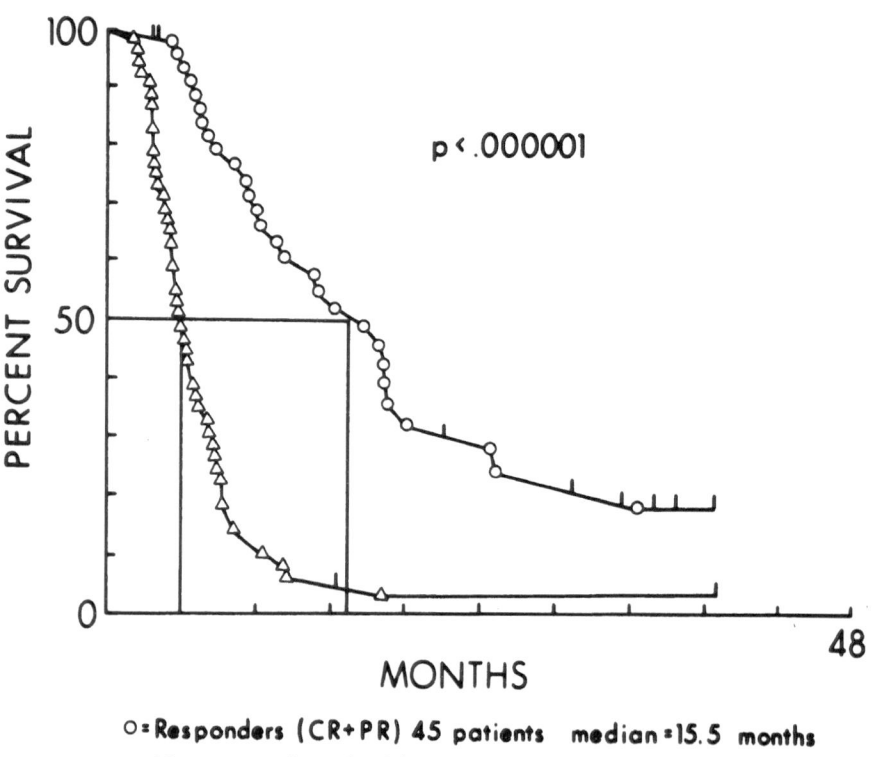

O = Responders (CR+PR) 45 patients median = 15.5 months
△ = Nonresponders (NR) 51 patients median = 4.7 months

*Figure 1.* Actuarial survival analysis of 45 patients with advanced metastatic melanoma who responded (CR + PR) to Bleomycin-Oncovin-Loumustine-DTIC (BOLD) (open circle) and 51 patients who did not (+). The median survival for the former was 15.5 months and for the latter 4.7 months. The difference has a statistical significance at p<0.000001.

Seigler et al. reported their experiences at Duke University with a four drug regimen containing bleomycin, lomustine, vincristine and DTIC with the acronym BOLD [130]. Seventy-two evaluable patients were treated between January 1977 and April 1978. Seven of these patients had complete responses and 22 partial responses of greater than 50% regression of their disease. Stabilization of disease (<50% regression of disease) was seen in 12 patients. The median response duration was 7.5 months and median survival was 16.5 months in responders compared to five months in nonresponders. Following this report an additional 57 patients have been treated with this regimen to date with response rates remaining at 40%. The major side effect from BOLD was nausea and vomiting. Moderate myelotoxicity noted in some patients was reversible. There had been no drug related deaths seen in the 129 patients. Figure 1 shows the updated survival curves for responders and nonresponders.

## Case reports

*Case I*

BL was a healthy 28-year-old woman until June of 1978 when she presented with a left heel lesion diagnosed and treated by a local dermatologist as a "plantar wart." The results of this therapy left a $2 \times 2$ cm ulcer and multiple satellite lesions. An excisional biopsy by another dermatologist showed the lesion to be a Clark's Level IV melanoma. During the month before surgery she had had a five- to eight-pound weight loss and a fullness in her left groin.

Chest X-ray and liver-spleen scan were normal and on July 14, 1978 she underwent radical excision of the lesions with split thickness skin graft on her left foot and a left groin dissection. No tumor was seen in the skin of the foot nor in 12 lymph nodes taken from the left groin. Three days after this surgery she began adjuvant immunotherapy consisting of 25 million, neuraminidase treated, irradiated melanoma cells and $0.1$ cm$^3$ BCG ($3-4 \times 10^4$ bacilli).

The patient received two further immunotherapy treatments and was closely followed. In March 1979 an excisional biopsy of a suspicious lesion on her left heel showed recurrent melanoma. Four additional immunotherapy injections were given. She remained free of clinical disease until September 11, 1979 when multiple recurrent lesions on her left thigh were found. Because of the extensiveness of her subcutaneous disease she was started on the four durg chemotherapy regimen (BOLD) discussed above. Chest x-ray and liver-spleen scan at this time did not show evidence of metastasis in those organs.

After she received two courses of chemotherapy, complete disappearance of all subcutaneous disease was noted. Since then she had been given a total of eight courses of BOLD with no major side effects other than severe nausea and vomiting requiring a strong antiemetic program [194]. She is now well, free of disease, and is not receiving any therapy 24 months from her last recurrence.

## Case II

VB was a 50-year-old woman whose past history of note included psoriasis treated with methotrexate and a hysterectomy in 1965. The patient was found to have a pigmented lesion on her left conjunctiva in June of 1973. She was referred to Duke Medical Center where she underwent an excisional biopsy of what was called a cancerous conjunctival melanosis with minimal invasion. The patient was readmitted in September of 1974 for another excisional biopsy of a recurrent lesion in the same location. Following excision she was started on adjuvant immunotherapy similar to that given to the patient in Case I. She received a total of five immunotherapy treatments and was followed closely. In July of 1977 she was found to have a large nodular density in the right mid-lung field. No other evidence of disease was found elsewhere. BOLD chemotherapy was begun in August 1977. She tolerated the therapy well with mild nausea and vomiting. When the patient returned for her third course of chemotherapy, the metastatic lung nodule in her chest x-ray completely disappeared. No new lesions developed during the subsequent follow-up until after her seventh course of chemotherapy in August 1978 when she experienced a series of focal seizures. Brain CAT scan showed a large lesion in the left parieto-occipital lobe and another in the right posterior frontal lobe. Further examination showed no other tumors outside her brain. Radiation therapy to the brain metastasis and phenytoin reduced the number of seizures. Her disease progressed rapidly from this point on and she died of her disease on February 6, 1979.

From these two patients illustrated above, chemotherapy caused disappearance of active tumors and had prevented the recurrence in the first patient for more than 24 months. The second patient had benefited from chemotherapy for about a year. Her recurrence in the brain, common in melanoma, demonstrated that this combination of drugs was ineffective in lesions in the central nervous system while it is effective for a lesion in the lung.

## Adjuvant chemotherapy

The addition of chemotherapy to surgery with curative intent has been tried to reduce the rate of recurrence in those patients in the high risk category. The rationale is based on animal data and the theory that small metastasis, which may be present beyond the area of surgery, could be eradicated by chemotherapy [149]. Results of the application of this strategy on human tumors (breast and sarcoma) [150, 151] have been controversial. In melanoma, literature and ongoing trials have also yielded insufficient or no evidence of benefit for the approach.

Two studies comparing values of adjuvant chemotherapy or chemoimmunotherapy regimens to historical controls (surgery alone) [152, 153] have shown no clear advantage to such addition.

A randomized prospective study comparing surgery alone with surgery and chemotherapy has been reported by Banzet et al. with sufficient numbers of Clarke's Level III–IV patients [154]. In this study a probable difference in disease free survival is said to exist between surgery and chemotherapy versus surgery alone (81% vs. 65%) at 24 months ($p = 0.3$). Other adjuvant studies reported did not compare surgery alone with their adjuvant treatments. They did however compare among various treatments with one another eg., postoperative chemotherapy versus chemotherapy and immunotherapy or immunotherapy alone.

Wood et al. [156] compared postoperative treatments using DTIC, BCG and the two combined. In 22 patients who received DTIC and BCG combined, no recurrences were noted at a median follow-up time of 12 months. In patients who received DTIC or BCG alone six of 20 and five of 28 recurrences respectively were observed.

El-Domeiri et al. [157] reported a study which compared 15 patients treated with BCG with 15 others treated with DTIC. At 24 months the disease free survival was not different between these two groups, although the BCG was naturally more easily tolerated by the patient than DTIC.

Quirt et al. [158] reported a randomized study comparing surgery with surgery followed by DTIC and BCG. Patients were further stratified into Stage I and Stage II diseases. In either subgroup survival was longer for those who received postoperative DTIC and BCG.

To determine differences in rates of recurrence Karakousis et al. [159], from Rosewell Park Memorial Institute, treated 84 patients (Stage I and II) with three regimens in a randomized manner. Twenty-eight patients (Group A) received surgery alone, 27 (Group B) received surgery and chemotherapy and 29 (Group C) received surgery and BCG. The chemotherapy program consisted of DTIC and estramustine phosphate. Preliminary results, in a mean follow-up of nine months showing three recurrences in Group A, four in Group B and five in Group C, indicate a lack of beneficial contribution by this chemotherapy or BCG following initial surgery.

The reports cited above fail to demonstrate clear superiority of adjuvant chemotherapy to curative surgery. The lack of benefit from these existing adjuvant treatments may be merely a reflection of absence of an effective form of therapy for melanoma. The factor of an unbalanced tumor–host interaction in favor of the tumor caused by chemotherapy might also play a role.


## Regional chemotherapy

Perhaps the best results of chemotherapy for melanoma are obtained in isolation treatment perfusion of primary or recurrent tumors of the extremities [171–176, 181, 182]. In these studies, patients with a limited disease in an extremity have had an approximately 85% cure rate and patients with stage II disease, however, have had a lower cure rate of 50%. For Stage I and II disease cure rates without perfusion treatment following operation are 60% and 30%, respectively. Chemotherapy by perfusion appears to add approximately 15–20% to the five-year survival rate. Isolation perfusion therapy in an enclosed system ("closed circuit") is often done by experts who have had extensive experience with the procedure and who have at their disposal a well-trained and experienced team. Moderate to severe morbidity, including loss of extremities may occur in the hands of inexperienced workers.

The other approach to regional chemotherapy has involved intra-arterial infusions ("open circuit"). Einhorn et al. [177] reported a 41% objective response rate in 17 patients with advanced regional disease with intra-aterial DTIC. Unfortunately, these responses were of short duration.

Savlov also treated a small number of patients (six) with DTIC intra-arterially [178]. He observed two responses, but felt that systemic therapy might be more appropriate as new lesions appeared away from the site of perfusion.

A 50% response rate in a very small number of patients (four) was reported by Pritchard et al. using intra-aterial cisplatin [179]. In contrast Calvo et al. also reported a series of 19 melanoma patients treated with intra-aterial cisplatin recently [180]. He observed two complete responses and eight partial responses for an overall response rate of 53%.


## Chemoimmunotherapy

Specific aspects of immunotherapy are discussed in another chapter of this monograph. This section will briefly discuss the combination of chemotherapy with immunotherapy in metastatic melanoma.

Many studies have explored the value of combinations of chemotherapy and immunotherapy. About one-third of the studies reviewed in this chapter used historical controls for comparison and these results should be viewed with caution because of the potential biases associated in this type of study [160–164].

Table 9 lists randomized studies comparing chemotherapy alone with chemotherapy combined with some form of immunotherapy. None of these studies reports any benefit from the addition of immunotherapy to chemotherapy.

## Future developments

There are many new experimental programs for the treatment of melanoma which are currently being studied. Several of the more promising are discussed below.

*Table 9.* Randomized trial of Chemo-immunotherapy

| References | ChemoRx | ImmunoRx | No patients | Responders | Observed response rate | Comments |
|---|---|---|---|---|---|---|
| 165 | DTIC CTX | | 29 | 8 | 28% | |
| | DTIC CTX | C. Parvum | 27 | 9 | 33% | No statistical difference |
| 166 | Procarb., VLB, Act-D | | 40 | 6 | 15% | No statistical difference |
| | Procarb., VLB, Act-D | Mer-BCG | 34 | 8 | 20% | |
| 167 | DTIC, Act-D | | 15 | 1 | 6.7% | |
| | DTIC Act-D | Mer-BCG | 13 | 1 | 7.7 | No statistical difference |
| 168 | Me-CCNU, VCR | | 26 | 6 | 23 | |
| | Me-CCNU, VCR | BCG | 24 | 4 | 17 | No statistical difference |
| 169 | DTIC, Hydrea, BCNU | | 75 | 21 | 28 | |
| | DTIC, Hydrea, BCNU | BCG | 87 | 25 | 29 | No statistical difference |
| 170 | DTIC | | 27 | 6 | 22 | No statistical difference |
| | DTIC | C. Parvum | 22 | 6 | 27 | |

One of the most publicized new agents tried in melanoma is human interferon. Retsas et al. [183] report the initial results of a Phase II study of human lymphoblastoid interferon in nine evaluable patients. One patient showed a partial response and another, stabilization of disease. In another study Nemoto et al. [184] reported the results of three patients who were given intralesional injections of human fibroblast interferon. Two of the three had a remarkable regression of the injected lesions. These are encouraging reports, but more studies must be done to define the optimal dose and schedule for interferon before its place in the treatment of melanoma is determined.

Levodopa in high doses has recently been found to be active against melanoma cells in vitro and in animals in vivo [185–189]. The combined application with the inhibitors of its catabolyzing enzyme (e.g., benserazide) magnifies its antimelanoma activity. The activity is selective because of greater incorporation of levodopa by the melanin-producing cells. Even the immediate metabolite, dopamine, has a growth inhibitory effect in B16 melanoma. The antimelanoma activity is believed to be associated with the suppression of DNA synthesis as measured by tritiated thymidine incorporation and with blockage of cells between G1 and S phases in the cell cycle. RNA and protein synthesis, however, are largely unaffected. Wick reported in 1980 that dopamine infused in patients with metastatic lesions caused an inhibition of melanoma growth by a tenfold reduction in labeling index as measured in the biopsied tumor. There was no change in the labeling index of bone marrow cells indicating a selective effect [189]. While the antimelanoma effect of levodopa combined with the inhibitor of its decarboxylase has been clearly shown in animal or human melanoma in tissue culture, its clinical application has just begun.

The authors of this chapter (VLS and ATH) have begun a Phase I study of levodopa and its decarboxylase inhibitor carbidopa (Sinemet, MSD). Side effects include moderate to severe agitation, mild to moderate postural-hypotension and severe insomnia requiring hypnotics. Dose escalation is often limited by one or more of these side effects. Therapeutic efficacy of this approach has not been ascertained at present. It is reasonable to assume that levodopa may eventually have a place in melanoma chemotherapy.

Fay et al. [190] recently reported the use of high dose carmustine (BCNU) and autologous marrow transplantation in melanoma. Thirty patients with widely metastatic melanoma were treated in this Phase I-II study. Doses ranged from $1050-2850$ mg/m$^2$ over three days followed by autologous marrow transplant. Five patients showed complete and nine patients had partial responses. Of note is that in three of ten patients with brain metastasis, lesions in the brain responded. Toxicity was, however, significant. Three drug related deaths were reported.

One of the more exciting new areas of research is extracoporeal immunoadsorption with protein A-bearing, formlin-fixed and heat-killed bacterium, *Staphylococcus aureus*. Infusion of filtered plasma through a column containing the killed bacteria or purified protein A via plasmapheresis unit or the usual phlebotomy is reported to cause an immediate tumor necrosis in a canine model [195]. The mechanism for the tumor regression induced by immunoadsorption with *Staphylococcus aureus* is not clear. Several theories might explain the observed response. Tumor regression might occur if circulating blocking factors are removed by protein A which binds to the Fc fragment of IgG. As suggested by Gupta et al. [191, 192] the immune complexes said to be present in patients with melanoma or other cancer may adversely affect cell-mediated immunity and affect the clinical course of the patient. These immune complexes may attach to the Fc receptors on effector lymphocytes, including natural killer cells, cells active in antibody-dependent cytotoxicity and subpopulations of T cells, and suppress their antitumor action. Treatment of patients' plasma with protein A in a column may cause a reactivation of these host defense mechanisms against the tumor. It has been recently reported that protein A may induce production of (lamda) interferon, which in turn activates natural killer lymphocytes [196].

The clinical application of this technique in many human tumors, begun at several institutions in the United States, has offered encouraging results. Side effects are transient and include marked pyrexia, hypertension, hypotension, chills and pain often in tumor-bearing areas. Most patients are well within 12–24 hours after the procedure. While responses have been reported in immune complex diseases (e.g., systemic lupus) and various tumors (e.g., breast and colon cancers), trials in melanoma are currently in progress.

## References

1. Bellet RE, Mastrangelo MJ, Berd D and Lustbader E: Chemotherapy of malignant melanoma. In: Brodsky I, Kahn SB and Conroy JF (eds) Cancer Chemotherapy III: The Forty-Sixth Hahnemann Symposium, pp 225–242. Grune & Stratton, New York, 1978.
2. Magnus K: Incidence of malignant melanoma of the skin in Norway 1955–1970. Cancer 32:1275, 1973.
3. Elwood JM and Lee JAH: Recent data on the epidemiology of malignant melanoma. Semin Oncol 2:149, 1975.
4. Cosman B, Heddle SB and Crikelair GF: The increasing incidence of melanoma. Plast Reconstr Surg 57:50, 1976.
5. Comis RL and Carter SK: Integration of chemotherapy into combined modality therapy of solid tumors. IV: Malignant melanoma. Cancer Treat Rev 1:285–304, 1974.
6. Comis RL: DTIC (NSC-45388) in malignant melanoma: a perspective. Cancer Treat Rep 60:165–176, 1976.
7. Einhorn LH, Burgess MA, Vallejos C et al: Prognostic correlations and response to treatment in advanced metastatic malignant melanoma. Cancer Res 34:1995–2004, 1974.

396

8. Ahmann DL, Hahn RG and Bisel HF: Evaluation of 1-(2-chloroethyl-3-4-methylcyclohexyl)-1-nitrosourea (methyl-CCNU, NSC-95441) versus combined imidazole carboxamide (NSC-45388) and vincristine (NSC-67574) in palliation of disseminated malignant melanoma. Cancer 33:615–618, 1974.

9. Wittes RE, Wittes JT and Golbey RB: Combination chemotherapy in metastatic malignant melanoma: a randomized study of three DTIC-containing combinations. Cancer 41:415–421, 1978.

10. Ahmann DL, Hahn RG, Bisel HF et al: Comparative study of methyl-CCNU (NSC-95441) with cyclophosphamide (NSC-26271) and 5-(3,3-dimethyl-1-triazeno) imidazole-4-carboxamide (NSC-45388) with vincristine (NSC-67574) in patients with disseminated malignant melanoma. Cancer Chemother Rep 59:451–453, 1975.

11. Costanza ME and Nathanson L: Combination DTIC and methyl CCNU vs single agents in disseminated malignant melanoma: preliminary report. Proc Am Assoc Cancer Res ASCO 15:173, 1974.

12. Young RC, Canellos GP, Chabner BA et al: Treatment of malignant melanoma with methyl CCNU. Clin Pharmacol Ther 15:617–622, 1974.

13. Tranum BL, Haut A, Rivkin S et al: Methyl CCNU in Hodgkin's disease and other tumors. Proc Am Assoc Cancer Res ASCO 15:171, 1974.

14. Firat D and Tekuzman G: Treatment of solid tumors and lymphomas with methyl-CCNU (NSC-95441). Proc Am Assoc Cancer Res ASCO 15:5, 1974.

15. Johnson RO, Bisel H, Andrews N et al: Phase I clinical study of 6-methylpregn-4-ene-3, 11, 20-trione (NSC-17256). Cancer Chemother Rep 50:671–673, 1966.

16. Ramirez G, Weiss AJ, Rochlin DB et al: Phase II study of 6-methylpregn-4-ene-3, 11, 20-trione (NSC-17256). Cancer Chemother Rep 55:265–268, 1971.

17. Pugh RP, Jacobs EM, Bateman JR et al: CCNU vs CCNU + vincristine in disseminated melanoma. Proc Am Assoc Cancer Res ASCO 16:246, 1975.

18. Cruz AB, Jr, Armstrong DM and Aust JB: Treatment of advanced malignancy with CCNU (1-[2-chloroethyl]-3-cyclohexyl-1-nitrosourea, NSC-79037): A Phase II cooperative study. Proc Am Assoc Cancer Res ASCO 15:184, 1974.

19. Ahmann DL, Hahn RG and Bisel HF: A comparative study of 1(2-chloroethyl)-3-cyclohexyl-1-nitrosourea (NSC-79037) and imidazole carboxamide (NSC-45388) with vincristine (NSC-67574) in the palliation of disseminated malignant melanoma. Cancer Res 32:2432–2434, 1972.

20. Hoogstraten B, Gottlieb JA, Caoili E et al: CCNU (1-[2-chloroethyl]-3-cyclohexyl-1-nitrosourea, NSC-79037) in the treatment of cancer: Phase II study. Cancer 32:38–43, 1973.

21. Broder LE and Hanson HH: 1-(2-chloroethyl)-3-cyclohexyl-1-nitrosourea (CCNU, NSC-79037): a comparison of drug administration at four-week and six-week intervals. Eur J Cancer 9:147–152, 1973.

22. DeConti RC, Hubbard SP, Pinch P et al: Treatment of advanced neoplastic disease with 1-(2-chloroethyl)-3-cyclohexyl-1-nitrosourea (CCNU; NSC-79037). Cancer Chemother Rep 57:201–207, 1973.

23. Perloff M, Muggia FM and Ackerman C: Role of a nitrosourea (CCNU, NSC-79037) in advanced nonhematologic cancer. Cancer Chemother Rep 58:421–424, 1974.

24. Ramirez G, Wilson W, Grage T et al: Phase II evaluation of 1,3-bis-(2-chloroethyl)-1-nitrosourea (BCNU; NSC-409962) in patients with solid tumors. Cancer Chemother Rep 56:787–790, 1972.

25. DeVita VT, Carbone PP, Owens AH, Jr et al: Clinical trials with 1,3-bis-2-chloroethyl)-2-nitrosourea, NCS-409962. Cancer Res 25:1876–1881, 1965.

26. Lessner HE: BCNU 1,3-bis-(2-chloroethyl)-1-nitrosourea. Effects on advanced Hodgkin's disease and other neoplasia. Cancer 22:451–456, 1968.

27. Benjamin RS, Keating MJ, Valdivieso M et al: Phase I–II study of piperazinedione in adults with solid tumors and acute leukemia. Cancer Treat Rep 63:939–943, 1979.

28. Presant CA, Bartolucci AA, Ungaro P and Oldham R: Phase II trial of piperazinedione in malignant melanoma: a report by the Southeastern Cancer Study Group. Cancer Treat Rep 63:1367–1369, 1979.
29. Al-Sarraf M, Thigpen T, Groppe CW et al: Piperazinedione in patients with advanced malignant melanoma: a southwest oncology group study. Cancer Treat Rep 62:1101–1103, 1978.
30. Stolinsky DC, Jacobs EM, Bateman JR et al: Clinical trial of trimethylcolchicinic acid methyl ether d-tartrate (TMCA; NSC-36354) in advanced cancer. Cancer Chemother Rep 51:25, 1967.
31. Strolinsky DC, Jacobs EM, Braunwald J et al: Further study of trimethylcolchicinic acid methyl ether d-tartrate (TMCA; NSC-36354) in patients with malignant melanoma. Cancer Chemother Rep 56:263–265, 1972.
32. Slack NH and Jones R: Single reversal trial of hydroxyurea (NSC-32065) in 91 patients with advanced cancer. Cancer Chemother Rep 54:53, 1970.
33. Cole DR, Beckloff GL and Rousselot LM: Clinical results with hydroxyurea in cancer chemotherapy. N Y State J Med 65:2132, 1965.
34. Creasey WA, Capizzi RL and DeConti RC: Clinical and biochemical studies of solid tumors with hydroxyurea (NSC-32065). Cancer Res 27:1843, 1967.
35. Bolton BH, Kaung DT, Lawton RL et al: Hydroxyurea (NSC-32065): a Phase I study. Cancer Chemother Rep 39:47, 1964.
36. Cassileth PA and Hyman GA: Treatment of malignant melanoma with hydroxyurea. Cancer Res 27:1843, 1967.
37. Gottlieb JA, Frei E and Luce JK: Dose-schedule studies with hydroxyurea in malignant melanoma. Cancer Chemother Rep 55:277, 1971.
38. Nathanson L and Hall TC: Phase II study of hydroxyurea (NSC-32065) in malignant melanoma. Cancer Chemother Rep 51:503, 1967.
39. Lerner HJ, Beckloff GL and Godwin MC: Hydroxyurea (NSC-32065) intermittent therapy in malignant diseases. Cancer Chemoth Rep 53:385, 1969.
40. Eilber FR and Isakoff W: High-dose methotrexate for disseminated malignant melanoma. Proc Am Assoc Cancer Res ASCO 17:262, 1976.
41. Fisher RI, Chabner BA and Myers CE: Phase II study of high-dose methotrexate in patients with advanced malignant melanoma. Cancer Treat Rep 63:147–148, 1979.
42. Karakousis CP and Carlson M: High-dose methotrexate in malignant melanoma. Cancer Treat Rep 63:1405–1407, 1979.
43. Ahmann DL, Bisel HF, Edmonson JH et al: Phase II study of VP-16-213 versus dianhydroglactitol in patients with metastatic malignant melanoma. Cancer Treat Rep 60:1681–1682, 1976.
44. Thigpen JT, Morrison F and Baker L: Phase II evaluation of dianhydroglactitol (DAG) in treatment of advanced sarcoma and malignant melanoma. Proc Am Assoc Cancer Res ASCO 18:240, 1977.
45. Thigpen JT, Al-Sarraf M and Hewlett JS: Phase II trial of dianhydroglactitol in metatastic malignant melanoma: a southwest oncology group study. Cancer Treat Rep 63:525–528, 1979.
46. Godfrey TE and Wilbur DW: Clinical experience with mitomycin C in large infrequent doses. Cancer 29:1647–1652, 1972.
47. Whittington RM and Close HP: Clinical experience with mitomycin C (NSC-26980). Cancer Chemother Rep 54:195–198, 1970.
48. Frei E, Franzino A, Shnider BI et al: Clinical studies of vinblastine. Cancer Chemother Rep 12:125, 1961.
49. Armstrong JG, Dyke RW, Fouts PJ et al: Hodgkin's disease, carcinoma of the breast and other tumors treated with vinblastine sulfate. Cancer Chemother Rep 18:49, 1962.

50. Acute Leukemia Group B and Eastern Cooperative Group: Neoplastic disease: treatment with vinblastine. Arch Intern Med 116:846, 1965.

51. Hill JM and Loeb E: Treatment of leukemia, lymphoma and other malignant neoplasms with vinblastine. Cancer Chemother Rep 15:41, 1961.

52. Faulkson G and Van Dyk JJ: The chemotherapy of malignant melanoma. S Afr Med J 42:89, 1968.

53. Wright TL, Hurley J, Korst DR et al: Vinblastine in neoplastic disease. Cancer Res 23:169, 1963.

54. Smart CR, Rochlin DB, Nahum AM et al: Clinical experience with vinblastine sulfate (NSC-49842) in squamous cell carcinoma and other malignancies. Cancer Chemother Rep 34:31, 1964.

55. Retsas S, Newton KA and Westbury G: Vindesine as a single agent in the treatment of advanced malignant melanoma. Cancer Chemother Pharmacol 2:257–260, 1979.

56. Smith IE, Hedley DW, Powles TJ and Mcelwain TJ: Vindesine: a Phase II study in the treatment of breast carcinoma, malignant melanoma and other tumors. Cancer Treat Rep 62:1427–1433, 1978.

57. Andrews NC, Weiss AJ, Ansfield FJ et al: Phase I study of dibromodulcitol (NSC-104800). Cancer Chemother Rep 55:61–65, 1971.

58. Phillips RW and Brook J: Clinical experiences with dibromodulcitol (NSC-104800) in solid tumors. Cancer Chemother Rep 55:567–573, 1971.

59. Bellet RE, Catalano RB, Mastrangelo MJ and Berd D: Positive Phase II trial of dibromo-dulcitol in patients with metastatic melanoma refractory to DTIC and a nitrosourea. Cancer Treat Rep 62:2095–2099, 1978.

60. Blum RH, Livingston RB and Carter SK: Hexamethylmelamine—a new drug with activity in solid tumors. Eur J Cancer 9:195–202, 1973.

61. Blum RH, Carter SK and Agre K: A clinical review of bleomycin: a new antineoplastic agent. Cancer 31:903, 1973.

62. Clinical Screening Co-operative Group of the European Organization for Research on the Treatment of Cancer: Study of the clinical efficiency of bleomycin in human cancer. Br Med J 2:643, 1970.

63. O'Bryan RM, Luce JK, Talley RW et al: Phase II evaluation of adriamycin in human neoplasia. Cancer 32:1, 1973.

64. Sieper WJ, Mastrangelo MJ and Bellet RE: Phase II study of adriamycin (NSC-123127) in patients with mestastatic melanoma. Cancer Chemother Rep 59:1181–1182, 1975.

65. Buckner CD, Rudolph RH, Fefer A et al: High-dose cyclophosphamide therapy for malignant disease: toxicity, tumor response, and the effects of stored autologous marow. Cancer 29:357, 1972.

66. Bergsagel DE and Levin WC: A prelusive clinical trial of cyclophosphamide. Cancer Chemother Rep 8:120, 1960.

67. Haar H, Marshall GJ, Bierman HR et al: The influence of cyclophosphamide upon neoplastic diseases in man. Cancer Chemother Rep 6:41, 1960.

68. Gottlieb JA, Mendelson D and Serpick AA: An evaluation of large intermittent intravenous doses of cyclophosphamide (NSC-26271) in the treatment of metastatic malignant melanoma. Cancer Chemother Rep 54:365, 1970.

69. Shnider BI, Gold GL, Hall T et al: Preliminary studies with cyclophosphamide. Cancer Chemother Rep 8:106, 1960.

70. Rundles RW, Laszlo J, Garrison FE et al: The antitumor spectrum of cyclophosphamide. Cancer Chemother Rep 16:407, 1962.

71. Mullins GM and Colvin M: Intensive cyclophosphamide (NSC-26271) therapy for solid tumors. Cancer Chemotherapy Rep 59:411, 1975.

72. Golomb FM, Solowey Ac, Postel A et al: Induced remission of malignant melanoma with actinomycin-D: immunologic implications. Cancer 20:656, 1967.

73. Moore GE, DiPaolo JA and Kindo T: The chemotherapeutic effects and complications of actinomycin-D in patients with advanced cancer. Cancer 11:1204, 1958.

74. Regelson W, Holland JF, Gold GL et al: 6-mercaptopurine (NSC-755) given intravenously at weekly intervals to patients with advanced cancer. Cancer Chemother Rep 51:277, 1967.

75. Fink DJ and Foye LV: 6-mercaptopurine (NSC-755) given intermittently in high doses: Phase II study. Cancer Chemother Rep 54:31, 1970.

76. Moore GE, Bross IDJ, Ausman R et al: Effects of 6-mercaptopurine (NSC-755) in 290 patients with advanced cancer. Cancer Chemother Rep 52:655, 1968.

77. Mckelvey EM, Hewlett JS, Thigpen T and Whitecar J: Cyclocytidine chemotherapy for malignant melanoma. Cancer Treat Rep 62:469–471, 1978.

78. Burke PJ, Owens AH, Colsky J et al: A clinical evaluation of a prolonged schedule of cytosine arabinoside (NSC-63878). Cancer Res 29:1325, 1970.

79. Frei E, Bickers JN, Hewlett JS et al: Dose schedule and antitumor studies of arabinosyl cytosine (NSC-63878). Cancer Res 29:1325, 1969.

80. Lopez R, Karakousis CP, Didolkar MS and Holyoke ED: Estramustine phosphate in the treatment of advanced malignant melanoma. Cancer Treat Rep 62:1329–1332, 1978.

81. Costa G, Hreshchyshyn MM and Holland JJ: Initial clinical studies with vincristine. Cancer Chemother Rep 32:39, 1962.

82. Gubisch NJ, Norena D, Perlia CP et al: Experience with vincristine in solid tumors. Cancer Chemother Rep 32:19, 1963.

83. Shaw RK and Bruner JA: Clinical evaluation of of vincristine (NSC-67574). Cancer Chemother Rep 42:45, 1964.

84. Reitemeier RJ, Moertel CG and Blackburn CM: Vincristine (NSC-67574) therapy of adult patients with solid tumors. Cancer Chemother Rep 34:21, 1964.

85. Smart CR, Ottoman RE, Rochlin DB et al: Clinical experience with vincristine (NSC-67574) in tumors of the central nervous system and other malignant diseases. Cancer Chemother Rep 52:733, 1968.

86. Brindley CO, Salvin LG, Potee KG et al: Further comparative trial of triethylene thiophosphoramide and mechlorethamine in patients with melanoma and Hodgkin's disease. J Chron Dis 17:19–30, 1964.

87. Holland JF and Regelson W: Studies of phenylalanine nitrogen mustard (CB 3025) in metastatic malignant melanoma of man. Ann N Y Acad Sci 68:1122, 1958.

88. Gumport SL, Wright JC and Golomb FM: The treatment of advanced malignant melanoma with triethylene thiophosphormide (Thio-TEPA or TSPA). Ann Surg 147:232, 1958.

89. Sykes MP, Karnofsky DA, Philips FS et al: Clinical studies on triethylene phosphoramide and diethylenephosphoramide, compounds with nitrogen mustard-like activity. Cancer 6:142, 1953.

90. Farber S, Appleton R, Downing V et al: Clinical studies on the carcinolytic action of triethylenephosphoramide. Cancer 6:135, 1953.

91. Tullis JL: Triethylenephosphoramide in the treatment of desseminated melanoma. J Am Med Assoc 166:37, 1958.

92. Moore GE, Bross IDJ, Ausman R et al: Effects of chlorambucil (NSC-3088) in 374 patients with advanced cancer. Cancer Chemother Rep 52:661–666, 1968.

93. Budman D, Currie V and Wittes R: Phase II trial of pyrazofurin in malignant melanoma. Cancer Treat Rep 61:1733–1734, 1977.

94. Bellet RE, Catalno RB, Mastrangelo MJ et al: Phase II trial of VM-26 in patients with metastatic malignant melanoma. Cancer Treat Rep 62:445–447, 1978.

95. Moore GE, Bross IDJ, Ausman R et al: Effects of 5-fluorouracil (NSC-19893) in 389 patients with cancer. Cancer Chemother Rep 52:641–653, 1968.

96. Bellet RE, Catalano RB, Danna VG et al: A study of the antitumor (Phase II) and Immunosuppressive effects of ICRF-159 (NSC-129943) in patients with metastatic melanoma. J Clin Pharmacol 16:433, 1976.

97. Du Priest RW, Huntington MC, Massy WH et al: Streptozotocin therapy in 22 cancer patients. Cancer 35:358, 1975.

98. Schein PS, O'Connell MJ, Blom J et al: Clinical antitumor activity and toxicity of streptozotocin (NSC-85998). Cancer 34:993, 1974.

99. Quagliana M, Constanzi J, O'Bryan R et al: A Phase II study of 5-azacytidine (5-azaC) in the treatment of solid tumors. Proc Am Assoc Cancer Res ASCO 15:121, 1974.

100. Weiss AJ, Stambaugh JE, Mastrangelo MJ et al: A Phase II study of 5-azacytidine (NSC-102816). Cancer Chemother Rep 56:413–419, 1972.

101. Ahmann DL, Frytak S, Kvois LK et al: Phase II study of maytansine and chlorzotocin in patients with desseminated malignant melanoma. Cancer Treat Rep 64:721–723, 1980.

102. Sullivan RD, Miller E, Zurek WZ et al: Re-evaluation of methotrexate as an anticancer drug. Surg Gynecol Obstet 125:819, 1967.

103. Vogler WR, Huguley CM and Kerr W: Toxicity and antitumor effect of divided doses of methotrexate. Arch Intern Med 115:285, 1965.

104. Zubrod CG, Schneiderman M, Frei E, III et al: Appraisal of methods for the study of chemotherapy of cancer in man: comparative therapeutic trial of nitrogen mustard and triethylene thiophosphoramide. J Chron Chron Dis 11:7–33, 1960.

105. Clifford P, Clift RA and Gillmore JH: Oral melphalan therapy in advanced malignant disease. Br J Cancer 17:381–390, 1963.

106. Hall BE, Willett FM and Hales DR: Observations on the effects of alkylating agents on human neoplastic disease. Ann Int Med 52:602–635, 1960.

107. Goodnight JE, Moseley HS, Eiber FR et al: Cis-dichlorodiammineplatinum (II) alone and combined with DTIC for treatment of disseminated malignant melanoma. Cancer Treat Rep 63:2005–2007, 1979.

108. Chary KK, Higby DJ, Henderson ES and Swinerton KD: Phase I study of high-sode cis-dichlorodiamineplatinum (II) with forced diuresis. Cancer Treat Rep 61:367–370, 1977.

109. Al-Sarraf M: Clinical trial of cis-platinum (NSC-119875): hydration with and without mannitol in patients with previously treated advanced melanoma: a southwest oncology group study. Proc Am Assoc Cancer Res ASCO 20:185, 1979.

110. Ahmann DL, Edmonson JH, Frytak S et al: Phase II study of ICRF-159 versus combination cis-dichlorodiammineplatinum (II) and DTIC in patients with disseminated malignant melanoma. Cancer Treat Rep 62:151–153, 1978.

111. Hath D, Robichaud K, Wooley PV et al: Phase II trial of chlorozotocin in metastatic malignant melanoma. Proc Am Assoc Cancer Res ASCO 20:413, 1979.

112. Van Amberg A, Ratkin G and Presant C: Complete responses in metastatic malignant melanoma with chlorozotocin in previously untreated patients. Proc Am Assoc Cancer Res ASCO 21:353, 1980.

113. Hall SW, Benjamin RS, Legha SS et al: AMSA: a new acridine derivative with activity against metastatic melanoma. Proc Am Assoc Cancer Res ASCO 29:372, 1979.

114. Constanza ME, Nathanson L, Lenhard R et al: Therapy of malignant melanoma with an imidazole carboxamide and bis-chloroethyl-nitrosourea. Cancer 30:1457–1461, 1972.

115. Gerner RE, Moore GE and Dickey C: Combination chemotherapy in disseminated melanoma and other solid tumors in adults. Oncology 31:22–30, 1975.

116. Costanza ME, Nathanson L, Schoenfeld D et al: Results with methyl-CCNU and DTIC in metastatic melanoma. Cancer 40:1010–1015, 1977.

117. Ahmann DL, Bisel HF, Edmonson JH et al: Clinical comparison of adriamycin and a combination of methyl-CCNU and imidazole carboxamide in disseminated malignant melanoma. Clin Pharmacol Ther 19:821–824, 1976.

118. Cohen SM, Greenspan EM, Weiner MJ et al: Triple combination chemotherapy of disseminated melanoma. Cancer 29:1489–1495, 1972.

119. Cohen SM, Greenspan EM, Ratner LH et al: Combination chemotherapy of malignant melanoma with imidazole carboxamide, BCNU and vincristine. Cancer 39:41–44, 1977.

120. Beretta G, Bonadonna G, Bajetta E et al: Combination chemotherapy with DTIC (NSC-45388) in advanced malignant melanoma, soft tissue sarcomas and Hodgkin's disease. Cancer Treat Rep 60:205–211, 1976.

121. Carter RD, Krementz ET, Hill GJ et al: DTIC (NSC-45388) and combination therapy for melanoma. I: studies with DTIC, BCNU (NSC-409962), CCNU (NSC-79037), vincristine (NSC-67574) and hydroxyurea (NSC-32065). Cancer Treat Rep 60:601–609, 1976.

122. Bellet RE, Mastrangelo MJ, Laucius JF et al: Randomized prospective trial of DTIC (NSC-45388) alone versus BCNU (NSC-409962) plus vincristine (NSC-67574) in the treatment of metastatic malignant melanoma. Cancer Treat Rep 60:595–600, 1976.

123. Carmo-Pereira J, Oliveira CF and Pimentel P: Combination cytotoxic chemotherapy for metastatic cutaneous malignant melanoma with DTIC, BCNU and vincristine. Cancer Treat Rep 60:1381–1383, 1976.

124. Beretta G, Bonadonna G, Cascineli N et al: Comparative evaluation of three combination regimens for advanced malignant melanoma: results of an international cooperative study. Cancer Treat Rep 60:33–40, 1976.

125. Mckelvey EM, Luce JK, Talley RW et al: Combination chemotherapy with bis-chloroethyl-nitrosourea (BCNU), vincristine and dimethyl triazeno imidazole carboxamide (DTIC) in disseminated malignant melanoma. Cancer 39:1–4, 1977.

126. Einhorn LH and Furnas B: Combination chemotherapy for disseminated malignant melanoma with DTIC, vincristine and methyl-CCNU. Cancer Treat Rep 61:881–883, 1977.

127. Costanzi JJ, Vaitkevicius VK, Quagliana JM et al: Combination chemotherapy for disseminated malignant melanoma. Cancer 35:342–346, 1975.

128. Mckelvey EM, Luce JK, Vaitkevicius VK et al: Bis-chloroethyl nitrosourea, vincristine, dimethyl triazeno imidazole carboxamide and chlorpromazine combination chemotherapy in disseminated malignant melanoma. Cancer 39:5–10, 1977.

129. Van Dyk JJ and Falkson G: A clinical trial of procarbazine plus vincristine plus bis-chloroethyl-nitrosourea plus imidazole carboxamide dimethyl triazeno in metastatic malignant melanoma. Med Pediatr Oncol 1:107–111, 1975.

130. Seigler HF, Lucas VS, Pickett NJ and Huang AT: A Phase II study of bleomycin, oncovin, loumustine and DTIC (Bold) in Stage IV metastatic melanoma. Cancer 43:2346–2348, 1980.

131. Dufour FD, Eilber FR and Morton DL: High-dose methotrexate combined with DTIC for metastatic melanoma. Proc Am Assoc Cancer Res ASCO 19:360, 1978 (meeting abstract).

132. Samson MK, Baker LH, Talley RW et al: Phase I-II study of intermittent bolus administration of DTIC and actinomycin-D in metastatic malignant melanoma. Cancer Treat Rep 62:1223–1225, 1978.

133. Ahmann DL, Hahn RG and Bisel HF: A comparative study of 1-(chloroethyl-3-cyclohexyl)-1-nitrosourea (NSC-79037) and imidazole carboxamide (NSC-45388) with vincristine (NSC-67574) in the palliation of disseminated malignant melanoma. Cancer Res 32:2432–2434, 1972.

134. Gerner RE, Moore GE and Didolkar MS: Chemotherapy of disseminated malignant melanoma with dimethyl triazeno imidazole carboxamide and dactinomycin. Cancer 32:756–760, 1973.

135. Samson MK, Baker LH, Izbicki RM et al: Phase I-II study of DTIC and cyclocytidine in disseminated malignant melanoma. Cancer Treat Rep 60:1369–1371, 1976.

136. Presant CA, Bartolucci AA and Balch C: Cyclophosphamide plus DTIC alone or with piperazinedione in melanoma. Proc Am Assoc Cancer Res ASCO 20:320, 1979.

137. Stolinsky DC, Bogdon DL, Soloman J et al: hexamethylmelamine (NSC-13875) alone and in combination with 5-(3,3-dimethyl-1-triazeno) imidazole-carboxamide (NSC-45388) in the treatment of advanced cancer. Cancer 30:654–659, 1972.

138. Ahmann DL, Hahn RG and Bisel HF: Evaluation of 1-(2-chlorethyl-3-4-methylcyclohexyl)-1-nitrosourea (methyl-CCNU, NSC-95441) versus combined imidazole carboxamide (NSC-45388) and vincristine (NSC-67574) in palliation of disseminated malignant melanoma. Cancer 33:615–618, 1974.

139. Ahmann DL, Edmonson JH, Frytack S et al: Phase II study of ICRF-159 versus combination cis-dichlorodiammineplatinum (II) and DTIC in patients with disseminated malignant melanoma. Cancer Treat Rep 62:151–153, 1978.

140. Karakousis CP, Getaz EP, Bjornsson S, et al: Cis-dichlorodiammineplatinum (II) and DTIC in malignant melanoma. Cancer Treat Rep 63:2009–2010, 1979.

141. Friedman MA, Kaufman DA, Williams JE et al: Combined DTIC and cis-dichlorodiammineplatinum (II) therapy for patients with disseminated melanoma: a Northern California oncology group study. Cancer Treat Rep 63:493–495, 1979.

142. Moon JH, Gailani S, Cooper MR, Hayes DM et al: Comparison of the combination of 1,3-bis-(2-chloroethyl)-1-nitrosourea (BCNU) and vincristine with two dose schedules of 5-(3,3-dimethyl-1-triazino) imidazole 4-carboxamide (DTIC) in the treatment of disseminated malignant melanoma. Cancer 35:368–371, 1975.

143. Perlin E, Engeler J, Reid JW et al: Treatment of malignant melanoma with vinblastine (NSC-49842), procarbazine (NSC-77213), and actinomycin-D (NSC-3053). Cancer Chemother Rep 59:767–768, 1975.

144. Contanzi JJ and Coltman CA: Combination chemotherapy using cyclophosphamide, vincristine, and methotrexate and 5-fluorouracil in solid tumors. Cancer 23:589–596, 1969.

145. Moon JH: Combination chemotherapy in malignant melanoma. Cancer 26:468–473, 1970.

146. Didolkar MS, Baffi RR, Catane R et al: Use of methyl-CCNU and procarbazine in advanced malignant melanoma resistant to DTIC therapy. Cancer Treat Rep 61:1738–1739, 1977 (letter).

147. De Wasch G, Bernheim J, Michel J, Lejeune F et al: Combination chemotherapy with three marginally effective agents, CCNU, vincristine and bleomycin, in the treatment of Stage III melanoma. Cancer Treat Rep 60:1273–1276, 1976.

148. Everall JD and Dowd PM: Use of combination chemotherapy with CCNU, bleomycin and vincristine in the treatment of metastatic melanoma in patients resistant to DTIC therapy. Cancer Treat Rep 63:151–155, 1979.

149. Schabel FM, Jr: Concepts for systemic treatment of micrometastases. Cancer 35:12–24, 1975.

150. Bonadonna G, Brusamolino E, Valagussa P et al: Combination chemotherapy as an adjuvant treatment in operable breast cancer. N Engl J Med 294:405–410, 1976.

151. Pratt C, Shanks E, Hustu O et al: Adjuvant multiple drug chemotherapy for osteosarcoma of the extremity. Cancer 39:51–57, 1977.

152. Paterson AH, McPherson TA and Willans DJ: Malignant melanoma (Stage IIIB): a pilot study of adjuvant chemo-immunotherapy. Cancer Treat Rep 62:571–573, 1978.

153. Alexander HG, Paterson T, McPherson A et al: Malignant melanoma: adjvant chemo-immunotherapy in Stage three and chemo-immunotherapy of Stage four. Proc Am Assoc Cancer Res ASCO 17:310, 1976 (meeting abstract).

154. Banzet P, Jacquillat C, Civatte J et al: Adjuvant chemotherapy in the management of primary malignant melanoma. Cancer 41:1240–1248, 1978.

155. Misset JL, Serrou C, Jeanne J et al: BCG vs chemotherapy followed by BCG as adjuvant treatment for malignant melanoma. Third International Conference on the Adjuvant Therapy of Cancer, abstract 27, March 18–21, 1981.

156. Wood WC, Cosimi AB, Carey RW et al: Randomized trial of adjuvant therapy for "high risk" primary malignant melanoma. Surgery 83:677–681, 1978.

157. El-Domeiri AA, Das Gupta TK, Trippon M et al: Adjuvant chemotherapy and immunotherapy in high risk patients with melanoma. Surg Gynecol Obstet 146:230–232, 1978.

158. Quirt I, Kersey M, Baker M et al: A comparison of adjuvant chemoimmuno therapy with observation alone in patients with poor prognosis primary malignant melanoma and completely resected recurent melanoma. Proc Am Assoc Concer Res ASCO 21:472, 1980.

159. Karakousis CP, Holtermann OA, Lopez J et al: Adjuvant therapy with BCG or DTIC + Estracyt in malignant melanoma. Proc Am Assoc Cancer Res ASCO 20:308, 1979.

160. Gutterman JU, Mavligit G, Gottlieb JA et al: Chemoimmunotherapy of disseminated malignant melanoma with dimethyl triazeno imidazole carboxamide and bacillus calmette-guerin. N Engl J Med 291:592-597, 1974.

161. Hall SW, Benjamin RS, Lewinski U et al: Actinomycin-D, levamisole chemoimmunotherapy of refractory malignant melanoma. Cancer 43:1195-1200, 1979.

162. Gutterman JU, Hersch EM, Mavligit GM et al: Chemoimmunotherapy of disseminated malignant melanoma with BCG: follow-up report. In: Terry WD and Windhorst D (eds) Progress in Cancer Research and Therapy, Vol 6, pp 103-111. Raven, New York, 1978.

163. McPherson TA, Paterson AH, Williams D et al: Malignant melanoma (Stage IIIB): a pilot study of adjuvant chemo-immunotherapy. In: Salmon SE and Jones SE (eds) Adjuvant Therapy of Cancer, pp 439-446. North-Holland, Amsterdam, 1977.

164. Schwarz MA, Gutterman JU, Burgess MA et al: Chemoimmunotherapy of disseminated malignant melanoma with DTIC-BCG, transfer factor plus melphalan. Cancer 45:2506-2525, 1980.

165. Presant CA, Bartolucci AA, Smalley RV et al: Effect of corynebacterium parvumon combination chemotherapy of disseminated malignant melanoma. In: Terry WD and Windhorst D (eds) Progress in Cancer Research and Therapy, Vol 6. Raven, New York, 1978.

166. Kostinas JE, Leone LA, Cuttner J et al: Procarbazine, vinblastine and actinomycin-D in Stage III and IV melanoma with or without methanol-extracted residue of bacillus calmette-guerin. Cancer Treat Rep 63:197-200, 1979.

167. Ramseur WL, Richards F, Muss HB et al: Chemoimmunotherapy for disseminated malignant melanoma: a prospective randomized study. Cancer Treat Rep 62:1085-1087, 1978.

168. Mastrangelo MJ, Bellet RE, Berd D et al: A randomized prospective trial comparing methyl-CCNU + BCG + allogenic tumor cell in patients with metastatic malignant melanoma. In: Terry WD and Windhorst D (eds) Progress in Cancer Research and Therapy, Vol 6, pp 95-102. Raven, New York, 1978.

169. Costanzi JJ: Chemotherapy and BCG in the treatment of disseminated malignant melanoma. In: Terry WD and Windhorst D (eds) Progress in Cancer Research and Therapy, Vol 6, pp 87-93. Raven, New York, 1978.

170. Clunie GJA, Gough IR, Dury M et al: A trial of imidazole carboxamide and corynebacterium parvum in desseminated melanoma clinical and immunologic results. Cancer 46:475-479, 1980.

171. Stehlin JS, Giovanella BC, De Ipolyi PD et al: Results of hyperthermic perfusion for melanoma of the extremities. Surg Gynecol Obstet 140:339-348, 1975.

172. Stehlin JS: Hyperthermic perfusion with chemotherapy for cancers of the extremities. Surg Gynecol Obstet 129:305-308, 1969.

173. McBride CM, Sugarbaker EV and Hickey RC: Prophylactic isolation perfusion as the primary treatment for invasive malignant melanoma of the limbs. Ann Surg 182:316-324, 1975.

174. Krementz ET and Ryan RF: Chemotherapy of melanoma of the extremities by perfusion: fourteen years clinical experience. Ann Surg 175:900-917, 1972.

175. McBride CM and Clark RL: Experience with 1-phenylalanine mustard hydrochloride in isolation-perfusion of extremities for malignant melanoma. Cancer 28:1293-1296, 1971.

176. Golomb FM: Perfusion of melanoma: 105 isolated perfusions in 92 patients. Oncology 26:197–205, 1972.

177. Einhorn LH, McBride CM, Luce JK et al: Intra-arterial infusion therapy with 5-(3,3-dimethyl-1-triazeno) imidazole-4-carboxamide (NSC-45388) for malignant melanoma. Cancer 32:749–755, 1973.

178. Savlov ED, Hall TC and Oberfield RA: Intra-arterial therapy of melanoma with dimethyl triazeno imidazole carboxamide (NSC-45388). Cancer 28:1161–1164, 1971.

179. Pritchard JD, Mavligit GM, Benjamin RS et al: Regression of regionally confined melanoma with intra-arterial cis-dichlorodiammineplatinum (II). Cancer Treat Rep 63:555–558, 1979.

180. Calvo DB 3D, Patt YZ, Wallace S et al: Phase I-II trial of percutaneous intra-arterial cis-diamminedichloroplatinum (II) for regionally confined malignancy. Cancer 45:1278–1283, 1980.

181. Shingleton WW: Perfusion chemotherapy for recurrent melanoma of extremity: progress report. Ann Surg 169:969–973, 1969.

182. Shingleton WW, Seigler HF, Stocks LH et al: Management of recurrent melanoma of the extremity. Cancer 35:574–579, 1975.

183. Retsas S, Priestman TJ, Newton KA et al: Evaluation of human lymphblastoid interferon (HLBI) in metastatic malignant melanoma (MMM): a Phase II study. Proc Am Assoc Cancer Res ASCO 22:371, 1981.

184. Nemoto T, Carter WA, Dolen JG et al: Human interferons and intralesional therapy of melanoma and breast carcinoma. Proc Am Assoc Cancer Res ASCO 20:246, 1979.

185. Wick M: L-DOPA methyl ester as a new antitumor agent. Nature 269:512–513, 1977.

186. Wick M: An experimental approach to the chemotherapy of melanoma. J Invest Derm 74:63–65, 1980.

187. Wick M, Beyers L and Frei E: L-DOPA: selective toxicity for melanoma cell in vitro. Science 197:468–469, 1977.

188. Wick M: Levodopa and dopamine analogs as DNA polymerase inhibitors and antitumor agents in human melanoma. Cancer Res 10:1414–1418, 1980.

189. Wick M: Inhibitory effect of dopamine on human malignant melanoma. Proc Am Assoc Cancer Res ASCO 21:328, 1980.

190. Fay JW, Levine MN, Phillips GL et al: Treatment of metastatic melanoma with intensive 1,3-bis-(2-chlorethyl)-1-nitrosourea (BCNU) and autologous marrow transplantation (AMTX). Proc Am Assoc Cancer Res ASCO 22:532, 1981.

191. Gupta RK, Golub SH and Morton DL: Correlation between tumor burden and anticomplementary activity in sera from cancer patients. Cancer Immunol Immunother 6:63–71, 1979.

192. Gupta RK, Theofilopoulous AN, Dixon FL et al: Circulating immune complexes as possible cause for anticomplementary activity in humans with malignant melanoma. Cancer Immunol Immunother 6:211–221, 1979.

193. Cowan FM, Klein DL, Armstrong GR et al: Neutralization of immune complex inhibition of antibody dependent cellular cytotoxicity in vitro by Staphylococcusaureus protein A. Biomedicine 30:23–27, 1979.

194. Laszlo J, Lucas VS, Hanson DC et al: Levonantradol For chemotherapy-induced emesis: Phase I-II oral administration. J Clin Pharmacol (in press).

195. Terman DS, Yamamoto T, Tillquist P et al: Tumoricidal responses induced by cytosine arabinoside after plasma perfusion over protein A. Science 209:1257–1259, 1980.

196. Catalona WJ, Ratliff TL and McCool RE: Interferon induced by S. aureus protein A augments natural killing and ADCC. Nature 291:77–79, 1981.

# 14. Dermatologic manifestations of melanoma

ROBERT S. GILGOR

## Introduction

There is a distinctive appearance to many of the early lesions of cutaneous malignant melanoma (CMM) which allows early diagnosis and surgical treatment. At present the only effective method of increasing the cure of CMM is with early surgical excision. Overall prognosis correlates best with anatomic level of invasion and tumor thickness [3]. As tumors invade more deeply into the dermis and fat, five-year survival diminishes [10]. The importance of early clinical diagnosis of CMM cannot be overemphasized, since this should lead to better cure rates. Indeed, primary CMM can be recognized clinically with inspection in over 90% of instances [2]. Earlier recognition and treatment may already have been responsible for an overall increase in survival when comparing patients treated prior to 1949 with those treated after 1960 [7]. Certainly, early recognition and treatment takes on even greater importance when one realizes there is an alarming increase in the incidence of melanoma reported in many, though not all [15], countries around the world [13, 14, 17, 19, 21, 23]. In spite of improvement in the one- and five-year survival rate over the last 30 years [23], it is estimated that there has been a doubling of the incidence of melanoma every ten to 15 years [1]. There has been a dramatic increase in melanoma on the neck and trunk among males and the lower extremity among females, but there has not been an increase in incidence of melanomas found in the eye or other noncutaneous areas [17]. It is somewhat alarming that the increase in incidence appears to be greatest in people under the age of 65 years and that the average age of patients dying from melanoma is falling. Patients born more recently have a higher incidence of and mortality from melanoma at all ages than those born previously [13].

In the older literature, descriptions of cutaneous melanoma have stressed terms such as enlarged, darkened, bleeding or ulcerated. However, these terms are descriptive of malignant melanomas which have invaded deeply [2] and carry a poor prognosis in spite of aggressive surgical treatment.

Publication No. 108, Division of Dermatology, Department of Medicine, Duke University Medical Center.

*Seigler, H. F. (ed.), Clinical Management of Melanoma. ISBN 978-94-009-7495-1*

Recognizing the symptoms and signs of early melanoma is obviously most important.

The types of CMM noted in 1130 cases [3] were superficial spreading melanoma (SSM) in 70%, nodular melanoma (NM) in 15%, melanoma of the hands and feet (acral melanoma: AM) in 8%, lentigo malignant melanoma (LMM) in 5% and indeterminant in 2%. The most common site for a melanoma to appear on the skin in both males and females in the United States is on the back. In males, the back, anterior torso, upper extremity, head and neck are the most common sites involved. In females, the back, the posterior aspect of the leg, upper extremities, head and neck are the most common sites involved. In 1187 patients from Queensland, Australia with CMM, the back, face and lower leg were involved in decreasing frequency in men, and the lower leg, upper arm and back in decreasing frequency in women [25].

The most common feature which draws patients' attention to a CMM is an increase in size [16]; this was noted in 67% of 160 patients [4]. Increased size was characterized either by centrifugal spread or elevation above the skin surface. Bleeding was noted in 44% of patients, change in color in 38%, itching in 35% and ulceration in 20%. Ulceration was usually intermittent with minimal bleeding and lasting only a few days. Changes in color which were noted by patients have been different shades of brown, blue, black, gray and pink. Patients have even noted dark moles changing to pink or amelanotic [25]. The changes in color or size or development of symptoms noted by patients and indicative of malignancy persisted or recurred over a few weeks to a few months [4].

The history and physical examination of the patient with a possible CMM should include more than the limited area of the tumor and its lymphatic drainage. Family history of melanoma, long exposures to sunlight with easy burning, a previous history of a melanoma or the presence of freckling, blue eyes, hazel eyes, reddish or fair hair are all of importance. Only 11% of Americans have a very fair complexion, yet 80% of patients with CMM fit this description [12, 16, 18, 20, 22]. The age of the patient is also of interest, since melanoma is rare until puberty, except in congenital giant nevi [24].

The physician should have a routine method for carefully examining the completely undressed patient. The back of the patient, the front of the patient, the scalp, toes, palms, soles, webs, intertriginous areas and genitalia should all be examined in bright light. A suspicious lesion should be examined with a magnifying lens, and the lesion should be side lighted to determine if it is elevated or flat and to demonstrate any irregularities in the surface of the lesion. The pigmented lesion should be gently pinched to see if it "dimples." Dimpling or umbilication with gentle pinching is characteristic of a pigmented dermatofibroma [76]. The lesion should be measured, since almost all benign nevocellular nevi are less than 10 mm in size. A lesion less than 7 mm (one that can be covered by an ordinary unused pencil eraser) is most likely a benign nevocellular nevus or at worst, a curable form of early CMM [5, 77]. Lesions greater than 10 mm in diameter should be examined with great care, since they are the ones most likely to be melanoma. The black and pigmented races should have their palms, soles, fingernail and toenail areas examined most carefully because of the increased tendency of melanomas to appear in these sites.

Ultimately the diagnosis rests on obtaining tissue. Small lesions should be excised with a thin rim of normal skin and examined histopathologically [6]. If the lesion is too large to easily excise and close primarily or if the lesion is so large or anatomically situated that excision would produce disfigurement, then a 4 mm punch biopsy or a small incisional biopsy should be done [11]. A policy of waiting and watching a suspicious lesion is incorrect. Ten-year survival for patients having a punch biopsy or incisional biopsy followed by standard surgical excision within one week is 65.4% versus 55.8% ten-year survival for patients having immediate surgical excision [8]. Apparently prior punch or incisional biopsy does not change survival as long as early proper surgery is performed. However, the number of patients studied in this manner are small.

Any biopsy should be done to show the depth of invasion and the particular type of melanoma one is dealing with, since prognosis depends upon both of these factors. Areas which are elevated or nodular or blue-black should be biopsied, since they are most likely to define the depth of invasion. The surrounding flatter area should tell the histopathologist whether the lesion is an SSM or LMM. When dealing with large lesions or questionable lesions, several biopsies may be needed. Large initial surgical excisions for diagnostic reasons should be avoided, since most black lesions on the skin are not melanoma [8]. Only 2.1% of 559 black lesions noted in a dermatology practice were CMM and 60% of the time an experienced dermatologist was incorrect in his diagnosis when a melanoma was suspected clinically [8]. Definitive surgery should be undertaken as soon after a biopsy of a CMM as possible, since if a delay of up to a month takes place before proper surgery is accomplished, the five-year cure rate is reduced considerably [9].

**Common types of melanoma** (see Table 1)

*Superficial spreading melanoma*

The most common type of CMM is superficial spreading melanoma (SSM) (68.9%). Fortunately, this often has a characteristic appearance which will permit early diagnosis while the tumor is still in the radial growth

Table 1.

|  | SSM | NM | LMM | AM |
|---|---|---|---|---|
| % of All melanomas | 63–71% | 12–15% | 4–10% | 5–9% (50% M of blacks) |
| Most common sites | Back - M & F Calf - F | Head, neck, back | Sun exposed (cheeks & nose) | Soles great toe, thumb |
| Sex predominance | F>M | M>F | F:M - 3:1 | ? M = F |
| Age at diagnosis | 35–55 yr | 45–55 yr | 50–70 yr | 55–65 yr |
| *Diagnostic features* |  |  |  |  |
| Duration RGP | 1–5 yrs (up to 14 yrs) |  | 5–30 yrs (up to 40 yrs) | 1–2 yrs |
| Border | Elevated, notched | Sharp, no radial growth | Flat, highly irregular | Flat, irregular |
| Color | Haphazard shades of red. white, blue | Blood blister, thunder cloud gray, blue-black | Haphazard; browns, blacks lines & spots "stain" | Variegate brown, brown-black "stain" |

phase, and therefore, there is a greater chance of surgical cure [27]. Approximately 70% of patients will have noted an increase in size or color change in the lesion which is helpful in making the clinical diagnosis [26].

The tumor occurs at any age after puberty, though most often in middle age. It may be slightly more common in women than men. SSM may occur anywhere on the body, but the most characteristic areas are the upper back in men and women and the posterior aspect of the leg in women. The lesions may be diagnosed clinically when 5–10 mm in size. The small lesions usually have a haphazard arrangement of tan, brown, black and blue-black colors. The color may be dark and clumped in one area, absent in another and lacey and fine in a third area. It is often necessary to examine these lesions with a magnifying lens in a bright light to appreciate this disarray of colors in a smaller lesion. Sidelighting, even at this early stage, may show loss of skin markings, especially in the center of the lesion. As the tumor increases in diameter over months to a few years, the complexity of color changes increases and more red, white and blue shades appear. Again, it is stressed that red, white and blue shades in any skin lesion should arouse strong suspicion that the tumor is a melanoma. Lesions over 10 mm in diameter often reveal the haphazard presence of blue, blue-gray, purple, white and shades of pink or red-brown admixed with tans, browns and black. These varied colors are a hallmark of SSM [28, 29, 78]. The presence of gray-white in the center of a pigmented lesion is another important finding very suggestive of SSM. Sometimes the white color surrounds the tumor as in a halo nevus, but the depigmentation differs from benign lesions by being asymmetric and irregular in outline, and the tumor is usually eccentrically placed within the depigmented skin.

The pink and red areas signify inflammatory response to the tumor; the white areas signify tumor regression; and the blue colors are due to melanin present deeper in the dermis. Besides the disarray of colors, the other features helpful in making a clinical diagnosis are surface changes and border abnormalities. Except for the occasional small lesion, the borders are almost always characterized by an irregular outline, prominent indentations or notching and sometimes a kidney-shaped outline. The irregular border is equated with irregular regression and spread of the tumor [26]. The notches in the border are quite characteristic and may be multiple and small or large. Not infrequently, one prominent notch is noted. The notching becomes more apparent as lesions increase in size. The third feature of SSM, irregular surface changes, is more difficult to appreciate clinically and may occur less often than the color changes or border abnormalities. Appreciation of the surface changes may be aided by shining a penlight obliquely at the tumor. One should look for irregular areas of scaling, irregular elevations and change in the surface markings. SSM usually presents with visibly or palpably elevated margins, as opposed to lentigo maligna (LM) which does not have elevated borders and is often noted to be similar to a stain. However, SSM on the back may have a flat border. The scaling may be diffuse or it may be focal or irregular. Scaling is noted especially on scalp lesions. Absence of the fine cross-hatched skin markings can be seen in early SSM lesions as well as advanced lesions, but this feature can also be noted in many benign conditions, such as nevocellualr nevi, dermatofibromas, pyogenic granulomas and blue nevi. Therefore, absence of fine skin lines in and of itself is not diagnostic of CMM, but must be considered along with the constellation of color changes, border abnormalities and other surface changes. Irregular elevations of the surface is another feature of SSM. With the beginning of the vertical growth phase (VGP), there may be a relatively sudden focal change in the surface elevation of the lesion. The tumor which develops nodules is usually $2\frac{1}{2}$ cm in diameter or greater. The nodule usually appears as a small uniformly blue-black, black, purple, brown or pink colored relatively rapidly growing, smooth surfaced papule or nodule. Frank hemmorrhage from the surface of these lesions is most unusual; ulceration and oozing of blood may occur. However, this is usually a late and ominous finding which means invasion to the deeper reticular dermis or fat [28].

The average SSM reaches 2.5 cm in diameter in size before patients seek medical care. It is quite unusual for a benign nevocellular nevus to be larger than 10 mm and therefore, size is another helpful finding in making the clinical diagnosis of CMM [27].

Most helpful features for clinical diagnosis of SSM:

1. History of change in color or size
2. Size: greater than 10 mm
3. Color: (early) 5–10 mm – haphazard tan, brown, black and blue-black; (later) greater than 10 mm – shades of red, white and blue with haphazard, variegate arrangement
4. Borders: irregular, notched
5. Elevation: irregular surface, irregular scaling, loss of skin markings
6. Use bright light, magnifying lens and sidelighting

*Lentigo malignant (LM) and lentigo malignant melanoma (LMM):*
*melanotic freckle of Hutchinson or circumscribed precancerous melanosis*
*of Dubreuilh*

LM is an intraepidermal melanoma which usually occurs as a single lesion in sun-exposed areas, especially the face and neck. It is most common in caucasians over the age of forty years (90%). It has, however, been noted as early as the third decade. The average age of onset is in the forties, though most patients don't seek help until the fifties to seventies [30–32]. To casual inspection, the initial lesion appears as a completely flat, tan, freckle-like stain on the skin. Early in its course the LM develops an irregular shape and a darker color [26–28]. Even in the early lesions one may appreciate a "play of colors" within the tan to brown to brown-black range. A magnifying lens more readily reveals the lines, flecks and reticulate deposits of irregular brown, dark brown, brown-black and black colors which extend to the margins of the lesions. A haphazard disarray of colors is noted. At the time of diagnosis the average lesion is 2.7 cm$^2$ (1–3 cm diameter most often), but lesions as large as 8 cm have been noted. The lesion extends and regresses irregularly over many years and may be present 40 to 50 years before developing vertical growth and invasive melanoma. Growth of the lesion is slow and erratic regarding both time and size. Borders become irregular and complex with indentations. Such areas extend with the characteristic fine flecks and lines of colors at the same time other sites regress with the appearance of white, gray, gray-white or bluish color [78]. Some lesions have been noted to completely resolve only to recur months or years later and sometimes with a nodule of lentigo meligna melanoma (LMM) [30, 32]. In general, the colors don't appear as rich as in SSM. Sometimes one gets the impression that a LM is moving around on the skin [26] and that the color is changing as well [30]. However, the overall tendency is for the lesion to expand in size. Patients are often aware of the lesions for years, but because of the slow changes they do not seek medical advice. When there is a more rapid increase in diameter, nodule development or marked increase in dark coloration in one site, patients will often become concerned and seek help [30]. Though LM is usually flat and appears as a stain on the skin, an occasional lesion will show epidermal hyperplasia. This verrucous component may involve either a localized area or the entire lesion similar to a seborrheic keratosis [28].

Dermal invasion has been noted in some LMs, while the lesion is still perfectly flat, and in one series only 15 of 45 patients with microscopic invasion of the dermis were noted clinically to have nodular lesions [30]. Lesions greater than 4 cm in diameter have the highest percentage of melanomas present, though most lesions with melanoma (about 50%) are in the 1–3 cm diameter range. The chances of LM developing into a LMM are greatest in the lesions found on the torso (12 of 16 patients) as compared to lesions on the head and neck (24 of 53 patients) [30]. The exact risk of developing invasive CMM in patients with LM is unknown, but once LMM develops mortality is between 10% and 15% [30, 32]. LMM has the best prognosis of all melanomas. Interestingly, there are reports of biopsy-proven LMM regressing spontaneously without any therapy.

With the onset of the verticle growth phase (VGP) and development of LMM, there may be a slight elevation in one area or occasionally more than one area. The color of these elevated portions is usually black but may be brown, blue-black or rarely flesh colored (amelanotic). The elevated areas may be shiny, scaly, hyperkeratotic, eroded or ulcerated, but they are not usually pedunculated [27, 28]. The diagnosis of LM and LMM rests on histologic examination, though it certainly may be suspected by the patient's age, location of the lesion in sun exposed sites, long duration of the LM and the clinical appearance. Several biopsies may be necessary to make the correct diagnosis. The areas most likely to show the atypical melanocytes of LM are the black specks or lines and the flat black areas rather than the tan or white. Elevated, infiltrated or papulo-nodular areas should be biopsied to rule out LMM. Lesions of LM on the torso should be biopsied in multiple sites to rule out LMM.

Most helpful features for the diagnosis of LM:

1. Color: haphazard arrangement of tans, browns, blacks with spots and lines of black

2. Flat: looks like a stain
3. Large size: 90% greater than 1 cm and 60% greater than 2 cm
4. Borders: markedly irregular
5. Age group: 90% over 40 years; average age at diagnosis 65 years
6. Site: mostly exposed areas especially face (cheeks and nose)
7. Evolution: usually over many years

*Nodular melanoma (NM)*

A nodular melanoma is a papule or nodule of melanoma cells with no significant radial growth phase (RGP) either clinically or histopathologically. The tumor from its inception appears to have only a VGP. Nodules of all melanomas are similar histologically. However, the skin surrounding the tumor allows the clinical and pathological categorization of the melanoma into different types (i.e., SSM, LMM, NM or ALM). NM is a much more aggressive tumor with a greater tendency to metastasize [26]. The initial lesion most commonly presents as a uniform blue-black, blue-gray, blue-red, blue-purple (thunder cloud gray), black, gray-black or red-brown dome-shaped papule or nodule that often resembles a blood blister or hemangioma. Rarely (less than 5% of NMs) [26] NM may start as an amelanotic flesh colored or pink lesion. There are usually areas of grayish blue hue within the amelanotic lesion, best noted in bright light. However, even amelanotic lesions have tiny flecks of black or blue-black at the base of the nodules. NM usually begins on uninvolved skin, but less commonly may arise from a nevocellular nevus. The early lesion is symmetrical and dome shaped with a smooth surface. Small lesions may become polypoidal with growth. Lesions grow rapidly, and they may ulcerate, crust or become scaly. There is usually a sharp border between the tumor and normal skin. Much less often the lesion presents as a blue-black or black plaque with an irregular surface containing nodules of different sizes. Certainly, the most outstanding feature of NM is the dark color resembling a blood blister [26–29, 78].

NM occurs more commonly on the head, neck and back of males. It occurs with equal frequency in males and females on the extremities. The most common time of onset is between 45 and 55 years of age [10].

The most helpful features in clinical diagnosis of NM:

1. Color: blood blister, thunder cloud gray, blue-black or black
2. Elevation: uniform, smooth papule or nodule
3. Rapid growth

*Acral melanoma and melanoma of periungual and subungual areas*

Acral melanoma refers to a melanoma occurring on the nonhair-bearing surfaces of the palms and soles and in the peri- and sub-ungual areas. NM and SSM can occur on palms and soles, but by far the most common type of melanoma occurring in these sites is the acral lentiginous melanoma (ALM). SSM on the palms and soles has most of the characteristics of SSM found in other locations. Marked color variation, irregular notched borders, distinct but slight elevation of the border, destruction of skin markings, hyperkeratosis and, later, nodulation may all be noted. The lesion is not as large nor as irregular in outline as ALM, and the surface is often irregular as compared to the smooth surface of ALM [29, 35]. NMs of the palms and soles usually appear as dark papules or nodules either brown-black, blue-black, blue or black. They may rarely be pink. They may be slightly raised or polypoidal and quite large. However, both SSM and NM are infrequently found in acral areas. The remainder of the discussion of acral melanoma will concern the ALM.

The ALM differs from the other lentiginous type melanoma, LMM, in several important aspects. The most important difference is that the ALM is a much more aggressive tumor with a great tendency to have nodal metastases and a high mortality. Level three and four invasion may be present with no or barely perceptible elevation of the lesion. No actinic damage is noted on histologic exam. The dysplastic melanocytic cells are found in the basal layer similar to a LM, rather than in a pagetoid fashion as in SSM. Similar lesions with a poor prognosis have been noted on mucous membranes, at the mucocutaneous junction of the oral and nasal cavities, and the anus. Early diagnosis and early surgical therapy for the ALM are the only means of improving the dismal prognosis [33–35]. Between 5% and 9% of all melanomas reported are in the volar–subungual sites; about 70% are volar and about 30% are subungual. Median age at diagnosis is usually between the late fifties and mid sixties; this diagnosis has been noted between the third and ninth decades [35, 36]. Patients in younger age groups seem to have a better prognosis [33]. The tumor tends to favor blacks [79–81], Orientals [82], Puerto Ricans [83] and natives of India [84]. While only 1% of all melanomas in the United States occurs in blacks, about 25% of melanomas on the soles and subungual areas of the toes occur in blacks [13, 85]. In one review, two-thirds of 27 patients with plantar lentiginous melanoma were black [33].

ALM (including peri- and sub-ungual lesions) may account for up to 50% of all melanomas in blacks [37]. ALM occurs more often on the soles than the palms [33, 34], while nail lesions occur with equal frequency on the hands and feet [27].

The palm and sole lesions begin as a "stain" on the skin with a haphaz-

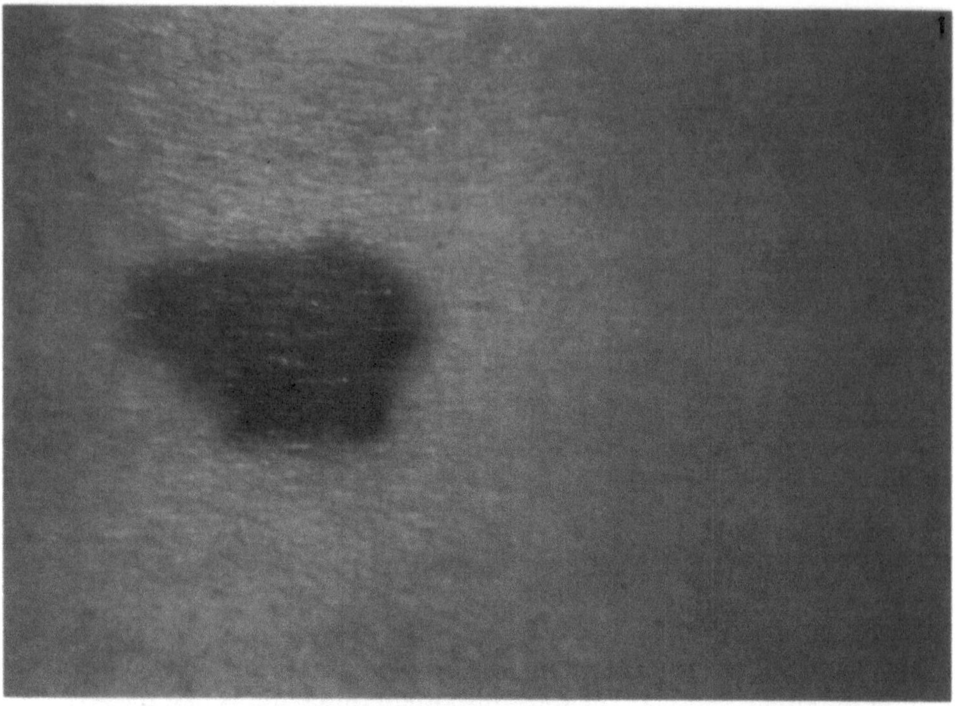

414

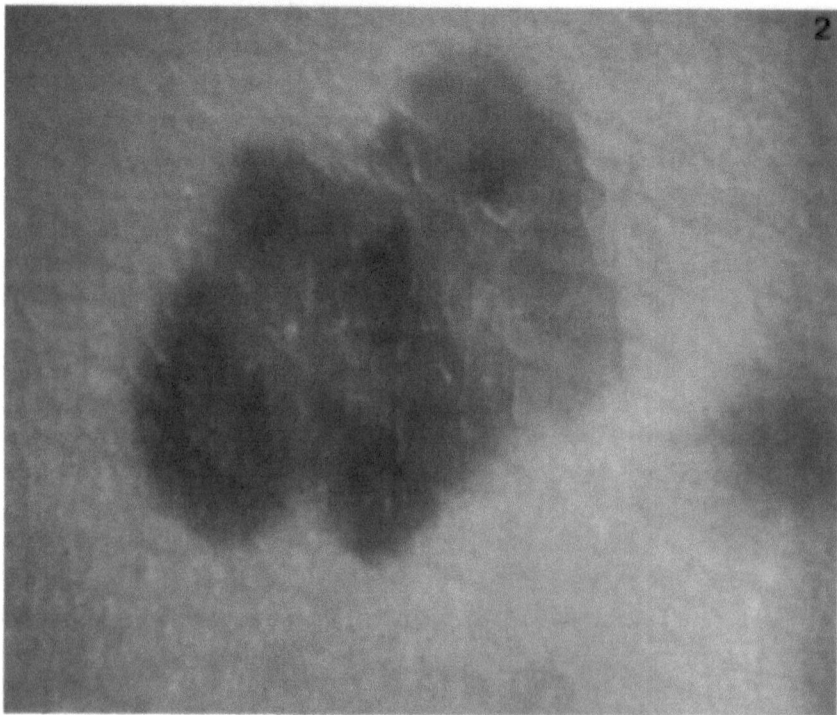

*Figure 1.* Early SSM, Level II. Note irregular outline, haphazard color. *Figure 2.* SSM: note notched borders, slight elevation and haphazard arrangement of pink, blue-black, brown and yellow-orange. Skin lines are different from surrounding skin.

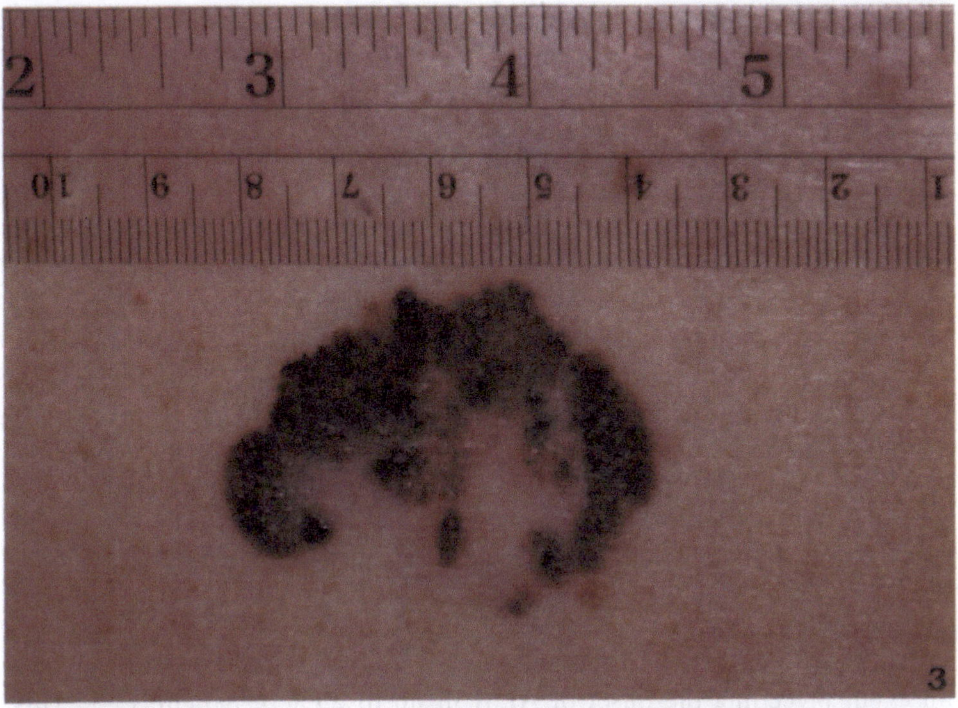

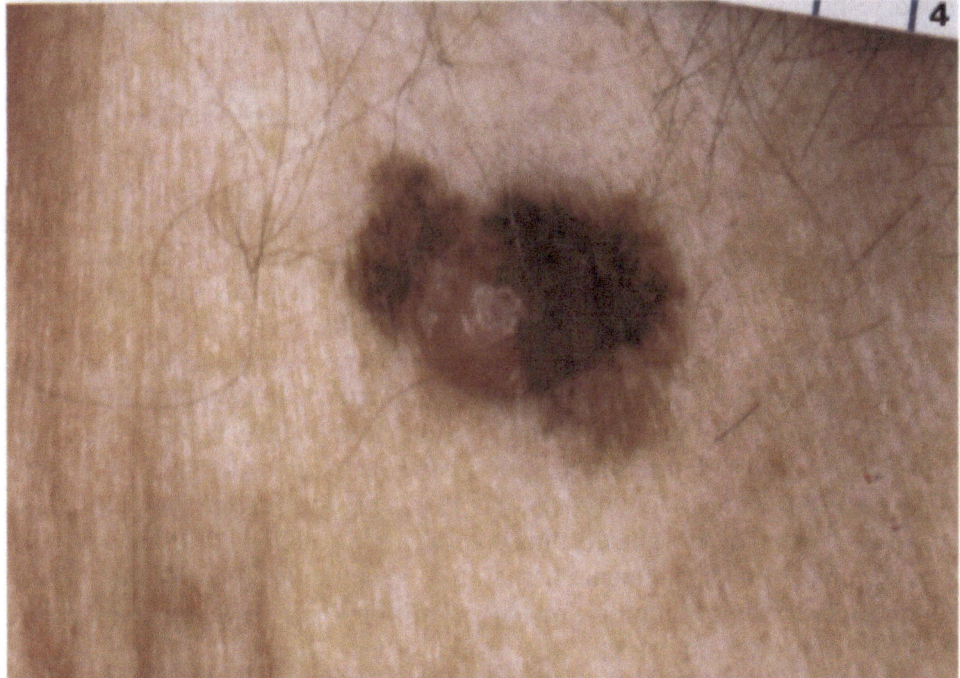

415

*Figure 3.* Large SSM, Level III. Note large and small notches of border. Striking color differences are seen with brown-black, pink, yellow, red, blue shades. Irregular elevation, loss of fine skin markings and irregular scaling can also be seen. *Figure 4.* SSM with Level IV nodule. Note notched border, irregular outline and color. Central nodule with irregular coloration.

ard and varied brown, brown-black color and an irregular border [35, 37, 40, 41]. Skin markings and print ridges are not disturbed. Lesions are usually flat at first. The average diameter at the time of diagnosis is about 2.7 cm, though they vary in size from 0.4 to 8 cm [33, 34]. The average duration prior to diagnosis is about two and a half years [33]. Peripheral growth is slow and irregular and bluish or depigmented areas occur. Lesions may attain a large size before the VGP develops, and there may be only minimal elevation of the lesion with level four invasion [26, 39]. The surface may become hyperkeratotic and even simulate the appearance of a resistant plantar verruca [38]. Ulceration may be common in neglected lesions and with time fungating masses may appear [33].

Since completely benign evenly pigmented acral lentigines occur in 20% to 40% of blacks [34], it is important to look carefully in black patients for a variegate and haphazard arrangement of colors and an irregular border to rule out ALM. If in doubt, a biopsy should be done. Sufficient incisional biopsy material should be taken, since the histology may show a gradation of dysplastic melanocytic cells [27, 37, 39].

Trauma or a history of regional corns or "blood blisters" may be noted as an event preceding the onset of ALM in up to 25% of patients [34]. This history should not dissuade the physician from allowing the physical findings of irregular borders, variegate colors, etc. to convince him to biopsy the varied colored acral lesion.

Subungual or periungual melanoma (SUM) or melanotic whitlow of Hutchinson is a rare type of melanoma, constituting only 72 of 2824 (2.6%) melanomas noted in one study [36] and 27 of 781 (3.4%) melanomas in another study [86]. Approximately one half occur under fingernails and half under toenails. SUM occurs with equal frequency in men and women and is most often diagnosed in the fifth, sixth and seventh decades (mean 57 years) [36]. SUM constitutes 15% to 20% of melanomas in blacks and 2% to 3% of melanomas in Caucasians [27]. Over two-thirds of SUMs involve the great toe or thumb. Over 40% of patients give a history of bleeding or some change in the nail following trauma. Many have been treated for benign conditions for months to years before a biopsy has been obtained. Up to one-third of patients with SUMs have enlarged regional lymph nodes when first seen. Unfortunately, many patients are followed for some time with the diagnosis of subungual hematoma. Up to 20% of SUMs are pink or flesh colored. Most patients have no symptoms and seek advice simply because of the appearance of a new lesion, or less often (25%), because of a change in color or enlargement of an old lesion. Occasionally patients have sought help because of distorted nail plates, swelling and bleeding from the nail bed, imgrowing toenail, paronychia, spontaneous ulceration, tumor presenting through the nail plate or pain [27, 29, 36, 86].

Early subungual melanomas may show brown to black discoloration in the nail bed and matrix with a rapid spread of pigment to involve the skin around the nail (Hutchinson's sign) and the nail plate [27, 86]. Bands or streaks of black or varying shades of brown, black, blue, tan and white are noted in the nail plate [27, 29]. These bands grow down the nail plate to the free margin at a variable rate. The nail plate may become detached from the nail bed and stop growing. Especially in the toenails, amelanotic tumors may closely resemble pyogenic granulomas. Thickening, distortion, destruction or splitting of the nail plate may occur with time and surrounding tissue may become inflamed and painful with secondary infection. The SUM may appear similar to several different benign or malignant conditions such as bacterial infection (felon), fungal infection, hematoma, Glomus tumor, Kaposi's sarcoma, pyogenic granuloma, epidermal inclusion cyst, bony exostosis, ingrown nail, foreign body reaction, nevocellular nevus, keratoacanthoma, Bowen's disease and squamous cell carcinoma [27]. It should be emphasized that SUMs involve the matrix, nail bed, nail plate and surrounding epidermis and involvement of the eponychium (Hutchinson's sign) is quite characteristic of this tumor [42].

Longitudinal bands of pigmentation in the nail plate are not uncommon in blacks and Orientals, while they are uncommon in Caucasians. They are probably not nevocellular in origin, but they are simply due to an increase in the number and activity of dopa positive melanocytes in the lower two to four layers of the nail matrix [43]. This benign pigmentation does not involve the surrounding epidermis nor the nail bed, and it does not distort the nail plate. These benign streaks generally are present for long periods of time without change as opposed to the rapid changes seen in SUMs.

The subungual hematoma is the most important benign lesion to differentiate from a SUM. The subungual hematoma may appear as a black lesion or a golden red-blue color in the nail bed or matrix, usually with, but sometimes without, a history of trauma. The hemorrhage is sharply localized, usually not parallel to the length of the nail plate and does not show pigmentation of adjacent skin. The demarcation of hemorrhage is usually sharp and with the margin usually parallel to the free edge of the nail plate. Variegate colors are not present [29]. If the diagnosis is in doubt, a large bore needle can be used to slowly drill a hole in the nail plate to reveal the blood. If the lesion is a subungual melanoma, tumor tissue may come through the small hole. A short period of two to three weeks of watchful waiting with pictures taken before and after may show the hematoma moving distally as the nail plate grows out. If there is any doubt of the diagnosis, an adequate incisional biopsy should be done of the nail bed and matrix [29].

Subungual glomus tumors usually appear as a blue varix under the nail plate. They are exquisitely tender to touch and sometimes sensitive to cold exposure. Sharp radiating pains are noted, either spontaneously or after trauma or cold exposure [36, 86].

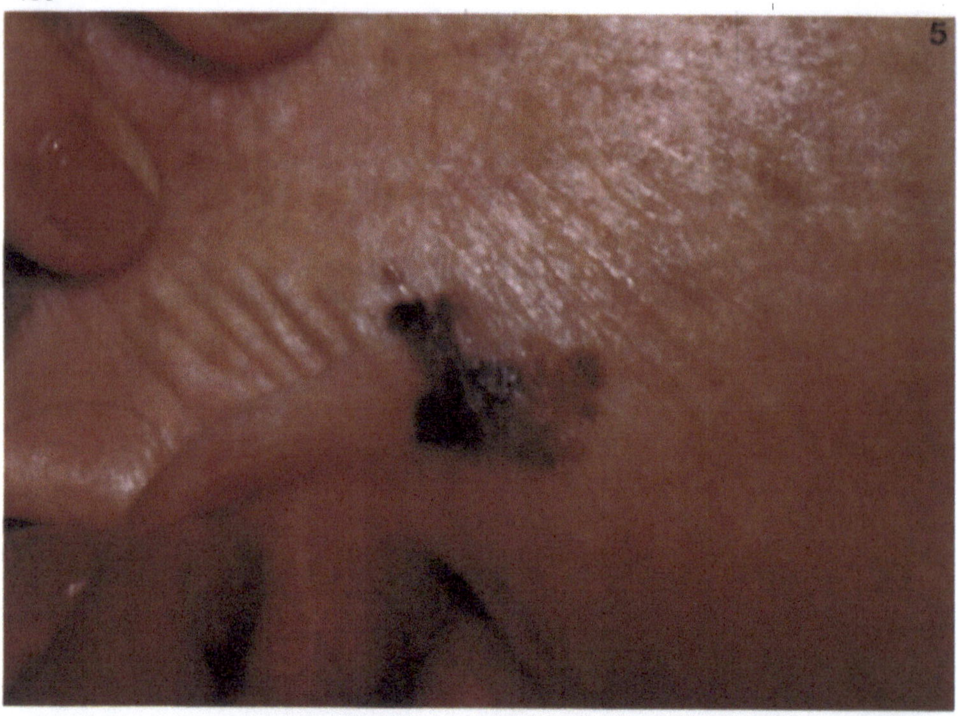

418

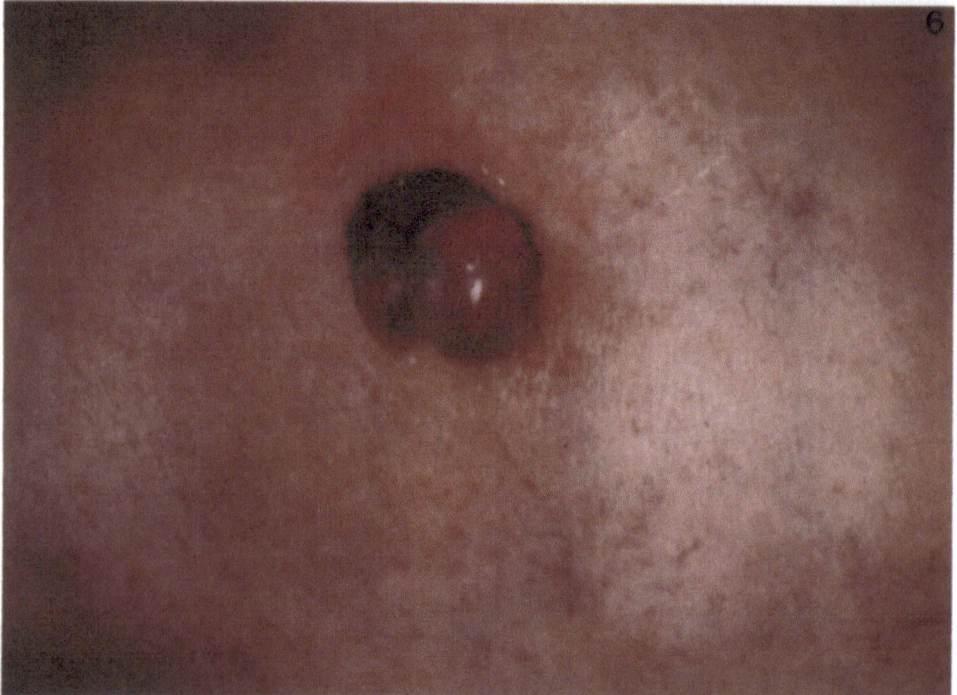

*Figure 5.* LMM, Level II: note markedly irregular outline to this preauricular lesion. Shades of tan, brown and brown-black are in disarray. *Figure 6.* Nodular melanoma with "blood blister" appearance. Red and dark brown colors are in haphazard arrangement.

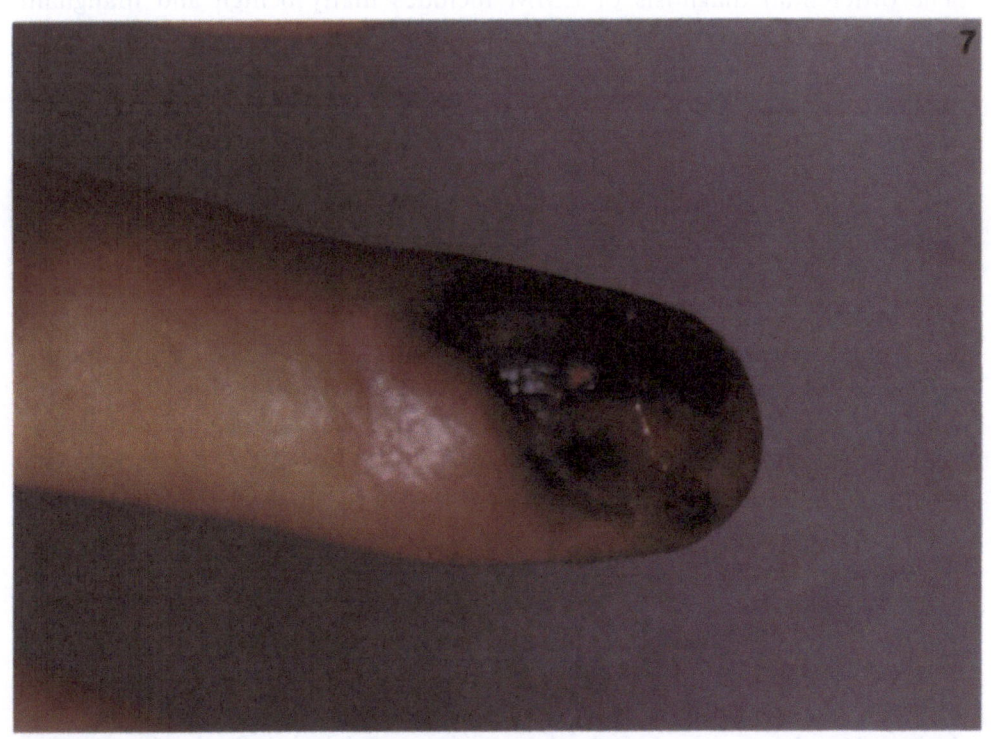

*Figure 7.* Subungual melanoma. Note spread of pigment to skin surrounding the nail plate (Hutchinson's sign). The nail plate is partially destroyed and irregularly colored.

Some SUMs are associated with pain, swelling and purulent discharge similar to a paronychia. However, most paronychia occur rather suddenly over a period of days and have no preceding nail pigment changes.

Pyogenic granulomas often occur in lateral nailfolds where ingrowing nail plates traumatize the skin. They are rapidly growing (over a period of weeks rather than months) pink to flesh colored, soft, friable and sharply marginated. They may be confused with amelanotic melanomas, although flecks of pigmentation are not seen at their base. Pyogenic granulomas should be examined histopathologically to assure their benign nature.

Most helpful clinical features of SUM:

1. Hutchinson's sign: pigmentation of skin next to the nail plate
2. Variably pigmented linear nail bands
3. Nail dystrophy

### Differential diagnosis of cutaneous malignant melanoma

The differential diagnosis of CMM includes many benign and malignant disorders, such as nevocellular nevus, BK moles, benign juvenile melanoma, halo nevus, blue nevus, pseudomelanoma (recurrent nevocellular nevus), plantar wart, pigmented BCE, dermatofibroma, seborrheic keratosis, vascular ectasia and hemangioma, pyogenic granuloma, pigmented actinic keratosis and pigmented Bowen's disease.

Nevocellular nevi rarely show the haphazard variegate pigmentation noted in SSM. They are usually tan to brown and show variations in shades of brown or orange-brown rather than pinks, blues, blacks and whites. Acquired nevi often first appear as flat junctional lesions between the ages of six months and one year. New lesions continue to arise late into the third decade. The radial growth is slow and color changes are also slow to take place. Nevi may darken or grow more rapidly during pregnancy or while patients are on anovulatory drugs. Symptoms do not often arise in nevocellular nevi. These benign lesions are almost always less than 10 mm in diameter. Their borders are usually regular and without notching. Generally their shape is regular, being round to oval. Diagnostic problems arise in nevi that are flat or slightly raised and have irregular borders and perhaps with some flecks of pigmentation or pink areas. These may closely resemble early SSM. If there is any doubt regarding the appearance or if there is any sudden physical change (over three months or less) or any symptoms, then the lesion should be excised. Indeed, any pigmented lesion 9 mm diameter or greater that has variegate color should be biopsied or excised [28, 29].

Intradermal nevi which are elevated or pedunculated and have melanin in the mid dermis may appear blue; they may be difficult to distinguish from nodular melanoma. These lesions are usually uniformly blue or light gray, and they are often present for a long period of time with slow growth as opposed to the rapid growth of NM.

Spindle cell nevi (Spitz nevi or benign juvenile melanoma, BJM) are benign lesions usually occurring on the face, upper extremities or trunk of children. Less often they occur in adults. They may have a sudden onset with rapid growth for nine to 12 months. They then stabilize or grow more slowly. Lesions are pink-tan and dome shaped, though they may be darker brown or even black. Diascopy or pressure with two glass slides to blanch out the pink, often reveals a tan-brown color. The color is usually uniform. Obviously, the rapid growth and pink color may resemble an amelanotic melanoma. However, NMs are quite rare in children and often show flecks of pigment at their base [26, 28, 29].

BK moles are discussed in more detail later in the chapter. BK moles are large, 5–15 mm irregularly outlined nevi, often multiple, with variable size and distribution. There may be less than ten to greater than a hundred present. They are most prominent in the "yoke area" of the trunk and upper extremities. They are haphazardly pigmented, often with pink, white, tan, brown and black areas. There are obvious resemblances to SSM. Indeed, BK moles have been associated with familial melanoma and the development of multiple melanomas which are usually SSM in type [28, 44, 45]. There are subtle differences often noted between SSMs and BK moles. The margins of a BK mole usually blend into the surrounding skin, rather than being elevated as in SSM. The skin markings are usually maintained in BK moles and often lost in SSMs. BK moles are minimally elevated in the center. New lesions may continue to develop throughout life.

Blue nevi are uniformly dark blue, flat or slightly elevated small lesions which are usually static in size. Their outline is usually uniform but can be irregular. Flat lesions should not be confused with SSM which has a play on colors. Elevated lesions may resemble a NM, though the uniform blue color and lack of smooth surface are not characteristic of NM [28].

Pigmented basal cell epitheliomas (BCEs) usually occur in one of two clinical presentations. The nodular BCE resembles NM with its black color. Examination with a magnifying lens often reveals within the nodule tiny black dots not usually seen in NM [28]. Pigmented BCEs do not have the rapid growth of NM. The second clinical picture is that of a flat or plaque-like pigmented BCE. This may resemble a SSM but often has a translucent thread-like border, or areas of translucency or black dots within the lesion itself. These features are best noted using a hand lens and sidelighting the tumor. Lesions may have scale, erythema, brown and bluish-black colors present. Telangiectasia typical of BCEs may sometimes be noted [27–29].

Pseudomelanoma or "recurrent melanocytic nevus following surgical removal" may occur within a few weeks of incomplete shave excision of intradermal nevocellular nevi in young adults [46, 87]. They are flat with slightly irregular borders and with "variegate pigmentation." They are usually stippled with jet black areas or may be uniformly black. Sometimes a scar may also be seen. History and histologic criteria will help differentiate this lesion from a SSM.

Large pigmented actinic keratoses (AKs) may resemble LM and may require biopsy for accurate diagnosis. The tan-brown color is usually more uniform than LM. The surface of AKs is often barely elevated and usually feels rough, while LMs are flat and smooth to the touch. Skin markings are abnormal in AKs while they are not interrupted in LMs. The border of a LM is more irregular than the border of an AK. Light reflects differently off the surface of an AK, being dull and flat.

Vascular ectasias and hemangiomas may be bluish or blue-black and globoid. They usually have the red-blue hue of blood or golden-purple hue of hemosiderin [29]. Pigmented Bowen's disease or superficial SCC may have the same irregular outline and variegate color as SSM, but these diseases usually have more hyperkeratosis than SSM. Lesions may be found anywhere on the body surface, but tend to favor the genitalia.

**BK mole syndrome and familial melanoma**

Familial malignant melanoma (FMM) is reported in at least 1% to 6% of patients with CMM [47, 48, 50, 88, 89, 90]. Patients with FMM have a tendency for their melanomas to occur earlier in life, for the development of multiple primary lesions and for an increased frequency of other types of malignancy, either in the patients or their families [50, 51, 88, 89]. Most of the patients are of Celtic or Northern-European descent [51]. Little or no consanguinity has been noted in the patients. In some instances no specific pattern of inheritance is found [51], while in several other studies an autosomal dominant type inheritance is noted [44, 45, 50, 52]. Many, but not all, patients with FMM present a distinctive phenotype called the BK mole syndrome [44] or the familial atypical multiple mole-melanoma syndrome [52]. In either case, whether part of the BK mole syndrome or not, relatives of patients with melanoma should be examined intermittently for melanomas, since they have a greater chance of developing CMM than the general population. In addition, patients and relatives should be screened for other types of malignancies such as breast, GI tract, sarcoma and lymphoreticular malignancies; the exact increase in risk for developing these problems has not been defined [50–52, 88, 89]. The patient with a single CMM, whether or not a familial pattern has been noted and whether or not he or she has the BK mole syndrome, has a much greater chance of developing a second primary melanoma than does someone from the general population [88]. Of patients who develop a second primary melanoma, most do so within five years of the first melanoma [91]. Patients with CMM require follow-up, not only to look for local recurrences and metastases, but also for a thorough evaluation of the entire skin surface for a second primary lesion. Multiple primary melanomas have been noted in 19% of patients with familial melanomas and 1% to 4% of patients without a family history [47–49]. The number of these malignancies is usually less than five.

The BK mole syndrome stands out as a unique disorder, characterized usually by a dominantly inherited syndrome of large and variably sized moles occurring mostly in the "horse collar" area above the breast and on the upper arms. Lesions can be found virtually anywhere on the body from the scalp to the feet, though they are infrequently noted on the lower extremities and buttocks. Nevocellular nevi, however, are quite rare on the buttocks and unusual on the lower extremities. BK moles are irregular in outline and have a haphazard arrangement of white, pink, tan, brown and black colors. There is great variability, not only in color, but in size when comparing several different lesions in an individual. They range from 5 to 15 mm in diameter and average about 10 mm. The edges of the lesions are flat, but the centers are slightly elevated. Some of these lesions have been noted photographically to develop into SSM [44].

The histology of the BK mole is also unique, showing atypical melanocytic hyperplasia, lymphocytic dermal infiltrate, delicate fibroplasia and new blood vessels occurring within a compound nevus or de novo [44, 45, 52].

Among six melanoma families, 15 of 17 patients examined with melanoma had the BK moles and of 41 relatives without melanoma, 22 had the BK moles. Ten of the fifteen with melanoma and BK moles had multiple primaries. Metastases and mortality were high [44]. In seven consecutive families with melanoma, the BK moles were noted in 18 of 20 patients (90%) with melanoma and 24 of 43 (56%) first degree relatives. This search led to the detection of early stage melanoma in six family members [45]. Familial melanoma in these two studies appears to be strongly linked with the BK mole syndrome. As many as 50% of relatives of patients with BK mole syndrome with CMM may have the same syndrome. A family search should be made in all patients with BK moles, since there will be a number of family members with early and curable CMMs. Patients with BK moles and family members both have to be followed closely. BK mole patients should be examined and pictures taken and compared three or four times yearly. Any suspicious lesions should be surgically excised.

## Leukoderma and melanoma

A variety of depigmentary phenomena may take place in patients with either primary CMM or metastatic melanoma or following several different treatments for melanoma. Most commonly, however, depigmentary phenomena are associated with completely benign disorders. Halos of depigmentation have been reported around nevocellular nevi (halo nevi), neural nevi, blue nevi and neurofibromas unassociated with any malignant disorder [60]. The pigment changes are best seen using Wood's light to accentuate the color changes within the epidermis. Halo nevus is the most common of these benign lesions, and it is not unusual to find vitiligo in the same patient [60]. Halo nevi occur most often in caucasian children and young adults (mean age about 17 years), especially on the trunk. They are usually small compound nevi, less than 7 mm in diameter, and they have a benign nevocellular histology with a dense lymphocytic infiltrate. The halo is usually quite regular and the nevus centrally placed, though on occasion eccentrically placed nevi and irregular borders have been noted. The nevocellular component usually disappears over years and less often the depigmented area may clear as well [59, 60].

Depigmentation may be noted in four setting in patients with CMM: 1) Halo nevi may occur in patients with CMM [27] or after removal of CMM [54] or coincident with the development of metastatic disease [57]. 2) Halos may occur around primary CMMs (halo melanomas) or metastases [61]. Most often these lesions show an eccentrically placed tumor with an irregular border and an irregularly shaped depigmented area. 3) Depigmented areas (areas of tumor regression) may occur within melanomas and may completely depigment the lesion [61]. 4) Widespread vitiligo and/or leukoderma have been noted at sites distant from halo melanomas [27], after chemotherapy [60] or vaccination therapy [55] of melanoma and coincident with metastatic melanoma [57].

Between one-third and 100% of patients [53, 56] with early CMM and virtually all resolving halo nevi patients [53] have significant titers of an IGG antibody directed against the cytoplasm of homologous melanoma cells. The cytoplasmic staining pattern of the halo nevus cells and CMM cells with this antibody are identical [58]. The anticytoplasmic antibodies have not been noted in patients with nevocellular nevi, vitiligo unassociated with halo nevi, nor in patients with BJM [53]. The first appearance of the antibody may coincide with the disappearance of nevus cells of the halo nevus and the melanocytes from the halo [53]. Within three to five months of excision of a halo nevus, and sometimes after the natural clearing of a halo nevus, the anticytoplasmic antibodies are no longer found in the circulation. A fall in antibody titer has been noted to precede the appearance of melanoma metastases. It has been speculated that a second antibody against the anticytoplasmic antibody may have caused this decrease in anti-cytoplasmic antibody. It has also been theorized that the loss of pigment and disappearance of the halo nevus may be an immunologic phenomenon brought about in part by the anticytoplasmic antibody directed against altered nevus cells that are undergoing malignant degeneration [53]. Clinically and histopathologically, halo nevi are benign lesions even though the cytoplasm of all of its nevus cells react with the cytoplasmic antibody, implying that all the nevocellular cells of the halo nevi have undergone some change from normal [54]. It may be that the appearance of the anti-cytoplasmic antibody can be used as a test in the early diagnosis of CMM and to note the onset of melanoma in giant congenital nevi or in high risk family groups [56].

Halo nevi have been noted following excision of a primary cutaneous melanoma [54]. The histology of these halo nevi has shown atypical, disintegrating melanocytes with pleomorphic and hyperchromatic nuclei adjacent to normal nevus cells. Only a sparse lymphocytic infiltrate was present as compared to the dense lymphocytic infiltrate in common halo nevi unassociated with the excisions of a primary cutaneous melanoma. Several of these patients have been noted to have marked in vitro cell mediated immune responses to the melanoma antigens; some patients had an overall increase in all intradermal tests applied [54]. The different roles the immune system is playing in CMM awaits further illucidation.

The exact incidence of halo nevi occurring in patients with primary CMM is not known, but this phenomenon may be more common than suspected. One should do a careful systemic, cutaneous examination looking for the presence of primary CMM in patients past puberty with vitiligo, halo nevi or other depigmenting phenomenon. A Wood's lamp may help accentuate some of the depigmented areas.

Development of depigmented areas temporally related to the onset of metastatic melanoma was noted in 11 of 64 patients. Four of the 11 with metastases had vitiligo. Four of 11 had halo nevi, and three of these four had six, eight, and over 50 halo nevus lesions, respectively. It was concluded that patients with halo nevi associated with malignant melanoma are more likely to have three or more halo nevi than patients who have halo nevi unassociated with melanoma. Five of 11 patients had a unique depigmenting event associated with metastatic CMM. They had a patchy distribution of irregularly marginated depigmented macules. The borders were distinctly different from those of vitiligo. The distribution of these lesions was not periorificial nor over areas of trauma or pressure points as in "benign" vitiligo. None of the pigmentary abnormalities correlated with the patient's age or sex or survival of the patient from time of diagnosis or onset of metastasis [57].

## Malignant melanoma in childhood and infancy

The transplacental metastasis of CMM has rarely been reported, though CMM is probably the most common malignancy to metastasize to the placenta [62, 63]. Seven of 18 placental metastases originated from maternal malignant melanoma.

Primary CMM in prepubertal children is rare, accounting for 0.5% of 3175 MM patients seen between 1944 and 1975 at the M.D. Anderson Hospital [64]. Four of 15 of these patients developed their melanoma in association with either a giant congenital nevus or meningeal melanocytosis. Other authors claim that as many as 40% of prepubertal melanomas develop in giant congenital nevi [65, 66]. Mortality in prepubertal CMM is approximately 60%. Perhaps the diagnosis is delayed because CMM is so unusual in children that it is not considered in the differential or because the lesion is difficult to distinguish from a benign growth such as a Spitz nevus [64]. Of 15 prepubertal melanoma patients, increasing size of the lesions was noted in seven, bleeding in three, change in color in two, subcutaneous mass in two, CNS symptoms in two, itching in one and regional lymphadenopathy in one. In only one instance was the clinical diagnosis made by a direct examination of the skin lesion.

At puberty the incidence of CMM starts to increase and continues to increase throughout the teenage years. Lesions are often noted first by the patient because of change in size (43%) or color (18%), bleeding (27%) or itching (12%) [64].

### Congenital lesions and melanoma

Lesions clinically compatible with pigmented nevi were noted on physical examination in about 2.5% of 200 newborn infants [67]. However, in newborn infants it is often impossible to differentiate nevocellular nevi from other types of pigmented lesions unless a biopsy is done. Of 1058 newborns examined in 1976, 41 (3.9%) had pigmented lesions compatible clinically with nevocellular nevi [68]. However, 2 mm punch biopsies of 34 of these 41 lesions showed only 11 (less than one-third of suspected nevi in newborns) were nevocytic nevi. In fact, then, the percentage of newborns with nevocellular nevi is closer to 1% (11 of 1058). Only two of these 11 had the histologic features of giant congenital nevus, a lesion with an increased potential for developing a melanoma [26, 27, 63, 65, 69, 72, 74]. Only four of the lesions noted were over 1.5 cm in largest diameter. Most of the 11 nevocellular nevi were compound nevi with junctional activity and nevus cells found only superficially in the papillary dermis and upper reticular dermis [68]. This is in contrast to what was noted in 60 larger congenital nevi excised and carefully examined histologically [70]. Fifteen percent of the 60 were less than 1.5 cm diameter, 40% were 1.5–4.9 cm in diameter, 32% were 4.9–9.9 cm in diameter and 13% were 10 cm in diameter or greater. Fifty-nine of these 60 lesions were noted to have nevus cells in the lower two-thirds of the dermis and 35 of 60 in the subcutaneous tissue. Nevus cells and spindle cells or fusiform cells were found between collagen bundles singly or in a single line of cells or both. Nevus cells also involved appendages, nerves, blood vessels and lymphatics in the lower two-thirds of the dermis and in the subcutaneous tissue. Most of these excisions were done on patients not in the neonatal period. It is conceivable that there is a different migration pattern of nevus cells in congenital nevi than acquired nevi. The nevus cells of congenital nevi may migrate more deeply into the skin and around its appendages over a period of time than do acquired nevus cells [71].

Congenital nevi at birth are similar in appearance to café au lait spots and are pale, tan and flat. During childhood they may become slightly elevated and form a plaque or fine papules may arise. They may develop small dark brown freckle-like lesions or may become uniformly dark brown (44%). Different shades of brown mixed with black are common (56%) and rarely gray and blue may be seen in these lesions. Coarse terminal hairs often arise (75%). Most of these lesions have been noted on the trunk (38%) and arms and legs (38%). The size of congenital nevi is often greater than that of acquired nevi [70], but all congenital nevocellular nevi are not greater than 1.5 cm. In addition, neither are all acquired nevocellular nevi less than 1.5 cm in diameter [70]. Seven of 11 biopsy-proven nevocellular nevi in neonates were less than 1.5 cm in diameter [68], while 85% of biopsy-proven congenital nevi noted in children were greater than 1.5 cm in diameter [70]. This discrepancy of size in congenital nevocellular nevi may suggest that congenital lesions grow larger than acquired nevocellular nevi, since the majority of congenital nevocellular nevi in the neonates are less than 1.5 cm diameter, while, in children, 85% of these lesions were greater than 1.5 cm in diameter.

The frequency with which small congenital nevi develop into malignant melanoma is not known. However, if the histopathologic picture of small congenital nevi is similar to that of giant congenital nevi, in which there is an increased risk of melanoma developing [65, 69], then there may be an increased risk for the smaller lesions as well. Indeed, remnants of congenital nevocytic nevi have been noted in some cutaneous malignant melanomas [69], and, in one study, one of 54 patients with a small congenital nevus developed a melanoma within the congenital nevus [70]. Some authors recommend that all congenital nevi "be viewed with suspicion" [65]. Whether or not there is an increased risk of developing melanoma within these smaller congenital nevi is not known at present. There are proponents for both the conservative approach to these lesions as well as proponents for the routine excision of all congenital nevi or congenital nevi over 1.5 cm in diameter [26, 27, 69]. If one plans to remove a congenital nevus for preventive reasons, and the resulting procedure will be difficult or the resulting scar might produce some cosmetic difficulties, then a 3 or 4 mm punch biopsy should be done first to define whether or not the lesion is indeed a congenital nevus. If the lesion is small and can easily be removed with good cosmetic results perhaps even superior to the appearance of the nevus itself, then suggesting or agreeing to the removal of such a lesion can be done in good conscience.

"Giant congenital nevi" (GCN, bathing trunk nevus, giant hairy nevus or garment nevus) are large congenital nevi not surgically resectable with a simple excision and primary closure without causing significant deformity [65]. Most of these lesions have been noted on the trunk in the dermatology literature [70, 74], while more are noted on the head and neck in the plastic surgery literature [72]. GCN have been reported to develop melanomas between 2% and 42% of the time with an average estimated at 12% to 15% [26, 27, 63, 65, 69, 72, 74]. These figures may be somewhat skewed, since patients with problems relating to GCN tend to have their unusual disease treated in large centers by physicians who report their findings. The greatest risk of melanoma developing in large lesions is within the first ten years of life [65, 72]. Of melanomas developing within GCN, 60% do so in the first decade, 10% in the second decade and 30% thereafter. The development of melanoma is often noted by nodulation or ulceration. The increased risk of melanoma developing may be due simply to an increase in the number of melanocytes in these large lesions, or an inherent tendency of congenital melanocytic lesions to become malignant. Certainly, melanoma does arise from the deep dermis of the GCN in some instances [65], and certain types of GCN may be more likely to develop into a melanoma. GCN with junctional activity or the histologic picture of a neural nevus or cellular blue nevus are reported more likely to develop into melanoma. Those GCN with a histology of superficial intradermal nevi may not have the same malignant potential [65]. Multiple biopsies have been recommended to help define the histologic types so as to determine whether there is an increased malignant potential [65]. However, melanoma has been reported to arise from a GCN with the histology of a benign looking compound nevus [72]. Regardless of this controversial finding, the consensus of opinions regarding treatment is for early aggressive, perhaps staged, excision and grafting of GCN because of the high risk of developing melanoma within the first decade. Early excision may help avoid psychic trauma and may be associated with better healing [26, 27, 63, 69, 72]. Unfortunately, excision is not always possible because of the size of the involved areas. Mesh grafts may be needed, which can compromise the cosmetic result.

Multiple procedures done over months to years puts a tremendous financial, physical and emotional strain on families. Obviously, an undertaking of this magnitude requires full detailed explanation to the patient's family of the risks involved, both with and without surgery.

Many of the giant lesions are associated with multiple smaller lesions scattered about the trunk and extremities [73], and these should be removed as well. They represent another problem in that they may interfere with grafting procedures. Lesions that are on the scalp or face or cover extremely large areas of skin present special technical and cosmetic problems. Early dermabrasion has been used in several of these patients with successful long-term clearing of pigment [71, 75]. Of interest is the fact that one patient had superficial nevus cells noted on biopsy at four and seven weeks of age, but deep dermal involvement at nine weeks. Dermabrasion at four and seven weeks was successful, but dermabrasion at nine weeks was followed by poor results [71]. Whether the nevus cells migrated to the deep dermis or were actually present at this depth at the biopsy site at birth is an unanswered guess. Whether or not this treatment will prove successful remains to be determined, but certainly dermabrasion offers the advantage of fewer and less difficult surgical procedures.

Meningeal melanocytosis, melanoma within the leptomeningeal melanocytes, communicating hydrocephalus due to impaired cerebrospinal fluid absorption and seizures have all been noted in patients with GCN. Patients with GCN of the scalp and neck are those most likely to have the central nervous system problems [27, 65, 74]. Also noted in association with GCN is an increase in other congenital abnormalities such as clubfeet, atrophy of an involved extremity and spina bifida occulta [74].

**Summary**

The clinical features of CMM have been described. Emphasis has been placed on the clinical characteristics of early SSM, LMM, NM and ALM, since early recognition should result in a higher cure rate. Any "suspicious lesion" should be excised when feasible or a biopsy taken when the lesion is too large to excise and close primarily. Important features of SSM, ALM and LMM in the early stages of development may include haphazard and variegate coloration, irregular and notched borders and irregular surface elevation. Nodular melanoma often appears as a "blood blister" or blue-black or "thunder cloud gray" lesion with rapid growth. After the diagnosis of CMM is made surgery should be accomplished without delay.

# References

1. Sober AJ, Fitzpatrick TB, Mihm MC, Wise TG, Pearson BJ, Clark WH and Kopf AW: Early recognition of cutaneous melanoma. J Am Med Assoc 242:2795-2799, 1979.

2. Mihm MC, Jr, Fitzpatrick TB, Lane, Brown MM, Raker JW, Malt RA and Kaiser JS: Early detection of primary cutaneous malignant melanoma. N Engl J Med 389:989-996, 1973.

3. Lopansri S and Mihm MC, Jr: Clinical and pathological correlation of malignant melanoma. J Cutan Pathol 6:180-194, 1979.

4. Milton GW: Clinical diagnosis of malignant melanoma. Br J Surg 55:755-757, 1968.

5. Clark WH, Jr: Clinical diagnosis of cutaneous malignant melanoma. J Am Med Assoc 236:484, 1976.

6. McGovern VJ, Mihm MC, Bailly C, Booth JC, Clark WH, Cochran AJ, Hardy EG, Hicks JD, Levene A, Lewis MG, Little JH and Milton GW: The classification of malignant melanoma and its histologic reporting. Cancer 32:1446-1457, 1973.

7. Cady B, Legg MA and Redfern AB: Contemporary treatment of malignant melanoma. Am J Surg 129:472-482, 1975.

8. Epstein E, Bragg K and Linden G: Biopsy and prognosis of malignant melanoma. J Am Med Assoc 208:1369-1371, 1969.

9. Pack GT, Gerber DM and Scharnagel IM: End results in the treatment of malignant melanoma. Ann Surg 136:905-911, 1952.

10. Everall JD and Dowd PM: Diagnosis, prognosis and treatment of melanoma. Lancet 2:286-289, 1977.

11. Harris MN and Gumport SL: Total excision biopsy for primary malignant melanoma. J Am Med Assoc 226:354-355, 1973.

12. Williams HM: Malignant melanoma. CA Cancer J Clin 18:151-155, 1968.

13. Elwood JM and Lee JAH: Recent data on the epidemiology of malignant melanoma. Semin Oncol 2:149-154, 1975.

14. Cosman B, Heddle SB and Crikelair GF: The increasing incidence of melanoma. Plast Reconstr Surg 57:50-56, 1976.

15. Resseguie LJ, Marks SJ, Winkelmann RK and Kurland LT: Malignant melanoma in the resident population of Rochester, Minnesota. Mayo Clin Proc 52:191-195, 1977.

16. McGovern VJ: Epidemiological aspects of melanoma: a review. Pathology 9:233-241, 1977.

17. Magnus K: Incidence of malignant melanoma of the skin in Norway, 1955-1970. Cancer 32:1275-1286, 1973.

18. Gellin GA, Kopf AW and Garfinkel L: Malignant melanoma, a controlled study of possibly associated factors. Arch Dermatol 99:43-48, 1969.

19. Devesa S and Silverman DT: Cancer incidence and mortality trends in the United States: 1935-74. J Natl Cancer Inst 60:545-571.

20. Pack GT, Davis J and Oppenheim A: The relation of race and complexion to the incidence of moles and melanomas. Ann N Y Acad Sci 100:719-729, 1963.

21. Wanebo HJ, Woodruff J and Fortner JG: Malignant melanoma of the extremities: a clinicopathologic study using levels of invasion (microstage). Cancer 35:666-676, 1975.

22. Pack GT, Davis J and Oppenheim A: The relation of race and complexion to the incidence of moles and melanomas. Ann N Y Acad Sci 100:719-729, 1963.

23. Cutler SJ, Myers MH and Green SB: Trends in survival rates of patients with cancer. N Engl J Med 293:122-124, 1975.

24. Teppo L, Parkanen M and Hakulinen T: Sunlight as a risk factor of malignant melanoma of the skin. Cancer 41:2018-2027, 1978.

25. Davis NC, McLeod GR, Beardmore GL, Little JH, Quinn RL and Holt J: Primary cutaneous melanoma: a report from the Queensland melanoma project. CA Cancer J Clin 26:80-107, 1976.

26. Sober AJ, Fitzpatrick TB and Mihm MC, Jr: Primary melanoma of the skin: recognition and management. J Am Acad Dermatol 12:179–200, 1980.
27. Malignant melanoma: a review. J Dermatol Surg Oncol 3:43–125, 1977.
28. Clark WH, Jr, Ainsworth AM and Mihm MC: The clinical manifestations of primary cutaneous malignant melanomas. In: Clark WH, Jr, Goldman Ll and Mastrangelo MJ (eds) Human Malignant Melanoma, pp 33–53.Grune & Stratton, New York, 1979.
29. Mihm MC, Jr, Clark WH, Jr and Reed RJ: The clinical diagnosis of malignant melanoma. Semin Oncol 2:105–118, 1975.
30. Wayte DM and Helwig EB: Melanotic freckle of Hutchinson. Cancer 21:893–911, 1968.
31. Pitman GH, Kopf AW, Bart RS and Casson PR: Treatment of lentigo maligna and lentigo maligna melanoma. J Dermatol Surg Oncol 5:727–737, 1979.
32. Clark WH, Jr and Mihm MC, Jr: Lentigo maligna and lentigo-maligna melanoma. Am J Pathol 55:39–54, 1969.
33. Arrington JH, III, Reed RJ, Ichinose H and Krementz ET: Plantar lentiginous melanoma: a distinctive variant of human cutaneous malignant melanoma. Am J Surg Pathol 1:131–143, 1977.
34. Coleman WP, III, Loria PR, Reed RJ and Krementz ET: Acral lentiginous melanoma. Arch Dermatol 116:773–776, 1980.
35. Clark WH, Jr, Bernardino EA, Reed RJ and Kopf AW: Acral lentiginous melanomas including melanomas of mucous membranes. In: Clark WH, Jr, Goldman LI and Mastrangelo MJ (eds) Human Malignant Melanoma, pp 109–124. Grune & Stratton, New York, 1979.
36. Pack GT and Oropeza R: Subungual melanoma. Surg Gynecol Obstet 124:571–582, 1967.
37. Taylor DR and South DA: Acral lentiginous melanoma. Cutis 26:35–36, 1980.
38. McBurney EI and Herron CB: Melanoma mimicking plantar wart. J Am Acad Dermatol 1:144–146, 1979.
39. Bart RS and Kopf AW: Tumor Conference # 10: a darkly pigmented lesion of a great toe (acral lentiginous melanoma). J Dermatol Surg Oncol 3:158–159, 1977.
40. Rippey JJ and Lewin JR: Acral lentiginous melanoma or Hutchinson's melanotic freckle of the extremities: a case report. S Afr Med J 53:1076–1077.
41. Decker AM and Chamness JT: Melanocarcinoma of the plantar surface of the foot. A review of twenty-five cases. Surgery 29:731–742, 1951.
42. Lupulescu A, Pinkus H, Birmingham DJ, Usndek HE and Posch JL: Lentigo maligna of the fingertip. Arch Dermatol 107:717–722, 1973.
43. Higashi N: Melanocytes of nail matrix and nail pigmentation. Arch Dermatol 97:570–574, 1968.
44. Clark WH, Jr, Reimer RR, Greene M, Ainsworth AM and Mastrangelo MJ: Origin of familial malignant melanomas from heritable melanocytic lesions: "the B-K Mole Syndrome." Arch Dermatol 114:732–738, 1978.
45. Reimer RR, Clark WH, Jr, Greene MH, Ainsworth AM and Fraumeni JF, Jr: Precursor lesions in familial melanoma. A new genetic preneoplastic syndrome. J Am Med Assoc 239:744–746, 1978.
46. Kronberg R and Ackerman AB: Pseudomelanoma: recurrent melanocytic nevus following partial surgical removal. Arch Dermatol 111:1588–1590, 1975.
47. Luce JK, McBride CM and Frei E, III: Melanoma. In: Holland FJ and Frei E, III (eds) Cancer Medicine, pp 1823–1843. Lea & Febiger, Philadelphia, 1973.
48. Pack GT, Scharnagel IM and Hillyer RA: Multiple primary melanoma: a report of sixteen cases. Cancer 5:1110–1115, 1952.
49. Beardmore GL and Davis NC: Multiple primary cutaneous melanomas. Arch Dermatol III:603–609, 1975.
50. Lynch HT and Krush AJ: Heredity and malignant melanoma: implications for early detection. Can Med Assoc J 99:17–21, 1968.

51. Wallace DC, Beardmore GL and Exton LA: Familial malignant melanoma. Ann Surg 177:15–20, 1973.
52. Lynch HT, Frichot BC and Lynch JF: Familial atypical multiple mole-melanoma syndrome. J Med Genet 15:352–356, 1978.
53. Copeman PWM, Lewis MG, Phillips TM and Elliott PG: Immunological associations of the halo naevus with cutaneous malignant melanoma. Br J Dermatol 88:127–137, 1973.
54. Epstein WL, Sagebeil R, Spitler L, Wybran J, Reed WB and Blois MS: Halo nevi and melanoma. J Am Med Assoc 225:373–377, 1973.
55. Roenigk HH, Jr, Deodhar S, St. Jacques R and Brudick K: Immunotherapy of malignant melanoma with vaccinia virus. Arch Dermatol 109:668–673, 1964.
56. Copeman PWM and Elliott PG: Melanoma cytoplasmic humoral antibody test: a diagnostic adjunct. Br J Dermatol 94:565–568, 1976.
57. Laucius JF and Mastrangelo MJ: Cutaneous depigmentary phenonema in patients with malignant melanoma. In: Clark WH, Jr, Goldman LI and Mastrangelo MJ (eds) Human Malignant Melanoma, pp 209–225. Grune & Stratton, New York, 1979.
58. Bennett C and Copeman PWM: Melanocyte mutation in halo naevus and malignant melanoma. Br J Dermatol 100:423–426, 1979.
59. Wayte DM and Helwig EB: Halo nevi. Cancer 22:69–90, 1968.
60. Kopf AW, Morrill SD and Silberberg I: Broad spectrum of leukoderma acquisitum centrifugum. Arch Dermatol 92:14–35, 1965.
61. Milton GW, McCarthy WH and Carlon A: Malignant melanoma and vitiligo. Aust J Dermatol 12:131–142, 1971.
62. Stephenson HE, Jr, Terry CW, Lukens JN, Shively JA, Busby WE, Stoeckle HE and Esterly JA: Immunologic factors in human melanoma "metastatic" to products of gestation (with exchange transfusion of infant to mother). Surgery 69:515–522, 1971.
63. Trozak DJ, Rowland WD and Hu F: Metastatic malignant melanoma in prepubertal children. Pediatr Clin 55:191–204, 1975.
64. Boddie AW, Jr, Smith J, Jr, McBride CM: Malignant melanoma in children and young adults: effect of diagnostic criteria on staging and end results. South Med J 71:1074–1078, 1978.
65. Kaplan EN: The risk of malignancy in large congenital nevi. Plast Reconstr Surg 53:421–428, 1974.
66. Fish J, Smith EB and Canby JP: Malignant melanoma in childhood. Surgery 59:304–315, 1966.
67. Pack GT and Davis J: The pigmented mole. Postgrad Med 27:370–382, 1960.
68. Walton RG, Jacobs AH and Cox AJ: Pigmented lesions in newborn infants. Br J Dermatol 95:389–396, 1976.
69. Kopf AW, Bart RS and Hennessey P: Congenital nevocytic nevi and malignant melanomas. J Am Acad Dermatol 1:123–130, 1979.
70. Mark GJ, Mihm MC, Liteplo MG, Reed RJ and Clark WH: Congenital melanocytic nevi of the small and garment type: clinical, histologic and ultrastructural studies. Hum Pathol 4:395–418, 1973.
71. Miller CJ and Becker DW, Jr: Removing pigmentation by dermabrading naevi in infancy. Br J Plast Surg 32:124–126, 1979.
72. Lanier VC, Jr, Pickrell KL and Georgiade NG: Congenital giant nevi: clinical and pathological considerations. Plast Reconstr Surg 58:48–54, 1976.
73. Greeley PW, Middleton AG and Curtin JW: Incidence of malignancy in giant pigmented nevi. Plast Reconstr Surg 36:26–37, 1965.
74. Reed WB, Becker SW, Becker SW, Jr and Nickel WR: Giant pigmented nevi, melanoma and leptomeningeal melanocytosis. Arch Dermatol 91:100–119, 1965.
75. Johnson HA: Permanent removal of pigmentation from giant hairy naevi by dermabrasion in early life. Br J Plast Surg 30:321–323, 1977.

76. Fitzpatrick TB and Gilchrest BA: Dimple sign to differentiate benign from malignant pigmented cutaneous lesions. N Engl J Med 296:1518, 1977.

77. Mihm MC, Jr and Fitzpatrick TB: Early detection of malignant melanoma. Cancer 37:597–603, 1976.

78. Mihm MC, Jr, Clark WH, Jr and From L: The clinical diagnosis, classification and histogenetic concepts of the early stages of cutaneous malignant melanomas. N Engl J Med 284:1078–1082, 1971.

79. Fleming ID, Barnawell JR, Burlison PE and Rankin JS: Skin cancer in black patients. Cancer 35:600–605, 1975.

80. Krementz ET, Sutherland CM, Carter RD and Ryan RF: Malignant melanoma in the American black. Ann Surg 83:533–542, 1976.

81. White JE, Strudwick WJ, Ricketts WN and Sampson C: Cancer of the skin in Negroes. J Am Med Assoc 178:845–847, 1961.

82. Seiji M, Mihm MC, Sober AJ et al: Malignant melanoma of the palmar-plantar-subungual-mucosal type: clinical and histopathologic features. Pigment Cell 5:95–104, 1979.

83. Pantoja E, Llobet RE and Roswit B: Melanomas of the lower extremity among native Puerto Ricans. Cancer 38:1420–1423, 1976.

84. Reddy CRRM, Yellama A, Satyanarayana BV and Sundareshwar B: Incidence and evolution of moles and the relationship to malignant melanoma in Eastern India. Int Surg 61:469–471, 1976.

85. Cosman B, Heddle SB and Crikelair GF: The increasing incidence of melanoma. Plast Reconstr Surg 57:50–56, 1976.

86. Rushforth GF: Two cases of subungual malignant melanoma. Br J Surg 58:451–453, 1971.

87. Hiss Y and Shafir R: "Pseudomelanoma" in a keloid. J Dermatol Surg Oncol 4:938–939, 1978.

88. Kopf AW, Mintzis M, Grier WRN, Silvers DN and Bart RS: Familial malignant melanoma. Cutis 17:873–876, 1976.

89. Frichot BC, III, Lynch HT, Guirgis HA, Harris RE and Lynch JF: New cutaneous phenotype in familial malignant melanoma. Lancet 1:864, 1977.

90. Anderson DE, Smith JL, Jr and McBride CM: Hereditary aspects of malignant melanoma. J Am Med Assoc 200:741–746, 1967.

91. Boland SL, Shaw HM and Milton GW: Multiple primary cancers in patients with malignant melanoma. Med J Aust 1:517–519, 1976.

# 15. Orthopaedic considerations in the treatment of malignant melanoma

JOHN M. HARRELSON

## Introduction

All organ systems are vulnerable to the metastatic spread of malignant melanoma. This chapter will examine the incidence, anatomic distribution, clinicopathological behavior, prognostic implications and treatment recommendations regarding melanoma metastatic to the skeletal system.

## Incidence

Though prior autopsy studies of patients with malignant melanoma have reported an incidence of osseous metastases from 0% to 49% [1–2], the true incidence of metastatic melanoma in bone is not known. The entire skeleton is not accessible for complete gross examination, as are other organ systems, and the reported incidence of osseous disease in autopsy series must therefore depend on the diligence of the prosector. It is not surprising therefore that the vertebrae, ribs and sternum are the most frequent sites of metastatic disease in such series, since these are the most available osseous structures. Further, metastatic tumor deposits in bone must destroy an estimated 50% of the mineral content of bone before radiographically appreciable lesions develop [4–6]. Thus, even autopsy series employing radiographic examination will probably underestimate the frequency of osseous metastasis.

Clinical detection of bony disease prior to death was made in 6.9% of 1677 patients with melanoma studied at the Duke University Medical Center from 1956 to 1976 [7]. Radionuclide bone imaging studies were employed only in the latter years of this study and both bone scan and skeletal roentgenograms were obtained only in response to complaints of bone pain. With the increased use of radionuclide scans in clinical practice, a more accurate picture of the incidence of osseous metastases should emerge.

Several observations suggest that metastasis of melanoma to bone is a late phenomenon in the course of this disease. Cochran [8], in a prospective study, found only one case of osseous metastasis in 73 patients with Stage I

*Seigler, H. F. (ed.), Clinical Management of Melanoma. ISBN 978-94-009-7495-1*
© *1982, Martinus Nijhoff Publishers, The Hague/Boston/London.*

disease while 58% of his patients with Stage III disease demonstrated positive bone scans. In our own study, only 3.1% of the total patient population experienced a bone metastasis as the first evidence of metastatic disease [7], a figure which correlates with the 2% incidence of a bony metastasis as the first evidence of metastatic disease as reported by Das Gupta and Brasfield [3].

Anatomically, the axial skeleton is the most frequent site of bony metastases comprising 70% of all lesions in our series and a similar frequency in other reports. No osseous structure is excluded in reports of metastatic melanoma with cases appearing in even the carpal and tarsal bones [3, 9].

In most series, the incidence of melanoma in females is slightly higher than in males. Also, most authors report a worse prognosis for males in terms of five-year survival [10]. In terms of skeletal metastases, 811 males (48.3%) in the series developed 58.6% of the osseous lesions. This is probably a further expression of the higher incidence of distant spread and corresponding bony disease observed in males.

## Clinicopathological features

Osseous metastases of melanoma occur late in the course of the disease. Presently, most skeletal metastases are discovered either as a result of complaints of bone pain leading to radiographic or radionuclide investigation or are seen in the ribs and dorsal vertebrae on routine chest roentgenograms. Despite the fact that most bony disease occurs in a setting of Stage II or Stage III disease, (metastatic disease remote to the primary site), it should be noted that 52 of 116 patients (44.8%) in our series developed bony metastatic disease as the *first* evidence of departure from Stage I classification. Further, five patients with bony metastases presented with no prior diagnosis of melanoma and diagnosis was established by biopsy of the skeletal lesions.

Not all skeletal deposits of melanoma produce pain. Particularly, lesions of the ribs, pelvis and scapulae may remain painless until structural defect or associated soft tissue tumor mass produces discomfort. Fifteen patients in our series had such painless bony metastases identified on incidental skeletal radiographs.

Neurological symptoms may be the initial complaint in patients with spinal metastatic disease. Seventy percent of the metastatic lesions in our series occurred in the axial skeleton. While the majority of these lesions were identified in the vertebral bodies (70 lesions), ten metastatic lesions were identified in the posterior vertebral arch. In all lesions presenting in the posterior arch, neurological symptoms occurred. Four patients developed a progressive cauda equina syndrome, two patients developed total paraplegia

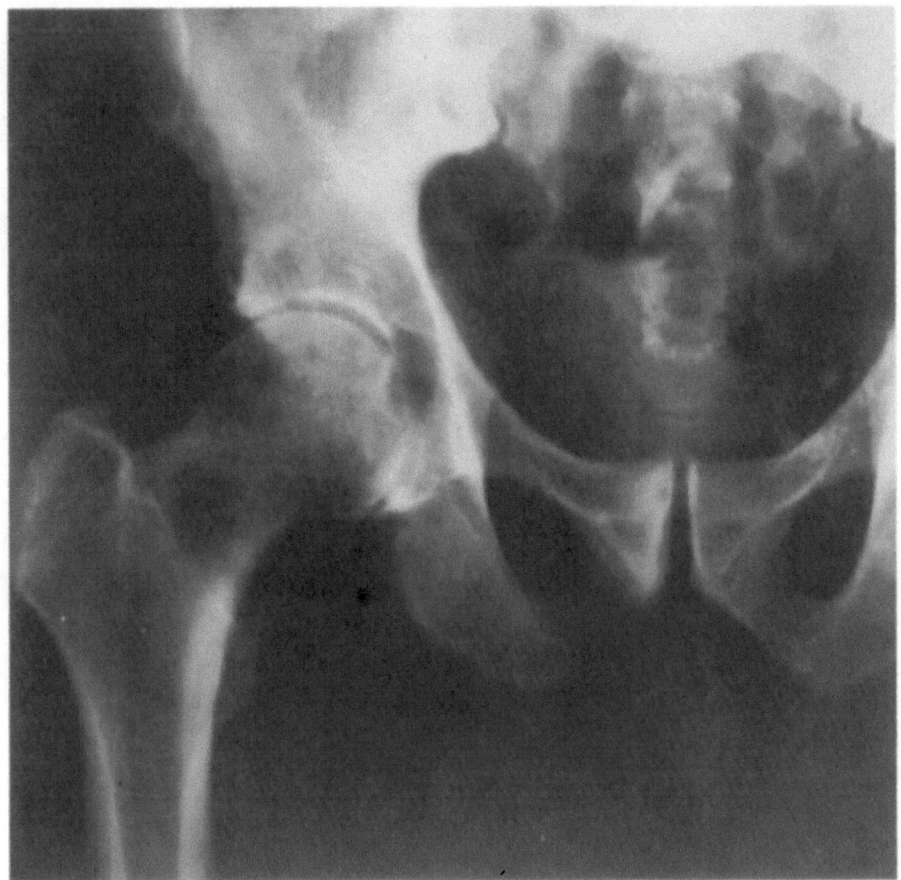

*Figure 1A.* AP view of the pelvis showing destruction of the pubic ramus in a geographic pattern.

at the midthoracic level, and four patients developed root compression syndromes from cervical or lumbar vertebral arch involvement.

Pathologic fracture is a common feature of metastatic melanoma to bone. However, the majority of these fractures occur in the vertebral bodies or ribs. Seventy-five patients in our series (64.7%) developed pathologic fracture but only six such fractures occurred in the appendicular skeleton. This is similar to the experience reported by Selby et al. who reported 15 spine or rib fractures and no long bone fracture in his study of 33 patients with metastatic melanoma to bone [5].

The radiographic appearance of skeletal deposits of melanoma has been well described by Selby and others [5, 11]. Such lesions are usually osteolytic in nature and may present patterns of geographic, permeative, or moth-eaten destruction as defined by Lodwick [6] (Figure 1). Expansion of the involved bone as may be seen with metastases from thyroid and renal cell carcinoma was not observed in any lesions due to melanoma. Lesions of the

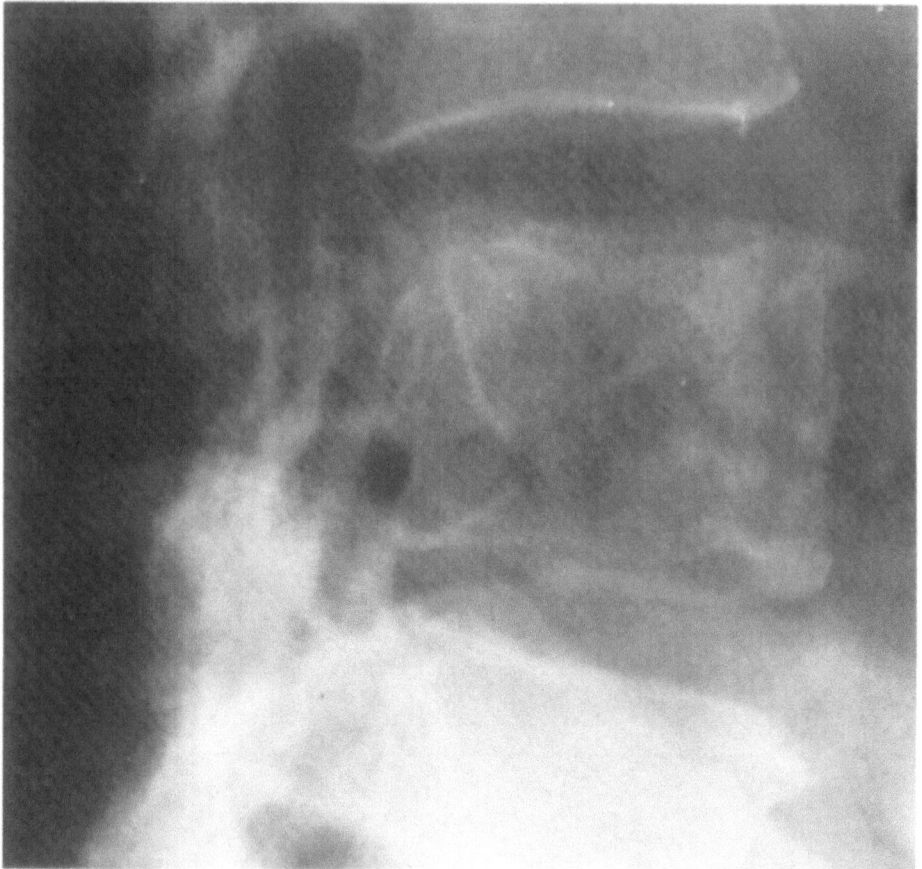

*Figure 1B.* Lateral view of the lumbosacral spine showing motheaten destruction of the vertebral body with preservation of disc spaces.

vertebral bodies tended to involve the entire vertebrae with preservation of adjacent intervertebral disc spaces and were often accompanied by compression fractures. Frequently, a paravertebral soft tissue mass could be identified in vertebral lesions on anteroposterior roentgenograms. In long bone metastases, the lesions tended to be oval, eccentric and associated with cortical destruction (Figure 2). Occasionally, we observed lesions arising in cortical bone without associated medullary destruction (Figure 3). Perilesional osteoblastic reaction (Figure 4) was occasionally observed in the absence of prior irradiation. Periosteal reaction was not observed in response to either medullary or cortical deposits of melanoma. Further, amorphous calcification was not seen either on plain roentgenograms or tomograms in either intraosseous lesions or associated soft tissue tumor mass.

The use of technetium-99m-labeled-phosphate compounds for bone imaging has aided in the detection of metastatic lesions of bone [12–14]. The sensitivity of this study for areas of osteoblastic collagen deposition and

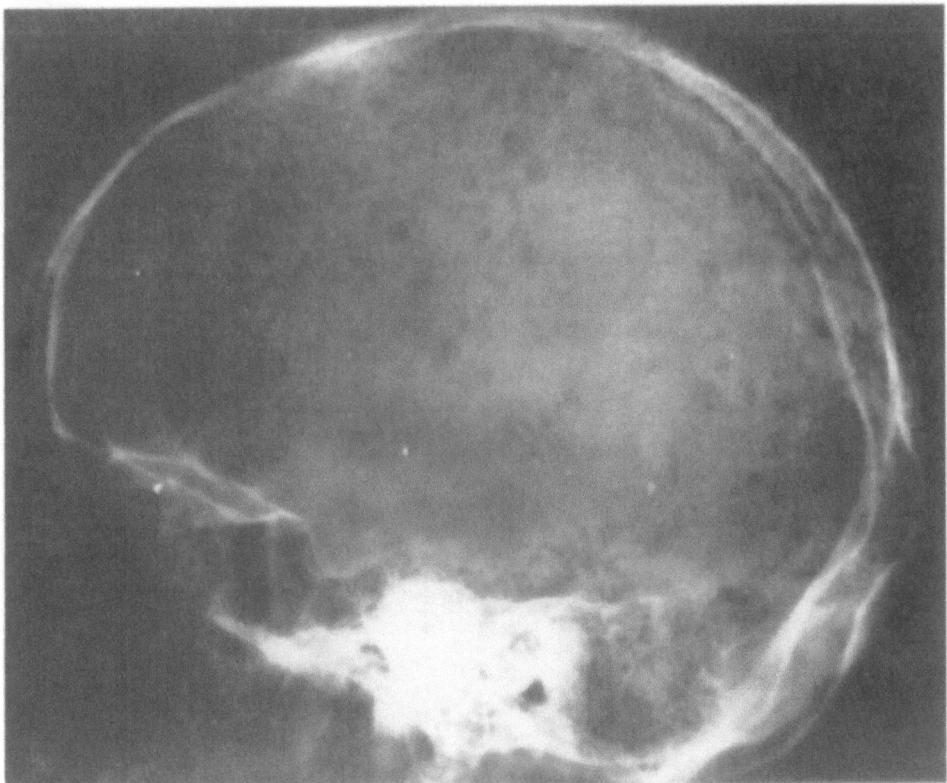

*Figure 1C.* Lateral view of the skull showing permeative destruction.

osteoid mineralization permits identification of lesions early in their course before sufficient bone destruction has occurred to allow identification by roentgenographic means. False positive studies may occur in response to degenerative joint disease, bone infarcts, trauma, infection and other benign un related conditions of bone. Correlation with clinical radiographs is mandatory. It is also recognized that false negative results may be obtained in certain malignant diseases, particularly thyroid carcinoma and myeloma. In 40 melanoma patients studied by bone scan and correlative radiographs, no false negative bone scans were encountered [7]. Where bone scan suggests the presence of a metastatic lesion and correlative roentgenograms or tomograms are inconclusive, we have found the use of computerized tomographic scanning to be of value. The density difference between a medullary deposit of metastatic tumor and adjacent normal marrow (usually fat in adult long bones) confirms the presence of a metastatic deposit. Perhaps the greatest value of radionuclide bone imaging lies in comparison studies at different intervals in time. A prior negative bone scan which subsequently becomes positive in the setting of known malignant disease may be of more diagnostic importance than a single positive study.

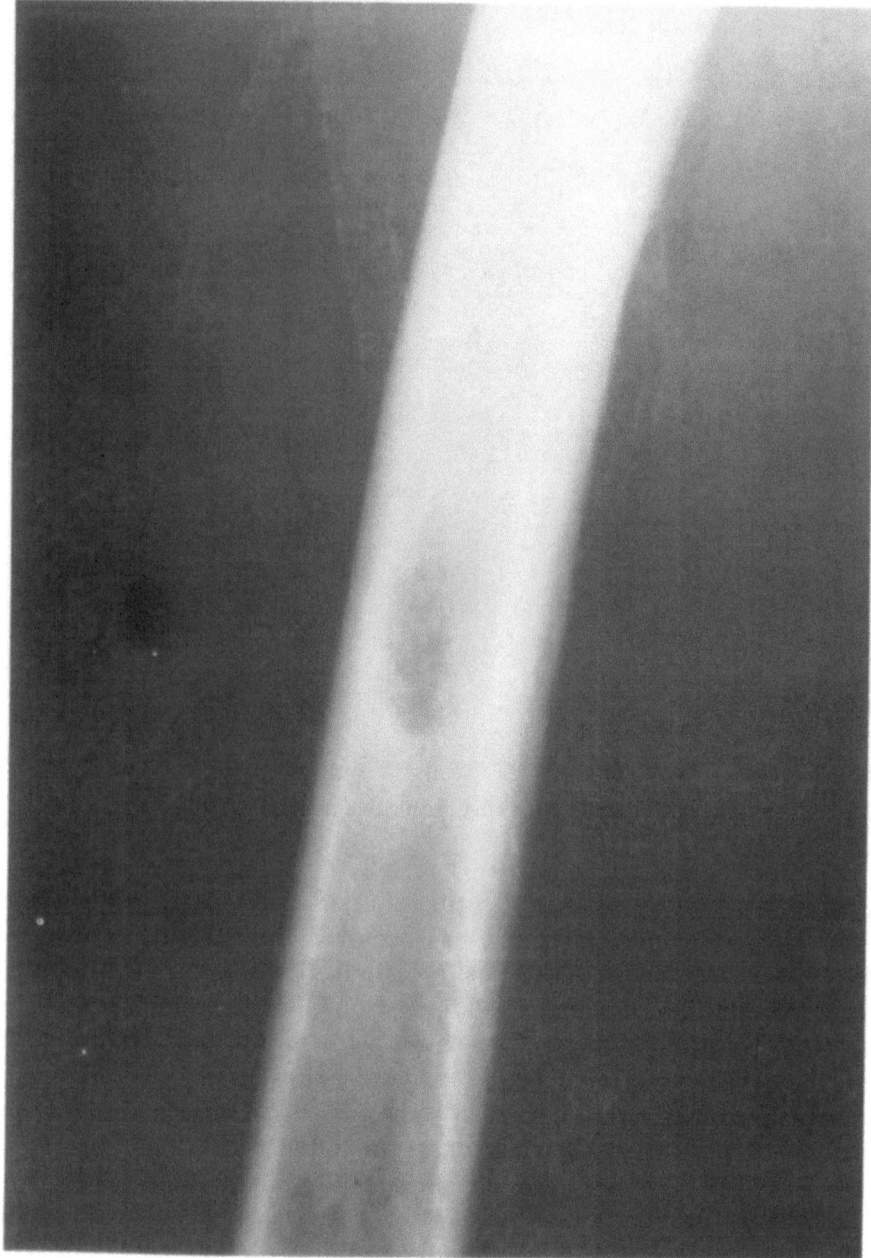

*Figure 2.* Lateral view of the femur showing oval, eccentric medullary and cortical destruction.

Unusual presentations of metastatic melanoma may occur. We have encountered two instances of metastatic melanoma to skeletal muscle, one occurring in the adductor muscles of the thigh and the other in the trapezius. In both instances, the patient's prior history of cutaneous melanoma

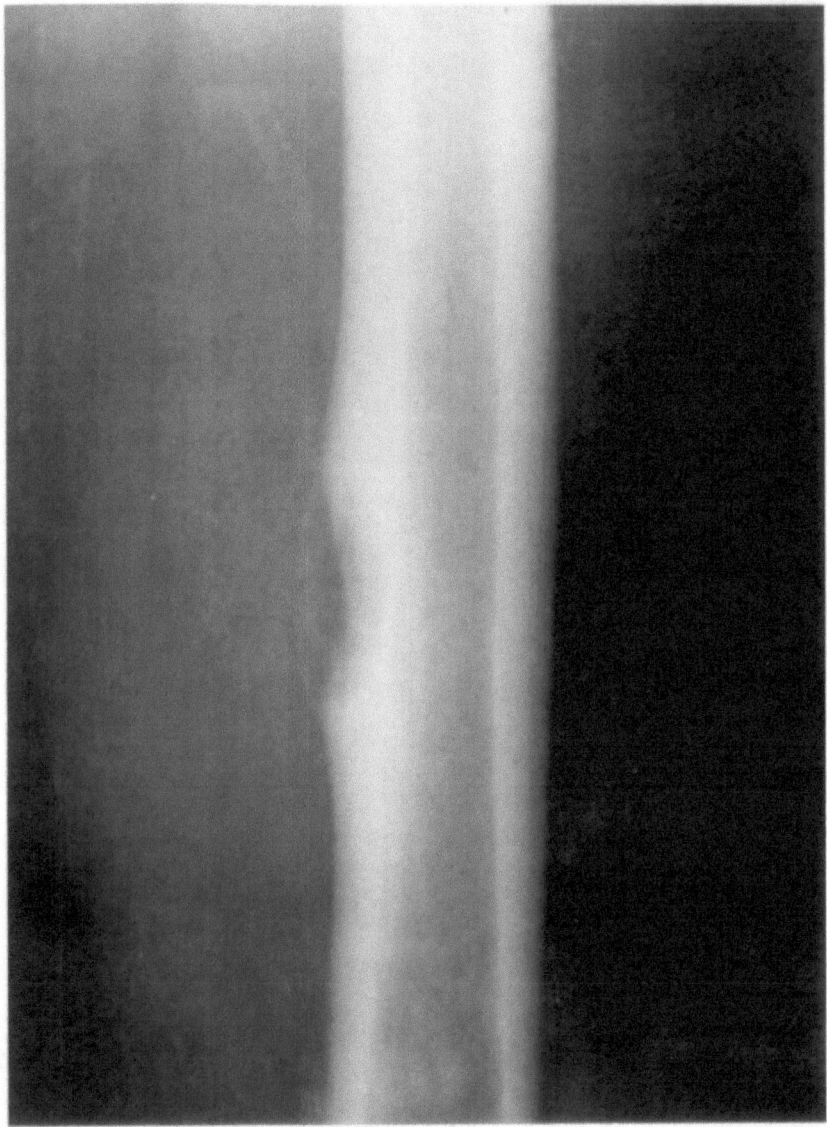

*Figure 3.* **AP** view of the femur showing superficial cortical metastasis without medullary involvement.

was remote and the clinical and radiographic features were similar in all respects to a primary soft tissue sarcoma (Figure 5). In a third individual with a history of melanoma of the scalp, a soft tissue tumor of the hamstring muscles proved to be a primary soft tissue sarcoma. It should not therefore be assumed that any intramuscular lesion presenting in a patient with known melanoma is metastatic. Muscular metastases are clearly uncommon and such lesions should be approached in the same manner employed for suspected primary soft tissue sarcomas.

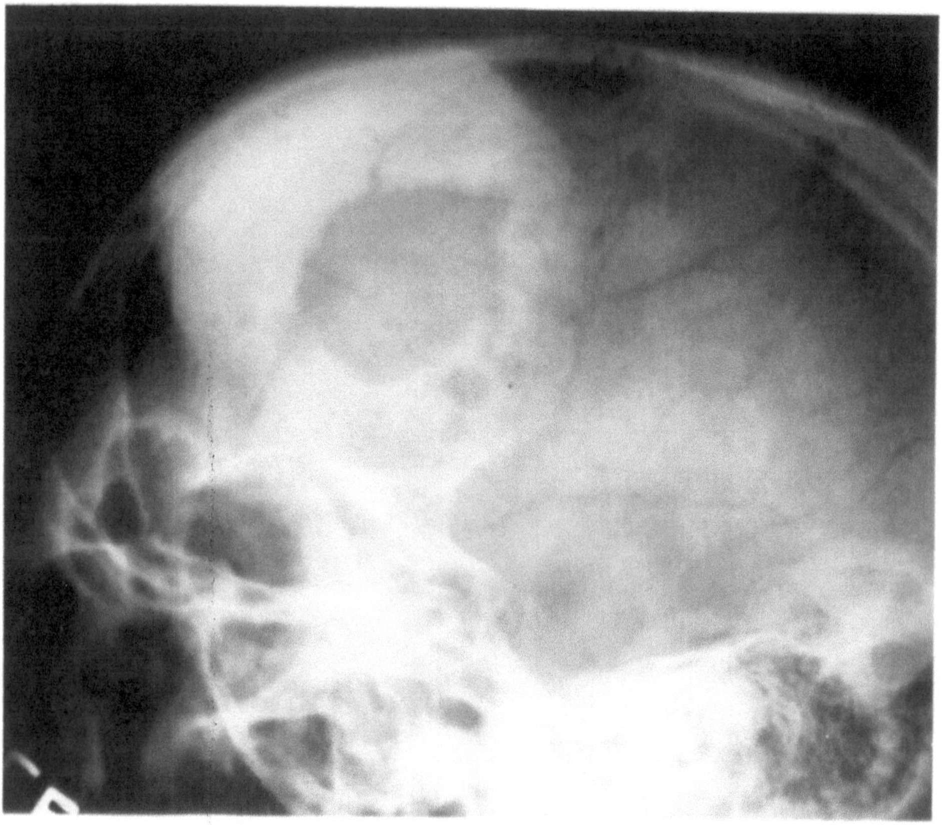

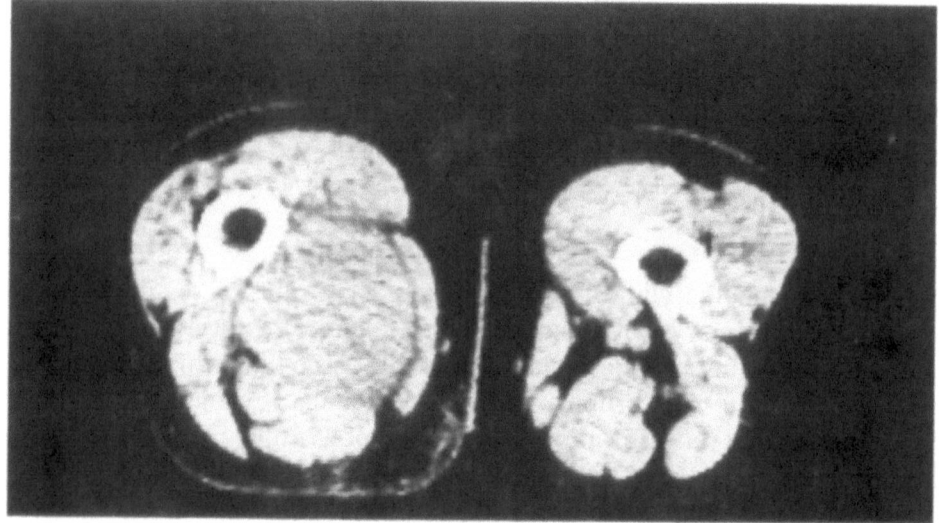

*Figure 4.* Lateral view of the skull showing central geographic destruction with surrounding osteoblastic response. This patient has not undergone radiation therapy.

*Figure 5.* CT scan of the thighs showing large mass in the adductor muscle group.

Of further orthopaedic interest are those primary lesions of melanoma which present in the foot. In reviewing 1749 cases over the past twenty-three years at this institution, 101 patients presented with primary foot lesions. While typical cutaneous lesions and subungual lesions do not present unusual diagnostic problems, these lesions may present atypically as ulcerative lesions and tend to obscure and delay diagnosis. It is recognized that survival of patients with primary melanoma of the foot is less than for primary lesions at other anatomic sites [15, 16]. Accordingly, we would recommend biopsy of any ulcerative foot lesion as a part of the routine diagnostic evaluation.

**Prognosis**

In our experience, survival of patients with osseous metastatic melanoma is extremely limited [7]. Despite one individual who survived 22 months from the time of skeletal metastasis, the mean survival for 116 patients with osseous melanoma was 3.6 months. This figure no doubt reflects the tendency of melanoma to spread to many organ systems simultaneously. Reclassification from Stage I to Stage III disease was made in 52 patients as a results of discovery of osseous metastases. The majority of these patients were found to have metastatic disease in other organ systems as well. Various modes of therapy employed at our institution over the past twenty-three years have not seemed to affect the survival of patients with skeletal metastases. This observation has led to a conservative approach in the surgical treatment of skeletal lesions. While survival tended to be better in females than in males, neither sex nor age was a statistically significant prognostic factor. Similarly, the site of the primary lesion and the site of skeletal metastases had no relationship to survival. The time interval between diagnosis of melanoma and the appearance of skeletal disease was quite variable. Five patients presented with metastatic bony disease as the first evidence of melanoma. One patient developed bony metastases 19 years following the original diagnosis of melanoma. The mean time from diagnosis of melanoma to the discovery of skeletal metastases for 116 patients was 21.6 months.

**Treatment**

Chemotherapy has been employed in various combinations at this institution (see Chapter 13) for the treatment of melanoma. Sixty five of 116 patients were receiving chemotherapy at the time osseous metastasis developed. Continued treatment of these patients and the institution of chemotherapy in patients who developed osseous metastases did not, in our experience, alter the progression of skeletal lesions when compared with patients not receiving chemotherapy (Figure 6). Few patients treated with chemotherapeutic agents subsequent to the development of osseous disease experienced significant pain relief as a result of their chemotherapy. Thus, with the agents presently available, institution of chemotherapy specifically for osseous disease does not seem to be indicated.

Immunotherapy for the treatment of malignant melanoma (see Chapter 17) has also been employed at this institution. Forty-three of 116 patients were receiving immunotherapy at the time of development of osseous metastasis. Neither pain relief nor alteration of bone destruction have been observed in response to immunotherapy. Presently, this modality of treatment seems more beneficial for cutaneous disease than for lesions in deeper anatomic locations.

Radiation therapy has been used regularly in the treatment of osseous metastatic lesions (see Chapter 11). Relief of pain has been a predictable result of radiation treatment [3, 7]. In the majority of cases, skeletal lesions do not alter their growth pattern in response to irradiation. However, we have observed several patients in whom the growth of the lesion either stopped or significantly slowed in response to radiotherapy (Figure 6). Thus, irradiation becomes the first line of defense in the treatment of a painful skeletal metastasis which would not be considered for surgical treatment. In several instances of long bone metastatic disease with impending pathologic fracture, surgery has been avoided by the use of radiotherapy which provided not only pain control, but prevented further progression of the lesion and, in one instance, partial healing of the lesion occurred.

Surgical treatment of skeletal metastatic disease has a limited but valuable role in the treatment of melanoma patients. Multiple factors influence the selection of patients for surgical treatment. The presence of extensive intra-cranial or pulmonary metastatic disease (the two most common causes of death in melanoma) may be strong contra-indications to major surgical procedures. The white blood cell count, platelet count and coagulation parameters, often altered by concurrent chemotherapy, should be carefully examined before surgical intervention.

The goals of surgical treatment are relief of pain and restoration or improvement of function. Successful surgical intervention may, therefore, reduce the amount of nursing care required and improve the quality of life in this group of patients with a fatal prognosis. As with other metastatic disease, achievement of these goals may allow the patient to return home when they would otherwise require continued hospitalization, thereby reducing ultimate expense for the patient.

The majority of axial metastases do not require surgery. However, lesions of the posterior vertebral arch characteristically produce neurologic deficits ranging from root compression signs to total paraplegia. In our experience, decompressive laminectomy and removal of soft tissue epidural tumor have been beneficial, resulting in varying degrees of neurologic improvement as well as relief from pain. The recovery from such surgery is rapid enough to

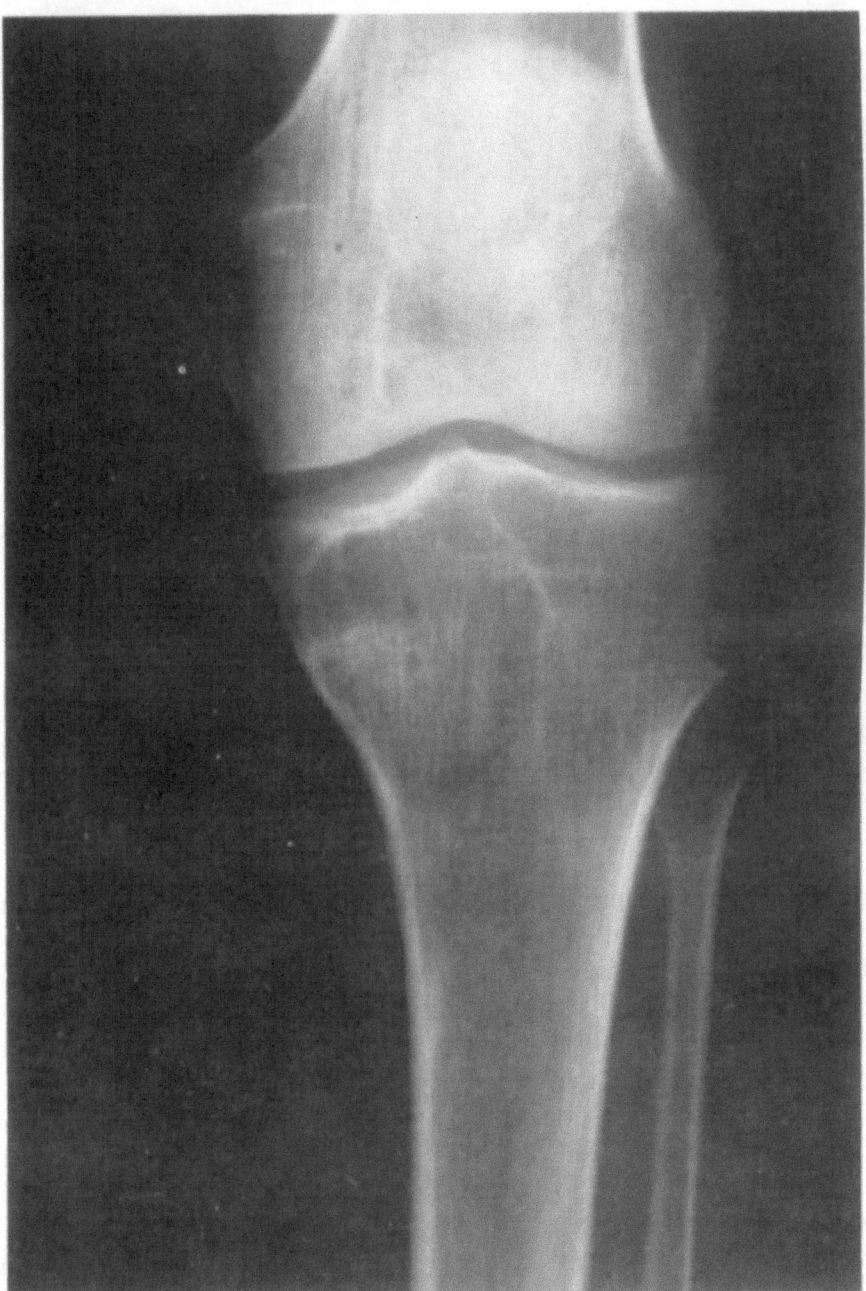

*Figure 6A.* AP roentgenogram of the tibia one year following irradiation for a medial metaphyseal lesion.

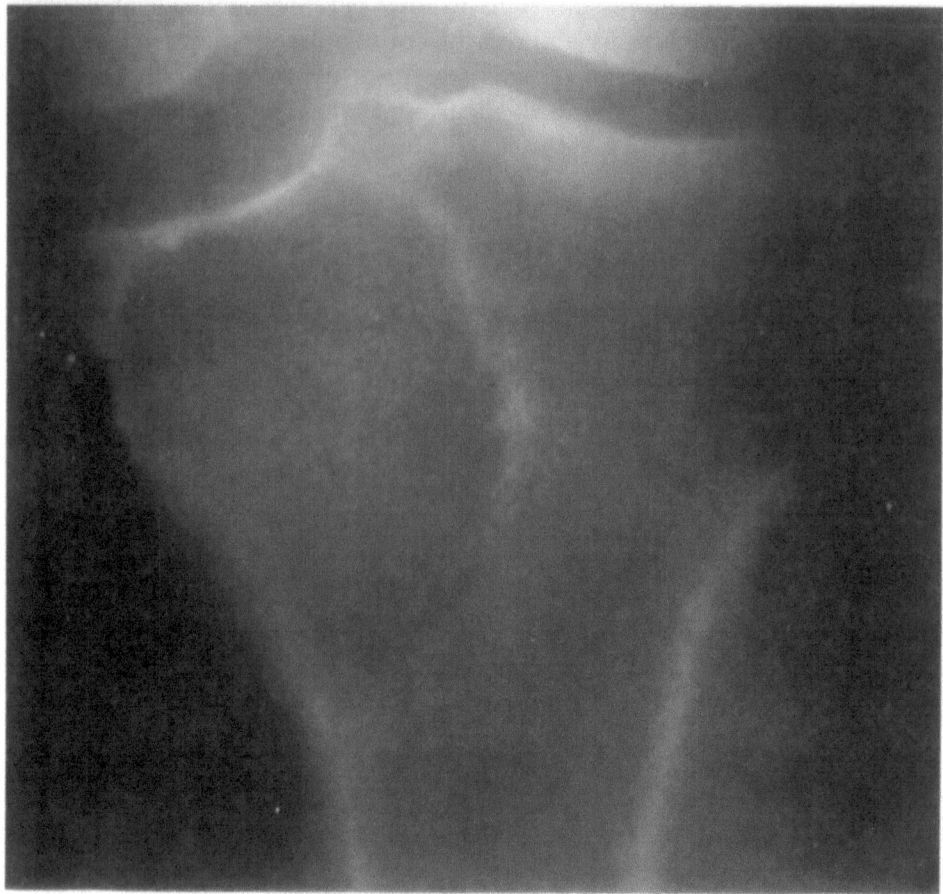

*Figure 6B.* Tomogram of the same lesion showing sclerotic border which developed in response to radiation therapy. There was no increase in the size of the lesion within the year following discovery.

justify its use despite projected survival. Occasionally, spinal stabilization may be required. In one patient with cervical vertebral body involvement and associated neurologic deficit, vertebral body resection, decompression of the anterior spinal canal and interbody bone graft resulted in neurologic improvement and stability sufficient to allow him to become ambulatory and to return home for the remaining seven months of his life. Posterior stabilization with Harrington rods or similar devices may also be considered. While we have not utilized this technique in a patient with melanoma, we have used the technique successfully in selected patients with spinal metastatic disease from other primary carcinomas.

Surgical stabilization of pathologic long bone fractures is indicated when there are no major contraindications to the anesthesia required. The techniques of long bone stabilization are well described in the literature [17–20] and no particular variation in accepted techniques is required in the treatment of metastatic melanoma. Where possible, intra-medullary fixation should be selected over plate fixation. Intra-medullary fixation distributes forces over a greater area and usually requires less surgical exposure. Further, the quality of bone proximal and distal to a major metastatic deposit is often not of sufficient quality to allow satisfactory screw fixation of a plate

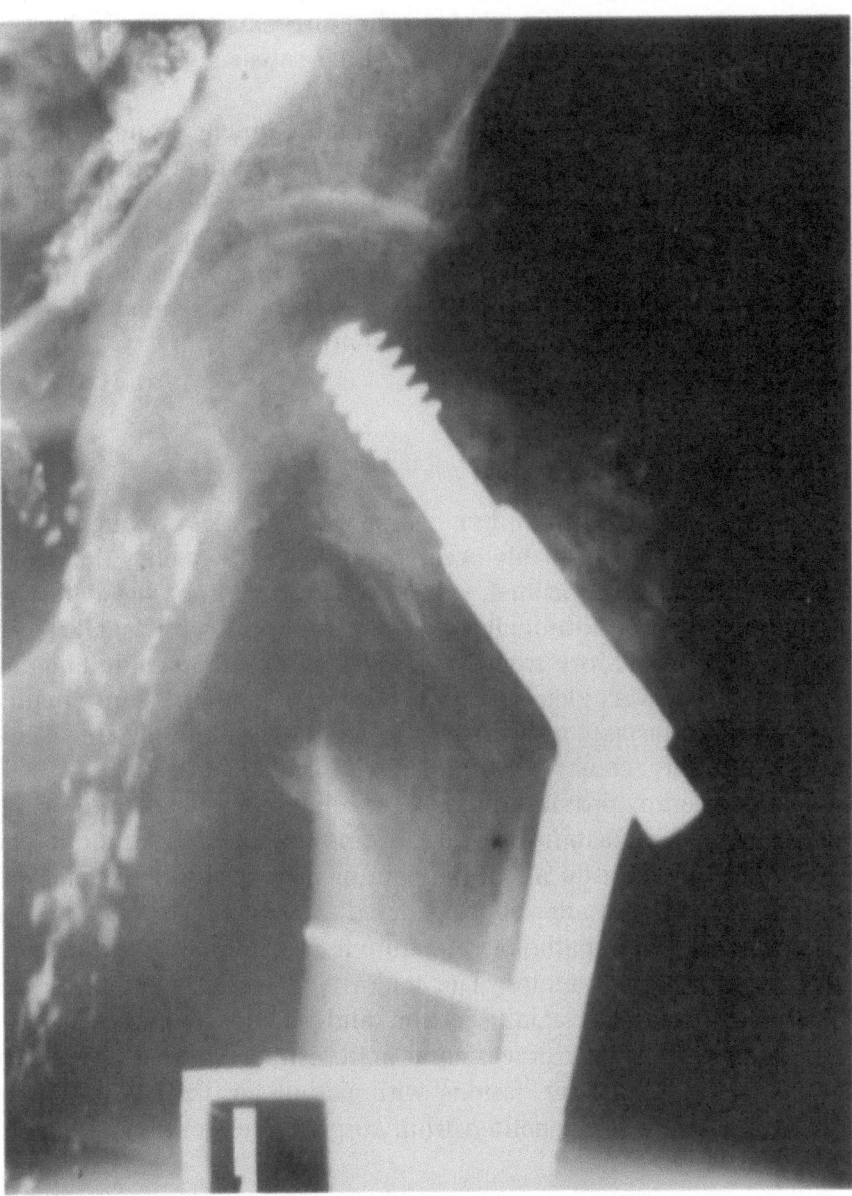

*Figure 7.* AP view of the proximal femur in a patient who had undergone prophylatic fixation of an impending fracture. This roentgeogram was obtained four months following chemotherapy and shows extensive destruction. The lesion was accompanied by a large soft tissue mass which ulcerated through to skin requiring hip disarticulation.

device. The additional use of methylmethacrylate has greatly improved the ability to achieve stable fixation [21].

Long bone metastases without pathologic fracture should be considered for surgical intervention when radiation therapy has failed to relieve pain or retard the growth of the lesion or when there is greater than 50% destruction of cortical bone. The guidelines for surgical treatment of these "incipient" fractures is the same as if pathologic fracture existed. Surgically treated lesions should undergo radiation therapy after satisfactory wound healing if no prior radiation has been given.

Rarely, amputation may be required in the treatment of metastatic melanoma [22]. Within the general guidelines for surgical treatment as described above, amputation should be considered when skeletal destruction is too extensive to permit ordinary reconstructive techniques or when the underlying skeletal lesion is accompanied by soft tissue tumor which has ulcerated to the skin. One such patient in our recent experience required hip disarticulation for a proximal femoral metastasis (Figure 7).

## Summary

While metastatic melanoma in bone is reported with less frequency than in other organ systems, it probably occurs with greater frequency than currently recognized and is associated with a poor prognosis. The detection of skeletal disease has traditionally resulted from radiographs taken in response to bone pain. More recent experience with radionuclide bone imaging suggests that earlier detection is possible not only in symptomatic but asymptomatic metastases as well, and regular scans should be considered as part of the routine evaluation of patients with melanoma.

While radiotherapy provides predictable relief of bone pain and occasional retardation of metastatic growth, chemotherapy and immunotherapy have not been observed to affect the pain or progression of skeletal metastases. Radiotherapy should be considered in osseous metastatic lesions where pain or incipient pathologic fracture is present and following surgical fixation of pathologic fracture. The majority of osseous metastases from melanoma occur in the axial skeleton and surgery therefore is seldom required. However, posterior vertebral arch lesions with associated neurologic deficit and long bone lesions with pathologic fracture or incipient pathologic fracture have benefited from surgical intervention.

# References

1. Willis RA: The Spread of Tumors in the Human Body. Butterworth, London, 1952.
2. Patel JK, Didolkar MS, Pickren JW et al: Metastatic pattern of malignant melanoma: a study of 216 autopsy cases. Am J Surg 135:807–810, 1978.
3. Das Gupta T and Brasfield R: Metastatic melanoma: a clinicopathological study. Cancer 17:1323–1339, 1964.
4. Wirth CR: Metastatic Bone Cancer: Current Problems in Cancer, p 336. Year Book Medical Publ, Chicago, 1979.
5. Selby HM, Sherman RS and Pack GT: A roentgen study of bone metastases from melanoma. Radiology 67:224–228, 1956.
6. Lodwick GS: Solitary malignant tumors of bone: the application of predictor variables in diagnosis. Semin Roentgenol 1:293–313, 1966.
7. Stewart WR, Gelberman RH, Harrelson JM and Seigler HF: Skeletal metastases of melanoma. J Bone Joint Surg 60(A):645–648, 1978.
8. Cochran AJ: Malignant melanoma: a review of ten years experience in Glasgow, Scotland. Cancer 23:1190–1199, 1969.
9. Gelberman RH, Stewart WR and Harrelson JM: Hand metastasis from melanoma. Clin Orthop Relat Res 136:264–266, 1978.
10. Franklin JD, Reynolds VH and Page DL: Cutaneous melanoma: a twenty-year retrospective study with clinicopathologic correlation. Plast Reconst Surg 56:277–285, 1975.
11. Meyer JE: Radiographic evaluation of metastatic melanoma. Cancer 42:127–132, 1978.
12. Loeffler RK, DiSimone RN and Howland WJ: Limitations of bone scanning in clinical oncology. J Am Med Assoc 234:1228–1232, 1975.
13. Lentle BC, Russell AS, Percy JS, Scott JR and Jackson FI: Bone scintiscanning updated. Ann Int Med 84:297–303, 1976.
14. Felix EL, Sindelar WF, Bagley DM, Johnston GS and Ketchum AS: The use of bone and brain scans as screening procedures in patients with malignant lesions. Surg Gynecol Obstet 141:867–869, 1975.
15. Cady B: Changing concepts in malignant melanoma. Med Clin North Am 59:301–308, 1975.
16. Keyhani A: Comparison of clinical behavior of melanoma of the hands and feet: a study of 283 patients. Cancer 40:3168–3173, 1977.
17. Harrington KD, Johnston JO, Turner RH and Green DL: The use of methylmethacrylate as an adjunct in the internal fixation of malignant neoplastic fractures. J Bone Joint Surg 54(A):1665–1676, 1972.
18. Koshinen EVS and Nieminen RA: Surgical treatment of metastatic pathological fractures of major long bones. Acta Orthop Scand 44:539, 1973.
19. Douglass HO, Shukla SK and Mindell E: Treatment of pathological fractures of long bones excluding those due to breast cancer. J Bone Joint Surg 58(A):1055–1061, 1976.
20. Ryan JR, Rowe DE and Salciccioli GG: Prophylatic internal fixation of the femur for neoplastic lesions. J Bone Joint Surg 58(A):1071–1074, 1976.
21. Harrington KD et al: Methylmethacrylate as an adjunct in internal fixation of pathological fractures. J Bone Joint Surg 58(A):1047–1055, 1976.
22. Frances KC: The role of amputation in the treatment of metastatic bone cancer. Clin Orthop Relat Res 73:61, 1970.

# 16. Melanomas of the eye and its adnexa

GORDON K. KLINTWORTH

## 1 Introduction

The ocular tissues contain two distinct melanin-containing types of cells: the melanocyte and the pigment epithelium. The melanocyte is of neural crest origin and, while being most abundant in the uvea (iris, choroid and ciliary body), also occurs in the conjunctiva, skin and less conspicuously in the sclera, meninges and orbital tissues. The pigment epithelium, which is of neural ectodermal origin, is located within the eye as the epithelial layers of the iris and ciliary body and as the retinal pigment epithelium. Malignant melanomas within the eye and its adnexa stem from melanocytes, or related cells, but interestingly the pigmented epithelia of neural ectodermal origin do not spawn malignant tumors.

## 2 Primary uveal melanomas

### 2.1 Incidence

Most noncutaneous melanomas (79%) arise in the eye [1] and uveal melanomas, the most common potentially fatal primary intraocular tumors, are estimated to have an annual average age-adjusted incidence rate in whites in the USA of 0.60 per 100 000 or one-tenth that of primary cutaneous melanomas [1]. In Denmark the estimated frequency of uveal melanomas is about the same (0.7/100 000/year) [2]. In the United States one can hence expect about 1320 new uveal melanomas per year. Melanomas arise most often from the choroid (77–93%) [2, 3], and less frequently from the ciliary body (2–9%) [2–6] and the iris (3–8%) [2, 3]. In the era before melanomas of the iris were treated by local excision or simple observation, melanomas in this location accounted for 0.9% to 1.3% of enucleated eyes [4, 7, 8].

Melanomas in all parts of the uvea are uncommon in children and young adults [9]. While less than 4% of patients with choroidal and ciliary body melanomas are younger than 30 years, a choroidal melanoma has been documented in a 2-year-old girl [10]. The average age at which uveal mela-

Seigler, H. F. (ed.), Clinical Management of Melanoma. ISBN 978-94-009-7495-1
© 1982, Martinus Nijhoff Publishers, The Hague/Boston/London.

nomas become diagnosed is in the sixth decade [1]. The incidence of choroidal melanomas increases steeply between from the ages of 30 and 70 and the tumor frequency remains high after persons reach their eightieth birthday [1] despite a clinical impression that the chances of a person developing a uveal melanoma become extremely low in advanced age.

While only about 10% of iris melanomas occur under the age of 20 years [11], melanomas have been documented in this part of the eye during the first decade of life [8, 12, 13] and the literature contains one that was present at birth [2]. Perhaps because abnormalities in the iris are more easily observed than in other parts of the uvea, the average age of subjects with iris melanomas is 10–20 years younger than subjects with melanomas elsewhere in the uvea [4, 7, 8]. Tapioca melanomas of the iris (see below) present at a younger age (average about 30 years) than the usual type of iris melanoma [7]. Despite the infrequency of iris tumors in childhood compared to adults, 41% of uveal melanomas found in childhood are located in the iris [12].

In some documented series there has been a preponderance of males or females [2] but as with cutaneous melanomas the incidence appears to be greater among females before 40 years of age and among males in persons 45 years or older [1].

Melanomas of the uvea develop predominantly in Caucasians [1, 14] and it is noteworthy that the black races, which have much more heavily pigmented uveal tissue than Caucasians, seldom develop uveal melanomas in the U.S.A. (0.07/100 000/year) [1] and in Africa [15, 16]. In a series of 2 535 uveal melanomas in the United States only 11 were from black patients [14], while another review limited to 125 iris melanomas included only two blacks [17]. Uveal melanomas are also rare in the Chinese [18] and Japanese [19].

## 2.2 Etiologic considerations

*2.2.1 Nevocellular nevi.* The prevalent concept that uveal melanomas can arise from nevi is an old one [20] and has received presumptive support from both clinical and histopathologic observations. Some ophthalmologists have had the rare clinical experience of observing an apparent nevus of the iris or choroid grow after a latent period into a malignant melanoma [21, 22]. More importantly small clusters of nevus-like cells occur beneath or at the periphery of about 70% of choroidal melanomas that are examined histologically [23–26]. This evidence is not watertight and in those exceptional cases where malignant transformation of nevi allegedly takes place according to clinical observations the nature of the original lesion is questionable, since it is not based on a histopathologic evaluation.

Even the nature of the alleged nevus cells which are found in association with most uveal melanomas is disputed. If these nevus-like cells do indeed represent nevi it is difficult to reconcile why they should occur at the base of metastatic or experimentally induced ocular melanomas which presumably do not arise from preexisting nevi [27, 28]. Even if choroidal nevi can evolve into malignant melanomas the risk is apparently low and one would only expect one in five thousand choroidal nevi to undergo this transformation annually in Caucasians [29]. With iris nevi the risk is so rare that it is insignificant.

Nevi of the uvea are not comparable to the junctional, compound and intradermal/subepithelial nevi of the skin and conjunctiva. Nevi of the choroid have been noted clinically in 1–9.5% of the general population [29] and in about 6.5–10% of eyes examined after death [30, 31]. Choroidal nevi are usually less than 4.5 mm in diameter and slightly thicker than the normal choroid. They range in color from jet black to a pale yellow with only specks of pigmentation and consist of a variety of cell types (plump polyhedral, slender spindle, plump spindle, fusiform, dendritic or balloon cells) [24]. While one cell type predominates in some choroidal nevi the entire spectrum of cells is present in others.

A specific nevus designated a melanocytoma (magnocellular nevus) is jet black and characterized by comparatively uniform plump polyhederal cells with abundant deeply pigmented cytoplasm and small round to oval nuclei without distinct nucleoli [32–34]. In such lesions the cytologic features can not be recognized until the pigment has been removed by bleaching. Although originally recognized in the optic nerve head this slowly growing nevus, which affects blacks more often than Caucasians, may occur in the choroid and ciliary body and even in the iris [35–40]. Melanocytomas rarely contain multinucleated and atypical cells as well as areas of necrosis [40]. Plump polyhedral cells resembling those in melanocytomas have been noted in eyes with uveal melanomas [39, 41] and this has led to the belief that melanocytomas can spawn melanomas on rare occasions.

Nevi are visible in the iris of about half of the adult population [42] and, although they have been suspected of being more frequent in histologic sections of eyes with choroidal melanomas [43, 44], this has not been substantiated clinically [42].

*2.2.2 Congenital ocular melanocytosis (melanosis oculi and oculodermal melanosis).* Some individuals are born with a unilateral grayish discoloration of the episclera and an increased pigmentation of the iris, ciliary body and choroid. This condition known as congenital ocular melanocytosis (melanosis oculi) is occasionally inherited usually in an autosomal dominant manner. The pigmentation results from the presence of an excessive number of melanocytes within the episclera, sclera, uveal tract and sometimes even in the eyelids and orbital tissues. Dermal melanosis of the lower eyelid at times with upper lid involvement (nevus of Ota) can occur alone or in association with melanosis oculi. Ever since Coats [45] drew attention to seven (26.9%) extrabulbar or choroidal melanomas among 26 patients with melanosis oculi, a high percentage of reported cases of ocular melanocytosis have had intraocular melanomas (1–25%) [26, 46–49]. Uveal melanomas have also occurred in association with the nevus of Ota [50–55]. This apparent higher incidence of melanomas in melanosis oculi than in the general population has suggested that melanocytes in this condition have an increased predisposition to malignancy. Several other observations support this view: (1) the rare event of two independent melanomas has been detected in an eye with melanosis oculi [56] and (2) at least two persons with oculodermal melanosis have developed the rare primary orbital malignant melanomas [57, 58].

However, the assertion that eyes with melanosis oculi have an increased susceptibility to malignant melanomas has been questioned for several reasons [48]: 1) The true incidence of malignant change in melanosis oculi is unknown as reported cases are biased towards subjects with ocular and adnexal tumors; 2) bilateral melanomas have not been documented in persons with bilateral melanosis oculi; and 3) melanomas have been observed in the blue eye of a patient with ocular melanocytosis in the fellow eye. Moreover, oculodermal melanocytosis is much more common in Orientals than Caucasians, yet uveal melanomas are rare in nonwhites and have not been documented in persons of these racial extractions who have melanosis oculi. Also, melanomas of the conjunctiva or eyelid have not been associated with melanosis oculi or the nevus of Ota.

*2.2.3 Heredity.* While there is no clear-cut inherited predisposition to ocular melanomas, several observations suggest that the genetic constitution of an individual may be important in the causation of uveal melanomas: (1) several familial uveal melanomas have been documented [46, 59–63]; (2) the unequal incidence of uveal melanomas among persons of different racial origin may reflect a genetic predisposition to the tumors or natural protection against them; and (3) persons with unusual inherited cutaneous nevi seem to develop melanomas more often than one would expect by chance.

In 1978 Clark et al. [64] drew attention to an unusual syndrome characterized by multiple large atypical cutaneous nevi of the upper trunk and extremities and an apparent increased susceptibility to malignant transformation. This so-called B-K mole syndrome (familial atypical mole syndrome) has an autosomal dominant mode of inheritance in some families, but cases may occur in the absence of a positive family history. Cutaneous melanomas develop at an early age in multiple sites from atypical melanocytic nevi. These nevi measure about 1 cm in diameter, are irregular in outline and range in number from ten to 100 or more. Primary choroidal melanomas have been documented in at least two individuals with this rare phenotype [65, 66]. Moreover, a uveal melanoma has been reported in a newborn child who had numerous cutaneous nevi like his mother [67].

Pigmented nevi of the choroid are common in von Recklinghausen's neurofibromatosis and uveal melanomas have been documented in several patients with this phakomatosis [26, 68–71]. However, it remains to be determined whether there is an increased incidence of malignant melanomas in this relatively common autosomal dominant disorder.

That some individuals may have an inherent susceptibility to cancer has been raised by the occurrence of more than one neoplasm in a particular person. While there is an increased incidence of certain occult or clinically apparent second primary malignant neoplasms in subjects with many different tumors [72, 73], coexistent tumors can result from several independent mechanisms. Some may represent independent cellular responses to carcinogenic agents, others form parts of inherited syndromes with multiple primary neoplasms. Choroidal melanomas have been documented in association with glioblastoma multiforme [74], leukemia [75, 76], cutaneous melanomas [65, 66, 77], carcinoma of larynx [78], breast [79, 80] and gastrointestinal tract [78, 80] as well as with other tumors [80]. In at least one documented patient [81] a uveal melanoma was associated with two other malignancies (scirrhous adenocarcinoma of the breast and papillary adenocarcinoma of the ovary) and at Duke University Medical Center one individual with a choroid melanoma was found to have independent coexistent adenocarcinomas of the breast and colon [82].

*2.2.4 Environmental factors.* The annual age-adjusted incidence of uveal melanomas is estimated to range from 2/100 000 among certain Asian countries to 10/100 000 in Scandinavia [83]. Whereas some of the difference in the incidence of uveal melanomas in various regions of the world probably represents inadequate reporting, part of it seems to reflect the occurrence of the tumor in Caucasians and its rarity in other racial groups. A vast amount of evidence implicates ultraviolet irradiation from the sun as a causal factor in cutaneous melanomas [84], but such evidence is lacking with melanomas in the uvea. For example, unlike skin melanomas there is no rising incidence of uveal melanomas in the U.S.A. as one passes from the North to the South [1] (Figure 1). Recently five choroidal melanomas (a statistically significant greater than expected occurrence) have been reported among present or former white workers of a chemical company [85]. Although specific carcinogens could not be implicated this finding of an increased risk for ocular melanomas in persons of a certain occupation, who also have an increased incidence of other malignant neoplasms, has opened new vistas in

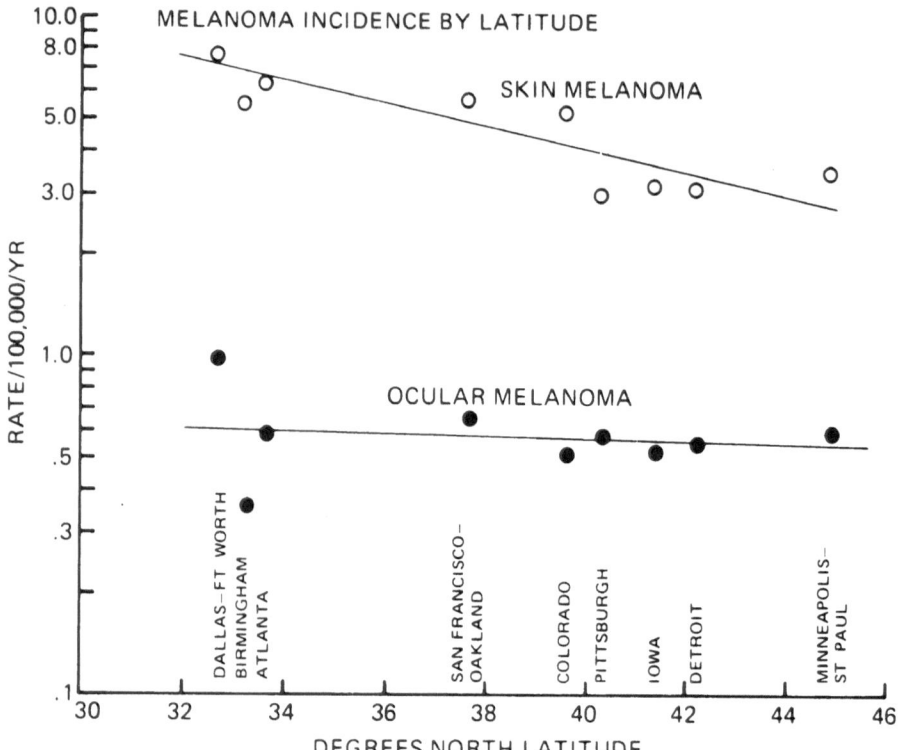

*Figure 1.* Incidence of uveal melanomas in the United States according to lattitude. Reproduced with permission from ref. [1].

the search for causes of ocular melanomas. While not comparable to the human tumor, melanomas have been induced experimentally in rats with intravitreal nickel subsulfide [85], and after oral ethionine and N-2-fluore-nylacetamide [86]. Pigmented tumors have been produced in dogs with radium, but these lesions seem to involve an abnormal proliferation of the retinal pigment epithelium [87].

## 2.3 Morphologic characteristics

The color of uveal melanomas varies from gray or light tan to brown or black depending on the amount of melanin. Whereas some melanomas are deeply pigmented, others contain no apparent pigmentation on gross or microscopic examination. Even the same melanoma sometimes varies in color with parts of it being heavily pigmented or virtually devoid of pigment (Figure 2). Some iris melanomas are amelanotic fleshy tumors with promi-nent superficial dilated blood vessels but most are darkly pigmented. Blood vessels are prominent 7% to 20% of iris melanomas [17] and may cause the tumor to clinically resemble a hemangioma [88–90]. Prominent dilated epi-scleral or bulbar conjunctival blood vessels are frequently engorged over ciliary body melanomas [46, 91–93] and the vascular pattern on the surface of 22% of melanomas is abnormal [93].

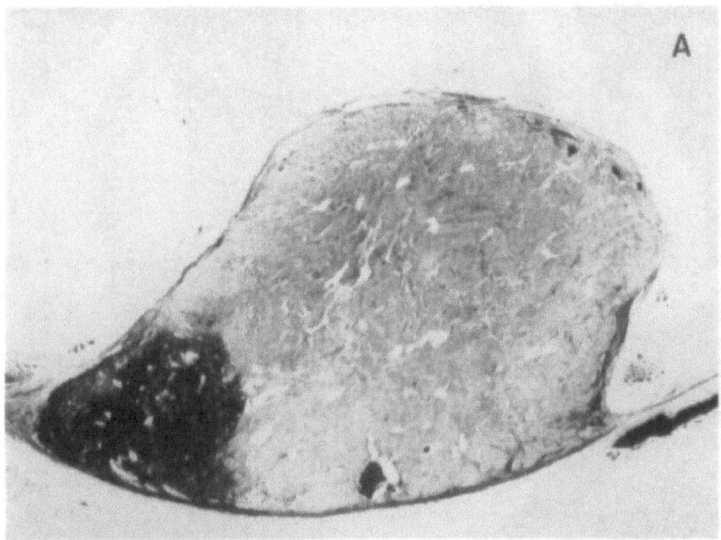

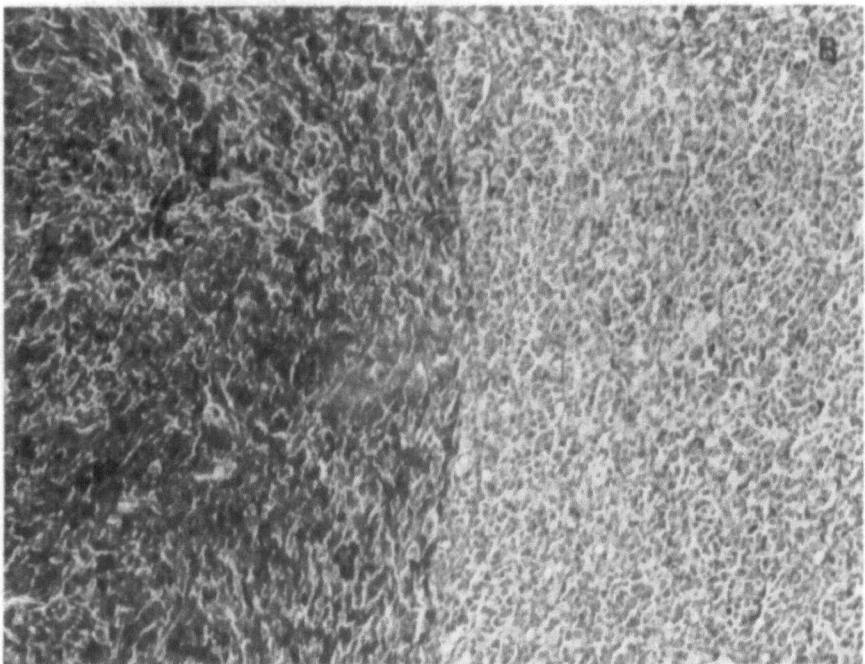

*Figure 2.* (A) While most uveal melanomas have a more or less homogeneous color, some contain heavily pigmented areas adjacent to amelanotic zones. Hematoxylin and eosin, × 6. (B) Higher magnification of tumor showing sharp line of demarcation between melanotic and amelanotic portions of tumor. Hematoxylin and eosin, × 100.

458

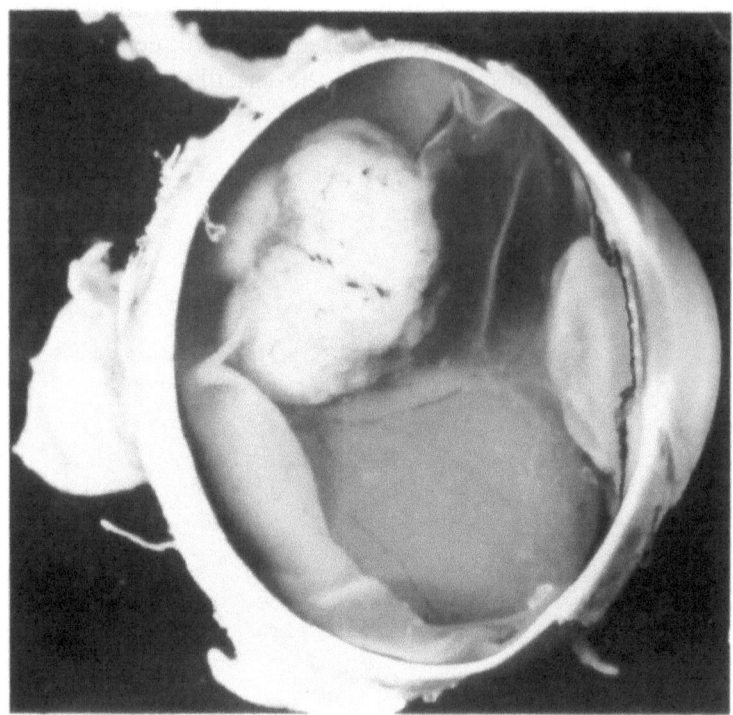

*Figure 3.* Mushroom-shaped melanoma of choroid displacing the retina towards the center of the eye. Reproduced with permission from Klintworth GK and Landers MB, III: The Eye: Structure and Function in Disease. Williams & Wilkins, Baltimore, 1976.

Primary uveal malignant melanomas are usually solitary discrete tumors, but on rare occasions they appear multifocally in the choroid [94–98] or iris [99] or arise in both eyes [76, 96, 100–102]. While most melanomas of the iris form a relatively flat mass within the stroma of the iris, some appear nodular and protrude into the anterior chamber. Most melanomas of the iris are situated inferiorly and especially in the midzone and peripheral iris [11, 17, 103]. A curious variant of the iris melanoma, but with similar histologic characteristics and prognosis to typical melanomas in this part of the uvea, is characterized by lightly pigmented, translucent nodules reminiscent of tapioca pudding or a cluster of fish eggs ("tapioca melanoma") [104]. The nodules lie within the iris stroma and are thought to represent multiple sites of primary growth rather than foci of implantation. Choroidal melanomas usually grow towards the center of the eye as localized globular or mushroom shaped masses (Figure 3), but about 5% of these tumors are flat and infiltrate the choroid without forming a definite mass or extending through Bruch's membrane (diffuse uveal melanomas) [105] (Figure 4). A unique diffuse uveal melanoma with extrascleral extension presented clinically as a ring-shaped amelanotic limbal tumor [106].

Although hemorrhage is not a feature of most uveal melanomas, some

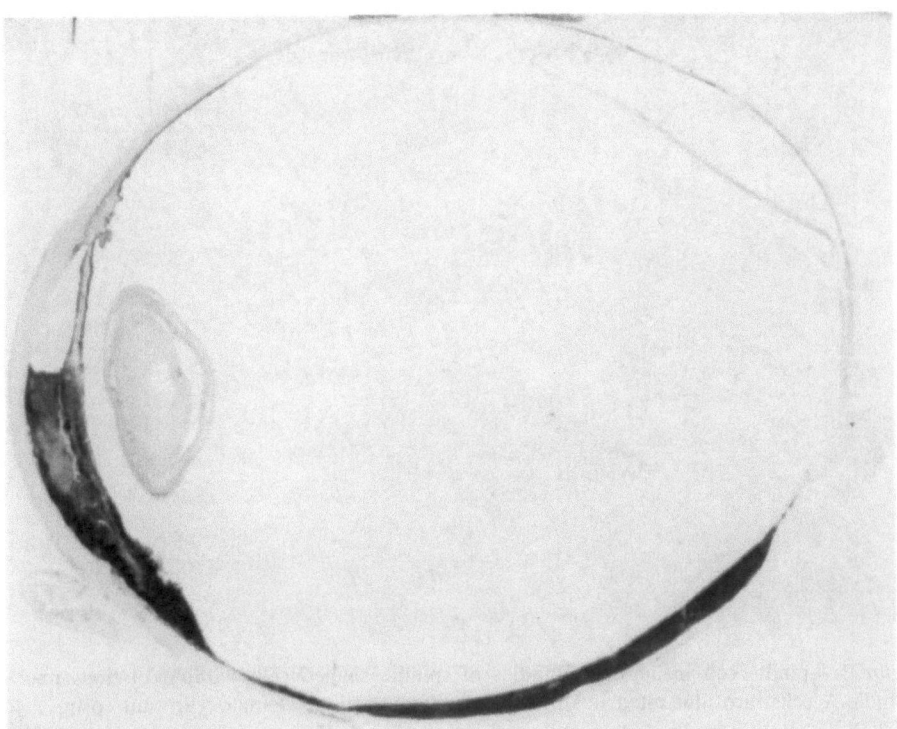

*Figure 4.* Diffuse uveal melanoma involving iris, ciliary body and choroid. Tumors cells have also sedimented in the anterior chamber. Hematoxylin and eosin, × 4.

necrotic melanomas bleed into the anterior chamber or vitreous and rarely this is the presenting sign of the tumor [107]. With choroidal melanomas hemorrhage occurs especially if the tumor ruptures through Bruch's membrane [93]. Iris melanomas sometimes bleed spontaneously into the anterior chamber (hyphema) [11, 17] and this may be the first evidence of tumor recurrence after previous excision [108].

Whereas a mild lymphocytic infiltrate surrounds many choroidal melanomas, a pronounced inflammatory reaction is provoked by necrotic melanomas especially in their vicinity. Rarely severe panophthalmitis ensues, sometimes accompanied by exophthalmos.

Almost 50 years ago Callender [109] drew attention to the fact that uveal melanomas are composed of three basic cell types: (1) small, slender spindle shaped cells with oval nuclei and ill-defined nucleoli (spindle-A cells) (Figure 5). Frequently a line or fold extends down the center of the nucleus in its long axis [110] due to a peculiar infolding of the nuclear membrane, (2) similar shaped cells with prominent nucleoli (spindle-B cells) and (3) relatively large polygonal cells of considerable variation in shape and size with large round to oval nuclei and one or two distinct nucleoli (epithelioid cells) (Figure 6).

460

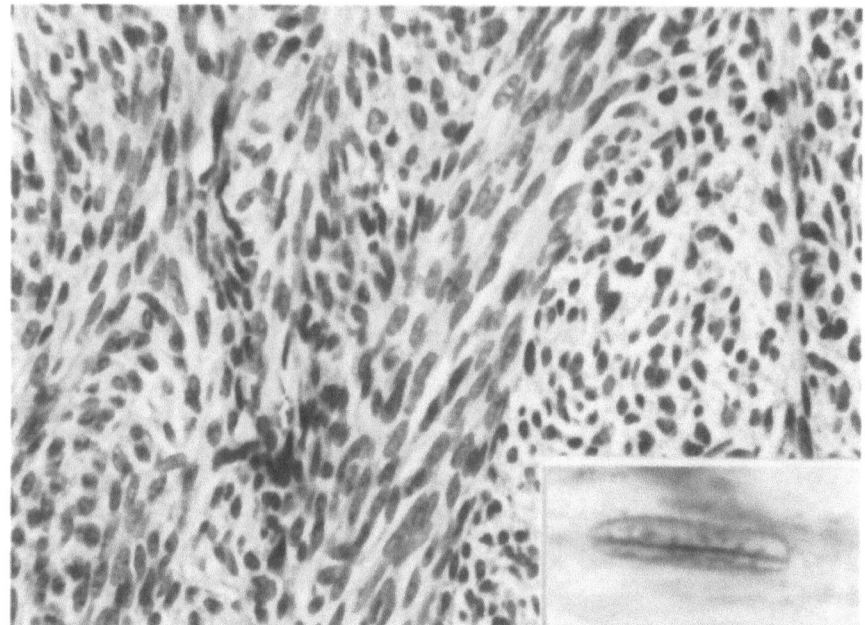

*Figure 5.* Spindle cell melanoma. Bundles of spindle shaped cells without obvious nucleoli (spindle-A cells) are illustrated in different planes of section. Hematoxylin and eosin, ×400. Inset shows prominent line down center of spindle-A cell. Hematoxylin and eosin, ×1700.

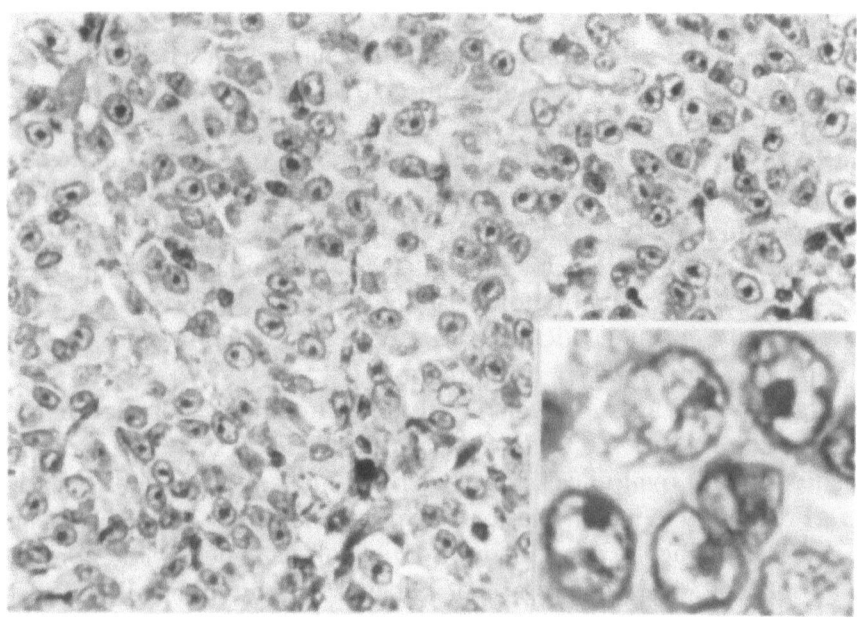

*Figure 6.* Epithelioid melanoma. In contrast to Figure 5, these tumor cells resemble epithelial cells and have prominent nucleoli. Hematoxylin and eosin, ×400. Inset shows epithelioid cells under higher magnification. Hematoxylin and eosin, ×1700.

Callender divided intraocular malignant melanomas into six types: spindle-A, spindle-B, fascicular, mixed, necrotic and epithelioid. Spindle-A melanomas are those composed almost exclusively of spindle-A cells, while spindle-B melanomas contain spindle-B cells (with or without spindle-A cells). Fascicular tumors derive their name from the ribbon or fascicular pattern which spindle-B cells sometimes form. Mixed cell melanomas are composed of both spindle and epithelioid cells, whereas epithelioid melanomas are made up almost exclusively of epithelioid cells. Sometimes the tumor is extensively necrotic and the cell type cannot be identified (necrotic melanoma) (Figure 7). Necrosis occurs most often with large choroidal tumors that have extended through Bruch's membrane. Pure spindle-A tumors are now regarded as nevi rather than malignant melanomas by some individuals.

Callender's classification of melanomas is still popular today despite several inherent shortcomings [111]: 1) the classification is based on one or a few random sections through the tumor and this is not necessarily representative of the entire tumor. While different cell types may be present in other portions of the tumor, it is not practical to cut serial sections of every melanoma; 2) the vast majority of melanomas consist of variable proportions of spindle-A, spindle-B and epithelioid cells and would be designated as mixed cell melanomas if the tumors were thoroughly sectioned; 3) all cells in uveal melanomas do not fall into one of Callender's morphologic

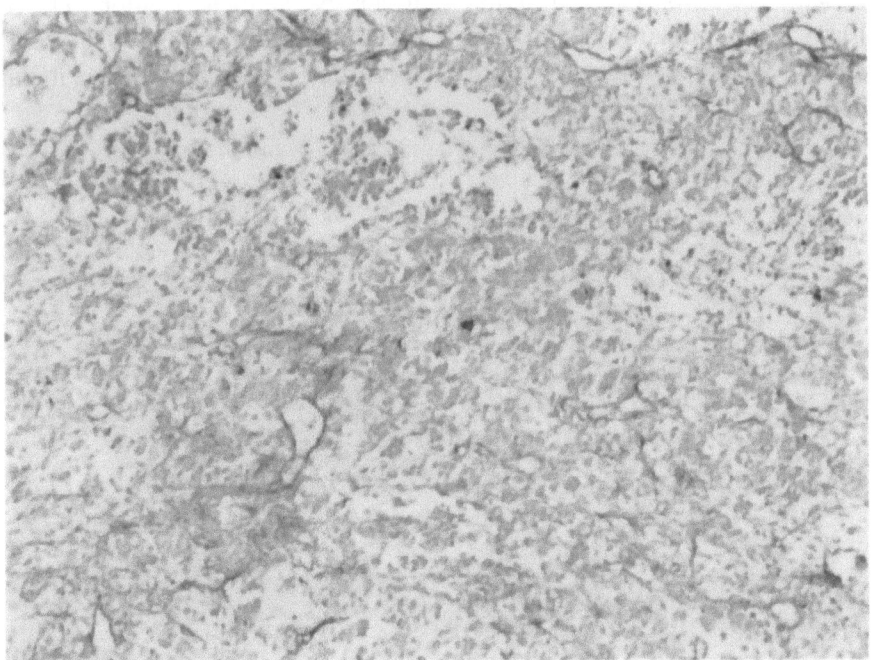

*Figure 7.* Necrotic melanoma. While parts of uveal melanoma often become necrotic, the entire tumor sometimes contains no recognizable viable cells. Hematoxylin and eosin, × 100.

subpopulations. For example, a single tumor may contain a variety of inter-mediate forms that can not be designated spindle-shaped or epithelioid and certain uveal melanomas contain lipid-laden cells (balloon cells) [112, 113]. Also, some tumors contain small anaplastic cells that are not epithelial-like in appearance and, rarely, the malignant cells possess a dentritic appearance (Figure 8); and 4) the classification of melanomas according to Callender's system varies to some extent with the whims and meticulousness of the classifier. This point is underscored by the study of Gass [114] who found that ophthalmic pathologists do not always classify a histologic section through the same tumor consistently. Also, in a re-evaluation of 105 so called spindle-A melanomas of the choroid and ciliary body that were ori-ginally classified at the United States Armed Forces Institute of Pathology, where Callender introduced his classification, McLean et al. [115] found only 15 of these tumors to consist entirely of spindle-A cells and that the rest contained variable numbers of spindle-B and/or epithelioid cells.

In the ciliary body and choroid the relative incidence of the various types of melanomas based on Callender's classification are about the same: spin-dle-A (5%), spindle-B (39%), epithelioid (3%), mixed (45%), and necrotic (7%). About 6% of uveal melanomas composed of spindle-B cells are arranged in a fascicular pattern [14]. In Jensen's [116] series of uveal mela-nomas extensive necrosis was associated with epithelioid cells and no tumors were so necrotic that a cell type could not be identified. This has also been our experience at Duke University Medical Center. The vast majority of iris melanomas are composed of spindle-A cells (90%) or spin-dle-B cells, while epithelioid cells are uncommon [7, 8, 11]. Tapioca melano-

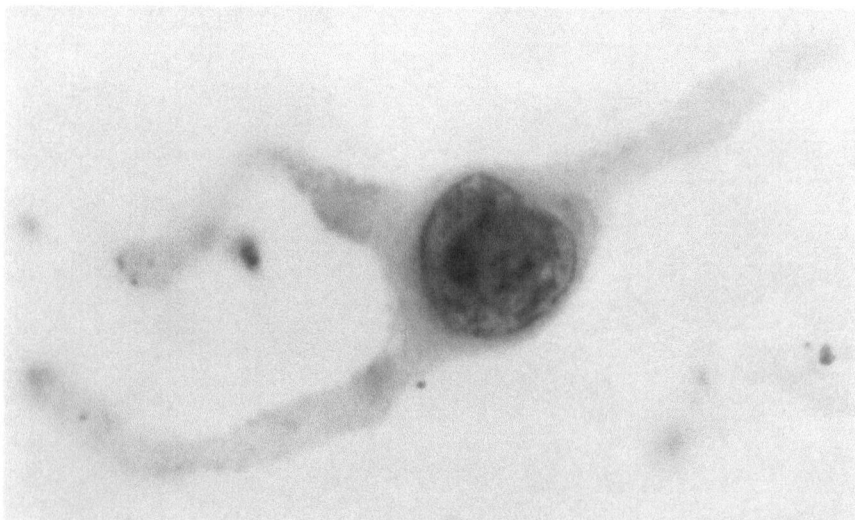

*Figure 8.* Microscopic appearance of dendritic-shaped melanoma cell on millipore filter. Papan-icolaou, × 3300.

mas of the iris are composed predominantly of spindle-A melanoma cells which contain little or no pigment [104, 117].

When viewed by transmission electron microscopy the appearance of individual tumor cells in uveal melanomas varies as it does by light microscopy (Figure 9). The fine structure varies with the cell type [118–122]. Nucleoli become larger and more prominent and free ribosomes and mitochondria appear more numerous as cells pass from the spindle-A end of the morphologic spectrum to epithelioid cells. A longitudinal invagination commonly occurs in the nuclear membrane of spindle-A cells [120] and this corresponds to the line that extends down the long axis of these cells when they are examined by light microscopy. Nuclear indentations tend to be more numerous in tumor cells of the spindle-B or epithelioid type and in cells of the latter variety the cytoplasm frequently protrudes into the nuclei

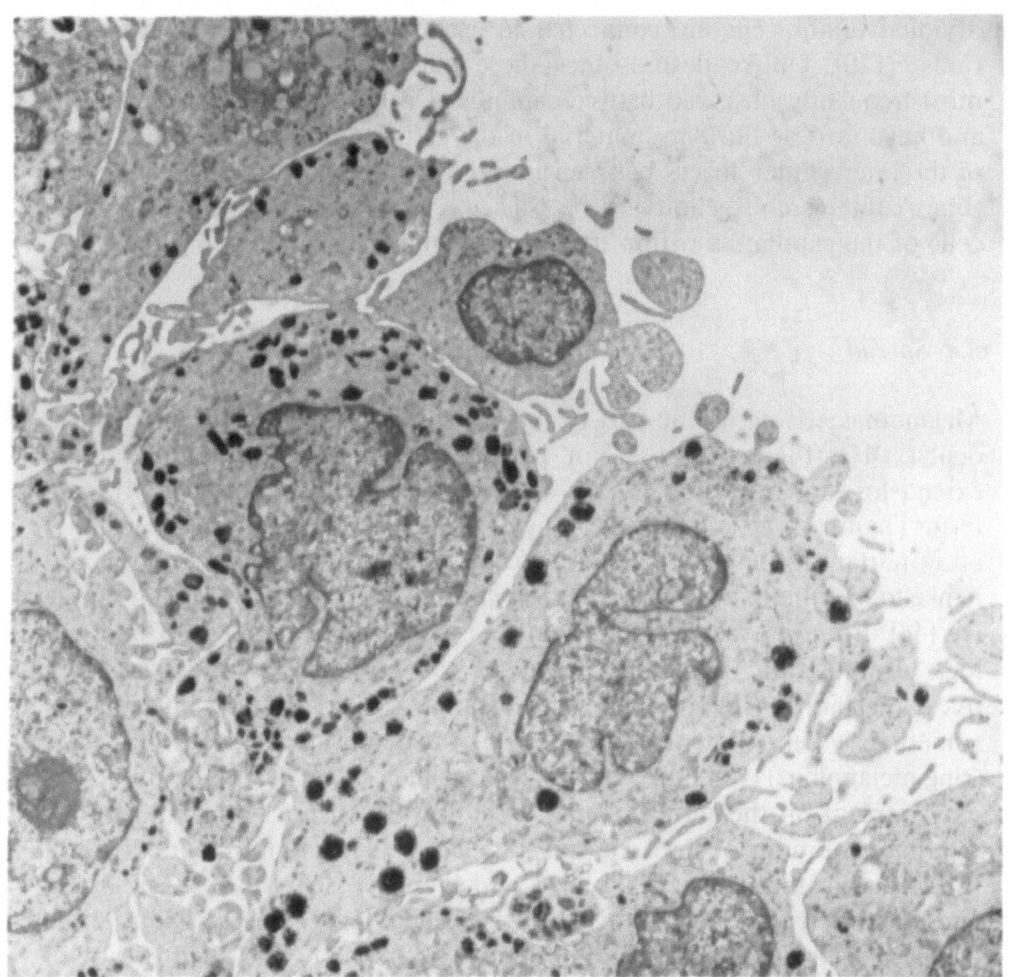

*Figure 9.* Transmission electron micrograph of melanoma cells of the epithelioid cell type. The cells contain abundant melanosomes but intercellular junctions are not prominent, × 10 200.

to form pseudonuclear inclusions. Rough-surfaced endoplasmic reticulum is particularly prominent in the spindle-B and epithelioid cell types and sometimes takes on a spiral or concentric arrangement [122]. Delicate cytoplasmic filaments having a morphology consistent with actin are especially numerous in spindle-shaped tumor cells. Although still present they are less evident in epithelioid cells and such cells react to antiserum to smooth muscle [123]. Amelanotic melanomas commonly contain premelanosomes or melanosomes by electron microscopy. It is noteworthy that in lightly pigmented melanomas melanin granules are often not abundant in the individual tumor cells and that those which are present are predominantly immature premelanosomes in various stages of development. Nevertheless, their presence can be of practical value in equivocal diagnostic situations. The cytoplasm of the tumor cells frequently contains abundant glycogen [119] and virus-like particles have occasionally been observed [122]. Individual tumor cells are connected to each other by "intermediate junctions" [120]. Unlike desmosomes these junctional complexes, which are most frequently observed between spindle-A cells, lack a central dense line and have far less fibrillary material in the associated cytoplasm. The width of the intercellular spaces between individual tumor cells varies and sometimes contains collagenous fibers. Like the choriocapillaris the endothelial cells of the capillaries within uveal melanomas are fenestrated [120].

*2.4 Spread*

Melanomas arising in one part of the eye sometimes spread to other intraocular sites (Figures 4, 10). For instance ciliary body melanomas often extend forward into the iris root or backward into the choroid [124], posterior chamber and vitreous. Seeding of melanoma cells into the aqueous is an important route of intraocular spread to the anterior chamber angle and hence to extrabulbar extension. Rarely choroidal melanomas implant on the iris [46]. From a practical standpoint the detection of tumor cells by cytologic examination in aspirated aqueous can establish the diagnosis of a uveal melanoma (Figure 8) [125]. Melanomas of the iris and ciliary body sometimes extend circumferentially along the major arterial circle of the iris (ring melanomas) [124] and under exceptional circumstances the tumor cells may implant on the surface of the optic nerve and in a retina [126].

A frequent mode of spread of uveal melanomas is into the orbit by way of the foramina through which nerves and blood vessels traverse the sclera, and very rarely, by direct invasion through the sclera (Figures 11, 12). Some degree of extrascleral extension occurs in 10–23% of enucleated eyes with melanomas of the choroid and ciliary body, and this is most frequently a manifestation of large epithelioid melanomas [127–130].

In contrast to retinoblastomas, which commonly invade the optic nerve, choroidal melanomas seldom extend out of the globe by this route and when this does take place the eyes are blind and the tumors are usually of the necrotic, mixed or epithelioid cell type and glaucoma is almost always

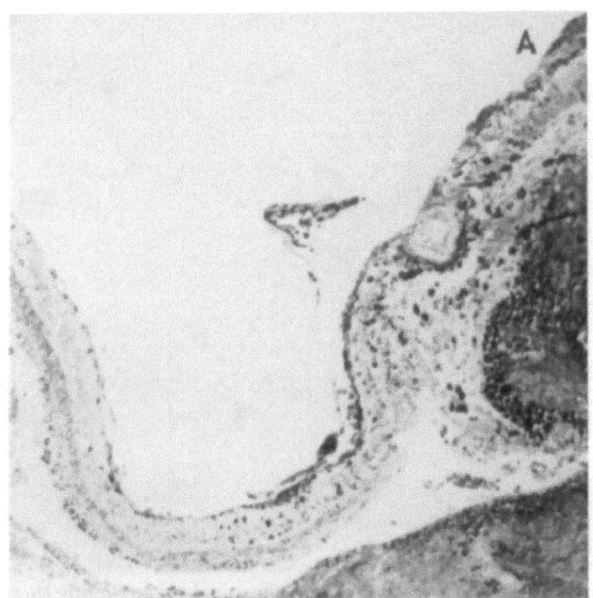

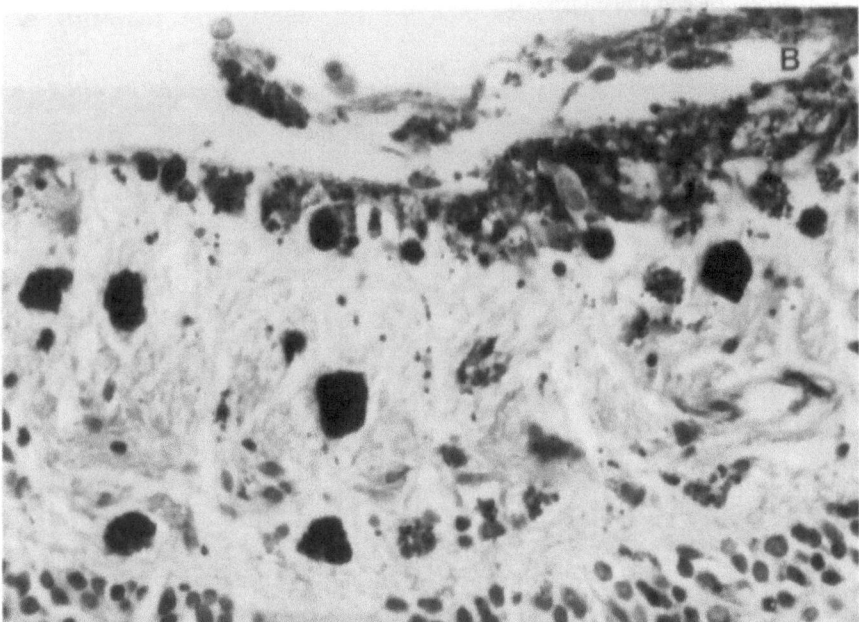

*Figure 10.* (A) On occasions choroidal melanomas invade the adjacent retina and grow on the surface of the retina. Hematoxylin and eosin, × 40. (B) Higher magnification of heavily pigmented cells of malignant melanoma are shown on the surface of the retina and within the inner retina. Hematoxylin and eosin, × 400.

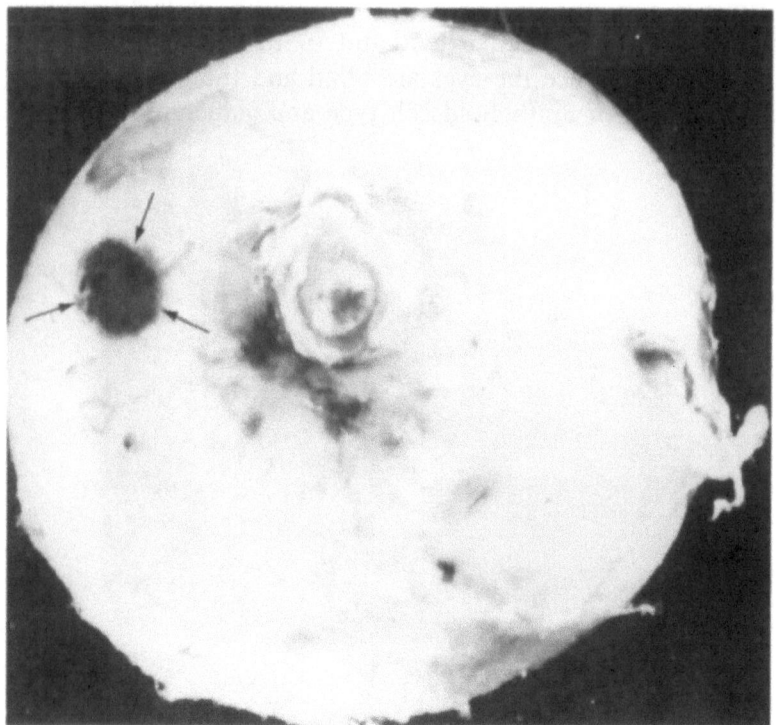

*Figure 11.* An Area of transcleral extension of a choroidal melanoma is shown on the posterior surface of an enucleated globe (arrows).

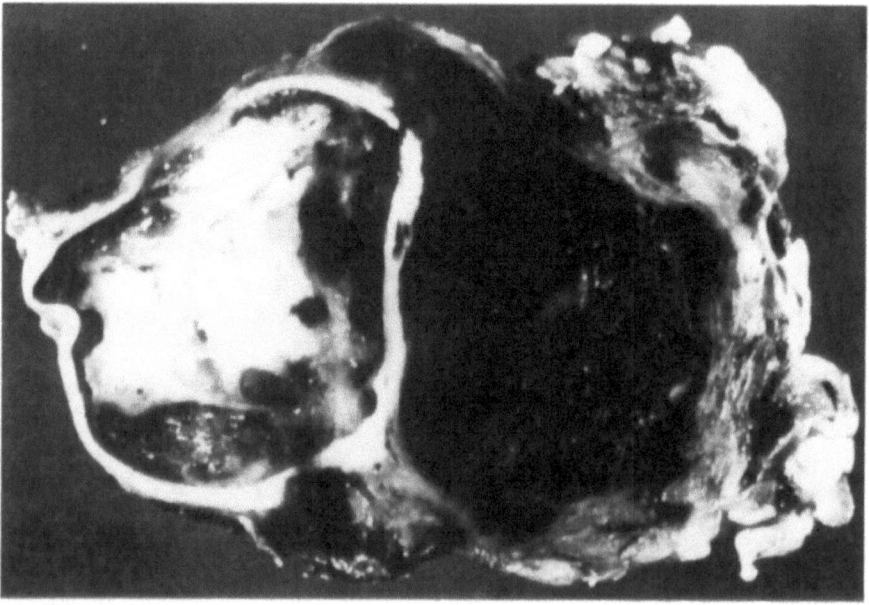

*Figure 12.* The orbital tissue behind a phthisical eye contains a melanomatous mass which arose from an intraocular melanoma, × 3.5.

associated [131-133]. In a review of 26 uveal melanomas extending around the optic nerve head (peripapillary choroidal melanomas) Shammas and Blodi [132] noted extension along the optic nerve and its meningeal sheaths in 21 cases (80.8%) [132]. A unique example of extraocular extension through the optic nerve from an iris and ciliary body melanoma without choroidal involvement has been documented [133].

Like the orbit the globe lacks lymphatic vessels because of an unexplained quirk of nature and uveal melanomas do not disseminate to regional lymph nodes. However, hematogenous dissemination to distant sites is an important mode of spread of all melanomas of the ocular tissues. It is noteworthy that distant metastases are exceedingly rare at the time of ocular presentation [134-136] and may not become clinically evident until many years after the eye with the melanoma is enucleated [2, 46, 137-139] (Table 1). The reason for the long latent period between uveal melanomas and metastases remains unknown. Since the malignant cells must have disseminated prior to, or during, the surgical removal, the metastatic implants presumably remain dormant for many years, as in other forms of cancer, because of immunologic, hormonal or other defense mechanisms of the host.

From the clinical standpoint metastases from uveal melanomas usually appear first in the liver [2, 138, 140] and are often limited to this location at the time of death [2]. In an autopsy series of 38 uveal melanomas Jensen [2] found metastases to be limited to the liver in 13 patients (34.2%). Einhorn et al. [138] found evidence of liver involvement in 22 of 25 (88%) patients with choroidal melanomas and metastatic disease and that in 15 (60%) of these cases the hepatic metastases were the sole initial clinical manifestation of metastatic disease. In a review of 12 uveal melanomas with metastatic disease Berd et al. [139] reported the liver to be initially involved in 11 cases and this was the sole site of metastatic disease in seven of these patients (58.3%). Uveal melanomas also frequently metastasize to the lungs, but less often to the central nervous system, bone, lymph nodes and other sites [2,

Table 1. Latent period between enucleation and metastatic disease

| Author | Series size | Longest latent period years | Latent period |
|---|---|---|---|
| Morton and Morton [37] | 18 | 32 | 10–32 years |
| Jensen [2] | 126 | 13 | 37 (29.4%), 5 years or longer 6 months–17 years; 43 months (median) |
| Einhorn et al. [138] | 25 | 17 | 8 (32%), 5 years or longer |
| Berd et al. [139] | 12 | 8¼ | 5 (41%), 5 years or longer |

Table 2. Distribution of commonest sites of metastases in patients dying of melanomas (postmortem series)

| SYSTEM | ORGANS | UVEAL MELANOMAS | | | NONOCULAR MELANOMAS | | | | | |
|---|---|---|---|---|---|---|---|---|---|---|
| | Reference | Einhorn et al. [138] | Jensen [2] | Total | Das Gupta and Brasfield [145] | Einhorn et al. [144] | Patel et al. [146] | Meyer [147] | Nathanson et al. [148] | Total |
| | Patient No. | 5 | 38 | 43 | 125 | 96 | 216 | 74 | 22 | 533 |
| Respiratory | Lungs | 4 (80%) | 13 (34%) | 17 (40%) | 88 (70%) | 84 (87%) | 154 (71%) | 56 (76%) | 18 (82%) | 400 (75%) |
| Gastrointestinal | Liver | 5 (100%) | 37 (97%) | 42 (98%) | 85 (68%) | 73 (76%) | 126 (58%) | 29 (54%) | 17 (77%) | 330 (62%) |
| | Peritoneum/mesentery/omentum | 1 (20%) | 4 (11%) | 5 (12%) | 17 (14%) | 26 (27%) | 92 (43%) | – | – | 135/437* (31%) |
| | Pancreas | 2 (40%) | 6 (16%) | 8 (19%) | 66 (53%) | 36 (38%) | 81 (38%) | 10 (32%) | 9 (41%) | 202 (38%) |
| | Small intestine | – | – | – | 73 (58%) | 25 (26%) | 77 (36%) | 25 (34%) | – | 200/511* (39%) |
| | Colon and cecum | – | 1 (3%) | 1 (2%) | 28 (22%) | 13 (14%) | 61 (28%) | 18 (24%) | 9 (41%) | 120/511 (23%) |
| | Stomach | 1 (20%) | 2 (5%) | 3 (7%) | 33 (26%) | 7 (7%) | 49 (23%) | 19 (26%) | 8 (36%) | 108/511 (21%) |
| | Biliary tract | – | 1 (3%) | 1 (2%) | 19 (15%) | 4 (4%) | 19 (9%) | 15 (20%) | – | 57/511 (11%) |
| Bone, soft tissue | Skin, subcutaneous muscle | 2 (40%) | 6 (16%) | 8 (19%) | 94 (75%) | 52 (54%) | 147 (68%) | – | 8 (36%) | 301/459 (66%) |
| | Vertebra/other bones | 2 (40%) | 3 (8%) | 5 (12%) | Unknown | 22 (23%) | 89 (49%) | 26 (35%) | 9 (41%) | 146/408 (36%) |
| Lymphoreticular | Lymph nodes | 2 (40%) | 8 (21%) | 10 (23%) | 81 (65%) | 71 (74%) | 121 (56%) | – | 16 (72%) | 289/459 (63%) |
| | Spleen | 1 (20%) | 3 (8%) | 4 (9%) | 45 (36%) | 41 (43%) | 66 (31%) | 20 (27%) | 8 (36%) | 180 (34%) |
| Nervous | Brain/meninges | 1 (20%) | 4 (11%) | 5 (12%) | 41/105 (39%) | 46/85 (54%) | 101 (49%) | 30 (40%) | 8 (36%) | 226/502 (45%) |
| Cardiovascular | Heart/pericardium | 3 (60%) | 9 (24%) | 12 (28%) | 62 (49%) | 53 (55%) | 102 (47%) | 30 (40%) | 9 (41%) | 256 (48%) |
| Endocrine | Adrenals | 1 (20%) | 3 (8%) | 4 (9%) | 63 (50%) | 52 (54%) | 77 (36%) | 38 (51%) | 8 (36%) | 238 (45%) |
| | Thyroid | 1 (20%) | 3 (8%) | 4 (9%) | 49 (39%) | 20 (21%) | 55 (26%) | 17 (23%) | 6 (27%) | 147 (28%) |
| Urogenital | Kidney | 2 (40%) | 2 (5%) | 4 (9%) | 56 (45%) | 56 (58%) | 79 (35%) | 28 (38%) | 10 (45%) | 229 (43%) |
| | Urinary bladder and ureter | – | – | – | 22 (18%) | 13 (14%) | 28 (13%) | 12 (16%) | – | 75/511 (15%) |

* Denominator is number examined

*Table 3.* Survival following clinical appearance of metastases from uveal melanomas

| Author | Series Size | Remarks |
| --- | --- | --- |
| Jensen [2] | 126 | 116 (92.1%) dead within 1 year of symptomatic metastases and all but 2 dead within 2 years. |
| Einhorn et al. [138] | 25 | Median survival 7 months (3–33 months) |
| Berd et al. [139] | 12 | Median survival 5 months (1–43 months) |

138, 141], and rarely to the other eye or orbit [2, 138, 142, 143]. The distribution of metastases with uveal melanomas differs strikingly from that of cutaneous melanomas [144–148 (Table 2). Lymph nodes and the lung are usually involved in most fatal cases of cutaneous melanoma, but they are much less often affected at postmortem examination with uveal melanomas. In contrast to uveal melanomas only 17% of patients with cutaneous melanomas have clinically detectable liver involvement when metastases become apparent [144]. The predisposition for liver metastases with uveal melanoma remains unexplained.

When uveal melanomas recur in the orbit, this often precedes by a year or more the development of distant metastases [2]. As with melanomas arising elsewhere, patients with uveal melanomas usually deteriorate rapidly once distant metastases appear and are usually dead in less than one year (Table 3).

## 2.5 Prognosis

Unfortunately most mortality figures on patients with uveal melanomas have included deaths from all causes or have assumed that fatalities due to widespread malignancies were due to metastatic melanoma even though postmortem examinations have seldom been performed. The mortality from all causes after ten or more years ranges from 27% to 74% [149] in different person's experience. In his well-studied series of 292 melanomas of the choroid and ciliary body with follow-ups of 13–23 years, Jensen found that 214 (73%) patients were dead with 154 (53%) of the cases dying with metastases [116].

Despite a considerable amount of effort by many investigators, the biological behavior of uveal melanomas remains unpredictable from the standpoint of specific individuals. Attempts have been made to correlate the prognosis of uveal melanomas with different parameters and more recently an effort has been made to relate the prognosis to combinations of these variables [150].

*2.5.1 Morphology of cells.* As might have been anticipated from basic principles of neoplasia, the morphologic appearance of tumor cells is an important prognostic indicator [149]. Despite its shortcomings Callender's classification of uveal melanomas is the best single indicator of the fate of persons with uveal melanoma [3, 14, 109–111, 116, 130, 151, 152]. Spindle-A melanomas have the best prognosis, while epithelioid melanomas have the least favorable outcome (Figure 13) notwithstanding the fact that some large melanomas with numerous epithelioid cells are apparently cured by enucleation. Fascicular tumors behave like other spindle-B melanomas.

*2.5.2 Tumor size.* While not as good an indicator of prognosis as cell type, the size of uveal melanomas reflects to some extent the eventual outcome and this is of clinical importance, since it can be detected in the living subject [151]. As might be expected the larger tumors have the worst prognosis [3, 111, 116, 130, 150, 152, 154]. Persons with a small epithelioid melanoma have a more unfavorable outlook than those with larger spindle cell tumors [150]. Most small choroidal melanomas have a much better prognosis than large tumors [151 and in individuals with such tumors early enucleation does not appear to influence the overall mortality rate when compared to subjects who are observed for some time prior to enucleation [155]. However, small choroidal melanomas may develop significant

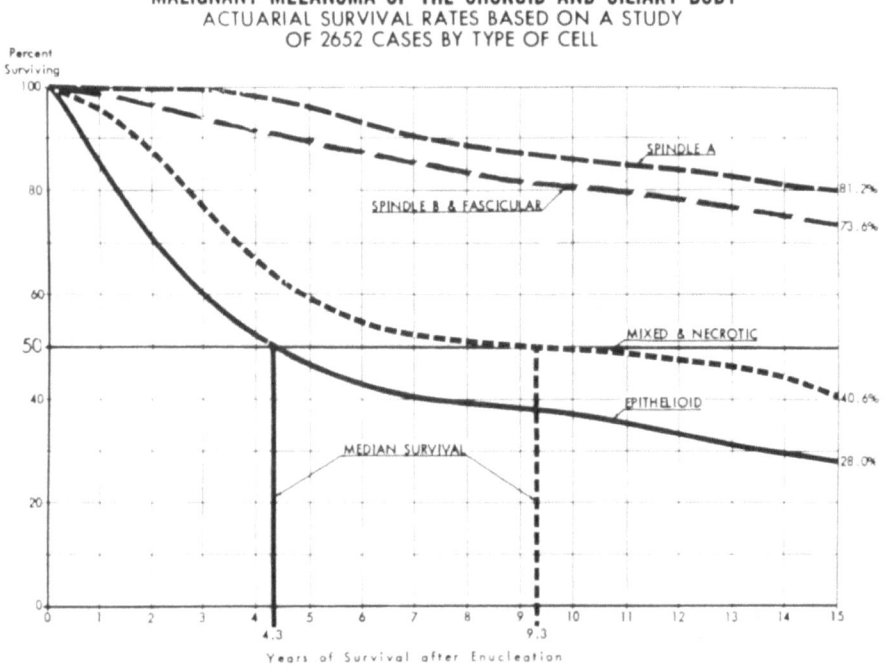

*Figure 13.* Mortality of patients with choroidal and ciliary body melanomas subdivided according to Callender's classification. Reproduced with permission from ref. [14].

extrascleral extension [156]. The mortality increases dramatically when the tumor has a volume greater than 1300 mm$^3$ [157] but the greatest single dimension of the melanoma is a more important prognostic indicator than the overall volume [150].

*2.5.3 Mitotic Index.* In uveal melanomas mitotic figures are exceedingly rare in spindle-A cells, uncommon in spindle-B cells but common in epithelioid cells. The mortality increases dramatically when more than two mitotic figures are detected when 40 high power fields are examined [150].

*2.5.4 Pigmentation.* Several investigators have noted a lower mortality in uveal melanomas of low pigment content (preciously called leucosarcomata) [3, 110, 111, 116, 130, 150, 152, 158]. Pigmented spindle cell uveal melanomas have a slightly higher mortality than lightly pigmented tumors of the same cell type [150]. Others have found the prognostic importance of the degree of pigmentation in uveal melanomas to be linked to the presence or absence of rupture through Bruch's membrane. Highly pigmented tumors only have a more lethal outcome when Bruch's membrane is ruptured [153].

*2.5.5 Tumor shape and pattern of growth.* Of the various shapes that uveal melanomas take, it is only the malignant melanoma which infiltrates the choroid without forming a definite mass (diffuse melanoma) that has a more unfavorable prognosis when compared to the usual nodular uveal melanomas [3, 23]. This probably reflects several factors: (1) diffuse melanomas of the choroid are difficult to diagnose clinically so that enucleation is delayed, (2) the tumors have frequently extended into the orbit by the time of diagnosis and (3) a high percentage of diffuse choroidal melanomas (85%) contain cells types of the more malignant variety according to Callender's classification [23]. The thickness of the tumor which reflects the tumor size, has been shown to correlate with the prognosis. The survival rate is best when the melanomas are less than 2 mm thick [153]. The mortality of uveal melanomas increases when Bruch's membrane has been ruptured [153] and this is probably a reflection of tumor size [157].

*2.5.6 Effect of treatment.* While untreated uveal melanomas can lead to death from widespread metastases [134] the innate behavior of populations of uveal melanomas without treatment is unknown. Until recently enucleation has been accepted a priori as the way to prevent metastases and to prolong life and this view is supported by animal studies [159]. However, Zimmerman and his collaborators [134, 149, 160–162] have recently challenged this assumption by suggesting that the tumor-related mortality rate in patients with melanomas who have undergone enucleation may be higher than in the natural history of the disease. This hypothesis originated from (1) their analysis of the mortality data published by Paul et al. [14] in which a rapid rise in mortality followed enucleation and then declined; (2) the fact that few patients with uveal melanomas have metastases before enucleation and (3) that patients whose eyes are not enucleated often have a high survival rate. They have pointed out that the peak mortality of patients with uveal melanomas occurs within three to four years of enucleation and that this surgical procedure may facilitate the dissemination of tumor emboli. Convincing as these arguments may appear the statistical analyses are questionable [135]. A large number of patients in Paul et al.'s series [14] were lost to follow-up causing sampling errors as well as the fact that patients of all ages were pooled in the analysis. Also, the method of computation of death rates used by Zimmerman et al. [160] makes rates in later years artifactually lower. Moreover, it is well known that the mortality of other forms of cancer is high in the early years after diagnosis and this is independent of the mode of therapy [135]. The high mortality shortly after diagnosis in uveal melanomas, as well as other forms of cancer, may well reflect an active phase of malignant growth which causes the patient to seek medical attention in the first place. The behavior of melanomas that are either asymptomatic or cause visual impairment while of a small size clearly cannot be compared with that of growing symptomatic tumors. The fact that widespread metastases from uveal melanomas are seldom present before diagnosis is not surprising, since most ocular melanomas cause symptoms when they are still relatively small. Also, the survival rate after enucleation for melanomas in patients more than 60 years of age is as good as their anticipated life expectancy [163]. Other arguments against the hypothesis of Zimmerman and colleagues have been raised [164, 165], but some of these are based on the disputable assumption that the growth of uveal melanomas follows an exponential curve [161]. The question of whether enucleation shortens the expected lifespan of persons with uveal melanomas is likely to remain unanswered until long-term follow-ups have been obtained in a prospective clinical study on sufficient age-matched patients with comparable ocular melanomas that are randomly treated by enucleation or allowed to progress unabatedly. Unfortunately, such an investigation is unlikely for ethical reasons.

While the validity of the assumption that the high postoperative mortality is iatrogenic remains debatable and unproven, it seems reasonable that the manner whereby eyes with ocular tumors are surgically enucleated may influence tumor spread. That enucleation may aid in the dissemination of tumor cells is supported by the observation that clumps of malignant cells are present in the peripheral blood stream during, or immediately after, enucleation in patients with choroidal melanomas [166]. Also it has been shown that ocular massage of experimentally induced intraocular tumors decreases longevity [167].

2.5.7 *Transcleral extension*. The prognosis of uveal melanomas worsens with transcleral extension into the orbit and this is related to the degree of scleral extension [116, 150, 152]. While the five-year survival rate of patients with uveal melanomas is 78% (without orbital extension), it is only 27% when orbital extension is associated [130]. This difference in survival, while significant, reflects in part the bias towards epithelioid and large melanomas. None of the 17 patients in Shammas and Blodi's [130] series of uveal melanomas with orbital extension survived five years without exenteration. On the other hand, with early exenteration the tumor recurred in the orbit in about 22% of cases and the five-year survival rate was 87%. With late exenteration the five-year survival rate dropped to 20% [130].

2.5.8 *Location of primary melanoma*. Irrespective of the morphologic appearance of the tumor cells primary melanomas of the iris usually follow a benign course and of all the documented melanomas arising in this part of the eye the overall mortality is about 3%. The 15-year mortality of iris melanomas is 2–5% whereas only 40–50% of persons with melanomas of the posterior uvea survive 15 years [2]. Melanomas originating in the iris rarely metastasize [2, 116, 125, 168, 169] and the literature contains almost 20 fatalities from metastatic iris melanomas [2, 8, 11, 12, 17, 103, 105, 116, 169]. Even following incomplete local resections of iris melanomas the tumor may not recur for many years [7] and in one case the postoperative latent period was 23 years [170]. The more favorable behavior of iris melanomas has been attributed to early detection, the smaller size and the resistance of the thick walled blood vessels of the iris to invasion by neoplastic cells. The degree of tumor vascularity is clearly not critical in this regard, since many iris melanomas contain numerous thin walled vascular channels [8]. Iridectomy for an iris melanoma does not seem to increase the incidence of the metastases [17] and, while epibulbar spread of melanomas in this location has followed this procedure [11], deaths from metastatic melanomas have not been reported [88, 105] despite some follow-ups for more than 20 years [105].

2.5.9 *Glaucoma*. Although not thoroughly investigated glaucoma, or surgical procedures to treat it, may adversely effect the survival of persons with melanomas [111, 171]. In one of the very few studies in which the relationship between glaucoma and survival was considered, not only was the mortality higher when associated with elevated intraocular pressure but the survival time following enucleations was shorter [111]. It is notewothy that three of the 11 documented deaths from iris melanomas occurred in persons who had undergone a glaucoma filtering procedure [11, 172]. Time will tell whether the apparent adverse effect of increased intraocular pressure is a reflection of the malignancy of the melanoma cells, a facilitation for metastatic spread caused by ocular hypertension or whether it merely mirrors the size of the melanoma.

*2.5.10 Other parameters.* An early morphologic study on uveal melanomas drew attention to an abundance of argentophile fibrils (reticulum, reticulin) about and between epithelioid cells [109]. Based on the relative content of argyrophilic fibers as demonstrated by the Wilder reticulum stain the amount of reticulum was classified as heavy, marked, medium, light or absent by Callender et al. [110] who found the mortality to be inversely related to the amount of reticulum. This impression has not stood the test of time and most pathologists agree that the reticulin (now known to represent collagen fibers of a finer diameter than usual) content of uveal melanoma is not of prognostic significance [150, 152]. In a series of small melanomas of the ciliary body and choroid, McLean et al. [150] found the mortality to be almost double if the tumor extended into the optic nerve. The prognosis for men is independent of age, but females below the age of 40 years had a better prognosis than older women in one series [116].

## 2.6 Effect on ocular structures

*2.6.1 Iris.* Melanomas arising in the iris or extending into it from the ciliary body, often distort the pupil and make it irregular in shape. The color of the iris may also be affected by tumors. Diffuse melanomas in the anterior uvea

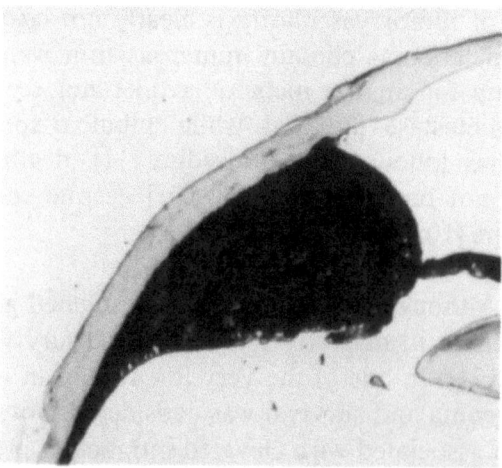

*Figure 14.* The angle of the anterior chamber is occluded by a melanoma originating in the ciliary body. Hematoxylin and eosin, × 6.

frequently cause the affected iris to become darker than the contralateral normal one (hyperchromic heterochromia iridis) [172]. In eyes with choroidal melanomas new vessels frequently form in the iris, especially on its anterior surface, and this so-called rubeosis iridis was detected in about 15% of such eyes in one series [91].

*2.6.2 Anterior chamber angle.* An anterior displacement of the iris by a melanoma in the ciliary body narrows the anterior chamber angle sometimes causing glaucoma. If the iris root, or the pars plicata and of the ciliary body, are displaced backwards by a melanoma of the ciliary body, the anterior chamber of the eye may become deeper than normal (Figures 14, 15).

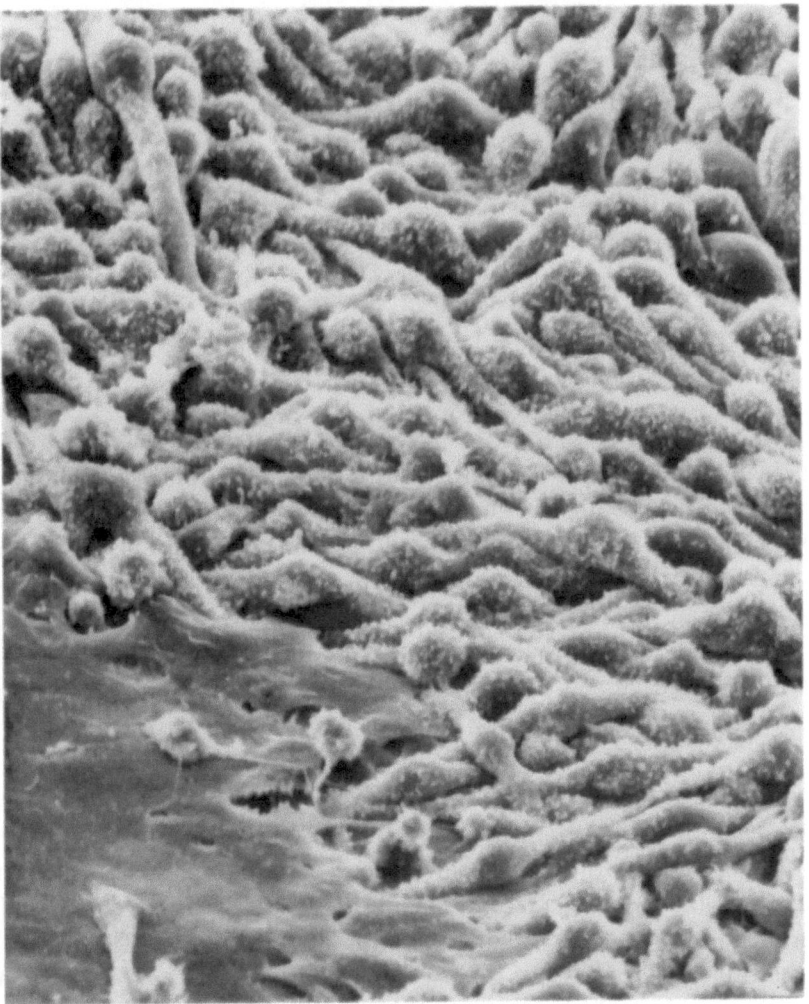

*Figure 15A.* Scanning electron micrograph of melanoma cells within angle of anterior chamber. Reproduced with permission from ref. [171], ×800.

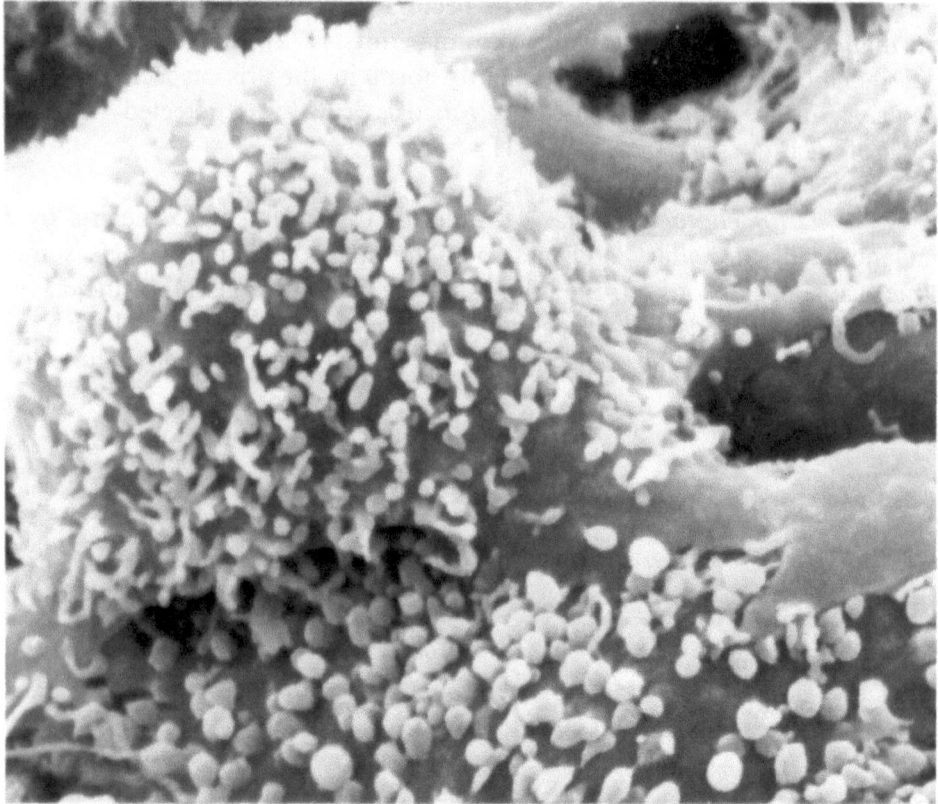

*Figure 15B.* Tumor cell at higher magnification, × 6200.

*2.6.3 Lens.* Melanomas of the iris and ciliary body, and some large choroidal melanomas, frequently encroach on the lens (Figure 16) and may opacify parts, or all, of it [11] (complicated cataract). Melanomas can even displace or sublux the lens when they are in apposition with it.

*2.6.4 Ciliary body.* With melanomas of the ciliary body the outer pigmented epithelium of the ciliary body sometimes separates from its inner nonpigmented epithelium to form an epithelial lined cyst [171, 173].

*2.6.5 Intraocular pressure.* Approximately 20% of eyes with uveal melanomas have glaucoma at the time of clinical presentation [174] and about one-third of eyes with choroidal melanomas are glaucomatous at the time of enucleation [46]. While glaucoma usually develops with large tumors [175], it complicates 14% of eyes with melanomas of the iris [11]. In the latter cases the intraocular pressure rises when such tumors extend into the anterior chamber angle and obstruct a sufficient amount of the trabecular meshwork [88, 171].

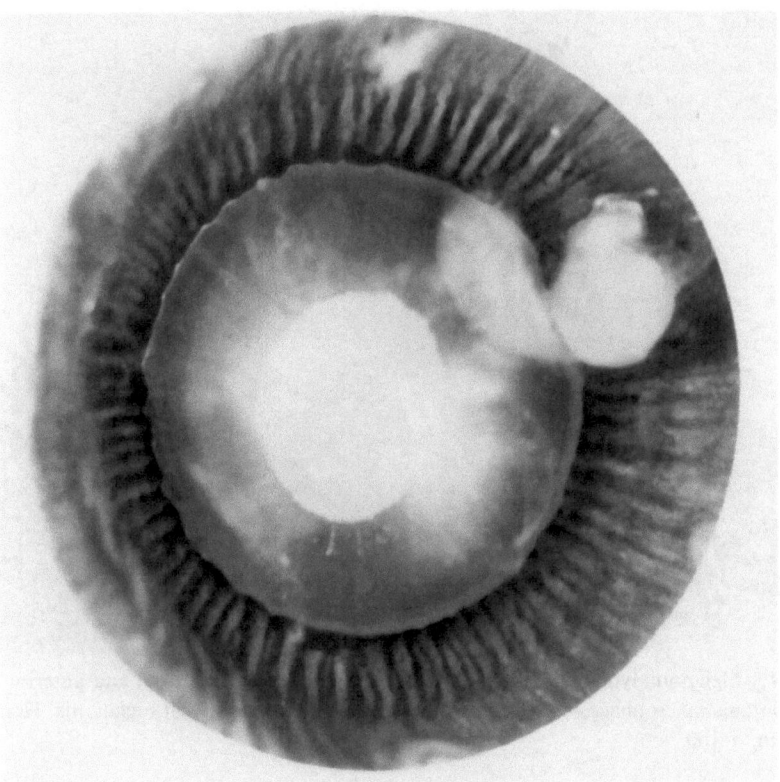

*Figure 16.* View of the crystalline lens and anterior uvea from behind showing melanoma of ciliary body. Reproduced with permission from ref. [171].

Uveal melanomas cause glaucoma by several mechanisms [124, 174, 176]. Often the tumor cells are shed into intraocular cavities and carried into the outflow system where they may occlude the trabecular meshwork and Schlemm's canal. With melanomas of the iris and ciliary body the invasion of these structures can occur by direct extension of the tumor into the angle of the anterior chamber. Melanomas especially of the anterior uvea, sometimes press the iris root against the trabecular meshwork and mechanically obstruct aqueous outflow. Melanin and other cellular debris released by necrotic melanomas becomes phagocytozed by macrophages which may obstruct the trabecular meshwork to produce a unilateral acute open angle glaucoma (melanomalytic glaucoma) [176] (Figure 17). Rubeosis iridis is a common sequel to uveal melanomas and this may lead to peripheral anterior synechiae and glaucoma.

The intraocular pressure in eyes with ciliary body melanomas is sometimes slightly lower than the fellow eye [92, 171, 175] and this pressure differential between the eyes presumably reflects the impaired secretion of aqueous by the abnormal ciliary body.

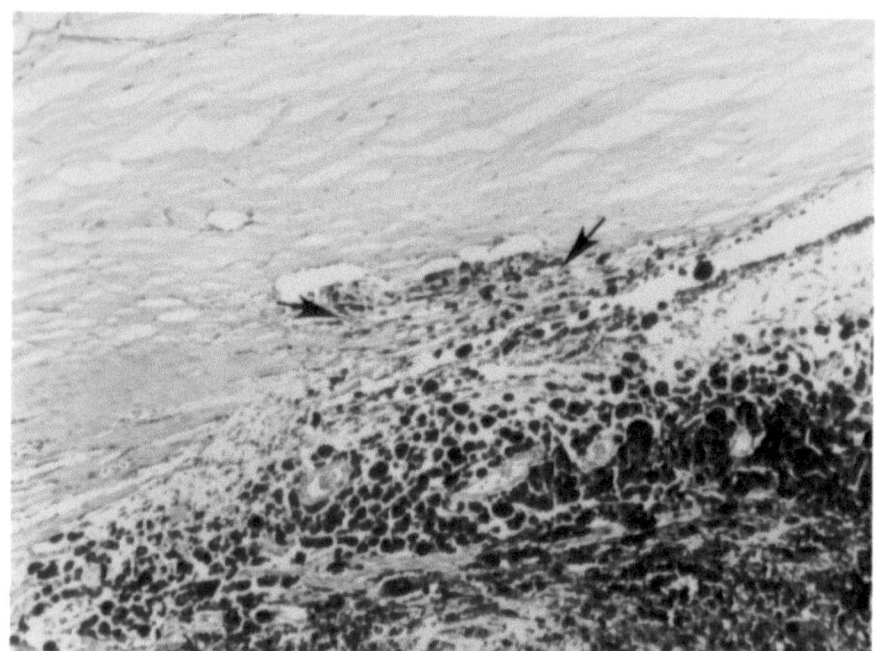

*Figure 17.* Melanomalytic glaucoma. The trabecular meshwork (arrows) and anterior chamber angle contains macrophages with necrotic debris derived from a uveal melanoma. Hematoxylin and eosin, × 100.

*2.6.6 Retina.* In persons with choroidal melanomas a protein rich fluid frequently separates the sensory retina from the retinal pigment epithelium [46, 177, 178], especially adjacent to and immediately over the tumor (Figure 18). This retinal detachment is often clinically significant and about 2 % of eyes with choroidal melanomas undergo surgical treatment for retinal detachment prior to enucleation [179]. Even a flat melanoma of the choroid

*Figure 18.* The sensory retina adjacent to choroidal melanomas frequently becomes detached from the retinal pigment epithelium by a protein-rich exudate. Hematoxylin and eosin, × 100.

may be accompanied by a total retinal detachment [180]. Some retinal detachments with melanomas of the choroid or ciliary body are associated with retinal tears which may be situated over the tumor or some distance from it [179, 181–186]. The sensory retina over choroidal tumors often degenerates and some retinal holes follow cystoid degeneration in the retina overlying the melanoma [181]. Cystoid macular edema sometimes forms in subjects with peripherally located choroidal melanomas [187, 188] and this may account for the presenting visual impairment.

Individual retinal pigment epithelial cells overlying a choroidal melanoma frequently become rounded and enter the subretinal space. Pigment with the histochemical and ultrastructural features of lipofuscin [189–191] sometimes appears in increased amounts within the retinal pigment epithelium overlying a choroidal melanoma, as well as within macrophages, situated within and beneath the overlying sensory retina (Figure 19). The presence of this pigment is of some clinical significance, since it rarely appears over other choroidal lesions, such as nevi, metastatic carcinomas and hemangiomas [192]. Aside from this, retinal pigment epithelial cells sometimes proliferate over malignant choroidal melanomas [193].

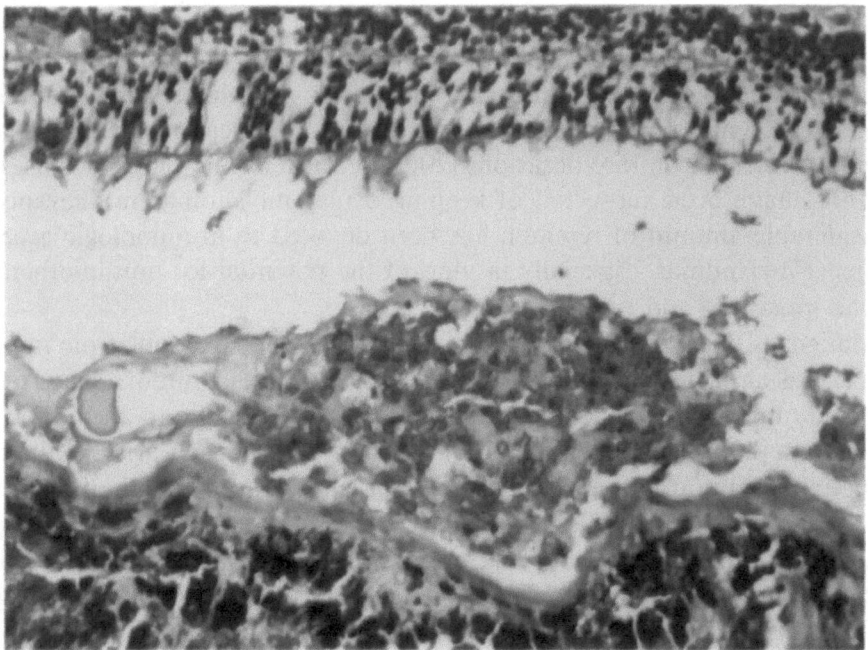

*Figure 19.* A cluster of lipofuscin filled cells is present between a choroidal melanoma and the sensory retina. Hematoxylin and eosin, ×250.

## 2.7 Clinical errors in diagnosis

The deep location within the eye of most uveal melanomas makes them inaccessible to safe biopsy so that ophthalmologists need to make clinical diagnoses of uveal melanomas without the benefit of a tissue diagnosis. It is hence not surprising that errors in clinical judgment sometimes culminate in the enucleation of eyes with benign lesions [194, 195]. The incidence of these errors is lower in teaching hospitals (5.6%) [196] than in series derived from the community at large (20%) [197, 198]. Aside from such unfortunate instances which often result in the unnecessary loss of sight, eyes with malignant melanomas are occasionally not suspected until late in the course of the disease with the result that treatment is delayed. Numerous ocular lesions simulate uveal melanomas clinically and a discussion of these conditions is beyond the scope of this chapter [2, 93, 156, 199–203]. It is partly because of such errors that ophthalmologists have become wary of enucleating eyes with small suspected melanomas without documented evidence of growth.

## 2.8 Immunopathology

Several observations have suggested that immunologic mechanisms are involved in the body's defense against ocular melanomas: (1) orbital or distal metastases often do not become evident until many years after enucleation of eyes with primary uveal melanomas [204], (2) areas of coagulative necrosis frequently occur in the immediate vicinity of blood vessels in uveal melanomas and lymphocytic infiltrates sometimes surround these tumors [205] and (3) spontaneous regressions of uveal melanomas have been documented on rare occasions [206]. Because immunologic defenses of the host have been suspected of keeping ocular melanomas in abeyance a considerable amount of research has been devoted to immunologic aspects of uveal melanomas. especially in view of the potential for immunotherapy in the treatment and prevention of metastases.

Malignant uveal melanomas contain both surface and cytoplasmic tumor-associated antigens [205, 207, 108] and, while different tumors share cytoplasmic tumor antigens, most surface antigens are specific to an individual melanoma [209]. Like melanomas of the skin those which arise in the eye sometimes contain two additional kinds of surface antigens: the first being specific to melanoma cells but shared with other tumors (i.e., histiotype-specific) and the other also being present on non-neoplastic cells of other tissues from several species. Elevated levels of carcinoembryonic antigen (CEA) have been detected in the plasma of some patients with choroidal malignant melanomas [210, 211], but this antigen has not been demonstrated in malignant melanoma cells by immunoperoxidase methods.

IgM and IgG antibodies which react with surface and cytoplasmic antigens of autologous and allogeneic melanoma cells have been demonstrated with indirect immunofluorescent techniques in the serum of some patients with uveal melanomas at the time of primary treatment [205, 207, 212, 213] and the choroidal melanomas may be relatively small [213]. The antibodies bind to and inhibit the growth of autochthonous and possibly allogeneic melanoma cells in vitro [205, 207, 212], are cytotoxic in short term cultures and, in the presence of complement, inhibit the synthesis of ribonucleic acid. The serum from many normal subjects and from persons with benign or malignant pigmented lesions of the uvea also contain low titers of "smooth muscle" antibodies which react with contractile elements of the cytoskeleton in melanoma cells, and other cells [123, 214]. As in some individuals with cutaneous malignant melanomas, melanoma-specific antinucleolar antibodies have been detected in the blood of persons with uveal melanomas [215]. Serum from patients with non-neoplastic eye diseases also appear to contain antibodies which react with (heterophile) antigens in the nucleoli of the melanoma cells.

Tumor-specific cytoplasmic antibodies tend to be absent or present in low titers in cases of uveal melanomas with clinical and histological hallmarks of a poor prognosis. The antibody levels increase after treatment by photocoagulation or radioactive cobalt [216]. Whereas melanoma-specific anticytoplasmic antibodies occasionally occur in low titers in the serum of normal persons, it has been claimed in one yet to be confirmed study that their presence in high concentrations is of both diagnostic and prognostic significance in subjects with uveal melanoma [216]. It is believed that circulating antibodies may play a role in preventing metastases from uveal melanomas but that cell-mediated defense reactions are more important in causing the regression or destruction of tumors [217, 218].

A normal percentage of T-lymphocytes are present in the peripheral blood of patients with uveal melanomas [219], and several functional attributes of these cells have been studied. Cell-mediated immunity in persons with primary localized uveal melanomas remains intact as evidenced by a normal cutaneous response to such antigens as tuberculoprotein (PPD), streptokinase-streptodornase, dermatophytin, as well as mumps and candida antigens. Some subjects with uveal melanomas manifest delayed hypersensitivity to a soluble or surface-membrane, antigen of uveal melanoma after intradermal injection [220], but the reaction is negative in many patients with histologically confirmed uveal melanomas and about 20% of persons with benign or non-neoplastic intraocular lesions also give a positive reaction [220]. The macrophage migration inhibition test has been used as a measure of the degree of cellular immunity in persons with uveal melanomas and a difference has been detected between certain subjects with choroidal melanomas and those with benign nevi, or metastatic carcinoma of the uvea using extracts of malignant uveal melanomas [220, 221]. Extracts of iris do not provoke this response suggesting that it is tumor-specific [221]. Lymphocytes from persons with malignant disease can be stimulated by a basic protein derived from the human brain (encephalitogenic factor) to release a macrophage-slowing factor which reduces mobility of guinea-pig macrophages in an electrical field. Rahi et al. [222] found that following incubation of lymphocytes from subjects with malignant melanomas of the choroid with basic myelin protein a macrophage slowing factor is released [222]. Lymphocytes from normal individuals do not usually give a positive reaction but can. While T-cell sensitization to melanoma-associated antigen is almost undetectable in individuals with intraocular melanomas, an unequivocal lymphoblast transformation response has been elicited in some patients with histologically established orbital spread [223]. Should this yet to be confirmed observation stand the test of time it may permit extraocular spread of uveal melanomas to be detected clinically. The lymphocytes of patients with uveal melanomas sometimes show cytotoxicity to melanoma cells in vitro [224] and produce lymphokines when exposed to extracts of these cells.

## 3   Primary malignant melanomas of eyelid

### 3.1  Types of melanomas

Malignant melanomas are uncommon in the eyelid and account for only 1 % of all malignant neoplasms on this part of the skin. As in other parts of the skin, melanomas of the eyelid can be divided into intraepithelial and invasive types [225–228].

*3.1.1 Lentigo maligna (Hutchinson's freckle, circumscribed precancerous melanosis of Dubreuilh).* Lentigo maligna appears as an uneven variably pigmented macule usually with a diameter of only a few centimeters. Individuals with fair skin that does not tan readily are prone to this lesion which is most frequently found on the face of elderly persons and almost exclusively on exposed surfaces of the body. The eyelids may be involved as they were in two of Hutchinson's original patients [229]. The spreading freckle-like lesions affect women almost three times as often as men and enlarge very slowly over many years, while sites within them often become depigmented [228, 230]. The abnormal skin, which is preceded by severe actinic elastosis, is composed of numerous irregularly arranged pleomorphic melanocytes in the epidermis. After a latent period which ranges from 15 months to 40 years [226, 230], about a third of these intraepithelial melanomas eventually invade the dermis and form a relatively benign type of melanoma known as a lentigo maligna melanoma.

*3.1.2 Superficial spreading melanoma (in situ pagetoid melanoma).* The superficial spreading melanoma begins at a younger age than lentigo maligna and affects middle-aged subjects (Figure 20). While nonexposed skin is usually affected, the eyelid is sometimes the site of this small elevated intraepithelial melanoma (less than 3 cm in diameter). This lesion, which contains large round melanocytes uniformly distributed throughout the epidermis, occasionally becomes invasive within a year. Superficial spreading melanomas account for about 70% of cutaneous melanomas.

*3.1.3 Nodular malignant melanoma.* The nodular malignant melanoma of the skin forms a small blue-black or gray smooth nodule especially in the fifth decade of life. It affects men twice as often as women and while the majority of these melanomas (80%) arise in the absence of an overt underlying lesion the remaining tumors arise from a nevocellular nevus. Large anaplastic cells predominate and involve both the epidermis and the dermis apparently from the outset. This type of melanoma grows more rapidly and invades the dermis more extensively than other varieties of cutaneous melanoma.

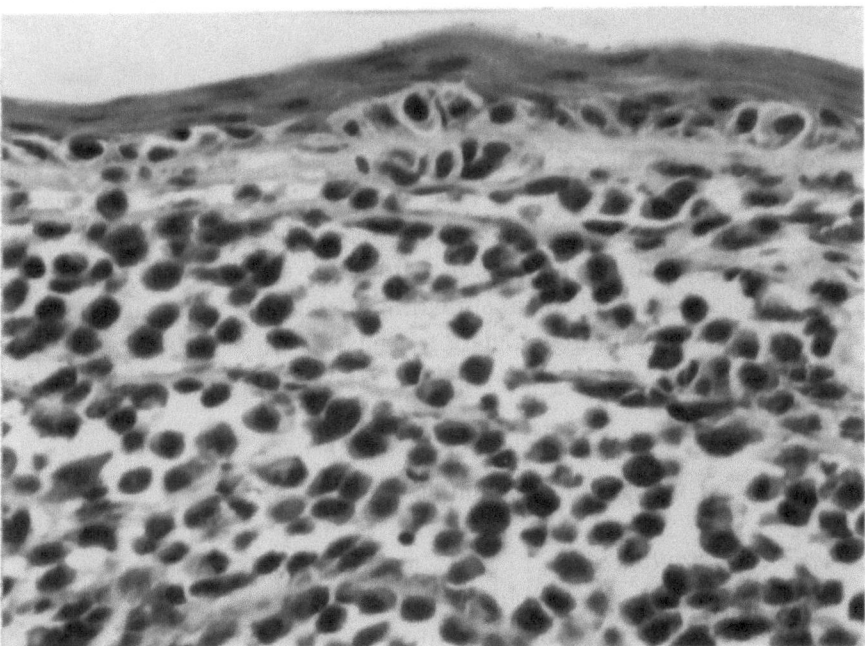

*Figure 20.* Melanoma of eyelid. The basal layer of the epithelium and the adjacent dermis contain pleomorphic rounded neoplastic cells. Hematoxylin and eosin, × 400.

484

Clark's classification of cutaneous melanomas into levels [226] based upon the depth of invasion by the neoplastic cells is applicable to the eyelid [231], but a large series of tumors in this location have not been studied from the viewpoint of this classification. According to Clark's classification primary melanomas of the skin are divided as follows: Level I, Confined to epidermis; level II, Invasion of the papillary dermis; Level III, filling of papillary dermis with abutment on reticular dermis; Level IV, invasion of the reticular dermis and Level V, invasion of the subcutaneous tissues.

## 3.2 Premalignant lesions

Like nevocellular nevi elsewhere in the skin, those of the eyelid are divided into intradermal, junctional and compound types, and variants include the balloon cell nevus and the benign juvenile melanoma. While it is widely believed that some nevi, especially junctional nevi, are premalignant the evidence for this is not good and some authorities believe that there is no formal histogenetic relation between moles and malignant melanomas [232]. Dermal melanocytomas (blue nevi) occasionally arise from melanocytes within the dermis of the eyelid and are usually dome shaped. The variant with deeply pigmented, plump and delicate spindle-shaped melanocytes known as the cellular blue nevus occasionally disseminate to lymph nodes, but death from widespread metastases has not been documented [232].

## 3.3 Prognosis

The prognosis of primary cutaneous melanomas is related to the depth of invasion [74, 230, 233] and to the type of melanoma. Lentigo maligna melanomas rarely metastazize and have a better prognosis than other types of melanoma level for level. They have a five-year survival rate of 89% compared with 68.5% for superficial spreading melanoma which frequently disseminates [226]. The nodular melanoma has the most unfavorable outlook and the five years mortality is 60% [230, 234, 235].

## 4  Conjunctival malignant melanomas

### 4.1 Types of melanomas

Although varying in shape and size, most malignant melanomas of the conjunctiva are flat and pigmented, and the majority are situated at the corneoscleral limbus. As with the skin the conjunctiva appears to spawn different types of melanomas, but, since melanomas of the conjunctiva are uncommon both the clinical features and the biological behavior of these different lesions are still not clearly defined. This is partly because of a confusing literature caused by different investigators classifying conjunctival melanomas in different ways. In a review of 218 ocular melanomas diagnosed at Duke University Medical Center, eight (3.8%) arose in the conjunctiva [82].

In view of histopathologic similarities between the conjunctiva and skin, several investigators have attempted to classify conjunctival melanomas in the same way as cutaneous melanomas [236, 237]. Melanomas comparable to the cutaneous lentigo maligna melanoma, superficial spreading melanoma and nodular melanoma of the skin occur in the conjunctiva [236, 138] (Figure 21).

*4.1.1 Lentigo maligna melanoma.* In conjunctival lentigo maligna melanomas the basal epithelium is hyperpigmented over a wide area with atypical melanocytes interspersed among normal melanocytes. In contrast to the superficial spreading malignant melanoma pagetoid spread is not a feature in the radial growth phase of this tumor.

*4.1.2 Superficial spreading melanoma of conjunctiva.* Like its cutaneous counterpart this form of melanoma contains nests of uniformly atypical

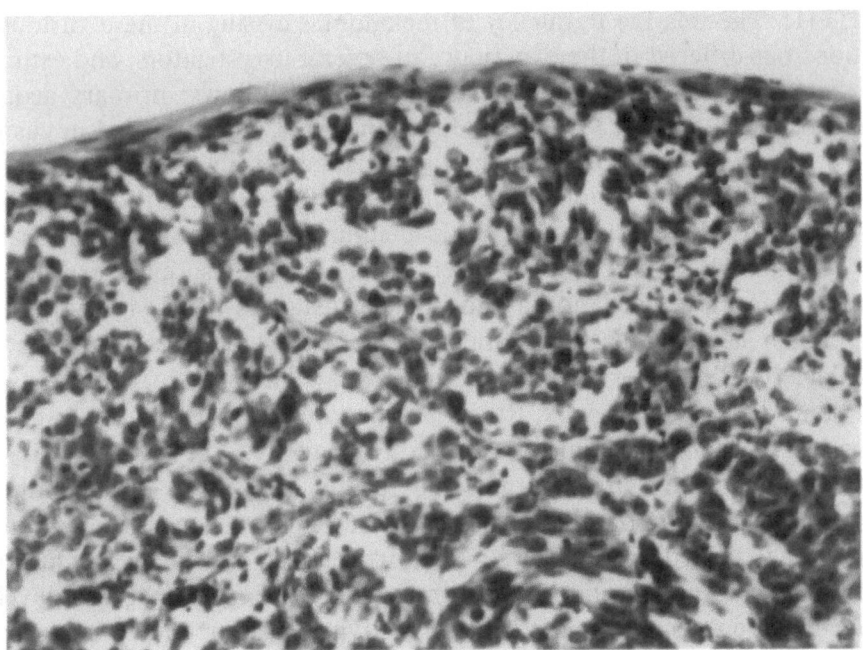

*Figure 21.* Conjunctival melanoma. A myriad of neoplastic cells are present within and beneath the conjunctival epithelium. Hematoxylin and eosin, × 250.

melanocytes associated with pagetoid spread of these cells into the more superficial epithelial layers in the radial growth phase. Invasion beyond the epithelial basement membrane appears early and in multiple sites. Superficial spreading melanoma of the conjunctiva, which is more common than lentigo maligna melanoma, contains multiple foci of darkly pigmented or nonpigmented thickened conjunctiva which are smaller than the foci of lentigo maligna melanoma.

*4.1.3 Nodular conjunctival melanomas.* Localized conjunctival melanomas analogous to the cutaneous nodular melanoma without a preceding or associated intraepithelial radial growth component are uncommon.

## 4.2 Premalignant lesions

While all conjunctival malignant melanomas stem from melanocytes, it has been suggested that some arise from preexisting melanocytic lesions. Some malignant melanomas of the conjunctiva are preceded by an acquired diffuse pigmentation of the conjunctiva (acquired conjunctival melanosis, precancerous melanosis). Localized conjunctival melanomas may also arise from preexisting nevi or from blemish-free conjunctiva ("de novo" melanoma). Melanomas arising from acquired conjunctival melanosis have been referred to as cancerous melanosis [46, 239, 240] and widespread melanoma [241]. The relative frequency of melanomas arising in these various situations has differed in the experience of several investigators, and estimates of the origin of conjunctival melanomas are as follows: primary acquired melanosis (17–50%) [239, 242, 243], a junctional or compound nevus (25–34%) and from normal conjunctival melanocytes in the absence of any apparent antecedent lesion (25–50%) [239, 242, 243]. A difficulty with the aforementioned assessments is that the actual origin in many cases cannot be determined with certainty. Often at the time of surgical excision the tumor is entirely a melanoma and in such instances the designation of the antecedent lesion is based on the clinical history, but this is not entirely reliable, since more or less nonpigmented nevi can spawn melanomas and yet be unsuspected clinically. Rarely a melanoma preceded by acquired conjunctival melanosis has coexisted with a melanocytic nevus [244].

Conjunctival nevi are common and readily subdivided in subepithelial, junctional and compound varieties. They resemble nevocellular nevi in the skin, but frequently contain cysts lined with goblet cells as well as a prominent surrounding lymphocytic infiltrate. A blue nevus sometimes develops from melanocytes within the subconjunctival tissue or underlying sclera.

Discoloration of the conjunctiva has many known causes and infrequently occurs for no apparent reason. Under the latter circumstances the condition is referred to as primary acquired conjunctival melanosis. Several investigators have proposed classifications of pigmented conjunctival lesions and have attempted to correlate the histologic pictures with the clinical behavior [237, 239, 245], but none of these classifications have received universal acceptance. Primary acquired conjunctival melanosis is a relatively uncommon pigmented lesion of the conjunctiva which appears in adulthood most often during the fifth decade of life. The condition affects women slightly more often than men and is characterized by a unilateral diffuse pigmentation of variable extent, which waxes and wanes. It has a prolonged course and, while sometimes remaining stationary, the lesions may enlarge yet remain histologically benign. They may also regress or become frankly malignant. The topic of primary acquired conjunctival melanosis is perplexing for several reasons: (1) the designation includes a variety of different histopathologic entities, (2) its natural history is poorly understood and (3) the nomenclature in the literature is confusing, and often inappropriate. Reese [239, 240, 246] subdivided primary acquired conjunctival melanosis into two varieties: precancerous melanosis (acquired junctional nevus) and cancerous melanosis (superficial melanocarcinoma). Further, he related precancerous melanosis to Hutchinson's melanotic freckle of the skin (now commonly referred to as lentigo maligna). It would appear from the histologic appearance of primary acquired conjunctival melanosis that the condition is heterogeneous. For example. some nonprogressive cases are characterized by increased pigmentation of the basal epithelial cells without increased numbers of basal melanocytes ("benign acquired conjunctival melanosis") [242]. Other cases contain an increased number of atypical melanocytes in the basal epithelium of the conjunctiva and are analagous to lentigo maligna, while further cases seem to represent intraepithelial superficial spreading melanomas of the conjunctiva.

## 4.3 Prognosis

The prognostic significance of several aspects of conjunctival melanomas have been investigated, viz., the underlying condition, the depth of invasion, the type of melanoma, the location of the tumor and the morphology of the tumor cells.

While some investigators have not detected a difference in the survival rates between conjunctival melanomas arising in apparently normal conjunctiva, from lentigo maligna or from a nevus [243], there is evidence that acquired conjunctival melanosis spawns a more ominous melanoma [239, 247]. Of Reese's series of 30 conjunctival melanomas arising in acquired conjunctival melanosis with follow-up periods of five years or longer, 14 (40%) died from metastases of the tumor 3–25 years from the time of onset [239] and the mortality is high regardless of treatment [247]. While some have also accepted the notion that "precancerous and cancerous melanosis" of the conjunctiva are the counterpart of the cutaneous lentigo maligna melanoma (Hutchinson's freckle) [242], this concept is difficult to reconcile with the poor prognosis of "cancerous melanosis", since lentigo maligna melanoma of the skin has a relatively good prognosis. Since many of these conjunctival lesions appear to parallel the behavior of cutaneous superficial spreading melanoma rather than cuteneous lentigo maligna melanoma, Bernardino et al. [244] suggest that "cancerous melanosis" may represent three forms of melanoma with an associated radial growth phase: lentigo maligna melanoma, superficial spreading melanoma and melanoma with unclassified radial growth phase. However, malignant melanomas arising in mucous membranes of the body may not behave like those of the skin [248–250].

Intraepithelial melanomas can eventually become invasive and metastasize and in this regard the localized variety appears to have a better prognosis (five-year and ten-year survivals, 83% and 78% respectively) than the widespread intraepithelial form (five-year and ten-year survivals, 76% and 50% respectively) [243]. Despite the fact that anatomical differences between the conjunctiva and skin makes an application of Clark's classification according to levels of invasion difficult, the depth of invasion is an important prognostic factor of conjunctival melanomas. In their series of 28 invasive conjunctival melanomas on file in the Algernon B. Reese Laboratory of Ophthalmic Pathology, Silvers et al. [237 ] reported that 43% died from the disease despite exenteration or local excision and irradiation (medium survival time being 4.1 years). These authors found that regardless of the extent of surgery, patients with invasion of the substantia propria of 1.5 mm or less survived (but they did not provide the survival time).

Lentigo maligna melanomas of the conjunctiva appear to have a better prognosis than other conjunctival melanomas and all four patients in Bernardino et al.'s [244] series with this type of conjunctival melanoma on whom follow-up data was available were alive and free from disease 8, 8, 16 and 20 years after their lesions were first diagnosed. In a study of ten superficial spreading melanomas of the conjunctiva Bernardino et al. [244] reported a 56% mortality from metastatic melanoma 4–11 years after diagnosis and repeated resections. In contrast to cutaneous nodular melanomas, localized limbal melanomas are reported to have a good prognosis [242, 243]. However, a patient with a nodular melanoma in the caruncle died six months after diagnosis from metastatic disease [246].

Other factors which may have an adverse effect on prognosis include involvement of the fornix and caruncle [237]. As with melanomas in the uvea those of the conjunctiva with a high proportion of epithelioid cells have the worst prognosis, while spindle cell melanomas have a more favorable outcome [243].

## 5 Primary corneal melanomas

The normal cornea lacks melanocytes even in persons of the black races and melanomas of the cornea are rare curiosities [251-254]. In the dark races and in pigmented animals, melanocytes may infiltrate between the epithelial cells [255-257] and such cells are presumably the ones that spawn melanomas on exceptional occasions. Melanomas of the cornea and conjunctiva need to be differentiated from pigmented squamous cell carcinomas [256] which sometimes develop in heavily pigmented individuals.

## 6 Primary orbital melanoma

Very rarely melanomas arise in the orbit in the absence of evidence of a primary tumor elsewhere [57, 58, 258-264]. In some instances the primary orbital melanoma develops in an individual with an underlying disorder of the melanocytic system such as neurocutaneous melanosis (multiple giant hairy nevi, especially when the head is involved), or oculodermal melanosis (nevus of Ota) [57, 58], but in other instances it arises without an apparent underlying abnormality. In the latter cases the melanoma presumably stems from ectopically located melanocytes within the orbit [261, 262]. It is noteworthy that a primary malignant melanoma of the orbit has been documented in a black individual notwithstanding the rarity of melanomas in the Negroid race [259]. Because they are so seldom encountered primary orbital melanomas may be unsuspected and misdiagnosed if a frozen section is performed at the time of surgical excision [258]. Moreover, they need to be distinguished from a cellular blue nevus which may occur within the orbit [263] or be localized to the sclera [202]. Since the orbit lacks lymphatics, melanomas of the orbit do not spread directly to lymph nodes.

## 7 Metastatic melanomas to eye and its adnexa

The vast majority of malignant melanomas found within the orbit are secondary to melanomas of the ciliary body and choroid. Much less commonly orbital melanomas arise in the conjunctiva [243] or are blood-borne metastases from distant primary sites. On rare occasions cutaneous melanomas metastasize to the eye and its adnexa [27, 265-268] and in only 1% of 125 fatal cases of cutaneous melanomas autopsied at Memorial Hospital in New York between 1935-1960 [145] was the eye the site of metastatic melanoma. However, the incidence of ocular metastases clearly depends upon the size of the metastases and the meticulousness with which the eyes are examined. In one series of 15 consecutive fatal cases of malignant melanomas of the

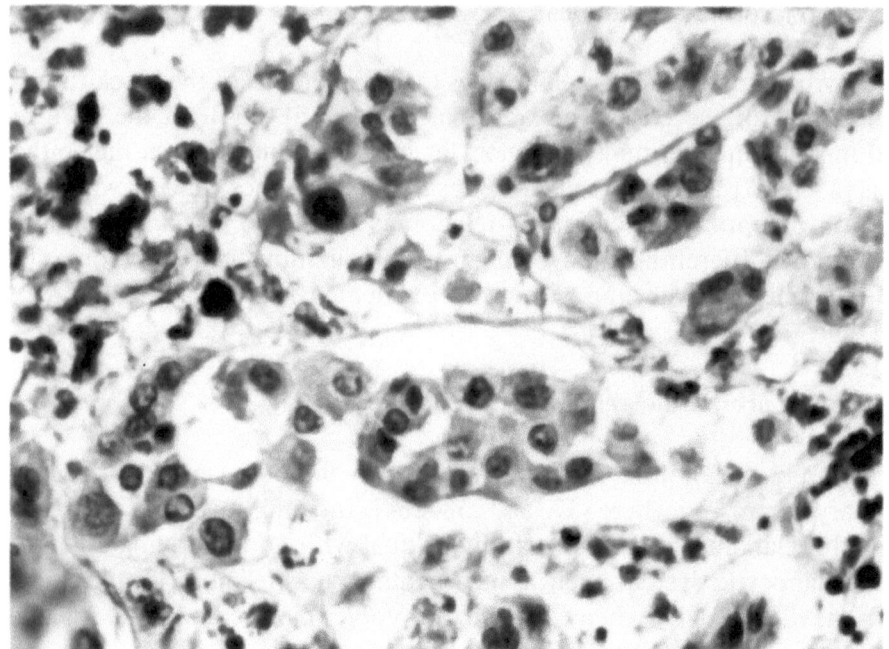

*Figure 22.* Metastatic melanoma in uvea of patient who died from a widely disseminated cutaneous melanoma. Nests of pleomorphic cells are present within the choroid. Hematoxylin and eosin, × 250.

skin asymptomatic microscopic ocular metastases were detected in a third of the patients [265]. Metastatic intraocular melanomas differ from primary uveal melanomas in several ways and there is no difficulty in distinguishing them from each other. Metastatic melanomas are usually small and multiple with little or no pigmentation. The tumor cells are epithelioid in type, and frequently affect the retina as well as the uve, and the lumens, and walls of blood vessels are often involved (Figure 22). The survival following diagnosis of ocular involvement is extremely short (average five months). In one series [253] the mean age was surprisingly younger (36.6 years) than the peak age for both primary uveal and skin melanomas.

## References

1. Scotto J, Fraumeni JF, Jr and Lee JAH: Melanomas of the eye and other noncutaneous sites: epidemiologic aspects. J Natl Cancer Inst 56:489–491, 1976.
2. Jensen OA: Malignant melanomas of the uvea in Denmark, 1943–1952: a clinical histopathological and prognostic study. Acta Ophthalmol Suppl 75:1–220, 1963.
3. Wright CJE: Prognosis in cutaneous and ocular malignant melanoma: a study of 222 cases. J Path Bact 61:507–525, 1949.
4. Kronenberg B: Topography and frequency of complications of uveal sarcoma. Arch Ophthalmol Suppl 20:290–298, 1938.

5. Duke-Elder S and Perkins ES: In: Duke-Elder S (ed), System of Ophthalmology: Diseases of the Uveal Tract, Vol 9, pp 852–854. CV Mosby, St. Louis, 1966.
6. Lawford JB and Collins ET: Sarcoma of the uveal tract, with notes of one-hundred and three cases. R London Ophthalmol Hosp Res 13:104–165, 1890–1893.
7. Ashton N: Primary tumours of the iris. Br J Ophthalmol 48:650–668, 1964.
8. Burki E: Über ein Sarkom der Iris im Sänglingsalter. Ophthalmologica 142:487–499, 1961.
9. Leonard BC, Shields JA and McDonald PR: Malignant melanomas of the uvea in children and young adults. Can J Ophthalmol 10:441–449, 1975.
10. Chaves E and Granville R: Choroidal malignant melanoma in a two-and-one-half-year-old girl. Am J Ophthalmol 74:20–23, 1972.
11. Arentsen JJ and Green WR: Melanoma of the iris: report of 72 cases treated surgically. Ophthalmol Surg 6:23–27, 1975.
12. Apt L: Uveal melanomas in children and adolescents. Int Ophthalmol Clin 2:403–410, 1962.
13. Lerner HA: Malignant melanoma of the iris in children. Arch Ophthalmol 84:754–757, 1970.
14. Paul EV, Parnell BL and Fraker M: Prognosis of malignant melanomas of the choroid and ciliary body. Int Ophthalmol Clin 2:387–402, 1962.
15. Templeton AC: Tumors of the eye and adnexa in Africans of Uganda. Cancer 20:1689–1698, 1967.
16. Oettle AG: Epidemiology of melanomas in South Africa. In: Della Porta G and Muhlbock O (eds) Structure and Control of the Melanocyte, pp 292–308. Springer-Verlag, Berlin, 1966.
17. Rones B and Zimmerman LE: The prognosis of primary tumors of the iris treated by iridectomy. Arch Ophthalmol 60:193–205, 1958.
18. Cummingham ER: Ocular tumours of West China: a statistical and clinical study. Trans Can Ophthalmol Soc 5:102–121, 1952.
19. Takahashi K, Hattori H, Ieb QS, Nagayama R and Kato T: Statistical observation on ocular tumors. Rinsho Ganka 23:295–300, 1969 (in Japanese).
20. Parsons JH: Pathology of the Eye, Vol 2, p 518. Hodder & Stoughton, London, 1905.
21. Hogan M: Melanomas of the uvea and optic nerve: clinical aspects, management and prognosis. In: Highlight of Ophthalmology, Vol 6, No 2, pp 146–166. Pan American Institute Ophthalmology, Panama, 1963.
22. Smolin G: Malignant change of a benign melanoma. Am J Ophthalmol 61:174–177, 1966.
23. Font RL, Spaulding AG and Zimmerman LE: Diffuse malignant melanoma of the uveal tract: a clinicopathologic report of 54 cases. Trans Am Acad Ophthalmol Otolaryngol 72:877–895, 1968.
24. Naumann G, Yanoff M and Zimmerman LE: Histogenesis of malignant melanomas of the uvea. I: histopathologic characteristics of nevi of choroid and ciliary body. Arch Ophthalmol 76:784–796, 1966.
25. Yanoff M and Zimmerman LE: Histogenesis of malignant melanoma of the uvea. II: relationship of uveal nevi to malignant melanoma. Cancer 20:493–507, 1967.
26. Yanoff M and Zimmerman LE: Histogenesis of malignant melanomas of the uvea. III: the relationship of congenital ocular melanocytosis and neurofibromatosis to uveal melanomas. Arch Ophthalmol 77:331–336, 1967.
27. Albert DM, Gaasterland DE, Caldwell JBH, Howard RO and Zimmerman LE: Bilateral metastatic choroidal melanoma, nevi and cavernous degeneration. Arch Ophthalmol 87:39–47, 1972.
28. Albert DM, Lahav M, Packer S and Yimoyines D: Histogenesis of malignant melanomas of the uvea: occurrence of nevus-like structures in experimental choroidal tumors. Arch Ophthalmol 92:318–323, 1974.

29. Ganley JP and Comstock GW: Benign nevi and malignant melanomas of the choroid. Am J Ophthalmol 76:19–25, 1973.

30. Hale PN, Allen RA and Straatsma BR: Benign melanomas (nevi) of the choroid and ciliary body. Arch Ophthalmol 74:532–538, 1965.

31. Naumann G: Pigmentierte Naevi der Aderhaut und des Ciliarkörpers. Fortschr Augenheilkd 23:187–272, 1970.

32. Shields JA: Melanocytoma of optic nerve head: a review. Int Ophthalmol 1:31-37, 1978.

33. Zimmerman LE: Melanocytes, melanocytic nevi and melanocytomas. Invest Ophthalmol 4:11–41, 1965.

34. Zimmerman LE and Garron LK: Melanocytoma of the optic disc. Int Ophthalmol Clin 2:431–440, 1962.

35. Bowers JF: Melanocytoma of the ciliary body. Arch Ophthalmol 71:649–652, 1964.

36. Howard GM and Forrest AW: Incidence and location of melanocytomas. Arch Ophthalmol 77:61–66, 1967.

37. Scheie HG and Yanoff M: Pseudomelanoma of the ciliary body. Arch Ophthalmol 77:81–83, 1967.

38. Shields JA and Font RL: Melanocytoma of the choroid clinically simulating a malignant melanoma. Arch Ophthalmol 87:396–400, 1972.

39. Barker-Griffith AE, McDonald PR and Green WR: Malignant melanoma arising in a choroidal magnacellular nevus (melanocytoma). Can J Ophthalmol 11:140–146, 1976.

40. Thomas CI and Purnell EW: Ocular melanocytoma. Am J Ophthalmol 67:79–86, 1969.

41. Roth AM: Malignant change in melanocytomas of the uveal tract. Surv Ophthalmol 22:404–412, 1976.

42. Michelson JB and Shields JA: Relationship of iris nevi to malignant melanoma of the uvea. Am J Ophthalmol 83:694–696, 1977.

43. Reese AB: Pigment freckles of the iris (benign melanomas): their significance in relation to malignant melanoma of the uvea. Am J Ophthalmol 27:217–226, 1944.

44. Wilder HC: Relationship of pigment cell clusters in the iris to malignant melanomas of the uveal tract. In: Miner RW (ed) The Biology of Melanomas, Vol 4, pp 137–142. Special publications of the New York Academy of Science, 1948.

45. Coats G: Unilateral diffuse melanosis of the uvea, with small elevations on the surface of the iris. Trans Ophthalmol Soc U K 32:165–171, 1912.

46. Reese AB: Tumors of the Eye, 3rd ed, pp 208–209. Harper & Row, Hagerstown, 1976.

47. Reese AB: Melanosis oculi: a case with microscopic findings. Am J Ophthalmol 8:865–870, 1925.

48. Blodi FC: Ocular melanocytosis and melanoma. Am J Ophthalmol 80:389–395, 1975.

49. Francois J: La melanose congenitale et benign de l'oeil. Arch Ophtalmol Paris 51:689–718, 1934.

50. Albert DM and Scheie HG: Nevus of Ota with malignant melanoma of the choroid. Arch Ophthalmol 69:774–777, 1963.

51. Font RL, Reynolds AM, Jr and Zimmerman LE: Diffuse malignant melanoma of the iris in the nevus of Ota. Arch Ophthalmol 77:513–518, 1967.

52. Frezzotti R, Guerra R, Dragoni GP and Bonanni P: Malignant melanoma of the choroid in a case of nevus of Ota. Br J Ophthalmol 52:922–924, 1968.

53. Halasa A: Malignant melanoma in a case of bilateral nevus of Ota. Arch Ophthalmol 84:176–178, 1970.

54. Roy PE and Schaeffer EM: Nevus of Ota and choroidal melanoma. Surv Ophthalmol 12:130–134, 1967.

55. Yamamoto T: Malignant melanoma of the choroid in the nevus of Ota. Ophthalmologica 159:1–10, 1969.

56. Sabates FN and Yamashita T: Congenital melanosis oculi: complicated by two independent malignant melanomas of the choroid. Arch Ophthalmol 77:801–803, 1967.

57. Hagler W and Brown C: Malignant melanoma of the orbit arising in a nevus of Ota. Trans Am Acad Ophthalmol Otolaryngol 70:817–822, 1966.

58. Jay B: Malignant melanoma of the orbit in a case of oculodermal melanosis (naevus of Ota). Br J Ophthalmol 49:359-363, 1965.

59. Bowen SF, Jr, Brady H and Jones VL: Malignant melanoma of eye occurring in two successive generations. Arch Ophthalmol 71:805–806, 1964.

60. Davenport RC: A family history of choroidal sarcoma. Br J Ophthalmol 11:443–445, 1927.

61. Duke-Elder WS: Textbook of Ophthalmology, Vol 3, pp 2478-2497. CV Mosby, St. Louis, 1941.

62. Lynch HT, Anderson DW and Krush AJ: Heredity and intraocular malignant melanoma. Cancer 21:119-125, 1968.

63. Tasman W: Familial intraocular melanoma. Trans Am Acad Ophthalmol Otolaryngol 74:955-958, 1970.

64. Clark WH, Reimer RR, Greene M, Ainsworth AM and Mastrangelo MJ: Origin of familial malignant melanomas from heritable melanocytic lesions. The B-K mole syndrome. Arch Dermatol 114:732–738, 1978.

65. Bellet RE, Shields JA, Soll DB and Bernardino EA: Primary choroidal and cutaneous melanomas occurring in a patient with the B-K mole syndrome phenotype. Am J Ophthalmol 89:567–570, 1980.

66. Rodriguez-Sains RS, Abramson DH and Rubman RH: B-K mole syndrome: cutaneous and ocular malignant melanoma. Invest Ophthalmol 19 (Suppl):108, 1980.

67. Greer CG: Congenital melanoma of the anterior uvea. Arch Ophthalmol 76:77–78, 1966.

68. Gartner S: Malignant melanoma of the choroid and von Recklinghausen's disease. Am J Ophthalmol 23:73–78, 1940.

69. Nordmann J and Brini A: Von Recklinghausen's disease and melanoma of the uvea. Br J Ophthalmol 54:641–648, 1970.

70. Strachov VP and Shepkalova VM: Von Recklinghausen's disease, neurinoma of the right orbit and melanosarcoma of the left choroid. Vestn Oftalmol 18:12–16, 1941.

71. Szekler R: Ein Uvealsarkom bei einem Mitglied einer Familie mit Reckinghausenscher Krankheit. Ophthalmologica Basel 126:248-251, 1953.

72. Schottenfeld D: The epidemiology of multiple primary cancers. CA Cancer J Clin 27:233–240, 1977.

73. Del Regato JA and Spjut HJ: Cancer: Diagnosis, Treatment and Prognosis, p 59. CV Mosby, St. Louis, 1977.

74. Asbury MK and Vail D: Multiple primary malignant neoplasms: report of a case of malignant melanoma of the choroid and glioblastoma multiforme of the right cerebral hemisphere. Am J Ophthalmol 48:650–668, 1964.

75. Nadbath RP and Bullwinkel HG: Coexistence of intraocular melanoma and lymphatic leukemia. Arch Ophthalmol 48:349-351, 1952.

76. Wiesinger H, Phipps GW and Guerry D: Bilateral melanoma of the choroid associated with leukemia and meningioma. Arch Ophthalmol 62:889-893, 1959.

77. Augsburger JJ, Shields JA, Mastrangelo MJ and Frank PE: Diffuse primary malignant melanoma after prior primary cutaneous malignant melanoma. Arch Ophthalmol 98: 1261-1264, 1980.

78. Nover A: Über das Vorkommen multipler maligner Primärtumoren. Graefes Arch Ophthalmol 157:237–259, 1956.

79. Henkind P and Roth MS: Breast carcinoma and concurrent uveal melanoma. Am J Ophthalmol 71:198-203, 1971.

80. Algan B, Peyresblanques J and Reny A: Les tumeurs primitives multiples a localisation ophtalmologique. Arch Ophtalmol Paris 25:705–722, 1965.
81. Morgan SS, Heidenry R and Bowen SF, Jr: Malignant melanoma of the iris and ciliary body as a third primary malignancy. Am J Ophthalmol 76:26–29, 1973.
82. Klintworth GK: Unpublished observations.
83. Haukulin T, Teppo L and Saxon E: Cancer of the eye. A review of trends and differentials. WHO Stat Q 31:143–158, 1978.
84. Kopf AW, Bart RS, Rodriquez-Sains RS and Ackerman AB: Malignant Melanoma, Masson, New York, 1979.
85. Albert DM, Puliafito CA, Fulton AB, Robinson NL, Zakov ZN, Dryja TP, Smith AB, Egan E and Leffingwell SS: Choroidal melanoma in chemical workers. Am J Ophthalmol 89:323–337, 1980.
86. Benson WR: Intraocular tumor after ethionine and N-2-fluorenylacetamide. Arch Pathol 73:404–406, 1962.
87. Taylor GN, Dougherty TF, Mays CW, Lloyd RD, Atherton DR and Jee WSS: Radium-induced eye melanomas in dogs. Radiat Res 51:361–373, 1972.
88. Makley TA: Management of melanomas of the anterior segment. Surv Ophthalmol 19:135–153, 1974.
89. Baghdassarian SA and Spencer WH: Pseudoangioma of the iris: its association with melanoma. Arch Ophthalmol 82:69–71, 1969.
90. Hamburg A: Iris melanoma with vascular proliferation simulating a hemangioma. Arch Ophthalmol 82:72–76, 1969.
91. Cappin JM: Malignant melanoma and rubeosis iridis: histopathological and statistical study. Br J Ophthalmol 57:815–824, 1973.
92. Foos RY, Hull SN and Straatsma BR: Early diagnosis of ciliary body melanomas. Arch Ophthalmol 81:336–344, 1969.
93. Reese AB: The differential diagnosis of malignant melanoma of the choroid. Arch Ophthalmol 58:477–482, 1957.
94. Bietti G and Vozza R: Melanoblastoma bilaterale della choroide. Clin Ocul 12:52–61, 1968.
95. Buschmann W and Goder G: Das doppelseitige maligne Melanoblastom der Aderhaut. Graefes Arch Ophthalmol 167:225–238, 1964.
96. Shammas HF and Watzke RC: Bilateral choroidal melanomas: case report and incidence. Arch Ophthalmol 95:617–623, 1977.
97. Tade AA: Bilateral primary melanoblastoma of the choroid. Vestn Oftalmol 4:30–35, 1960 (in Russian).
98. Uliesinger H, Phipps GW and Guerry D: Bilateral melanoma of the choroid associated with leukemia and meningioma. Arch Ophthalmol 62:889–893, 1959.
99. Diamond S, Borley WE and Miller WW: Partial iridocyclectomy for chamber angle tumors. Am J Ophthalmol 57:88–94, 1964.
100. Volcker HE and Naumann GOH: Multicentric primary malignant melanomas of the choroid: two separate malignant melanomas of the choroid and two uveal naevi in one eye. Br J Ophthalmol 62:408–413, 1978.
101. Tade AA: Bilateral primary melanoblastoma of the choroid. Vestn Oftalmol 4:30, 1960 (Excerpta Medica XII, 16:957, 1962).
102. Lubin JR, Gragoudas ES, Albert DM and Weichselbaum RR: Bilateral malignant choroidal melanomas. Int Ophthalmol Clin 20(2):103–115, 1980.
103. Cleasby GW: Malignant melanoma of the iris. Arch Ophthalmol 60:403–417, 1958.
104. Reese AB, Mund ML and Iwamoto T: Tapioca melanoma of the iris. Part I: clinical and light microscopy studies. Am J Ophthalmol 74:840–850, 1972.
105. Reese AB and Howard EM: Flat uveal melanomas. Am J Ophthalmol 64:1021–1028, 1967.

106. Spaulding AG, Green WR and Font RL: Ring-shaped limbal tumor, secondary to unrecognized diffuse malignant melanoma of the uvea. Arch Ophthalmol 77:76–80, 1967.

107. Gass JDM: Hemorrhage into vitreous, a presenting manifestation of malignant melanoma of choroid. Arch Ophthalmol 69:778–779, 1963.

108. Kurz GH and Zimmerman LE: Spontaneous hyphema and acute glaucoma as initial signs of recurrent iris melanoma. Arch Ophthalmol 69:581–582, 1963.

109. Callender GR: Malignant melanotic tumors of the eye: a study of histologic types in 111 cases. Trans Am Acad Otolaryngol 36:131–142, 1931.

110. Callender GR, Wilder HC and Ash JE: Five hundred melanomas of the choroid and ciliary body followed five years or longer. Am J Ophthalmol 25:962–967, 1942.

111. MacRae A: Prognosis in malignant melanoma of choroid and ciliary body. Trans Ophthalmol Soc UK 73:3–30, 1953.

112. Riley FC: Balloon cell melanoma of the choroid. Arch Ophthalmol 92:131–133, 1974.

113. Rodrigues MM and Shields JA: Malignant melanoma of the choroid with balloon cells. A clinicopathologic study of three cases. Can J Ophthalmol 11:208–216, 1976.

114. Gass JDM: Problems in the differential diagnosis of choroidal nevi and malignant melanomas. Am J Ophthalmol 83:299–323, 1977.

115. McLean IW, Zimmerman LE and Evans RM: Reappraisal of Callender's spindle-A type of melanoma of choroid and ciliary body. Am J Ophthalmol 86:557–564, 1978.

116. Jensen OA: Malignant melanomas of the human uvea: recent follow-up of cases in Denmark, 1943–1952. Acta Ophthalmol 48:1113–1128, 1970.

117. Iwamoto T, Reese AB and Mund ML: Tapioca melanoma of the iris. Part 2: electron microscopy of the melanoma cells compared with normal iris melanocytes. Am J Ophthalmol 74:851–861, 1972.

118. Berard-Badier M and Cesarini JP: Melanomas malius de l'uvée: étude anatomopathologique et ultrastructurale. Ann Ocul 204:1244–1245, 1971.

119. Bierring F and Jensen OA: Electron microscopy of melanosomes of the human uveal tract: the ultrastructure of four malignant melanomas of the mixed cell type. Acta Ophthalmol 42:665–671, 1964.

120. Iwamoto T, Jones IS and Howard GM: Ultrastructural comparison of spindle-A, spindle-B, and epithelioid cells in uveal malignant melanomas. Invest Ophthalmol 11:873–889, 1972.

121. Kroll AJ and Kuwabara T: Electron microscopy of uveal melanoma: a comparison of spindle and epithehoid cells. Arch Ophthalmol 73:378–386, 1965.

122. Jensen OA and Povlsen A: Melanomas of the choroid. In: Johannessen JV (ed) Electron Microscopy in Human Medicine, Vol 6, pp 346–368. McGraw Hill, New York, 1979.

123. Rahi AHS, Garner A and Malaty AHA: Contractile protein antigens in the cells of malignant melanoma of the choroid and their diagnostic significance. Br J Ophthalmol 62:394–401, 1978.

124. Hopkins RE and Carriker FR: Malignant melanomas of the ciliary body. Am J Ophthalmol 45:835–843, 1958.

125. Hogan MJ: Clinical aspects, management and prognosis of melanomas of the uvea and optic nerve. In: Boniuk M (ed) Ocular and Adnexal Tumors: New and Controversial Aspects, pp 203–302. CV Mosby, St. Louis, 1964.

126. Samuels SL and Payne BF: Malignant melanoma of the iris: mode of extension and dissemination. Am J Ophthalmol 55:629–631, 1963.

127. Starr HJ and Zimmerman LE: Extrascleral extension and orbital recurrence of malignant melanomas of the choroid and ciliary body. Int Ophthalmol Clin 2:369–385, 1962.

128. Byers WGM and MacMillan JA: Treatment of sarcoma of the uveal tract. Arch Ophthalmol 14:967–973, 1935.

129. Pawel E: Beitrag zur Lehre von dem Choroidealsarkom. Graefes Arch Ophthalmol 49:71–124, 1900.

130. Shammas HF and Blodi FC: Orbital extension of choroidal and ciliary body melanomas. Arch Ophthalmol 95:2002-2005, 1977.
131. Spencer WH: Optic nerve extension of intraocular neoplasms. Am J Ophthalmol 80:465-471, 1975.
132. Shammas HF and Blodi FC: Peripapillary choroidal melanomas: extension along the optic nerve and its sheaths. Arch Ophthalmol 96:440-445, 1978.
133. Spencer WH and Iverson HA: Diffuse melanoma of the iris, with extrabulbar extension via the optic nerve. Surv Ophthalmol 10:365-371, 1965.
134. Zimmerman LE, McLean IW and Foster WD: Does enucleation of the eye containing a malignant melanoma prevent or accelerate the dissemination of tumor cells? An unanswered question. In: Jakobiec FA (ed) Ocular and Adnexal Tumors, pp 31-38. Aesculapius, Birmingham, 1978.
135. Seigel D, Myers M, Ferris F, III and Steinhorn SC: Survival rates after enucleation of eyes with malignant melanoma. Am J Ophthalmol 87:761-765, 1979.
136. Zimmerman LE and McLean IW: Metastatic disease from untreated uveal melanomas. Am J Ophthalmol 88:524-534, 1979.
137. Morton JJ and Morton JH: Cancer as a chronic disease. Ann Surg 137:683-685, 1953.
138. Einhorn LH, Burgess MA and Gottlieb JA: Metastatic patterns of choroidal melanoma. Cancer 34:1001-1004, 1974.
139. Berd D, Mastrangelo MJ and Bellet RF: Metastatic uveal melanoma. In: Clark WH, Jr, Goldman LI and Mastrangelo MJ (eds) Human Malignant Melanoma, pp 489-496. Grune & Stratton, New York, 1979.
140. Char DH: Metastatic choroidal melanoma. Am J Ophthalmol 86:76-80, 1978.
141. Chopra JS and Chander K: Bilateral breast metastases from malignant melanoma of the eye. Aust N Z J Surg 42:183-185, 1972.
142. Velhagen C: Ueber den Befund von zwei Choroidealsarkomen in einem Augapfel. Klin Monatsbl Augenheilkd 64:252-255, 1920.
143. Foster J, Henderson W, Cowie JW and Harriman DSF: Choroidal sarcoma with a metastasis in the opposite orbit. Br J Ophthalmol 41:42-47, 1957.
144. Einhorn LH, Burgess MA, Vallejos C, Bodey GP, Sr, Gutterman J, Mavligit G, Hersh EM, Luce JK, Frei E, III, Freireich EJ and Gottlieb JA: Prognostic correlations and response to treatment in advanced metastatic malignant melanoma. Cancer Res 34:1995-2004, 1974.
145. Das Gupta T and Brasfield R: Metastatic melanoma: a clinicopathological study. Cancer 17:1323-1339, 1964.
146. Patel JK, Didolkar MS, Pickren JW and Moore RH: Metastatic pattern of malignant melanoma: a study of 216 autopsy cases. Am J Surg 135:807-810, 1978.
147. Meyer JE: Radiographic evaluation of metastatic melanoma. Cancer 42:127-132, 1978.
148. Nathanson L, Hall TC and Farber S: Biological aspects of human malignant melanoma. Cancer 20:650-655, 1967.
149. Zimmerman LE and McLean IW: A comparison of progress in the management of retinoblastomas and uveal melanomas. In: Nicholson DH (ed) Ocular Pathology Update, pp 191-212. Masson, New York, 1980.
150. McLean IW, Foster WD and Zimmerman LE: Prognostic factors in small malignant melanomas of choroid and ciliary body. Arch Ophthalmol 95:48-58, 1977.
151. Warren RM: Prognosis of malignant melanomas of the choroid and ciliary body. In: Blodi FC (ed) Current Concepts in Ophthalmology, Vol 4, pp 158-166. CV Mosby, St.Louis, 1974.
152. Packard RBS: Pattern of mortality in choroidal malignant melanoma. Br J Ophthalmol 64:565-575, 1980.
153. Shammas HF and Blodi FC: Prognostic factors in choroidal and ciliary body melanomas. Arch Ophthalmol 95:63-69, 1977.

154. Davidorf FH and Lang JR: The natural history of malignant melanoma of the choroid: small vs. large tumors. Trans Am Acad Ophthalmol Otolaryngol 79:310–320, 1975.

155. Raivio I: Uveal melanoma in Finland: an epidemiological, clinical, histological and prognostic study. Acta Ophthalmol Suppl 133:1–64, 1977.

156. Canny CLB, Shields JA and Kay ML: Clinically stationary choroidal melanoma with extraocular extension. Arch Ophthalmol 96:436–439, 1978.

157. Flocks M, Gerende JH and Zimmerman LE: The size and shape of malignant melanomas of the choroid and ciliary body in relation to prognosis and histologic characteristics: a statistical study of 210 tumors. Trans Am Acad Ophthalmol Otolaryngol 59:740–758, 1955.

158. Benjamin B, Cumings JN, Goldsmith AJB and Sorsby A: Prognosis in uveal melanoma. Br J Ophthalmol 32:729–738, 1948.

159. Burns RP, Fraunfelder FT and Klass AM: A laboratory evaluation of enucleation in treatment of intraocular malignant melanoma. Arch Ophthalmol 67:490–500, 1962.

160. Zimmerman LE, McLean IW and Foster WD: Does enucleation of the eye containing a malignant melanoma prevent or accelerate the dissemination of tumour cells? Br J Ophthalmol 62:420–425, 1978.

161. Zimmerman LE: Bowman lecture: uveal melanoma. Trans Ophthalmol Soc U K, 1980.

162. McLean IW, Foster WD, Zimmerman LE and Martin DG: Inferred natural history of uveal melanoma. Invest Ophthalmol Vis Sci 19:760–770, 1980.

163. Westerveld-Brandon ER and Zeeman WPC: The prognosis of melanoblastoma of the choroid. Ophthalmologica 134:20–29, 1957.

164. Gass JDM: Changing concepts of natural course and management of uveal melanomas. In: Nicholson D (ed) Ocular Pathology Update, pp 227–234. Masson, New York, 1980.

165. Manschot WA and Peperzeel HA: Choroidal melanoma—enucleation or observation? A new approach. Arch Ophthalmol 98:71–77, 1980.

166. Stanford GB and Reese AB: Malignant cells in the blood of eye patients. Trans Am Acad Ophthalmol Otolaryngol 75:102–109, 1971.

167. Fraunfelder FT, Boozman FW, Wilson RS and Thomas AH: No-touch technique for intraocular malignant melanomas. Arch Ophthalmol 95:1616–1620, 1977.

168. Zakka KA, Foos RY and Sulit H: Metastatic tapioca iris melanoma. Br J Ophthalmol 63:744–748, 1979.

169. Sunba MSN, Rahi AHS and Morgan G: Tumors of the anterior uvea. I. metastasizing malignant melanoma of the iris. Arch Ophthalmol 98:82–85, 1980.

170. Freyler H: Malignes Melanom der Iris: 23 Jahre nach unvollständiger Entfernung des Tumors. Klin Monatsbl Augenheilkd 166:704–709, 1975.

171. Shields MB and Klintworth GK: Anterior uveal melanomas and intraocular pressure. Ophthalmology 87:503–517, 1980.

172. Rones B and Zimmerman LE: The production of heterochromia and glaucoma by diffuse malignant melanoma of the iris. Trans Am Acad Ophthalmol Otolaryngol 61:447–463, 1957.

173. Shaw H: Melanoma of ciliary body. Am J Ophthalmol 38:104–105, 1954.

174. Yanoff M: Glaucoma mechanisms in ocular malignant melanomas. Am J Ophthalmol 70:898–904, 1970.

175. Dunnington JH: Intraocular tension in cases of sarcoma of the choroid and ciliary body. Arch Ophthalmol 20:359–363, 1938.

176. Yanoff M and Scheie HG: Melanomalytic glaucoma: report of a case. Arch Ophthalmol 84:471–473, 1970.

177. Lincoff H and Kreissig I: Patterns of non-rhegmatogenous elevation of the retina. Br J Ophthalmol 58:899–906, 1974.

178. Rones B and Linger HT: Early malignant melanoma of the choroid. Am J Ophthalmol 38:163–170, 1954.

179. Boniuk M and Zimmerman LE: Occurrence and behavior of choroidal melanomas in eyes subjected to operations for retinal detachment. Trans Am Acad Ophthalmol Otolaryngol 66:642–658, 1962.

180. Kolb H and Vollmer F: Beitrag zum flachenhaften malignen Melanom der Choroiidea. Graefes Arch Ophthalmol 191:45–52, 1974.

181. Berson E, Bigger JF and Smith ME: Malignant melanoma, retinal hole and retinal detachment. Arch Ophthalmol 77:223–225, 1967.

182. Bierman EO: Retinal tears associated with tumors. Am J Ophthalmol 46:74–75, 1958.

183. Manschot WA: Ring melanoma. Arch Ophthalmol 71:625–632, 1964.

184. Manschot WA: Retinal hole in a case of choroidal melanoma. Arch Ophthalmol 73:666–668, 1965.

185. McGraw JL: Malignant melanoma associated with retinal hole. Arch Ophthalmol 46:666–667, 1951.

186. Morgan OG: Some problems arising in a case of malignant melanoma of the choroid. Trans Ophthalmol Soc U K 76:649–657, 1956.

187. Browstein S, Orton R and Jackson WB: Cystoid macular edema with equatorial choroidal melanoma. Arch Ophthalmol 96:2105–2107, 1978.

188. Newsom WA, Hood CI, Horwitz JA, Fine SL and Sewell JH: Cystoid macular edema: histopathologic and angiographic correlations. Trans Am Acad Ophthalmol Otolaryngol 76:1005–1009, 1972.

189. Font RL, Zimmerman LE and Armaly MF: The nature of the orange pigment over a choroidal melanoma: histochemical and electron microscopic observations. Arch Ophthalmol 91:359–362, 1974.

190. Wallow IHL and Tso MOM: Proliferation of the retinal pigment epithelium over malignant choroidal tumors: a light and electron microscopic study. Am J Ophthalmol 73:914–926, 1972.

191. Shields JA, Rodrigues MM, Sarin LK, Tasman WS and Annesley WH, Jr: Lipofuscin pigment over benign and malignant choroidal tumors. Trans Am Acad Ophtalmol Otolaryngol 81:OP871–OP881, 1976.

192. Smith LT and Irvine AR: Diagnostic significance of orange pigment accumulation over choroidal tumors. Am J Ophthalmol 76:212–216, 1973.

193. Wallow IHL and Tso MOM: Proliferation of the retinal pigment epithelium over malignant choroidal tumors: a light and electron microscopic study. Am J Ophthalmol 73:914–926, 1972.

194. Ferry AP: Lesions mistaken for malignant melanoma of the iris. Arch Ophthalmol 74:9–18, 1965.

195. Howard GM: Erroneous clinical diagnoses of retinoblastoma and uveal melanoma. Trans Am Acad Ophthalmol Otolaryngol 73:199–203, 1969.

196. Blodi FC and Roy PE: The misdiagnosed choroidal melanoma. Can J Ophthalmol 2:209–211, 1967.

197. Ferry AP: Lesions mistaken for malignant melanoma of the posterior uvea: a clinicopathologic analysis of 100 cases with ophthalmoscopically visible lesions. Arch Ophthalmol 72:463–469, 1964.

198. Shields JA and Zimmerman LE: Lesions simulating malignant melanoma of the posterior uvea. Arch Ophthalmol 89:466–471, 1973.

199. Davies WS: Malignant melanomas of the choroid and ciliary body: a clinicopathological study. Am J Ophthalmol 55:541–546, 1963.

200. Kirk HQ and Petty RW: Malignant melanoma of the choroid: correlation of clinical and histological findings. Arch Ophthalmol 56:843–860, 1956.

201. Minckler D, Font RL and Shields JA: Non-melanoma ocular lesions with positive $P^{32}$ tests. In: Jakobiec F (ed) Ocular and Adnexal Tumors, pp 245–256. Aesculapius, Birmingham, 1978.

202. Smith TR and Brockhurst RJ: Cellular blue nevus of the sclera. Arch Ophthalmol 94:618–620, 1976.

203. Rycroft BW: Choroidal detachment. Br J Ophthalmol 27:283–291, 1943.

204. Newton FH: Malignant melanoma of choroid: report of a case with clinical history of 36 years and follow-up of 32 years. Arch Ophthalmol 73:198–199, 1965.

205. Rahi AHS: Autoimmune reactions in uveal melanoma. Br J Ophthalmol 55:793–807, 1971.

206. Jensen AO and Andersen SR: Spontaneous regression of a malignant melanoma of the choroid. Acta Ophthalmol 52:173–182, 1974.

207. Wong IG and Oskvig RM: Immunofluorescent detection of antibodies to ocular melanoma. Arch Ophthalmol 92:97–102, 1974.

208. Rahi AHS: Immunological aspects of malignant melanoma of the choroid. Trans Ophthalmol Soc U K 93:79–91, 1973.

209. Rahi AHS: The immunological aspects of ocular tumours. In: Perkins ES and Hill DW (eds) Scientific Foundations of Ophthalmology, pp 119–124. Heinemann, London, 1977.

210. Michelson JB, Felberg NT and Shields JA: Carcinoembryonic antigens: its role in the evaluation of intraocular malignant tumors. Arch Ophthalmol 94:414–416, 1976.

211. Michelson JB, Felberg NT and Shields JA: Evaluation of metastatic carcinoma to the eye. Carcinoembryonic antigen and gamma glutamyl transpeptidase. Arch Ophthalmol 95:692–694, 1977.

212. Federman JL, Lewis MG, Clark WH, Jr, Igerer I and Sarin LK: Tumor-associated antibodies in the serum of ocular melanoma patients. Trans Am Acad Ophthalmol Otolaryngol 78:OP784–OP794, 1974.

213. Browstein S, Sheikh KM and Lewis MG: Tumor associated antibodies in the serum of patients with uveal melanoma. Can J Ophthalmol 11:147–154, 1976.

214. Malaty AHA, Rahi AHS and Garner A: Ostensible antimelanoma antibodies in patients with non-malignant eye diseases. In: Silverstein AM and O'Connor GR (eds) Immunology and Immunopathology of the Eye. Masson, New York, 1979.

215. Rahi AHS and Agarwal PK: Prognostic parameters in choroidal melanomata. Trans Ophthalmol Soc U K 97:368–372, 1977.

216. Federman JL, Felberg NT and Shields JA: Effect of local treatment on antibody levels in malignant melanoma of the choroid. Trans Ophthalmol Soc U K 97:436–439, 1977.

217. O'Connor GR: The uvea annual review. Arch Ophthalmol 89:505–518, 1973.

218. The TH, Eibergen R and Lamberts HB: Immune phagocytosis in vivo of human malignant melanoma cells. Acta Med Scand 192:141–144, 1972.

219. Char DH: Immunological mechanisms in choroidal melanoma. Trans Ophthalmol Soc U K 97:393, 1977.

220. Char DH, Hollinshead A, Cogan DG, Ballintine EJ, Hogan MJ and Herberman RB: Cutaneous delayed hypersensitivity reactions to soluble melanoma antigen in patients with ocular malignant melanoma. N Engl J Med 291:274–277, 1974.

221. Manor RS, Livni E, Joshua H and Ben-Sira I: Inhibition of macrophage migration by choroidal malignant melanoma-associated antigens in patients with uveal melanoma. Invest Ophthalmol Vis Sci 17:684–687, 1978.

222. Rahi AHS, Otiko F and Winder AF: Evaluation of macrophage electrophoretic mobility (MEM) test as an indicator of cellular immunity in ocular tumours. Br J Ophthalmol 60:589–593, 1976.

223. Noor Sunba MS, Rahi AHS, Morgan G and Holborow EJ: Lymphoproliferative response as an index of cellular immunity in malignant melanoma of the uvea and its correlation with the histological features of the tumor. Br J Ophthalmol 64:576–590, 1980.

224. Unsgaard B and O'Toole C: The influence of tumour burden and therapy on cellular cytotoxicity responses in patients with ocular and skin melanoma. Br J Cancer 31:301–316, 1975.

225. Kopf AW, Bart RS and Rodriguez-Sains RS: Malignant melanoma: a review. J Dermatol Surg Oncol 3:41–125, 1977.

226. Clark WH, Jr, From L, Bernardino EA, and Mihm MC: The histogenesis and biological behavior of primary human malignant melanomas of the skin. Cancer Res 29:705–727, 1969.

227. Lever WF and Schaumberg-Lever G: Histopathology of the Skin, 5th Ed. JB Lippincott, Philadelphia, 1975.

228. McGovern VJ, Mihm MC, Jr, Bailly C, Booth JC, Clark WH, Jr, Cochran AJ, Hardy EG, Hicks JD, Levene A, Lewis MG, Little JH and Milton JW: The classification of malignant melanoma and its histologic reporting. Cancer 32:1446–1457, 1973.

229. Hutchinson J: Lentigo-melanosis: a further report. Arch Surg London 5:253–256, 1894.

230. Clark WH, Jr and Mihm MC, Jr: Lentigo maligna and lentigo-maligna melanoma. Am J Pathol 55:39–67, 1969.

231. Naidoff MA, Bernardino VB, Jr and Clark WH, Jr: Melanocytic lesions of the eyelid skin. Am J Ophthalmol 82:371–382, 1976.

232. Clark WH, Jr and Mihm MC, Jr: Moles and malignant melanoma. In: Dermatology in General Medicine, pp 491–511. McGraw-Hill, New York, 1979.

233. Wanebo HJ, Fortner JG, Woodruft J, MacLean B and Binkowski E: Selection of optimum surgical treatment of Stage I melanoma by depth of microinvasion. I: use of the combined microstage technique (Clark-Breslow). Ann Surg 182:302–315, 1975.

234. Huvos AG, Mike V, Donnellan MJ, Seemayer T and Strong FW: Prognostic factors in cutaneous melanoma of the head and neck. Am J Pathol 71:33–47, 1973.

235. McGovern VJ: The classification of melanoma and its relationship with prognosis. Pathology 2:85–98, 1970.

236. Bernardino VB, Jr, Naidoff MA and Clark WH, Jr: Malignant melanomas of the conjunctiva. Am J Ophthalmol 82:383–394, 1976.

237. Silvers DN, Jakobiec FA, Freeman TF, Lefkowitch JH and Ellie RC: Melanoma of the conjunctiva: a clinicopathologic study. In: Jakobiec FA (ed) Ocular and Adnexal Tumors. Aesculapius, Birmingham, 1978.

238. McGovern VJ and Lane-Brown MN: The Nature of Melanoma, pp 92–116. Charles C. Thomas, Springfield, 1969.

239. Reese AB: Precancerous and cancerous melanosis. In: Boniuk M (ed) Ocular and Adnexal Tumors, pp 19–23. CV Mosby, St. Louis, 1964.

240. Reese AB: Precancerous and cancerous melanosis of the conjunctiva. Am J Ophthalmol 39:96–100, 1955.

241. Jay B: Pigmented lesions of the conjunctiva. I. Br J Ophthalmol 51:862–863, 1967.

242. Zimmerman LE: Pigmented tumors of the conjunctiva. In: Boniuk M (ed) Ocular and Adnexal Tumors, pp 24–30. CV Mosby, St. Louis, 1964.

243. Jay B: Naevi and melanomata of the conjunctiva. Br J Ophthalmol 49:169–204, 1965.

244. Bernardino VB, Jr, Naidoff MA and Clark WH, Jr: Malignant melanoma of the conjunctiva. In: Clark WH, Jr, Goldman LI and Mastrangelo MJ (eds) Human Malignant Melanoma. Grune & Stratton, New York, 1979.

245. Zimmerman LE: Criteria for management of melanosis. Letter to the editor. Arch Ophthalmol 76:307–308, 1966.

246. Reese AB: Precancerous melanosis and diffuse malignant melanoma of the conjunctiva. Arch Ophthalmol 19:354–365, 1938.

247. Lederman M: Discussion of pigmented tumors of the conjunctiva. In: Boniuk M (ed) Ocular and Adnexal Tumors, pp 32–40. CV Mosby, St. Louis, 1964.

248. McGovern VJ: Melanoma: growth patterns, multiplicity and regression. In: McCarthy WH (ed), Melanoma and Skin Cancer, pp 95–106. VCN Blight, Sidney, 1972.

249. Clark WH, Jr, Ainsworth AM, Bernardino EA, Yang C-H, Mihm MC, Jr and Reed RJ: The developmental biology of primary human malignant melanomas. Semin Oncol 2:83–103, 1975.
250. Takagi M, Ishikawa G and Mori W: Primary malignant melanoma of the oral cavity in Japan. Cancer 34:358–370, 1974.
251. Darabos G: Primäres Melanom der Hornhauthinterflache. Klin Monatsbl Augenheilkd 145:529–534, 1963.
252. Lamers WPMA: Malignant melanoma of the cornea. Ophthalmologica 146:353–354, 1963.
253. Stallard HB: Primary malignant melanoma of the cornea. Br J Ophthalmol 46:40–44, 1962.
254. Welsh NH and Jhavery Y: Malignant melanoma of the cornea in an African patient. Am J Ophthalmol 72:796–800, 1971.
255. Henkind P: Migration of the limbal melanocytes into the corneal epithelium of guinea pigs. Exp Eye Res 4:42–47, 1965.
256. Jauregui H and Klintworth GK: Pigmented squamous cell carcinoma of cornea and conjunctiva: a light microscopic, histochemical and ultrastructural study. Cancer 38:778–788, 1976.
257. McCracken JS and Klintworth GK: Ultrastructural observations on experimentally produced melanin pigmentation of the corneal epithelium. Am J Pathol 85:167–182, 1976.
258. Coppeto JR, Jaffe R and Gillies CG: Primary orbital melanoma. Arch Ophthalmol 96:2255–2258, 1978.
259. Drews R: Primary malignant melanoma of the orbit in a Negro. Arch Ophthalmol 93:335–336, 1975.
260. Jakobiec FA, Ellsworth R and Tannenbaum M: Primary orbital melanoma. Am J Ophthalmol 78:24–39, 1974.
261. Rottino A and Kelly AS: Primary orbital melanoma: case report with review of the literature. Arch Ophthalmol 27:934–949, 1942.
262. Wolter JR, Bryson JM and Blackhurst RT: Primary orbital melanoma. Eye Ear Nose Throat Mon 45(8):64–67, 1966.
263. Speakman JS and Phillips MJ: Cellular and malignant blue nevus complicating oculodermal melanosis (nevus of Ota syndrome). Can J Ophthalmol 8:539–547, 1973.
264. Foster J: An encapsulated orbital melanoma. Br J Ophthalmol 28:293–296, 1944.
265. Fishman ML, Tomaszewski MM and Kuwabara T: Malignant melanoma of the skin metastatic to the eye: frequency in autopsy series. Arch Ophthalmol 94:1309–1311, 1976.
266. Font RL, Naumann G and Zimmerman LE: Primary malignant melanoma of the skin metastatic to the eye and orbit: report of ten cases and review of the literature. Am J Ophthalmol 63:738–754, 1967.
267. Radnot M: Metastatisches Melanosarkom des Strahlenkorpers. Klin Monatsbl Augenheilkd 121:352–354, 1952.
268. Szeps J and Patterson TD: Metastatic malignant melanoma of ciliary body and choroid from a primary melanoma of the skin. Can J Ophthalmol 4:394–399, 1969.

# 17. Immunotherapy of melanoma

## HILLIARD F. SEIGLER

Physicians have long noted that there is a wide spectrum of response of patients to their malignant disorder. In some incidences, patients will live in relative harmony with their malignant disease for a number of years. At the opposite end, some patients will develop a neoplastic process and will die secondary to their disease in a matter of days to weeks. All levels of response between these clinical courses have been repetitively documented. In some patients, spontaneous tumor regression, complete or patial, has been described by numerous authors [1, 2]. At times the tumor regression has been associated with a serious infection. This observation has led some investigators to suspect that the host immune response to the infection was also responsible for the tumor regression. It was this background that led Coley [3], at the turn of the century, to evaluate bacterial toxins in patients with malignant tumors and he extended his observations to include a more successful response if the toxin was introduced directly into the tumor site. With the development of immunology as a science, a clinical application of vaccination for the prevention of infectious diseases gained an important role in medical science throughout the first half of this century. Ghose and Bleir [4] applied these techniques in a rodent system to demonstrate that animals could be protected from tumor take by immunization against particular methylcholanthrene tumors. More recently investigators have observed that animals can be immunized with either intact tumor cells, tumor cell membrane preparations, purified solubilized tumor antigen extract, unaltered or attenuated oncogenic virus and be rendered immune to tumor challenges. Specific immunologic techniques, including transfer factor, immune RNA, adoptive transfer of immune lymphocytes, infusion of hyperimmune globulin, interferon induction, genetic engineering of tumor cells and plasma absorption with staphylococcal purified protein-A continue to undergo investigation as a means of altering the tumor–host relationship.

Both animal and human experiments would suggest that the host–tumor interaction in man should be evaluated in terms of the antigenic profile expressed on tumor cell membranes and the complexity of the various immune responses to these antigens. Normal adult mammalian cells express both blood group antigens, histocompatibility antigens and, in some concentration, fetal antigens. Human tumor cells express these same blood

*Seigler, H. F. (ed.), Clinical Management of Melanoma. ISBN 978-94-009-7495-1*
© *1982, Martinus Nijhoff Publishers, The Hague/Boston/London.*

group antigens and HLA alloantigens but also express fetal antigens, differentiation antigens and tumor associated antigens that are both cross-reactive and individually specific. Utilizing cell fusion experiments, recent studies [5] have shown that human cells fused with mouse myeloma cells have been successful in producing hybrids that are deficient in the C6 human chromosome and thus do not express the serologically detectable HLA antigens, but do express tumor associated antigens. The antigens associated with the Dr system are undergoing intensive investigation. These antigens have been reported to be important in both cell–cell interactions and for control of cell proliferation. The Dr antigens have been detected on human melanoma cells [6], and they might indeed be important in terms of the gross characteristics of these tumor cells and offer some explanation as to their escape from immune destruction in tumor-bearing patients. Galloway et al. [7] have studied melanoma associated antigens shed into spent culture medium and have described two glycoproteins with molecular weights of 240 000 and 94 000. The 240K is present only on melanoma cells, whereas the 94K molecular species was also found on other malignant cells and on fetal melanocytes. Utilizing mouse–mouse fusions, Koprowski has produced monoclonal antibodies that react with human melanoma cells. Both Dr antigens and melanoma associated antigens were detected by these studies. Mitchell et al. [8] have described three distinct human melanoma surface antigens detected by monoclonal antimelanoma antibodies. One antigen was expressed on all melanoma cells and on certain astrocytoma cells but not on any other kind of normal or tumor cell tested. A second antigen was expressed on many, but not all, melanomas and was identified as the antigenic product of the HLA-D locus, the Dr antigen. A third protein antigen was not found on any normal cell tested but did occur on some, but not all, tumors of different origins.

Peter et al. [9] have studied cell mediated cytotoxicity in vitro of human lymphocytes against tissue cultured melanoma cell lines. These investigators were able to show both cell mediated cytotoxicity and antibody dependent cytotoxicity using cells obtained from melanoma patients. Both of these activities could be blocked by preincubation of the effector cells in aggregated IgG. Depletion of B cells from the cell population increased the killing activity, whereas depletion of T cells removed the cell killing capability. Mavligit et al. [10] have evaluated cell mediated immunity to human solid tumors using a lymphoblastogenic assay. These authors suggested that cell mediated immunity to human solid tumors could be demostrated in vitro by the lymphocyte blastogenesis method. They were able to show blastogenic responses to unseparated autochthonous tumor cells in most of the patients that they studied. Treves et al. [11] have completed experimental studies in a rodent model that would suggest an in vivo effect of lymphocytes sensitized in vitro against tumor cells. These investigators have developed and analyzed a mouse model for immunotherapy of lethal tumor metastasis by lymphocytes sensitized in vitro against tumor cells. The population of T lymphocytes in an enlarged spleen in the tumor-bearing animal was found to exert an enhancing effect on tumor growth. This effect was based on their action as suppressor cells against host reactivity to the tumor. These investigators found that lymphocytes sensitized in culture on monolayers of target tumor cells manifested specific antitumor cytotoxicity when tested in vitro and when injected into syngeneic animals from which the primary tumor graft was removed seven days after implantation, and conferred protection against lethal lung metastases. Lotze and co-workers [12] have studied human T lymphocytes grown in T cell growth factor for cytotoxic activity against both autologous and allogeneic target tumor cells. They have shown that T cell growth factor can be used to expand cytotoxic human T cells in tissue culture for possible use in immunotherapy. They were able to expand cytotoxic T cells from 500 to 20 000-fold and to assay these cells in a chromium release model. Their studies indicated that these cultured lymphocytes display significant cytotoxicity against fresh normal lymphoid cells while lymphocytes cultures in autologous serum had the greatest cytotoxic effect.

Using present day monoclonal antibody technology, we are able to study human pan T lymphocytes, inducer cells, cytotoxic T cells and suppressor cells. This advanced technology should permit us to alter host response in such a way that suppressor cells are specifically reduced and specifically cytotoxic T lymphocytes are expanded as a means of altering the tumor–host interaction in such a way as to immunologically mediate specific tumor cell destruction by the host.

A number of biologic modulators have been utilized in an effort to potentiate the immune response of the host against his tumor. These agents include Bacillus Calmettte-Guerin (BCG), Corynebacterium parvum, vaccina, levamisole and oncofetal antigen. The original observations of Morton et al. [13] suggested that most cutaneous metastatic melanoma lesions regressed following intralesional injection with BCG. The BCG injections were not directly toxic to tumor cells as tumor regressions were not seen unless a delayed cutaneous hypersensitivity response to the BCG was generated by the patient. These results led these investigators [14] to study the role of adjuvant immunotherapy for control of occult metastasis in Stage II melanoma patients. The patients who received BCG showed a marked reduction in recurrence rate. Overall, 63% of immunotherapy patients remain free of disease compared to 36% of those who were treated by operation alone. Ashley et al. [15] have reported their results concerning studies of conditions required for eradication by immunization of lymph node metastasis which remained after surgical removal of an intradermally transplanted hepatoma. Guinea pigs that received no postsurgical treatment all died with progressive growing lymph node metastases. The growth of these metastases could be permitted in a significant portion of the animals by postsurgical treatment with vaccines containing BCG admixed with irradiated tumor cells. Vaccines containing living tumor cells cured most of the guinea pigs but produced tumors at the vaccine sites in a few animals. Irradiated tumor cells were not tumorigenic but required more tumor cells for successful therapy. Therapy was dependent both on the dose of tumor cells and on the BCG. Animals rendered tumor-free by postsurgical vaccine therapy rejected a subsequent intradermal challenge with living tumor cells. Hanna and Peters [16] have also reported on an experimental study of specific immunotherapy of established visceral micrometastasis by utilization of a BCG-tumor cell vaccine. Their studies demonstrate that, under defined conditions of vaccine preparation and regimen, the BCG-tumor cell vaccine did produce cure in the majority of the animals with otherwise lethal visceral metastases. Histopathologically, Hanna was able to show that immunization with the vaccine prevented the progressive growth of pulmonary micrometastatic foci of approximately 0.1 mm in diameter. No protection against antigenically distinct tumors was realized. The tumor cell vaccine was also effective in curing guinea pigs of minimal disseminated tumor burden when administered after surgery of an established skin tumor and draining lymph node. Seigler and co-workers [17] have reported an extensive experience with specific active immunotherapy for melanoma in humans. Clark's Level III patients with Stage I disease experienced an 88% survival at four years, while 47 Stage II patients had an observed survival of 82% during the same time period. Very similar statistics were observed for 124 Stage I, Clark's Level IV patients and 70 Stage II patients. Nineteen and 26 Clark's Level V patients with Stage I and Stage II disease realized a 100% and 55% observed survival at four years respectively. In both experimental models and Phase I clinical trials, Juilliard [18–20] has demonstrated a positive and systemic effect of either tumor cell vaccine alone or tumor cell vaccine plus BCG when administered via the endolymphatic route. This new and novel approach might indeed improve the observed beneficial effect of specific active immunotherapy. Further study is clearly warranted. Other experimental studies as well as clinical trials using levamisole, Corynebacterium parvum and vaccina have had similar results to BCG when used alone. Blume et al. [21] have reported their usage of adjuvant immunotherapy of high risk Stage I melanoma patients with transfer factor. One hundred patients with Clark's Level III, IV and V primaries and exceeding 1 mm in Breslow's thickness were treated with transfer factor. Actuarial nonfailure rate in this series was reported to be 90% and survival rate 99% at five years. 46 patients with comparable risk treated by surgery alone had a failure rate of 63% and a survival rate of 69%. These authors suggest that transfer factor immunotherapy may be a valuable adjuvant in the treatment of patients with high risk Stage I melanoma. Dorval and co-workers suggest that the addition of transfer factor to patients that have previously been low or poor responders to other biologic modulators might indeed increase their immunologic reactivity to these modulators and be associated with increased disease-free intervals and prolonged survival times [22].

Different types of antibodies have successfully been raised that react specifically with either differentiation-type antigens or tumor associated antigens present on the surface of human melanoma cells. Polyclonal antibodies have been raised in a number of different species as well as in patients hyperimmunized with melanoma tumor cells [23-24]. Most of the monoclonal antibodies reactive with human melanoma cells have been prepared by immunizing mice against human melanoma cells and fusing the immune lymphocytes with mouse myeloma cells. Resultant hybridoma cells producing the antimelanoma antibodies are cloned and maintained in tissue culture.

We have recently demonstrated specific in vivo localization of antibodies reactive with human melanoma cell membrane tumor associated antigens in an athymic nude mouse model growing subcutaneous human melanoma tumor xenografts. Antimelanoma antibody sources included human alloantibody obtained from melanoma patients immunized against allogeneic melanoma cells, a monkey antiserum raised by immunization against a single human melanoma tissue culture cell line and a murine monoclonal antimelanoma antibody-secreting hybridoma cell line. Localization of these radiolabeled antibodies and of control IgG preparations to tumor tissue was determined by whole body scintigraphy and by differential tissue counting. Compared with the different control IgG preparations, each of the antimelanoma IgG preparations exhibited significant specific accumulation within the melanoma tissue. This technique for tumor localization is very promising and has obvious potential application, both in terms of diagnosis as well as possible therapy [25]. Currie et al. [26] have demonstrated lysis of cultured human melanoma cells using polyclonal xenoantibodies to melanoma associated antigens. They have additionally demonstrated a significant increase in susceptibility to immune lysis following treatment with puromycin. Jones and co-workers [27] have reported prolonged survival for melanoma patients with elevated IgM antibody to oncofetal antigen. This study was designed to see if there was an effect of tumor growth by a positive or negative correlation with antibody levels in convalescent patients with Stage II melanoma. A positive correlation with disease-free interval and survival was detected among patients who had high levels of IgM class of antibody before and shortly after surgery for Stage II disease. The IgG class of antibody over the period measured did not correlate consistently with tumor recurrence. These data suggested that immunity to fetal antigens expressed on the tumor cells might indeed play a role in host–tumor interaction. Imal et al. have successfully characterized a number of monoclonal antibodies to human melanoma associated antigens [28]. These monoclonal antibodies recognize antigenic determinants maximally expressed on cultured human melanoma cells as well as freshly explanted melanoma cells. These monoclonal reagents could mediate antibody-dependent cellular cytotoxicity of cultured melanoma cells, but none could mediate complement dependent cytotoxicity. This work has been confirmed by other investigators. In our own laboratory we have observed inhibition in the growth of melanoma in nude mice by both polyclonal antibody and monoclonal antibody reactive with human melanoma cell. Our experimental results do provide an approach for the study of immunotherapeutic possibilities for antimelanoma antibodies in humans.

Antibody-linked cytotoxic agents for the treatment of malignancy holds some promise. Antibodies against tumor cell membrane associated antigens have been used to selectively direct anticancer agents which themselves lack such specificity. Ghose has recently reviewed a number of other toxic agents that have been linked to antitumor globulins and these agents include alkylating drugs, antibiotics, antimetabolites, cell surface agents, protein synthesis inhibitors and unconventional anticancer agents that selectively convert nontoxic arsenicals or halides into cytocidal derivatives [4]. A number of investigators are presently testing experimental models using the very toxic diphtheria A fragment or ricin conjugated to monoclonal antimelanoma antibody. It is suggested that antibody-linked cytotoxic agents might be most efficient when dealing with micrometastatic disease after patients have had their tumor burdens surgically eradicated.

There is an increasing body of literature suggesting that circulating antigen or immune complexes plays an important role in inhibiting the host response against a spontaneously developed malignancy. Elevated immune complexes have been demonstrated in a variety of malignancies and have been described as blocking factors present in tumor-bearing patient serum. Injection of serum blocking factor as been reported to promote tumor growth in vivo [29]. These observations have suggested that removal of the blocking factors might indeed allow the expression of a host antitumor response. Isreal et al. attempted this initially using plasmaphoresis [30]. This study, as well as others, met with only limited success and stimulated a more specific method for removal of possible blocking factors using plasma absorption with purified protein-A obtained from Cowan I strain of staphylococci. The protein-A specifically binds to the Fc portion of IgG, and to a lesser extent, IgM of humans and certain other animals [31]. Using canine and feline experimental models, a number of investigators [32–34] have shown a marked tumorocidal response using this plasma immunoabsortion technique. Terman et al. [35] have also found that infusion of cytosine arabinoside after the immunoabsortions gave a much stronger antitumor response than either treatment alone. This investigator and his colleagues have recently extended their observations in a Phase I-type trial involving humans with advanced breast adenocarcinoma [36]. They completed plasma absorption in three such patients that developed exquisite pain in tumor sites within a matter of minutes after infusion of the absorbed plasma. There was a resultant increase in tumor temperature, hyperemia followed within two days by frank necrolysis. After a number of treatments, each of the patients realized significant regression and healing of visible tumorous areas with little in the way of attendant toxic side effects. Young et al. [37] have characterized the hemodynamic response during extracorporeal plasma absorption with staphlyococcus protein-A. Their observed hemodynamic responses were interpreted to result from simultaneous or sequential activity of multiple immune reactants or mediators liberated during tumor necrolysis. It must be stressed that at this time it is not at all clear if this technique is to have a clinical or simply research application. It might well be that the protein-A immunoabsorption effect is due not to a removal of plasma components, but rather to activation of factors needed for effective tumor lysis. The role that the activated complement cascade plays in the observed phenomenon has not been elucidated. Additionally, staphylococcus purified protein-A is both a T cell and B cell mitogen [38, 39] and can augment natural killer cell activity, possibly by induction of interferon [40]. A potential synergistic effect of completing plasma absorption using protein-A and following this with infusion of monoclonal antimelanoma antibody should be evaluated in a experimental model and, if warranted, extended to clinical trials.

It is not evident from either experimental trials or early human usage if interferon is to play an effective role in the management of patients with melanoma. Reid et al. [41] have reported their studies concerning the influence of interferon on the growth and metastasis of tumor cells. They speculate that interferon is the principle regulatory molecule governing the athymic mouse. Human tumor tissue shows enhanced growth if the animals are treated with anti-interferon antibody or antilymphocyte serum. They suggest that these results are consistent with the view that interferon might be important in restricting the growth, invasiveness, and metastasis of tumor cells by acting indirectly through components of the immune system, such as NK cells. Bart and co-workers have reported inhibition in the growth of B16 murine melanoma using exogenous interferon. They interpret their findings to suggest that the in vivo inhibition of the growth of B16 melanoma cells realized in both animals treated with interferon inducers as well as those treated with exogenous interferon result, at least in part, from a direct effect of interferon on the tumor cells themselves [42].

The greatest success that clinicians have had in managing different neoplastic disorders is in the treatment of choriocarcinoma. It has been suggested that these results are because this tumor is indeed partially histoincompatible with the host. Most spontaneous malignancies express all or most of the antigenic profile of the patient. Choriocarcinomas additionally express those antigens that are contributed by the father to the placenta. Experimental models would support the thesis that histoincompatible tumors are more immunogenic to the host than are histocompatible tumors. Efforts to alter the antigenicity or immunogenicity of spontaneous human tumors continues to stimulate investigators in the field of cancer research. The failure of human tumors to precipitate a significant rejection reaction must play an important role in the human tumor–host relationship. A very different observation has been made when considering tumors induced by viruses. Surface antigens induced by viruses are quite immunogenic and, by virtue of their cell membrane location, can become targets for immune attack by the host. Wallack et al. have reported on the use of vaccina oncolysates in the treatment of recurrent Stage II malignant melanoma [43]. These investigators have utilized a live vaccina virus augmented tumor cell vaccine as a specific, active immunotherapeutic agent. No patient realized an adverse reaction to the vaccine, and early results indicate that this regimen might serve as a potent immune mechanism stimulator. Iglehart and co-workers have utilized retrovirus infection of human tumor cells for the addition of virion antigens onto tumors as they grow in situ in the host animal [44]. The C-type viruses introduced strong transplantation antigens onto murine tumors both in vivo and in vitro. These viruses are virtually nonpathogenic in animals and give rise to a strong immune response [44]. When present on the cell surface, the tumor-producing capability of several classes of tumor cells is significantly decreased or abolished [44, 45]. Furthermore, certain retroviruses given to animals bearing lethal, nonvirus producing tumors are able to seek out the tumor cells in the animal and specifically infect them [44, 45]. These in vivo infected tumor cells are converted to a highly immunogenic state and express high levels of virion coated antigens. A number of investigators have shown success in experimental models utilizing administration of antiviral antiserum by passive administration of antibody prepared against purified surface components of the virion agents [46–49]. A combination of in vivo antigenic modification using infectious viruses followed by either specific antiviral antibody, antimelanoma antibody, or the two antibodies simultaneously, might act synergistically toward controlling otherwise highly lethal tumors refractory to immunologic control.

# References

1. Koop CE, Kiesewetter WB and Horn RC: Neuroblastoma in childhood. Surgery 38:27, 1955.
2. Everson TC and Cole WH: Spontaneous Regression of Cancer, pp 560. WB Saunders, Philadelphia and London, 1966.
3. Coley WB: Some clinical evidence in favor of the extrinsic origin of cancer. Surg Gynecol Obstet 59:353, 1925.
4. Ghose T and Blair AH: Antibody-linked cytotoxic agents in the treatment of cancer: current status and future prospects. J Natl Canc Inst 61:657–676, 1978.
5. Koprowski H, Steplewski Z, Herlyn D and Herlyn M: Study of antibodies against human melanoma produced by somatic cell hydrids. Proc Natl Acad Sci 75:3405–3407, 1978.
6. Winchester RJ, Wang C-Y, Gibofsky A, Kunkel, Lloyd KO and Old LJ: Expression of Ia-like antigens on cultures human malignant melanoma cell lines. Proc Natl Acad Sci 75:6235–6239, 1978.
7. Galloway DR, McCabe RP, Pellegrino MA, Ferrone S and Reisfeld RA: Tumor-associated antigens in spent medium of human melanoma cells: immunochemical characterization with xenoantisera. J Immunol 126:62–66, 1981.
8. Mitchell KF, Fuhrer JP, Steplewski Z and Koprowski H: Biochemical characterization of human melanoma cell surfaces: dissection with monoclonal antibodies. Proc Natl Acad Sci 77:7287–7291, 1980.
9. Peter HH, Pavie-Fischer J, Fridman WH, Aubert C, Cesarini JP, Roubin R and Kourilsky FM: J Immunol 115:539–548, 1975.
10. Mavligit GM, Gutterman JU, McBride CM and Hersh EM: Cell-mediated immunity to human solid tumors: in vitro detection by lymphocyte blastogenic responses to cell-associated and solubilized tumor antigens. Natl Canc Inst Monogr 37:167–176, 1980.
11. Treves AJ, Cohen IR, Schechter B and Feldman M: In vivo effects of lymphocytes sensitized in vitro against tumor cells. Ann N Y Acad Sci 150:165–175, 1980.
12. Lotze M, Strausser J and Rosenberg SA: Human lymphocytes grown in T cell growth factor (TCGF): cytotoxicity against autologous an allogeneic tumor. Proc Am Assoc Cancer Res 21:216, 1980.
13. Morton DL, Eilber FR, Malmgren RA and Wood WC: Immunological factors which influence response to immunotherapy in malignant melanoma. Surgery 68:158–164, 1970.
14. Eilber FR, Morton DL, Holmes EC, Sparks FC and Ramming KP: Adjuvant immunotherapy with BCG in treatment of regional lymph node metastases from malignant melanoma. N Engl J Med 294:237–240, 1976.
15. Ashley MP, Zbar B, Hunter JT, Rapp HJ and Sugimoto T: Adjuvant-antigen requirements for active specific immunotherapy of microscopic metastases remaining after surgery. Cancer Res 40:4197–4203, 1980.
16. Hanna MG, Jr and Peters LC: Specific immunotherapy of established visceral micrometastases by BCG-tumor cell vaccine alone or as an adjuvct to surgery. Cancer 42:2613–2625, 1978.
17. Seigler HF, Cox E, Mutzner A, Shepherd L, Nicholson E and Shingleton WW: Specific active immunotherapy for melanoma. Ann Surg 190:366–372, 1979.
18. Juilliard GJF et al: Regional intralymphatic infusion (ILI) of irradiated tumor cells with evidence of distant effects. Cancer 39:126–130, 1977.
19. Juilliard GJF, Boyer PJJ and Snow HD: Intralymphatic infusion of autochthonous tumor cells in canine lymphoma. Int J Radiat Oncol Biol Phys 1:497–503, 1976.
20. Juilliard GJF, Boyer PJJ and Yamashiro CH: A Phase I study of active specific intralymphatic immunotherapy. Cancer 41:2215–2225, 1978.

21. Blume MR, Rosenbaum EH, Cohen RJ, Gershow J, Glassberg AB and Shepley E: Adjuvant immunotherapy of high risk Stage I melanoma with transfer factor. Cancer 47:882–888, 1981.
22. Dorval G, Mankiewicz E, Wilkinson R, Shibata HR, Marquis G and Milne K: Levamisole/BCG-transfer factor in Stage II malignant melanoma patients unresponsive to BCG-tine: program and abstracts of the 2nd International Conference on the Adjuvant Therapy of Cancer, March 28–31, Tucson, 1979.
23. Mutzner PA, Stuhlmiller GM and Seigler HF: Characterization of melanoma cell membrane tumor-associated antigens using xenoserum, alloserum and autoserum. I: immunofluorescence. J Surg Oncol 14:367–377, 1980.
24. Reisfeld RA, David GS, Ferrone S, Pellegrino MA and Holmes EC: Approaches for the isolation of biologically functional tumor-associated antigens. Cancer Res 37:2860–2865, 1977.
25. Stuhlmiller GM, Sullivan DC, Vervaert C, Croker BP, Harris CC and Seigler HF: In vivo tumor localization utilizing tumor specific monkey xenoantibody, alloantibody and murine monoclonal xenoantibody. Ann Surg (in press).
26. Curry RA, Quaranta V, Pellegrino NA and Ferrone S: Lysis of cultures human melanoma M10 cells by polyclonal cenoantibodies to melanoma associated antigens. Cancer Res 41:463–466, 1981.
27. Jones PC, Sze LL, Liu PY, Morton DL and Irie RF: Prolonged survival for melanoma patients with elevated IgM antibody to oncofetal antigen. J Natl Cancer Inst 66:249–254, 1981.
28. Imal K, Ng AK and Ferrone S: Characterization of monoclonal antibodies to human melanoma-associated antigens. J Natl Cancer Inst 66:489–496, 1981.
29. Hellstrom KE and Hellstrom I: Immunologic enhancement of tumor growth in mechanisms of tumor immunity. In: Green I, Cohen S and McCluskey RT (eds) Growth in Mechanisms of Tumor Immunity, pp 209–277. John Wiley, New York.
30. Isreal I, Edelstein R, Mannoni P, Rhadal E and Greenspan EM: Plamsapheresis in patients with disseminated cancer: clinical results and correlation with changes in serum protein. Cancer 40:3146–3154, 1977.
31. Steele G, Ankerst J and Sjogren HO: Alteration of in vitro antitumor activity of tumor-bearer sera by absorption with Staphylococcus aureus, Cowan I. Int J Cancer 14:83–92, 1974.
32. Terman DS: Tumoricidal responses in spontaneous canine neoplasm after extracorporeal perfusion over immobilized protein-A. Fed Proc 40, 1980.
33. Terman DS, Yamamoto T, Mattioli M, Cook G, Tillquist R, Henry H, Passer R and Daskal Y: Extensive necrosis of spontaneous canine mammary adenocarcinoma after extracorporeal perfusion over Staphylococcus aureus, Cowan I. J Immunol 124:795–805, 1980.
34. Bansal SC, Bansal BR, Rhoads JE, Cooper DR, Roland JR and Mack R: Ex vivo removal of mammallian immunoglobulin G: method and immunological alterations. Int J Art Organs 2:94–103, 1978.
35. Terman DS, Yamamoto T, Tillquist RL, Henry JF, Cook GL, Silvers A and Shearer WT: Tumoricidal response induced by cytosine arabinoside after plasma perfusion over protein-A. Science 209:1257–1259, 1980.
36. Terman DS, Shearer WT, Ayus JC, Lehane D and Young JB: Necrotizing tumoricidal response after plasma perfusion over immobilized protein-A: initial experience in human breast adenocarcinoma. AFCR Oncol 29:378, 1981.
37. Young JB, Ayus JC, Miller LK, Miller RR and Terman DS: Prospective characterization of unique hemodynamic responses during extracorporeal immunotherapy of human breast adenocarcinoma. AFCR Oncol 29:253A, 1981.

38. Sirianni AC, Pandolf F, Aiuti F and Wigzell H: Protein-A positive staphylococci serve as a selective B cell mitogen for lymphocytes from primary immunodeficiency patients. Clin Exp Immunol 36:107, 1979.
39. Ringden O and Rynnel-Dagoo B: Activation of human B and T lymphocytes by protein-A of Staphylococcus aureua. Eur J Immunol 8:47, 1978.
40. Catalona WJ, Ratliff TL and McCool RE: Characterization of interferon induced by human lymphocytes by staphylococcal protein-A. Am Assoc Cancer Res 21:238, 1980.
41. Reid LM, Minato N, Gresser I, Holland J, Kadish A and Bloom BR: Influence of antimouse interferon serum on the growth and metastasis of tumor cells persistently infected with virus and of human prostatic tumors in athymic nude mice. Proc Natl Acad Sci 78:1171–1175, 1981.
42. Bart RS, Porzio NR, Kopf AW, Vilcek JT, Cheng EH and Farcet Y: Inhibition of growth of B16 murine malignant melanoma by exogenous interferon. Cancer Res 40:614–619, 1980.
43. Wallack MK, Mayer M, Bourgoin A and Leftheriotis E: The use of vaccinia oncolysates in the treatment of recurrent Stage II malignant melanoma. Medical oncology: abstracts of the 5th Annual Meeting of the Medical Oncology Society, December 1–3, Nice, France, 1979.
44. Iglehart JD, Ward EC et al: J Natl Cancer Inst (in press).
45. Iglehart JD, Weinhold K et al: J Natl Cancer Inst (in press).
46. Schwarz H, Fischinger PJ et al: Virology 93:159–174, 1979.
47. Schafer W, Schwarz H et al: Virology 75:401–418, 1976.
48. DeNornoha F, Schafer W et al: Virology 85:617–621, 1978.
49. DeNornoha F, Baggs R et al: Nature 267:54–56, 1977.

# INDEX